Thyroid Disorders

Syed Khalid Imam • Shamim I. Ahmad
Editors

Thyroid Disorders

Basic Science and Clinical Practice

Springer

Editors
Syed Khalid Imam
Internal Medicine
Al-Mouwasat Hospital
Jubail
Saudi Arabia

Shamim I. Ahmad
School of Science and Technology
Nottingham Trent University
Nottingham
UK

ISBN 978-3-319-25869-0 ISBN 978-3-319-25871-3 (eBook)
DOI 10.1007/978-3-319-25871-3

Library of Congress Control Number: 2016933871

Springer Cham Heidelberg New York Dordrecht London

Printed on acid-free paper

Springer International Publishing AG Switzerland is part of Springer Science+Business Media (www.springer.com)

The editor (SKI) wishes to dedicate this book to his parents, Ahmad Imam and Mah Jabeen, for their constant support, patronage, and guidance in his career; his children, Abdullah, Maham, and Ebadullah, whose voices and gestures were never boring and from them he has learned to love and enjoy the flavor of life; his wife, Uzma, the key family member, who lifted his heart and encouraged him a lot because of her spiritual wholeness, inexhaustible hope, and strong personality. Lastly, to all patients who have been suffering from various kinds of illnesses and fight against the ailment with great courage and hope.

The editor (SIA) wishes to dedicate this book to his wife, Riasat Jan, for her patience, love, and persistent encouragement during the production of this book and to his children, Alisha Ahmad and Arsalan Mujtaba Ahmad, who have been giving him so much pleasure with their innocent interceptions and resulting recovery from the loss of energy. Also dedication goes to the caregivers, nurses, and medics who painstakingly look after the patients throughout their suffering period.

Preface

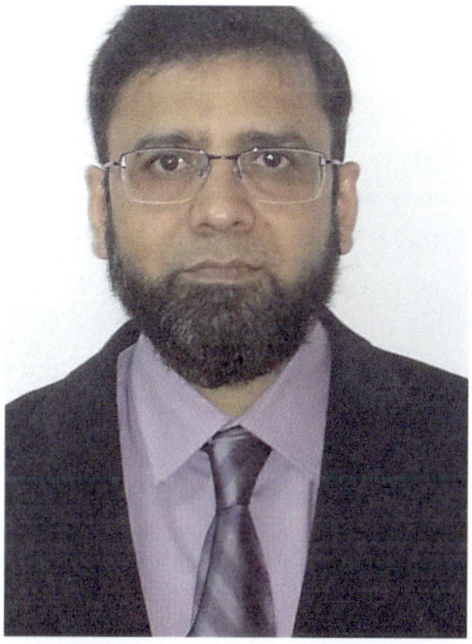

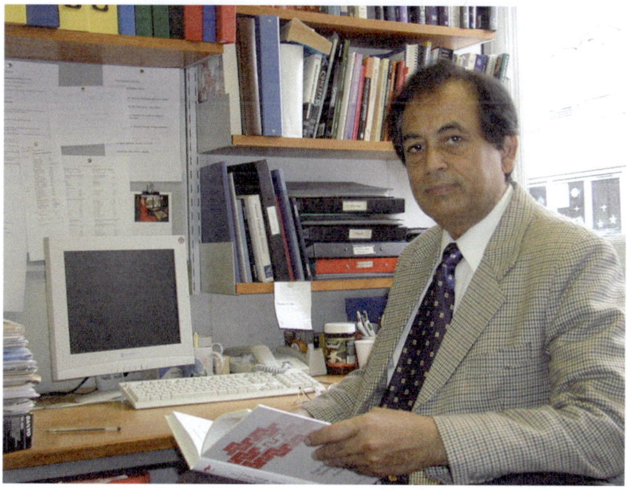

Endocrinology is the study of one of the most exciting hormonal diseases covering a plethora of information on thyroid disorders, which are among the most prevalent of medical conditions. In general population, the prevalence of thyroid dysfunction ranges from 1 to 10 %. In the United Kingdom, 1–2 % of the adult population is found to have thyroid disorders. It is interesting to note that thyroxine is the sixth most commonly prescribed drug in Scotland.

Virtually all studies report higher prevalence of thyroid diseases in women and mostly with those undergoing advancing age.

The incidence of thyroid disorders has been increasing with time and varies between localities. Their manifestations vary considerably from area to area and are determined principally by the availability of iodine in the diet. Almost one-third of the world's population lives in areas of iodine deficiency. Populations living particularly in remote mountainous areas in South-East Asia, Latin America, and Central Africa risk more of suffering from this disease.

Globally, wherever population lives in iodine-deficient regions, due to the sub-optimal amount of iodine intake from the natural sources such as sea vegetables, potatoes, cranberries, etc., the prevalence of hypothyroidism is higher than in iodine-efficient regions. It is important to note that most persons with thyroid disorders have one or more autoimmune disease such as Hashimoto's thyroiditis, primary atrophic hypothyroidism, and thyrotoxicosis caused by Graves' disease. Moreover, suppressed thyroid-stimulating hormone levels have been associated with decreased bone density and with an increased risk of atrial fibrillation and premature atrial beat. It has been known for decades that overt hypothyroidism contributes to elevated serum cholesterol levels and cardiovascular risk, and recent studies suggest this may also be true with subclinical hypothyroidism. Abnormal thyroid functions have important public health concerns.

Medical researches on thyroid diseases have been persistently reporting, in a wide range of journals and literatures, materials relevant to endocrinology, pediatrics, nuclear medicine, and surgery, making it more challenging for clinicians to keep abreast of new developments. Therefore, the objective of this publication is to provide an updated review on thyroid gland and its functional impairments and to highlight the recent trends in the management of thyroid diseases. Pregnancy-related thyroid disorders are also covered in this book.

The Contents list can basically be divided into three sections: Part I providing the basic information on thyroid glands, Part II largely focusing on important and common thyroid dysfunctions and their clinical management, and Part III addressing thyroid dysfunction during pregnancy, a commonly ignored area.

The book on thyroid disorders is meant to be read by a wide range of readers including physicians, endocrinologists, dietitians, researchers, industries involved in developing and manufacturing thyroid drugs, postgraduate and undergraduate medical students, and may help to update knowledge of non-specialist in the diagnosis and management of thyroid diseases.

The editors are certain that this book will provide core basic and clinical knowledge to all those who are attached with the health care and also involve in managing various kinds of diseases related to thyroid disorders. We hope that appropriate diagnosis and clinical application of the basic and advance knowledge provided in this book would ultimately benefit patients.

Jubail, Kingdom of Saudi Arabia — Syed Khalid Imam, FCPS, FACE
Nottingham, UK — Shamim I. Ahmad, MSc, PhD

Acknowledgments

The editors cordially acknowledge various authors of this book for their contribution of the chapters with in-depth knowledge and highly skilled presentation. Without their input, it would not have been possible to produce this book on such an important subject and complicated disease. We would also like to acknowledge the hard work, friendly approach, and patience of the staff, especially of Ms Julia Megginson, of Springer Publications for efficient and highly professional handling of this project.

Editors

Dr. Syed Khalid Imam is an Assistant Professor of Medicine and Consultant Endocrinologist. He acquired Fellowship in Internal Medicine from College of Physicians and Surgeons Pakistan (CPSP) and Fellowship in Endocrinology from American College of Endocrinology (ACE). He was trained as a Clinical Fellow in Endocrinology at Liaquat National Hospital and Medical College, Karachi-Pakistan, one of the biggest private tertiary care hospitals of the country. He has been affiliated with this organization for more than 15 years and accomplished postgraduate training and professional and career growth from this renowned health care industry. He fulfilled his responsibilities for several years as Head of the Department of Diabetes, Endocrinology and Metabolism, Program Director of Internal Medicine Residency Training, Chairman of Research and Ethics Committee, and Supervisor of Endocrinology Fellowship at College of Physicians and Surgeons, Pakistan.

He is a member of the American Association of Clinical Endocrinologists (AACE), member, Pakistan Chapter of AACE, member of an executive advisory panel of International Foundation for Mother and Child Health (IFMCH), and an executive member of Pakistan Endocrine Society and served as the General Secretary of the society as well.

He has several publications including review articles in national and international journals and participated in many conferences as invited speaker. Obesity, diabetes, and thyroid are his areas of special interest and research.

Shamim I Ahmad after obtaining his master's degree in Botany from Patna University, Bihar, India, and his Ph.D. in Molecular Genetics from Leicester University, England, joined Nottingham Polytechnic as grade 1 lecturer and subsequently promoted to Senior Lecturer. Nottingham Polytechnic subsequently became Nottingham Trent University where after serving for about 35 years, he took early retirement yet still serving as a part-time Senior Lecturer. He is now spending much of his time producing/writing medical books. For more than three decades, he researched on different areas of molecular biology/genetics including thymineless death in bacteria, genetic control of nucleotide catabolism, development of anti-AIDS drug, control of microbial infection of burns, phages of thermophilic bacteria, and microbial flora of Chernobyl after the accident at nuclear power station. But his main interest, which started about 30 years ago, is DNA damage and repair specifically by near ultraviolet light specially through the photolysis of biological compounds, production of reactive oxygen species, and their implications on human health including skin cancer. He is also investigating near ultraviolet photolysis of nonbiological compounds such as 8-metoxypsoralen and mitomycin C and their importance in psoriasis treatment and in Fanconi anemia. In collaboration with the University of Osaka, Japan, in his recent research publication, he and his colleagues were able to show that a number of naturally occurring enzymes were able to scavenge the reactive oxygen species. In 2003, he received a prestigious "Asian Jewel Award" in Britain for "Excellence in Education." He has been the Editor for the following books published by Landes Bioscience/Springer publication: *Molecular Mechanisms of Fanconi Anemia, Molecular Mechanisms of Xeroderma Pigmentosum; Molecular Mechanisms of Cockayne Syndrome; Molecular Mechanisms of Ataxia Telangiectasia; Diseases of DNA Repair;* and *Neurodegenerative Diseases, Diabetes: an Old Disease a New Insight* and also co-author for the book *Diabetes: A Comprehensive Treatise for Patients and Caregivers* and a co-editor for the book *Obesity: A Practical Guide.*

Contents

Contributors

Editors

Syed Khalid Imam, FCPS, FACE Department of Internal Medicine, Al Mouwasat Hospital, Jubail, Kingdom of Saudi Arabia

Shamim I. Ahmad, MSc, PhD School of Science & Technology, Nottingham Trent University, Nottingham, UK

Authors

Javed Akram, MRCP, FRCP, FACC, FACP, FASIM Department of Endocrinology, Shaheed Zulfiqar Ali Bhutto Medical University, PIMS, Islamabad, Pakistan

Zakir Alavi National Medical Center, Defense Housing Authority, Karachi, Pakistan

Muhammad Zaman Khan Assir, MBBS, FCPS Department of Medicine, Allama Iqbal Medical College, Lahore, Pakistan

Anilza Bonelo-Perdomo, BSc, MSc, Ph.D Division of Basic Immunology and Biomedical Sciences, University of Valle, Cali-Valle, Colombia

Nishanth Dev, MD Department of Medicine, ESIC Medical College and Hospital, Faridabad, India

Elnasser Elmaghraby, MRC Psych Military Medical Academy, Cairo, Egypt

Alan J. Hargreaves Interdisciplinary Biomedical Research Centre, School of Science & Technology, Nottingham Trent University, Nottingham, UK

Asim Hassan, MRCP, FRCP, SCE/MRCP(Diab, Endo) University Diabetes Center, King Saud University, Riyadh, Saudi Arabia

Syed Khalid Imam, FCPS, FACE Department of Internal Medicine, Al Mouwasat Hospital, Jubail, Kingdom of Saudi Arabia

Dania Idriss Marrakchi Department of Molecular Biology, University Manar 2 of Tunis, Tunis, Tunisia

Ali Jawa, MD, MPH, DABIM, DABIM (Endo), FACE, DABPNS Department of Endocrinology, Allama Iqbal Medical College, Lahore, Pakistan

Salem Kachboura Cardiology Department, Abderrahman Mami Hospital, Ariana, Tunisia

Ikram Kammoun Cardiology Department, Abderrahman Mami Hospital, Ariana, Tunisia

Faouzi Kanoun Endocrinology Department, La Rabta Hospital, Tunis, Tunisia

Henrique Vara Luiz, MD Department of Endocrinology and Diabetology, Hospital Garcia de Orta, Avenida, Almada, Portugal

Isabel Manita, MD Department of Endocrinology and Diabetology, Hospital Garcia de Orta, Avenida, Almada, Portugal

Sonia Marrakchi Meziou, MD Cardiology Department, Abderrahman Mami Hospital, Ariana, Tunisia

Ivonne Meza-Cabrera, MD Laboratory of Pathology, Hospital Universityario San José, Popayán-Cauca, Colombia

Jorge Portugal, MD Department of Endocrinology and Diabetology, Hospital Garcia de Orta, Avenida, Almada, Portugal

Syed Abbas Raza, MD, FACE Department of Internal Medicine, Shaukat Khanum Hospital and Research Center, Lahore, Pakistan

Syed Hunain Riaz, MBBS, FCPS Department of Endocrinology, Allama Iqbal Medical College, Lahore, Pakistan

Jhuma Sankar, MD Department of Pediatrics, All India Institute of Medical Sciences, New Delhi, India

Aqiba Sarfaraz Department of Diabetes and Endocrinology, Liaquat National Hospital and Medical College, Karachi, Pakistan

Aisha Sheikh, MBBS, FCPS Section of Endocrinology, Department of Medicine, The Aga Khan University Hospital, Karachi, Pakistan

Carlos Hernán Sierra-Torres, Ph.D Division of Genetic and Molecular Epidemiology, University of Cauca, Popayán-Cauca, Colombia

Hernando Vargas-Uricoechea, MD, MSc, Ph.Dc Division of Endocrinology and Metabolism, Internal Medicine Department, University of Cauca, Popayán-Cauca, Colombia

M.V. Vinay, MD Department of Pediatrics, All India Institute of Medical Sciences, New Delhi, India

Part I

Fundamental Concepts

Thyroid: A General Overview

1

Syyed Khalid Imam

Abstract

Thyroid gland is one of the largest endocrine organs and releases triiodothyronine and thyroxine. These hormones play a key role in fuel metabolism and energy homeostasis and essential for normal growth and development. Iodine is required for thyroid hormone synthesis and its imbalance affect thyroid hormone function. Thyroid dysfunction is quite common in the general population and contributes to significant health issues. Therefore, it is prudent to early diagnose and treat so as to prevent complications arising from its imbalance.

Introduction

Thyroid gland is a highly vascular endocrine organ and plays a key role in energy metabolism, growth and maturation of human body. These effects are mediated by the thyroid hormones, thyroxine (T4) and triiodothyronine (T3). Thyroid hormones stimulate diverse metabolic activities, leading to an increase in basal metabolic rate. One consequence of this activity is to increase body heat production, which seems to result, at least in part, from increased oxygen consumption and rates of ATP hydrolysis [1].

The thyroid hormones act on nearly every cell in the body. They act to increase the basal metabolic rate (BMR), affect protein synthesis, help regulate long bone growth (synergy with growth hormone) and neural maturation, and increase the body's sensitivity to catecholamines (such as adrenaline) by permissiveness. The thyroid hormones are essential to proper development and differentiation of all cells of the human body. These hormones also regulate protein, fat, and carbohydrate metabolism, affecting how human cells use energetic compounds. They also stimulate vitamin metabolism. Numerous physiological and pathological stimuli influence thyroid hormone synthesis. A detail account of thyroid hormone functions is given in Chap. 2.

Thyroid hormone dysregulation causes a significant change in body homeostasis, not only in adults but also in children where it can affect mental and growth development to a significant level. Therefore, it is important to identify the thyroid hormone deficiency as early as possible

S.K. Imam, FCPS, FACE
Department of Internal Medicine, Al Mouwasat Hospital, Jubail, Kingdom of Saudi Arabia
e-mail: docimam@yahoo.com

S.K. Imam, S.I. Ahmad (eds.), *Thyroid Disorders: Basic Science and Clinical Practice*,
DOI 10.1007/978-3-319-25871-3_1

to initiate desired treatment. This chapter will provide a concise overview of structure of thyroid gland, disease burden in community, health issues related to its dysfunction and screening strategy and recommendations.

Thyroid Gland: Basic Structure

The thyroid gland is a highly vascular butterfly-shaped brownish red organ and is composed of two cone-like right and left lobes connected via the isthmus. Each lobe is about 5 cm long, 3 cm wide and 2 cm thick. The organ is situated on the anterior side of the neck, lying against and around the larynx and trachea, reaching posteriorly the esophagus and carotid sheath (See Fig. 1.1). It starts cranially at the oblique line on the thyroid cartilage (just below the laryngeal prominence, or 'Adam's Apple'), and extends inferiorly to approximately the fifth or sixth tracheal ring [2, 3].

The thyroid is one of the largest endocrine glands, weighing 2–3 g in neonates and 18–60 g in adults, and size is increased in pregnancy. Occasionally, in 28–55 % of population a third pyramidal lobe may be present, also known as Lalouette's pyramid. It is of conical shape and extends from the upper part of the isthmus, up across the thyroid cartilage to the hyoid bone. The pyramidal lobe is a remnant of the fetal thyroid stalk, or thyroglossal duct [4]. The thyroid is supplied with arterial blood from the superior thyroid artery, a branch of the external carotid artery, and the inferior thyroid artery, a branch of the thyrocervical trunk, and sometimes by the thyroid ima artery, branching directly from the subclavian artery. The venous blood is drained via superior thyroid veins, draining in the internal jugular vein, and via inferior thyroid veins, draining via the plexus thyroideus impar in the left brachiocephalic vein. Lymphatic drainage passes frequently the lateral deep cervical lymph nodes and the pre- and paratracheal lymph nodes. The gland is supplied by parasympathetic nerve input from the superior laryngeal nerve and the recurrent laryngeal nerve [5].

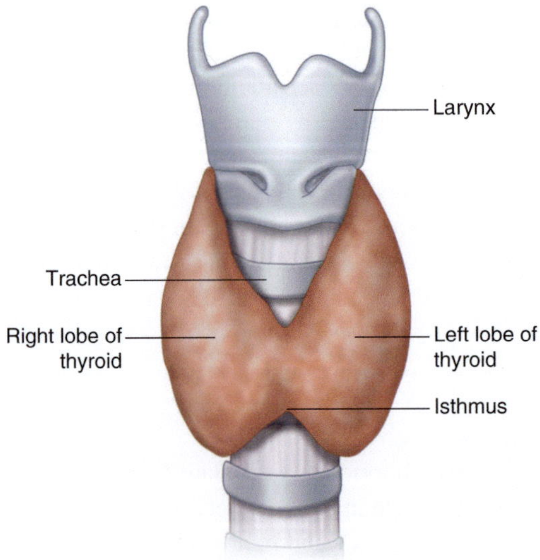

Fig. 1.1 Thyroid gland

Gross examination of thyroid gland will reveal four light-colored small nodules placed on its surface. These are known as parathyroid glands. The structure of a parathyroid gland is distinctly different from a thyroid gland. The cells that synthesize and secrete parathyroid hormone are arranged in rather dense cords or nests around abundant capillaries.

The microscopic structure of the thyroid is quite distinctive. Thyroid epithelial cells are arranged in spheres called thyroid follicles. Follicles are filled with colloid, a proteinaceous depot of thyroid hormone precursor. In addition to thyroid epithelial cells, the thyroid gland houses one other important endocrine cell, nestled in spaces between thyroid follicles, called as parafollicular or C cells which secrete the hormone calcitonin.

Thyroid Dysfunction: Distribution and Burden

Thyroid disorders are amongst the commonest endocrine diseases and there is a tremendous burden in general population, and in Indian subcontinent, it is reported to be the most common among all endocrine diseases [6]. It is quite evident from western literature that approximately 50 % of people in the community have microscopic nodules, 15 % develops palpable goiters, 10 % shows an abnormal thyroid-stimulating hormone level, and 5 % of women have overt hypothyroidism or hyperthyroidism and 3.5 % demonstrate occult papillary carcinoma [7].

As we know that iodine plays an important role in thyroid hormone regulation and nearly one-third of the world's population lives in areas of iodine deficiency [8]. In areas where the daily iodine intake is 50 mg, goiter is usually endemic, and when the daily intake falls 25 mg, congenital hypothyroidism is seen. The prevalence of goiter in areas of severe iodine deficiency can be as high as 80 %. Populations at particular risk tend to be remote and live in mountainous areas in South-East Asia, Latin America and Central Africa [9]. Iodization programmes are of proven value in reducing goiter size and in preventing goiter development and cretinism in children, but it should be remembered that iodization programmes can also induce thyrotoxicosis, especially in those aged more than 40 years with nodular goiters [10]. In iodine-sufficient areas, most persons with thyroid disorders have autoimmune disease, ranging from primary atrophic hypothyroidism, Hashimoto's thyroiditis to hyperthyroidism caused by Graves' disease [10]. Data from screening large US population Samples have revealed differences in the frequency of thyroid dysfunction and serum thyroid antibody concentrations in different ethnic groups [11, 12]. Whereas studies from Europe have revealed the influence of dietary iodine intake on the epidemiology of thyroid dysfunction [13]. See chapter 'Iodine and thyroid' for further detail.

Hyperthyroidism and hypothyroidism are common conditions that have lifelong effects on health. About 5 % of U.S. adults report having thyroid disease or taking thyroid medication [11, 12]. In a population that has been screened previously, the incidence of new cases of thyroid dysfunction is the most important factor in determining the yield of a second round of screening. In a 20-year follow-up of the Whickham population, the annual incidence of overt thyroid dysfunction was 4.9 per 1000 in women (4.1 hypothyroid and 0.8 hyperthyroid) and 0.6 per 1000 in men (all hypothyroid) [14]. In most other studies, the incidence of hyperthyroidism is 0.3–0.4 per 1000 in women and 0.01–0.1 per 1000 in men [7]. Within a given geographic region, older age, an elevated TSH level, antithyroid antibodies, and female sex are the strongest risk factors for developing overt hypothyroidism. In the Whickham survey, for a 50-year-old woman who has a serum TSH level of 6 mU/L and positive antithyroid antibodies, the risk for developing overt hypothyroidism over 20 years is 57 %; for a serum TSH of 9 mU/L, the risk is 71 % [14].

It is presumed that a 50-year-old woman who has a normal TSH and negative antibody test carries a risk for only 4 % over 20 years. The risk for progression is not evenly distributed throughout the follow-up period. Nearly all women who developed hypothyroidism within 5 years had an initial serum TSH greater than 10 mU/L.

Classification of Thyroid Dysfunction

Thyroid dysfunction is a graded phenomenon, and progresses from early to more advanced forms. As better biochemical tests have come into use, classification of the grades of thyroid dysfunction has changed dramatically. Historically, clinical, biochemical, and immunologic criteria have been used to classify patients with milder degrees of thyroid dysfunction [15, 16]. Today, the most common approach is to classify patients according to the results of thyroid function tests. In this classification, "overt hypothyroidism" refers to patients who have an elevated TSH and a low thyroxine (T4) level. "Overt hyperthyroidism" refers to patients who have a low TSH and an elevated T4 or triiodothyronine (T3).

The terms "subclinical hypothyroidism" and "mild thyroid failure" refer to patients who have an elevated TSH and a normal thyroxine level. The term "subclinical hyperthyroidism" is used to describe conditions characterized by a low TSH and normal levels of circulating thyroid hormones (thyroxine and triiodothyronine). Subclinical hyperthyroidism has the same causes as overt hyperthyroidism [17].

Thyroid Dysfunction and Health Issues

Advocates of screening for subclinical hyperthyroidism argue that early treatment might prevent the later development of atrial fibrillation, osteoporotic fractures, and complicated overt hyperthyroidism. Other potential benefits of screening are earlier treatment of neuropsychiatric symptoms and prevention of the long-term consequences of exposure of the heart muscle to excessive stimulation from thyroid hormones [18–21].

Thyroid function regulates a wide array of metabolic parameters. Thyroid function significantly affects lipoprotein metabolism as well as some cardiovascular disease (CVD) risk factors, thus influencing overall CDV risk [11, 22, 23]. The best-studied potential complications of hypothyroidism are hyperlipidemia, atherosclerosis, symptoms, and (for subclinical disease) progression to overt hypothyroidism [24–26]. In pregnancy, subclinical hypothyroidism confers additional risks to both mother and infant. Beyond their effect on lipid profile thyroid hormones can equally affect a number of other metabolic parameters related to CVD risk. Indeed, thyroid function can influence adipocyte metabolism and the production of adipokines [27–29]. Hyperthyroidism has been associated with increased levels of adiponectin, whereas hypothyroidism is not associated with significant changes in adiponectin [27, 29]. Insulin resistance is also correlated with thyroid function [30–33]. TSH is positively associated with fasting and postprandial insulin concentration and negatively with insulin sensitivity Moreover, low normal FT4 levels are significantly associated with increased insulin resistance. Oxidative stress is also affected by thyroid function with studies however showing controversial outcomes [34]. Furthermore, endothelial and cardiac function as well as atherosclerosis have been positively associated with thyroid hormone dysfunction [35]. A positive association between TSH and body mass index (BMI) or waist circumference has also been described [36, 37].

Thyroid hormone excess causes left ventricular thickening, which is associated with an increased risk of heart failure and cardiac-related death. Thyrotoxicosis has been associated with dilated cardiomyopathy, right heart failure with pulmonary hypertension, and diastolic dysfunction and atrial fibrillation [38]. See chapter 'arrhythmia and thyroid dysfunction' for further details. An increase in the rate of bone resorption occurs. Bone loss, measured by bone mineral densitometry, can be seen in severe hyperthyroidism at all ages and in both sexes. In mild subclinical disease, however, bone loss has been convincingly shown only in postmenopausal women.

Screening for Thyroid Disorders

Screening is defined as the application of a test to detect a potential disease or condition in a person who has no known signs or symptoms of that condition [39]. By this definition, screening with thyroid function tests may identify asymptomatic individuals as well as patients who have mild and nonspecific symptoms such as cold intolerance or feeling a little tired.

Accuracy of Screening Tests

Screening for thyroid dysfunction can be done using a history and physical examination, antithyroid antibodies, or thyroid function tests, including various assays for TSH and T4. Today, the TSH test is usually proposed as the initial test in screening because of its ability to detect abnormalities before serum thyroxine and triiodothyronine levels are abnormal. When used to confirm suspected thyroid disease in patients referred to an endocrine specialty clinic, the sensitive TSH has a sensitivity above 98 % and a specificity greater than 92 % for the clinical and functional diagnosis [40].

In screening programs and in the primary care clinic, many patients found to have an abnormal TSH revert to normal over time. In one randomized trial, for example, mildly elevated TSH levels reverted to normal in 8 of 19 patients given placebo [41].

In older subjects, only 59 % (range, 14–87 %) of patients with an undetectable TSH on initial screening had an undetectable TSH level when the TSH was repeated [42, 43].

In the Framingham cohort, screening identified 41 people with an undetectable serum TSH (≤0.1 mU/L) and a normal serum T4 level (<129 nmol/L) [44]. After 4 years of follow-up, when 33 of these people were retested, 29 had higher serum TSH levels (>0.1 mU/L). Nonthyroidal illness is an important cause of false positive TSH test results. In a recent systematic review of screening patients admitted to acute care and geriatric hospitals, the positive predictive value of a low serum TSH (<0.1 mU/L) was 0.24, meaning that approximately 1 in 4 patients proved to have hyperthyroidism. For hypothyroidism, the predictive value of a serum TSH between 6.7 and 20 mU/L was 0.06. In 1996, the United States Preventive Services task Force (USPSTF) recommended against routine screening for thyroid disease in asymptomatic adults but recommended screening based on the higher prevalence of disease and the increased likelihood that symptoms of thyroid disease will be overlooked [45].

The USPSTF: Summary of Recommendation

The USPSTF found fair evidence that the thyroid-stimulating hormone (TSH) test can detect subclinical thyroid disease in persons without symptoms of thyroid dysfunction, but poor evidence that treatment improves clinically important outcomes in adults with screen-detected thyroid disease. Although the yield of screening is greater in certain high-risk groups (e.g., postpartum women, persons with Down syndrome, and the elderly), the USPSTF found poor evidence that screening in these groups leads to clinically important benefits. There is the potential for harm caused by false-positive screening tests; however, the magnitude of harm is not known. There is good evidence that overtreatment with levothyroxine occurs in a substantial proportion of patients, but the long-term harmful effects of overtreatment are not known. As a result, the USPSTF could not determine the balance of benefits and harms of screening asymptomatic adults for thyroid disease.

Recommendations of Other Authorities

The American Thyroid Association recommends measuring thyroid function in all adults beginning at age 35 years and every 5 years thereafter, noting that more frequent screening may be appropriate in high-risk or symptomatic individuals [46].

The Canadian Task Force on the Periodic Health Examination recommends maintaining a high index of clinical suspicion for nonspecific symptoms consistent with hypothyroidism when examining perimenopausal and postmenopausal women [47].

The American College of Physicians recommends screening women older than 50 with one or more general symptoms that could be caused by thyroid disease [48].

The American Association of Clinical Endocrinologists recommends TSH measurement in women of childbearing age before pregnancy or during the first trimester [49].

The American College of Obstetricians and Gynecologists recommends that physicians be aware of the symptoms and risk factors for postpartum thyroid dysfunction and evaluate patients when indicated [50].

The American Academy of Family Physicians recommends against routine thyroid screening in asymptomatic patients younger than age 60 [51].

Conclusion

Thyroid gland is a highly vascular organ and performs various important metabolic functions and is necessary for normal growth and development, all these effects mediated by thyroid hormones. Thyroid gland dysfunction is quite common in the community and contributing a significant disease burden globally. Iodine plays an important role in thyroid hormone synthesis and its nutrition should be ensured to all individual at risk of deficiency. Although, Iodization programmes are of proven value in reducing goiter size and in preventing goiter development and cretinism in children, but it should be remembered that iodization programmes can also induce hyperthyroidism, especially in those aged more than 40 years with nodular goiters. Due to lack of resources and insufficient data, routine screening for thyroid dysfunction is generally not recommended by many authorities, however, it should be considered for those at high risk of developing thyroid dysfunction. TSH is the best screening test to order with a sensitivity of over 98 % and has the ability to detect thyroid dysfunction in asymptomatic phase. Thyroid dysfunction carries significant degree of morbidity and mortality and early diagnosis and treatment are essential to avert long term complications.

References

1. Klaudia B, Dagmar F, Heike B. Molecules important for thyroid hormone synthesis and action – known facts and future perspectives. Thyroid Res. 2011;4 Suppl 1:S9.
2. Cummings CW, et al. Thyroid anatomy. In: Cummings CW, editor. Otolaryngology – head and neck surgery. 3rd ed. Mosby: St. Louis; 1998. p. 2445–9.
3. Williams PL, Bannister LH, et al. Gray's anatomy. 38th ed. New York: Churchill Livingstone; 1995. p. 1891–6.
4. Kim DW, Jung SL, Baek JH, et al. The prevalence and features of thyroid pyramidal lobe, accessory thyroid, and ectopic thyroid as assessed by computed tomography: a multicenter study. Thyroid. 2013;23(1):84–91.
5. Dorland. Dorland's. Illustrated medical dictionary. 32nd ed. Philadelphia: Elsevier Saunders; 2012. p. 999.
6. Kochupillai N. Clinical endocrinology in India. Curr Sci. 2000;8:1061–7.
7. Wang C, Crapo LM. The epidemiology of thyroid disease and implications for screening. Endocrinol Metab Clin North Am. 1997;26(1):189–218.
8. Zimmerman MB. Iodine deficiency. Endocr Rev. 2009;30:376–408.
9. Vanderpump MP. The epidemiology of thyroid disease. Br Med Bull. 2011;99:39–51.
10. Vanderpump MP. The epidemiology of thyroid diseases. In: Braverman LE, Utiger RD, editors. Werner and Ingbar's the thyroid: a fundamental and clinical text. 9th ed. Philadelphia: JB Lippincott-Raven; 2005. p. 398–496.
11. Canaris GJ, Manowitz NR, Mayor G, et al. The Colorado thyroid disease prevalence study. Arch Intern Med. 2000;160:526–34.
12. Hollowell JG, Staehling NW, Flanders WD, et al. Serum TSH, T4, and thyroid antibodies in the United States population (1988 to 1994): National Health and Nutrition Examination Survey (NHANES III). J Clin Endocrinol Metab. 2002;87:489–99.
13. Laurberg P, Bulow Pedersen I, Knudsen N, et al. Environmental iodine intake affects the type of nonmalignant thyroid disease. Thyroid. 2001;11:457–69.
14. Vanderpump MP, Tunbridge WMG, French JM, et al. The incidence of thyroid disorders in the community: a twenty-year follow-up of the Whickham survey. Clin Endocrinol (Oxf). 1995;43:55–68.
15. Helfand M, editor. Screening for thyroid dysfunction: Rationale, strategies, and cost-effectiveness. St. Louis: Mosby-Year Book, Inc.; 1992.
16. O'Reilly DS. Thyroid function tests-time for a reassessment. BMJ. 2000;320:1332–4.
17. McDermott MT, Ridgway EC. Subclinical hypothyroidism is mild thyroid failure and should be treated. J Clin Endocrinol Metab. 2001;86:4585–90.
18. Sawin C, Geller A, Wolf P. Low serum thyrotropin concentrations as a risk factor for atrial fibrillation in older persons. N Engl J Med. 1994;331:1249–52.
19. Parle JV, Maisonneuve P, Sheppard MC, Boyle P, Franklyn JA. Prediction of all-cause and cardiovascular mortality in elderly people from one low serum thyrotropin result: a 10-year cohort study. Lancet. 2001;358:861–5.
20. Uzzan B, Campos J, Cucherat M, et al. Effects on bone mass of long term treatment with thyroid hormones: a meta-analysis. J Clin Endocrinol Metab. 1996;81:4278–89.
21. Faber J, Galloe AM. Changes in bone mass during prolonged subclinical hyperthyroidism due to L-thyroxine treatment: a meta-analysis. Eur J Endocrinol. 1994;130:350–6.
22. Duntas LH. Thyroid disease and lipids. Thyroid. 2002;12:287–93.

23. Friis T, Pedersen LR. Serum lipids in hyper- and hypothyroidism before and after treatment. Clin Chim Acta. 1987;162:155–63.
24. Johnston J, McLelland A, O'Reilly DS. The relationship between serum cholesterol and serum thyroid hormones in male patients with suspected hypothyroidism. Ann Clin Biochem. 1993;30:256–9.
25. Valdemarsson S, Hansson P, Hedner P, Nilsson-Ehle P. Relations between thyroid function, hepatic and lipoprotein lipase activities, and plasma lipoprotein concentrations. Acta Endocrinol. 1983;104:50–6.
26. Elder J, McLelland A, O'Reilly DS, et al. The relationship between serum cholesterol and serum thyrotropin, thyroxine, and tri-iodothyronine concentrations in suspected hypothyroidism. Ann Clin Biochem. 1990;27:110–3.
27. Iglesias P, Diez JJ. Influence of thyroid dysfunction on serum concentrations of adipocytokines. Cytokine. 2007;40:61–70.
28. Viguerie N, Millet L, Avizou S, Vidal H, Larrouy D, Langin D. Regulation of human adipocyte gene expression by thyroid hormone. J Clin Endocrinol Metab. 2002;87:630–4.
29. Hsieh CJ, Wang PW. Serum concentrations of adiponectin in patients with hyperthyroidism before and after control of thyroid function. Endocr J. 2008;55:489–94.
30. Crunkhorn S, Patti ME. Links between thyroid hormone action, oxidative metabolism, and diabetes risk? Thyroid. 2008;18:227–37.
31. Fernandez-Real JM, Lopez-Bermejo A, Castro A, et al. Thyroid function is intrinsically linked to insulin sensitivity and endothelium-dependent vasodilatation in healthy euthyroid subjects. J Clin Endocrinol Metab. 2006;91:3337–43.
32. Chubb SA, Davis WA, Davis TM. Interactions among thyroid function, insulin sensitivity, and serum lipid concentrations: the Fremantle diabetes study. J Clin Endocrinol Metab. 2005;90:5317–20.
33. Roos A, Bakker SJ, Links TP, Gans RO, Wolffenbuttel BH. Thyroid function is associated with components of the metabolic syndrome in euthyroid subjects. J Clin Endocrinol Metab. 2007;92:491–6.
34. Faure P, Oziol L, Artur Y, Chomard P. Thyroid hormone (T3) and its acetic derivative (TA3) protect low-density lipoproteins from oxidation by different mechanisms. Biochimie. 2004;86:411–8.
35. Auer J, Berent R, Weber T, Lassnig E, Eber B. Thyroid function is associated with presence and severity of coronary atherosclerosis. Clin Cardiol. 2003;26:569–73.
36. De Pergola G, Ciampolillo A, Paolotti S, Trerotoli P, Giorgino R. Free triiodothyronine and thyroid stimulating hormone are directly associated with waist circumference, independently of insulin resistance, metabolic parameters and blood pressure in overweight and obese women. Clin Endocrinol (Oxf). 2007;67:265–9.
37. Knudsen N, Laurberg P, Rasmussen LB, et al. Small differences in thyroid function may be important for body mass index and the occurrence of obesity in the population. J Clin Endocrinol Metab. 2005;90:4019–24.
38. Dahl P, Danzi S, Klein I. Thyrotoxic cardiac disease. Curr Heart Fail Rep. 2008;5:170–6.
39. Eddy D. How to think about screening. In: Eddy D, editor. Common screening tests. Philadelphia: American Coll Physicians; 1991. p. 1–21.
40. Helfand M. Screening for subclinical thyroid dysfunction in nonpregnant adults: a summary of the evidence for the U.S. Preventive Services Task Force. Ann Intern Med. 2004;140(2):128–41.
41. Jaeschke R, Guyatt G, Gerstein H, et al. Does treatment with L-thyroxine influence health status in middle-aged and older adults with subclinical hypothyroidism? J Gen Intern Med. 1996;11:744–9.
42. Parle J, Franklyn J, Cross K, Jones S, Sheppard M. Prevalence and follow-up of abnormal thyrotropin (TSH) concentrations in the elderly in the United Kingdom. Clin Endocrinol (Oxf). 1991;34:77–83.
43. Sundbeck G, Jagenburg R, Johansson P-M, et al. Clinical significance of a low serum thyrotropin concentration by chemiluminometric assay in 85-year-old women and men. Arch Intern Med. 1991;151:549–56.
44. Sawin CT, Geller A, Kaplan MM, et al. Low serum thyrotropin (Thyroid-Stimulating Hormone) in older persons without hyperthyroidism. Arch Intern Med. 1991;151:165–8.
45. U.S. Preventive Services Task Force. Screening for thyroid disease. Guide to clinical preventive services. Baltimore: Williams & Wilkins; 1996.
46. Ladenson PW, Singer PA, Ain KB, et al. American Thyroid Association guidelines for detection of thyroid dysfunction [published erratum appears in Arch Intern Med 2001;161:284]. Arch Intern Med. 2000;160:1573–5.
47. Canadian Task Force on the Periodic Health Examination. The Canadian Guide to clinical preventive health care. Ottawa: Canada Communication Group; 1994. p. 611–8.
48. Clinical guideline, part 1. Screening for thyroid disease. American College of Physicians. Ann Intern Med. 1998;129:141–3.
49. Baskin HJ, Cobin RH, Duick DS, et al. American Association of Clinical Endocrinologists medical guidelines for clinical practice for the evaluation and treatment of hyperthyroidism and hypothyroidism. Endocr Pract. 2002;8:457–69.
50. American College of Obstetricians and Gynecologists. ACOG Practice Bulletin. Clinical management guidelines for obstetricians-gynecologists. Number 37, August 2002. Obstet Gynecol. 2002;100:387–96.
51. American Academy of Family Physicians. Summary of policy recommendations for periodic health examinations. Accessed 25 Feb 2004, at: http://www.aafp.org/PreBuilt/PHErev54.pdf.

2 Functions of Thyroid Hormones

Nishanth Dev, Jhuma Sankar, and M.V. Vinay

Abstract

Thyroid hormones (THs) play critical roles in growth, differentiation and metabolism. They are important for optimal functioning of almost all tissues with major effects on metabolic rate and oxygen consumption. The thyroid gland secretes two biologically active thyroid hormones: thyroxine (T4) and 3,5,3′-triiodothyronine (T3). TH synthesis and secretion is exquisitely regulated by a negative-feedback system that involves the hypothalamus, pituitary, and thyroid gland (the HPT axis). Some of the important functions of the thyroid hormones include- neural growth and differentiation, myocardial contractility, regulation of bone formation and resorption, development and function of brown and white adipose tissue, cholesterol metabolism and synthesis, and in-utero they are important for fetal growth and differentiation. Thus, given their pleotropic effects, thyroid hormones are critical for survival and optimal functioning of the human body.

Introduction

Thyroid hormones (THs) play critical roles in growth, differentiation and metabolism. They are important for optimal functioning of almost all tissues with major effects on metabolic rate and oxygen consumption. Therefore, it is not surprising that, thyroid gland disorders are among the most common endocrine disorders. Thyroid dysfunction affects several hundreds of people worldwide. Therefore it is important to understand its functions so as to clinically correlate with conditions causing deficiency or excess of the hormones.

N. Dev, MD (✉)
Department of Medicine, ESIC Medical College and Hospital, Faridabad, India
e-mail: devnishant@gmail.com

J. Sankar, MD • M.V. Vinay, MD
Department of Pediatrics, All India Institute of Medical Sciences, New Delhi, India

Thyroid Hormone Synthesis

Thyroid gland is a chief endocrine gland in the body situated in the anterior triangle of neck in front of thyroid cartilage. The thyroid gland

S.K. Imam, S.I. Ahmad (eds.), *Thyroid Disorders: Basic Science and Clinical Practice*,
DOI 10.1007/978-3-319-25871-3_2

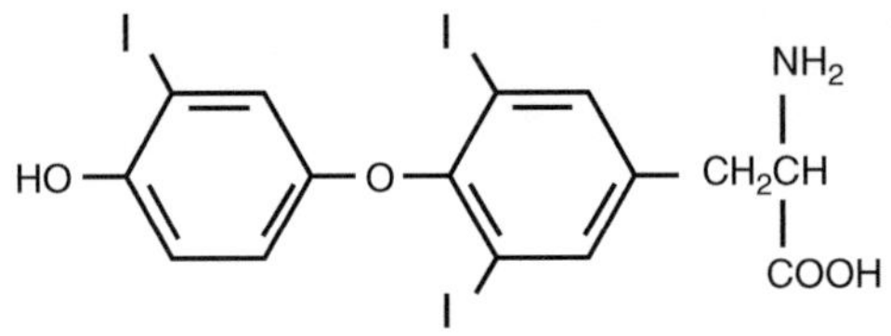

3,3′5-Triiodo-L-Thyronine
(T_3)

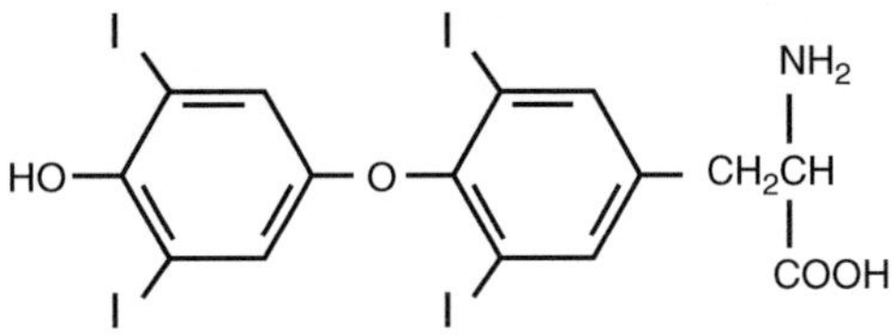

Thyroxine
(T_4)

Fig. 2.1 Structure of thyroid hormones

secretes two biologically active thyroid hormones: thyroxine (T4) and 3,5,3′-triiodothyronine (T3) (Fig. 2.1). They are composed of a phenyl ring attached via an ether linkage to a tyrosine molecule. Both have two iodine atoms on their inner tyrosine ring. The difference between the two is that, T4 has two iodine atoms on its phenyl (outer) ring, whereas T3 has only one. The compound formed if an iodine atom is removed from the inner ring of T4 is 3,3′,5′-triiodothyronine (reverse T3, rT3), which has no biological activity [1].

Steps Involved in Synthesis of Thyroid Hormones

TH synthesis and secretion is exquisitely regulated by a negative-feedback system that involves the hypothalamus, pituitary, and thyroid gland [hypothalamic/pituitary/thyroid (HPT) axis] [2].

- Thyrotropin releasing hormone (TRH) is a tripeptide (PyroGlu-His-Pro) synthesized in the paraventricular nucleus of the hypothalamus. It is transported via axons to the median eminence and then to the anterior pituitary via the portal capillary plexus.
- TRH binds to TRH receptors in pituitary thyrotropes, a subpopulation of pituitary cells that secrete thyroid stimulating hormone (TSH). TRH stimulation leads to release and synthesis of new TSH in thyrotropes [3, 4].
- TSH is a 28-kDa glycoprotein composed of α- and β-subunits designated as glycoprotein hormone α- and TSH β-subunits. Both TRH and TSH secretion are negatively regulated by TH and described in detail in the section under 'central regulation of thyroid hormone function' below. An important mechanism for the negative regulation of TSH is probably the intrapituitary conversion of circulating T4 to T3 by type II deiodinase.
- TSH is the primary regulator of TH release and secretion. It also has a critical role in thyroid growth and development. TSH binds to the TSH receptor (TSHr), which also is a seven-transmembrane spanning receptor coupled to Gs. A number of thyroid genes, including Na+/I− symporter (NIS), thyroglobulin (Tg), and thyroid peroxidase (TPO), are stimulated by TSH and promote the synthesis of TH [2].
- Iodide is actively transported and concentrated into the thyroid by NIS. The trapped iodide is oxidized by TPO in the presence of hydrogen peroxide and incorporated into the tyrosine residues of a 660-kDa glycoprotein, Tg. This iodination of specific tyrosines located on Tg yields monoiodinated and diiodinated residues (MIT, monoiodo-tyrosines; DIT, diiodo-tyrosines) that are enzymatically coupled to form T4 and T3 [5].
- The iodinated Tg containing MIT, DIT, T4, and T3, then is stored as an extracellular storage polypeptide in the colloid within the lumen of thyroid follicular cells.
- The secretion of THs requires endocytosis of the stored iodinated Tg from the apical surface of the thyroid follicular cell. The internalized Tg is incorporated in phagolysosomes and undergoes proteolytic digestion, recapture of MIT and DIT, and release of T4 and T3 into the circulation via the basal surface. The majority of released TH is in the form of T4, as

total serum T4 is 40-fold higher than serum T3. Only 0.03 % of the total serum T4 is free (unbound), with the remainder bound to carrier proteins such as thyroxine binding globulin (TBG), albumin, and thyroid binding prealbumin. Approximately 0.3 % of the total serum T3 is free, with the remainder bound to TBG and albumin. It is the free TH that enters target cells and generates a biological response.

- While T4 is solely produced by thyroid gland, T3 is a product of the thyroid as well as all tissue in which it is produced by deiodination of T4. Only 20 % of circulating T3 is synthesized in the gland and rest is generated by peripheral conversion of T4 by the deiodinase present in 3 forms : type 1 deiodinase (D1), preferentially expressed in the liver and also expressed in the kidney, thyroid, and pituitary; D2, present in the CNS, anterior pituitary, brown adipose tissue, and placenta; and D3 in the CNS, placenta, skin, and fetal tissue. D1 and D2 are activating forms while D3 is the inactivating form. These are seleno enzymes and selenium deficiency is associated with decreased activity. D2 is the primary activator enzyme causing rapid increase in intracellular T3 and thereby regulate the effects in human tissues [6, 7].
- In addition to the classical thyroid hormones, thyroid gland also secretes non- classical thyroid hormones namely thyronamines, tetrac, triac, di-iodothyronine and reverse T3. The functions and actions of these molecules are still under research.

> Only 0.03 % and 0.3 % of total serum T4 and T3 respectively is free (unbound). It is the free TH that enters target cells and generates a biological response

Role of Iodine in Thyroid Hormone Synthesis and Function

Iodine is the chief elemental composition of thyroid hormones and its deficiency is a major cause of hypothyroidism in the developing world. Iodine is absorbed from the GI tract in the form of iodide which circulates in the plasma with a half-life of 24 h. About 75–80 % of the total body iodine gets concentrated in the thyroid tissue with the help of NIS (basolateral sodium iodide symporter) across a concentration gradient of 20–50 times. Iodide is excreted mainly by the kidney within 24–48 h after consumption [1, 5, 6]. There are various methods of iodine estimation namely calorimeter using spectrophotometry (most common), iodine specific electrode, neutron activation analysis and mass spectrometry.

Wolff- Chiakoff Effect

In response to increasing doses of iodine above the optimum level, the rate of thyroid hormone synthesis and release decreases due to its inhibitory action on the process of 'organification'. This acute inhibition of organification secondary to high concentration of plasma iodode levels is termed as Wolff Chiakoff effect (thyroid constipation). The underlying mechanism is probably due to inhibition of peroxidase enzyme and down regulation of NIS transporter [8]. The methods to estimate burden of iodine deficiency in field survey are :

1. Palpatory method : In areas of moderate to severe iodine deficiency, size of goiter will give an estimate of prevalence iodine deficiency.
2. Spot UI (urinary iodine) concentration: More than 90 % of iodine is eliminated by kidney and hence the median of UI in spot urine sample will give an estimate of recent intake of iodine.
3. Thyroglobulin levels: In iodine deficiency, thyroglobulin levels increase due to greater TSH stimulation and thyroid mass.

Central Regulation of Thyroid Hormone Synthesis: The 'Hypothalamic –Pituitary-Thyroid Axis'

The hypothalamic-pituitary-thyroid (HPT) axis primarily functions to maintain normal, circulating levels of thyroid hormone that is essential for the biological function of all tissues. Important among these functions are regulation of food intake and energy expenditure among others [1, 2, 6].

Production of TRH

This regulatory system contains a group of neurons that reside in the hypothalamic paraventricular nucleus (PVN), produce TRH, and integrate a wide variety of humoral and neuronal signals to regulate the HPT axis. The TRH synthesizing neurons are present in several brain regions, but only hypophysiotropic TRH neurons located in the PVN are involved in the central regulation of the HPT axis. This nucleus is a critical vegetative center of the hypothalamus and is located symmetrically at the upper third of the third ventricle. The PVN contains a magnocellular and a parvocellular division. The magnocellular division houses oxytocin and vasopressin neurons that project to the posterior pituitary. The parvocellular division is further divided into anterior, periventricular, medial, ventral, dorsal, and lateral parvocellular subdivisions. In humans, the PVN also contains a large population of TRH neurons, especially in its medial part, but the location of hypophysiotropic TRH neurons is not yet known [9, 10].

Hypophysiotropic and Non-hypophysiotropic Neurons

Hypophysiotropic TRH neurons are functionally different from the nonhypophysiotropic TRH neurons in the PVN. Only hypophysiotropic TRH neurons project to the external zone of the median eminence, where their axon terminals release TRH into the extracellular space of this blood brain- barrier -free circumventricular organ. TRH is then conveyed to the anterior pituitary via the hypophysial portal circulation where TRH regulates the secretion of TSH from thyrotrophs and prolactin from lactotrophs. In addition to TRH, hypophysiotropic neurons also express a second neuropeptide, cocaine and amphetamine regulated transcript (CART) [2]. CART is simultaneously released into the hypophysial portal circulation and has been shown to inhibit the effect of TRH on prolactin secretion, but it has no effect on TRH induced release of TSH. Hypophysiotropic TRH neurons also express the vesicular glutamate transporter 2, establishing the glutamatergic phenotype of these cells but its physiological significance is unknown [9, 10].

In contrast to the hypophysiotropic TRH neurons, non-hypophysiotropic TRH synthesizing neurons are widely distributed in the central nervous system. However, there is little information available on the anatomy and physiologic effects of these neurons.

Role of Autonomic Nervous System in Regulation of Thyroid Function

In addition to the stimulation of TSH secretion of the anterior pituitary by TRH, the central nervous system can also regulate thyroid function via the autonomic nervous system [11, 12]. The thyroid gland is innervated by both adrenergic nerve fibers of the sympathetic nervous system and the cholinergic axons originating from the vagus nerve. Both sympathetic and parasympathetic nerves densely innervate the blood vessels of the thyroid gland, but axon terminals of these autonomic systems can also be found around the thyroid follicles, indicating that not only the blood flow, but also the activity of thyroid follicles could be under direct control of autonomic inputs. Unfortunately, relatively little data are available about how these to the thyroid gland regulate thyroid function. However, the sympathetic input seems to have an inhibitory action because electrical stimulation of the cervical sympathetic trunk decreases thyroid blood flow. Noradrenaline also inhibits the stimulatory effect of TSH on the thyroid cells in vitro and decreases thyroid hormone secretion in vivo. In contrast, electric stimulation of the thyroid nerve, which carries parasympathetic inputs to the thyroid gland, results in increased thyroid blood flow that can be prevented by atropine pretreatment. In addition to the classical transmitters, the neuropeptides, NPY and vasoactive intestinal peptide are also present in axons innervating the thyroid gland. NPY is present in the sympathetic innervation of the thyroid gland and inhibits thyroidal blood flow. In contrast, vasoactive intestinal

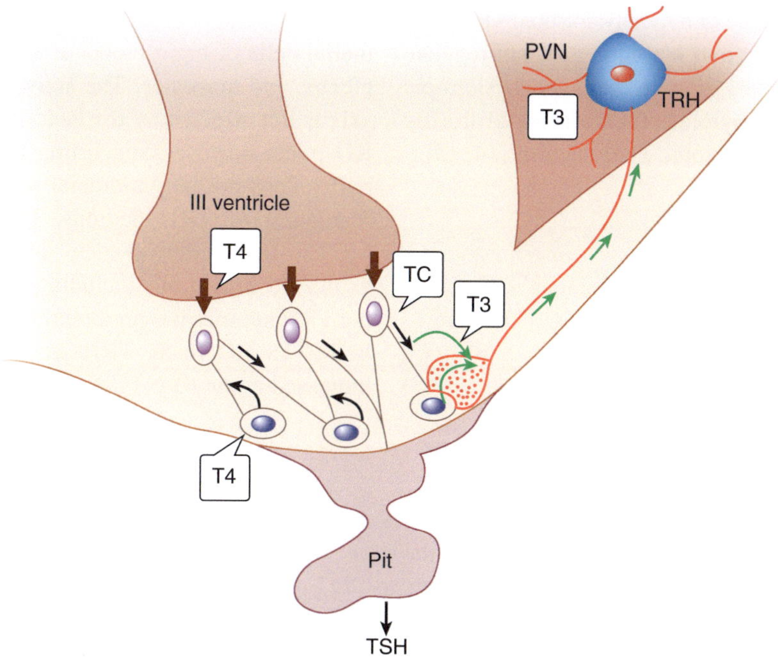

Fig. 2.2 Schematic representation of the negative feedback regulation of the Hypothalamic-pituitary-thyroid axis by thyroid hormones. *TC* Tanycyte, *TSH* thyroid stimulating hormone, *TRH* Thyrotropin releasing hormone, *PVN* paraventricular nucleus, *Pit* pituitary

peptide increases the thyroid blood flow and thyroid hormone secretion [11, 12].

Inactivation of Secreted TRH

Inactivation of secreted TRH in the brain is primarily catalyzed by a membrane bound ectoenzyme, pyroglutamyl peptidase II (PPII). PPII is a type II integral membrane protein comprised of a small, N-terminal, intracellular region and a large, extracellular domain containing the active site of the enzyme. PPII produces the dipeptide HisProNH from TRH, which is further degraded by dipeptidyl aminopeptidase IV, or spontaneously cyclizes to His-Pro diketopiperazine. PPII is primarily synthesized by neurons, but it is also produced by tanycytes, a specialized glial cell type, in the hypothalamus. Inhibition of PPII activity markedly increases the amount of TRH released from brain tissue slices, supporting the importance of thispeptidase in the metabolism of TRH. In serum, TRH is degraded by a soluble enzyme that was formerly called thyroliberinase, but was subsequently shown to be a product of the PPII gene produced in the liver by proteolytic cleavage of membrane bound PPII . Two broad specificity cytosolic peptidases, pyroglutamyl peptidase- I and prolyl endopeptidase, can also degrade TRH. However, because there is no evidence for the presence of these enzymes in the extracellular space it appears that these enzymes do not play a major role in the inactivation of released TRH [9, 11, 13].

Negative Feedback Regulation of Hypophysiotropic TRH Neurons

Negative feedback regulation of hypophysiotropic TRH neurons is an important regulatory mechanism in ensuring stable thyroid hormone levels (Fig. 2.2). When circulating thyroid hormone levels are increased, TRH gene expression is decreased in hypophysiotropic neurons and vice versa. Regulation of TRH transcription by thyroid hormone is relatively rapid because the exogenous administration of thyroid hormone can suppress transcription of the TRH gene in the PVN within 5 h [14]. This regulatory mechanism is a unique feature of hypophysiotropic TRH neurons because thyroid hormone does not regulate TRH gene expression in nonhypophysiotropic TRH neurons. Thyroid hormone is sensed directly by the hypophysiotropic TRH neurons [14, 15].

> Thyroid hormones regulate transcription of TRH gene rapidly. This is unique to hypophysiotropic TRH neurons as THs are sensed directly by these neurons.

Deiodinases and Their Role in Negative Feedback Regulation

The concept that the circulating level of T3 is solely responsible for negative feedback regulation of hypophysiotropic TRH by acting directly on these neurons has been challenged. It has been seen that restoration of circulating levels of T3 to normal levels in hypothyroid rats without the administration of T4 did not normalize TRH gene expression in the PVN. Only if very high hyperthyroid levels of T3 were achieved in the circulating blood was it possible to decrease TRH mRNA levels in the PVN into the normal, euthyroid range. These data indicate that in addition to T3, circulating T4 is also necessary for appropriate feedback control of hypophysiotropic TRH neurons. However, because T4 functions primarily as a prohormone, its conversion to T3 within the central nervous system must be an essential part of the feedback regulatory mechanism [16, 17].

> Circulating T4 is as important for appropriate feedback control of TRH neurons as T3

Role of Thyroid Hormone Transporters in Secretion of Ths

Several transporters contribute to the uptake of TH into the peripheral tissue, including organic anion-transporting polypeptides (OATPs), L-type amino acid transporters, monocarboxylate transporters (MCT), and bile acid transporter. OATP1C1 has a similar high affinity for T3 and T4 and is abundantly expressed in endothelial cells of brain blood vessels, the choroid plexus, and tanycytes. The activity of the HPT axis is not affected by the lack of OATP1C1 in KO mice, however, suggesting that this transporter does not play a crucial role in feedback regulation of TRH neurons. In contrast, the MCT8 transporter, which is preferentially expressed in neurons including hypophysiotropic TRH neurons has preferential affinity for T3. In MCT8 KO mice, TRH gene expression is increased in the PVN [18].

> **The key points to remember about the Hypophysiotropic TRH axis are**
> - The Hypophysiotropic TRH neurons secrete TRH
> - Under basal conditions, the activity of hypophysiotropic TRH neurons is regulated by the negative feedback effects of thyroid hormone
> - This involves complex interactions between hypophysiotropic TRH neurons and the vascular system, cerebrospinal fluid, and specialized glial cells called tanycytes.
> - Hypophysiotropic TRH neurons also integrate other humoral and neuronal inputs that can alter the setpoint for negative feedback regulation by thyroid hormone.
> - This mechanism facilitates adaptation of the organism to changing environmental conditions, including the shortage of food and a cold environment.
> - The thyroid axis is also affected by other adverse conditions such as infection, but the central mechanisms mediating suppression of hypophysiotropic TRH may be pathophysiological.

Thyroid Hormones- Mechanism of Action

The thyroid hormones mediate their actions through two mechanisms: genomic and non genomic.

Genomic Pathways

Genomic pathways acts through nuclear receptors (TRs) wherein the hormones, similar to steroid hormones, after entering the cell bind to the receptors inside the nucleus which homodimerise with the transcription factors and regulate the transcription. The mechanism in detail is as follows: TRs homodimerize or interact with other nuclear receptors such as the retinoic X receptor. They belong to a large family of ligand-dependent transcription factors such as vitamins, xenobiotics, and sex steroids. They are termed as TRa and TRb and are encoded by two genes (a and b) located on two different chromosomes that express differently in developing and adult tissues. The expression of Tra1 is highest in the brain, with lower levels in the kidney, skeletal muscle, lungs, heart, and liver, whereas the expression of Trb1 is mainly in the kidneys and liver, and lower in brain, heart, thyroid, skeletal muscle, lungs, and spleen. TRb isoforms are involved in lipid metabolism as it has been found that TRb disruption in mice impairs fatty acid (FA) oxidation even in the presence of TRa over expression. TRb agonists have approximately tenfold greater affinity for TRb than TRa, with major effect on the liver and are very efficient in lowering of cholesterol [19, 20].

> TRb isoforms are involved in lipid metabolism. TRb agonists such as KB141 have therefore been seen to reduce cholesterol in primates and may have future potential as a cholesterol lowering agent in humans as well

The expression of thyroid hormones and its functions also depend on co-regulators. Co-activators that facilitate thyroid hormone functions are steroid receptor co activator, p160 family, cAMP responsive elements (CREB) and PGC a1 acting through acetylation of histones and transcription upregulators. Co-repressors like NCoR and SMRT down regulate action of thyroid hormones by deacetylation. Although T3 exerts many of its actions through canonical transcriptional regulation, an increasing amount of evidence shows that many of T3 effects are initiated outside the nucleus. These effects are mediated by what are called the non-genomic pathways [21, 22].

Non-genomic Pathways

Non genomic actions are mediated through second messenger systems like Calcium-ATPase, PI3K(phosphor-inositol 3 kinase) and AMPK(AMP activated protein kinase). However, the nongenomic processes overall are poorly understood but emerge as important accessory mechanisms in TH actions. They have been observed at the plasma membrane, in the cytoplasm, cytoskeleton, and in organelles.

For example, on the cell surface through non-genomic actions, THs trigger the serine–threonine kinase (MPK/ERK) pathway via the integrin receptor initiating complex cellular events. In the cytoplasm, THs activate PI3K and thereby downstream gene transcription of specific genes. T3 also activates PI3K from the integrin avb3 hormone receptor site. Calcium is a second messenger regulated by THs through the modulation of a Ca2C-ATPase. Here again through short-term nongenomic effects THs act on intracellular calcium by modulating plasma membrane and mitochondrial pathways in rat pituitary GH3 cells. Their cellular actions involving Akt/protein kinase B and AMP-activated protein kinase (AMPK) (in mice) are well documented. In rat skeletal muscle, T3 stimulates FA and glucose metabolism through rapid activation of AMPK and Akt/protein kinase B signal transduction [21–23].

> Thyroid hormones exert their action through genomic and non-genomic pathways. In genomic pathways the THs bind to thyroid hormone receptors inside the nucleus and mediate transcription. In non-genomic pathways they mediate their actions through second messenger systems such as Calcium-ATPase, PI3K and AMPK

Table 2.1 Effect of thyroid hormones on various organs and tissues of the body

Organ/tissue	Function of thyroid hormones
1. Brain	Organization and function throughout life
	Synaptogenesis, neurogenesis, migration, plasticity and myelination
	Effect cholinergic and **seretonergic activities**
	T3 is the predominant form acting on brain
2. Myocardium	Essential for aerobic metabolism and prevention lactic acidosis
	Upregulate beta adrenergic receptors and have inotropic and vasodilatory properties
	Effect intracellular homeostasis of ionized calcium
	Medical and surgical conditions may decrease T3 and T4 and increase reverse T3. This phenomenon is called 'Euthyroid sick syndrome' (ESS)
	ESS causes stunned myocardium and may cause cardiogenic shock in extreme cases.
3. Bone	Important for bone growth and development
	Involved in both bone formation and resorption
	Hyperthyroidism causes increased porosity and decreased cortical thickness
4. Adipose tissue (fat)	Important in development and function of BAT and WAT
	In WAT THs regulate basal oxygen consumption, lipogenesis, lipolysis
	TRα-1 gene is the predominantly expressed TR isoform in Ob17 cells
	Expression of these genes is modulated by high carbohydrate diet, insulin and cAMP
5. Liver	Stimulates enzymes regulating lipogenesis and lipolysis
	Regulate expression of important proteins and enzymes involved in cholesterol metabolism
	Deficiency causes hypercholesterolemia with elevated intermediate and LDL cholesterol
	TRβ-1 is the predominant isoform in liver
	Regulate gene expression of cellular pathways such as gluconeogenesis, lipogenesis, insulin signaling, cell proliferation and apoptosis
6. Pituitary	Regulate transcription of thyrotropin, prolactin mRNA
	Regulate TSH synthesis

Thyroid Hormone Functions

The Thyroid hormones are crucial for metabolism of almost all tissues in the body and play a critical role in development of CNS of fetus and infant. Thyroid hormones regulate the metabolic processes necessary for normal growth and development. The effect of thyroid hormones on various tissues and organs are described in detail here and summarized in Table 2.1.

Role in Brain Development

Thyroid hormones are vital for brain organization and function throughout life. T3 is implicated in multiple processes like neurogenesis, synaptogenesis, migration, plasticity and myelination. *Thyroid dysfunction is associated with neurological and behavioural disorders*. The subgranular zone(SGZ) of the hippocampal dentate gyrus and the subventricular zone(SVZ) are the two main neurogenic niches which produce new neurons from neural stem cells(NSC). T3 acts on SGZ and SVZ at the step where progenitor nerve cells enter the committed step in the process of forming mature neuron/neuroblast respectively influencing the progenitor proliferation and differentition. It is also hypothesised that TH may have a role on stem cells of hypothalamus [23–27].

T3 also has effect on seretonergic and cholinergic activities in the brain, contributing to psychomotor symptoms. They also have an effect on cognition and neurodegeneration. The predominant form of thyroid hormone acting in brain is the T3 and its activity is controlled by de-iodinase 2. De-iodinase 3 is the deactivating enzyme and acts as the regulating enzyme [25–27]. A detail account of role of thyroid hormone in neural development is given in Chapter 4.

THs have important role in the critical step of maturation of neuron. T3 affects neurogenesis, synaptogenesis, migration, plasticity, myelination and also has effect on cholinergic and seretonergic activities in the brain. Thyroid dysfunction is therefore associated with neurological and behavioural disorders, psychomotor symptoms, cognitive disturbances and neurodegeneration

Effect on Myocardium

Thyroid hormones are essential for proper aerobic mitochondrial function, generation of high energy phosphates, prevention of lactic acidosis, upregulation of beta adrenergic receptors and have important role in intracellular homeostasis of ionised calcium. THs affect excitation contraction coupling, have inotropic properties and are strong vasodilators of systemic arteries including coronary arteries [28–30]. The acute changes in TH levels in the form of decreased T3 & T4 along with increased reverse T3 following acute pathogenic event(medical,surgical, traumatic) is called euthyroid sick syndrome(ESS) [31]. The ESS often depresses the myocardiun transiently and is sometimes referred to as 'stunned myocardium' [32]. The term is used in conditions where there is regional or global ischemia. The effect may vary from mild hemodynamic compromise to cardiogenic shock [33]. According to current consensus, no thyroid hormone replacement is given in patients with ESS. Recent evidences however, have shown rewarding results in 3 conditions where ESS and myocardial stunning coexist: (a) transient regional myocardial ischemia and reperfusion (b) transient global myocardial ischemia in patients undergoing cardiac surgery/bypass (c) transient inadequate global myocardial perfusion in brain dead potential organ donors. Under all these conditions, administration of T3/T4 rapid reversal of myocardial perfusion was found [28].

Effect on Bone

TH is important for normal bone growth and development. Hypothyroidism can cause short stature and delayed closure of the epiphyses. THs are involved in both bone formation and resorption [34–36]. Both osteoblast and osteoclast activities are stimulated by TH. It has been observed that there is enhanced calcification and bone formation coupled to increased bone resorption in hyperthyroid patients. There also is marked increase in porosity and decreased cortical thickness in cortical bone in hyperthyroid patients. TH may act on bone via TH stimulation of growth hormone and insulin-like growth factor I (IGF-I) or by direct effects on target genes. Recent studies have shown that T3 also can directly stimulate IGF-I production in osteoblasts and enhance T3 stimulation of [3H]proline incorporation, alkaline phosphatase, and osteocalcin [36].

Although TH increases the activities of osteoblasts and osteoclasts in vivo and in culture, little is known about its effects on the transcription of target genes in these cells. There are a number of osteoblast proteins that are stimulated by TH. These include proteins involved in matrix formation such as alkaline phosphatase, osteocalcin, and collagen. Additionally, IGF-I and IGF-binding protein-2 mRNA are stimulated by T3 in rat primary cultures. However, it is not known whether TH directly regulates transcription of these target genes. The T3stimulation of IGF and IGFBPs suggests that TH may participate in osteoblast differentiation and proliferation by regulating growth factor synthesis and action [36, 37].

Effect on Adipose Tissue

THs plays important roles in the development and function of brown and white adipose tissue (BAT and WAT) [38]. In experimental studies it has been found that T3 not only induced intracellular lipid accumulation and various adipocyte-specific markers such as malic enzyme and glycerophosphate dehydrogenase, but also stimulated adipocyte cell proliferation and fat cell cluster formation [39].

Studies in the adult rat have shown that T3 plays important roles in regulating basal oxygen consumption, fat stores, lipogenesis, and lipolysis [40]. In WAT, T3 induces key lipogenic enzymes such as acetyl CoA carboxylase, malic enzyme, glucose-6-phosphate dehydrogenase, fatty acid synthase, and spot 14 [41]. The mechanism(s) by which T3 induces WAT differentiation currently is not known but likely involves transcriptional regulation of important target genes by TRs. Both TRα-1 and TRβ-1 are expressed in Ob17 cells, with the TRα-1 as the predominantly expressed TR isoform. The expression of these genes is also modulated by other factors such as high-carbohydrate diet, insulin, and cAMP [40]. Additionally, T3 also regulates lipolysis in a coordinate manner with lipogenesis. Thus TH stimulation of lipolysis may activate other nuclear hormone receptor systems, and thereby promote differentiation [40].

Moreover, enzymes of the lipogenic pathway, ATP-citrate lyase, malic enzyme, and fatty acid synthase, are induced by T3 in differentiating adipocytes, suggesting T3 promotes the acquisition of differentiated functions in white adipocyte tissue [40, 41].

Recently it has been shown that both TRα and TRβ-1 are differentially expressed during the development of brown adipose tissue (BAT) [42], a major contributor to facultative thermogenesis in rodents. Facultative thermogenesis occurs in response to cold exposure or overeating and depends on T3 and adrenergic stimulation of mitochondrial uncoupling protein (UCP) synthesis. It is not known whether these effects are directly mediated by T3 or via downstream signals such as free fatty acids generated by lipolysis. *The stimulation of UCP synthesis increases thermogenesis by uncoupling oxidative phosphorylation resulting in energy dissipation as heat.* Interestingly, BAT also contains a type II deiodinase whose activity increases in response to cold, thereby enabling BAT to have the important ability to regulate intracellular T3 concentration in a tissue-specific manner. This increase in T3 concentration likely saturates nuclear TRs and enhances norepinepinephrine stimulation of UCP [43, 44]. The adrenergic stimulation in BAT is predominantly, mediated by brown fat specific adrenergic β3-receptors. The dual regulation of UCP by the type II deiodinase and the adrenergic system suggests convergence of nuclear- and membrane-signaling systems in the transcriptional regulation of these important target genes in BAT, but the precise relative contributions and interplay between these regulatory systems is not yet clear [42–44].

Several human studies have shown that chronic hypo- and hyperthyroidism as well as acute T3 treatment did not affect serum leptin levels. However few have also shown that increased leptin levels correlated with adiposity and that T3 can decrease leptin levels but the mechanism is not clear [45].

Effect on Liver

TH causes stimulation of enzymes regulating lipogenesis and lipolysis as well as oxidative processes [46]. As described above (effect on fat) some of the lipogenic enzymes that are regulated are malic enzyme, glucose-6-phosphate dehydrogenase, and fatty acid synthase [46, 47]. Of these, malic enzyme has been extensively studied. Malic enzyme has been shown to be stimulated by direct action of T3 as well as secondary effect due to stimulation by other gene products that are regulated by T3. In rats it has been seen that a number of lipogenic enzymes may be regulated by growth hormone, which is induced by T3. Malic enzyme is very sensitive to T3 in the liver, but it is unresponsive in the brain, suggesting that tissue-specific factors are important in determining T3-mediated stimulation of transcription. T3 regulation of malic enzyme gene transcription also can be regulated by carbohydrate intake, insulin, and cAMP. For example, it has been seen that T3 effects on malic enzyme gene transcription are minimal in fasted animals but are most pronounced in animals fed a sucrose-containing fat-free (lipogenic) diet [46, 48]. Similar interactions between T3 and dietary carbohydrate also occur in the gene regulation of other lipogenic enzymes. Another T3-regulated gene expressed in liver that has been studied extensively has been the one encoding S14 protein [47]. Its mRNA is rapidly induced by T3 after 20 min in hypothyroid rats and precedes the expression of lipogenic enzymes [41]. Additionally, it is coregulated by carbohydrate similar to lipogenic enzymes. Its tissue distribution is similar to those of lipogenic enzymes as it is expressed in liver, white and brown fat, and lactating mammary tissue [41].

It is well known that hypothyroidism is associated with hypercholesterolemia with elevated serum intermediate and low-density lipoprotein (LDL) cholesterol concentrations [49]. The major mechanism for these effects may be lower cholesterol clearance resulting from decreased LDL receptors. Also, the genotype of the LDL receptor gene may influence the elevation of serum LDL cholesterol concentrations in hypothyroid patients and their response to thyroxine treatment. Apart from this, it has been seen that hepatic lipase activity is decreased in hypothyroidism which decreases conversion of intermediate-density lipoproteins to LDL and high-density lipoprotein metabolism. It is not known whether these effects are mediated directly or indirectly by THs [50]. THs also have been shown to regulate the expression of several important proteins and enzymes involved in cholesterol metabolism and synthesis such as the LDL receptor, cholesterol ester hydrolase, and cholesterol acyltransferase. TRβ-1 is the predominant isoform expressed in liver, whereas TRα-1 is the major isoform expressed in heart. These differences in TR isoform expression have made it difficult to develop isoform- specific TH analogs that may have cholesterol-lowering effects but minimal cardiac toxicity [51, 52].

There is ongoing research activity in identifying various hepatic target genes. TH has been shown to regulate gene expression of a diverse range of cellular pathways and functions such as gluconeogenesis, lipogenesis, insulin signaling, adenylate cyclase signaling, cell proliferation, and apoptosis [53]. Thus gene therapy may hold promise in future in all these metabolic pathways related to thyroid.

Effect on Pituitary

THs have been shown to stimulate the transcription of GH mRNA and GH synthesis in rats. THs also can negatively regulate thyrotropin (TSH) transcription by direct and indirect mechanisms. T3 can also downregulate prolactin mRNA. TH hormone also can negatively regulate TSH by decreasing transcription of the glycoprotein hormone α-subunit (common to TSH, luteinizing hormone, follicle-stimulating hormone, and human chorionogonadotropic hormone) and the TSHβ subunit genes [54]. Recent cotransfection and knockout studies suggest that TRβ-2 isoform may be playing the predominant role in regulating TSH. In situ hybridization and immunostaining studies have shown that TRβ-2 is highly expressed in thyrotropes in the pituitary [55]. Additionally, RXRγ isoform appears to be selectively expressed in thyrotropes, suggesting that it also may play a functional role in the regulation of TSH via isoform-specific TR/RXR complexes or RXRγ homodimers [56].

Effect on Fetal Growth and Maturation

The role of thyroid hormones on fetal growth depends on various factors like

1. placental transfer of thyroid hormones
2. the maturation of hypothalamo-pituitary thy roid axis of the developing fetus
3. the peripheral conversion of T4 to more active T3 and
4. the maturation of intracellular thyroid receptors.

It has been seen that plasma T4 concentrations are correlated positively to the body weight of the fetus and newborn. The availability of these hormones in utero regulates fetal growth by acting as a signal of the nutrient and oxygen supply to the fetus. Fetal thyroid hormones are required for both accretion of fetal mass and differentiation of specific cell types. However the placental transfer of thyroid hormones are sufficient enough and compensate for the fetal thyroid deficiency. This is attributed to their role in regulating the somatotropic axis and local tissue expression of the IGFs (insulin like growth factors) which have major role in fetal tissue accretion [57–60].

Effect on Growth

The effect of low thyroid hormones on fetal growth is evidenced by studies on thyroidectomised fetal animals. It is shown that the protein content of fetal tissues such as the heart, lung, and skeletal muscle is reduced by fetal thyroidectomy. The growth restriction is asymmetrical in the sense that greater effects are seen on the weight of soft tissues than on the length of bones. The appendicular skeleton is more adversely affected than the axial skeleton. The effect on bone metabolism is affected by reducing the osteocalcin, a marker of bone deposition rather than altering the calcium homeostasis in the body.

Effect on Fetal Metabolism (Oxygen (O_2) Consumption)

THs increase O_2 consumption by fetal tissues upto 28 % and increase umbilical blood flow. This is by inducing oxidative mechanisms by changing expression and activity of the electrogenic Na–K ATPase pump or by acting on the mitochondrial electron transport chain (ETC) and oxidative phosphorylation. These hormones are necessary for normal developmental increments in hepatic glycogen and gluconeogenic enzymes. They have an important role in maturational effects of thermogenic capacity of brown adipose tissue as has been described earlier in the text (*see adipose tissue*).

Effect on Fetal Tissue Maturation

Thyroid hormones also facilitate maturation and differentiation of fetal tissues evidenced by activation of physiological processes essential for survival immediately at birth such as pulmonary gas exchange, adaptations in cardiac function, hepatic glucogenesis and thermogenesis [60, 61].

Effect on Lung Maturation

THs tend to increase the expression of pulmonary b-adrenergic receptors and apical Na channels in the fetus thereby facilitationg lung fluid absorption at birth. It is shown that they also facilitate production of surfactant by synergistic action along with cortisol [62].

Effect on Fetal Heart and Cardiovascular System

THs promote a switch from proliferation to hypertrophy and differentiation of the cardiac myocytes by playing an important role in the perinatal switch from b- to a-myosin heavy chains in the sacromeres [63].

Other Important Effects

Effect on mitochondria*:* The mitochondria are important target for THs. They modulate mitochondrial activity through two ways: direct or indirect. In the direct pathway, the hormone enters the cell and binds to binding sites of organelles. These organelles are responsible for regulation of mitochondrial transcription apparatus. One of these binding sites, termed p43, has been identified as a bona fide TR (nuclear receptor) that binds to the D-loop region that contains the promoters of the mitochondrial genome. Thus, THs play important role in regulation of the mitochondrial transcription apparatus. In the indirect pathway, the THs act through increased, nuclear TR-dependent transcription of factors that modulate the expression of mitochondrial genes [64].

Conclusion

Thyroid hormones (THs) play critical roles in growth, differentiation and metabolism. They are important for optimal functioning of almost all tissues with major effects on metabolic rate and oxygen consumption. The thyroid gland secretes two biologically active thyroid hormones: thyroxine (T4) and 3,5,3′-triiodothyronine (T3). TH synthesis and secretion is exquisitely regulated by a negative-feedback system that involves the hypothalamus, pituitary, and thyroid gland (the HPT axis). Iodine is the chief elemental composition of thyroid hormones and its deficiency is a major cause of hypothyroidism in the developing world. Thyroid hormones exert their action through genomic and non-genomic pathways. Thyroid hormones have important functions in regulating neuronal differentiation, maturation, migration, in cholinergic pathways in the brain. In the heart and peripheral vessels they are essential for aerobic mitochondrial function, prevention of lactic acidosis, have inotropic and vasodilatory properties. THs are involved in both bone formation and resorption. They have important role in the development and function of brown and white adipose tissue and T3 plays important role in regulating lipogenesis and lipolysis. They have important role in cholesterol metabolism and synthesis and their deficiency is known to be associated with hypercholesterolemia. THs regulate transcription of thyrotropin, prolactin mRNA and TSH synthesis in the pituitary. In the developing fetus, THs are required for both accretion of fetal mass and differentiation of specific cell types. They have important roles in maturation and differentiation of vital organs such as lungs and heart. Thus, given their pleotropic effects, thyroid hormone functions are critical for survival and optimal functioning of the human body.

References

1. Kopp P. Thyroid hormone synthesis. In: Braverman LE, Utiger RD, editors. The thyroid: fundamental and clinical text. 9th ed. Philadelphia: Lippincott Williams and Wilkins; 2005. p. 52.
2. Fekete C, Lechan RM. Central regulation of hypothalamic-pituitary-thyroid axis under physiological and pathophysiological conditions. Endocr Rev. 2014;35:159–94.
3. Persani L. Hypothalamic thyrotropin releasing hormone and thyrotropin biological activity. Thyroid. 1998;8:941–6.
4. Harris AR, Christianson D, Smith MS, et al. The physiological role of thyrotropin releasing hormone in the regulation of thyroid stimulating hormone and prolactin secretion in the rat. J Clin Invest. 1978;61:441–8.
5. Spitzweg C, Heufelder AE, Morris JC. Thyroid iodine transport. Thyroid. 2000;10:321–30. Review.
6. Taurog A. Hormone synthesis. In: Braverman L, Utiger R, editors. Werner and Ingbar's the thyroid. Philadelphia: Lippincott-Raven; 1996. p. 47–81.
7. Kohrle J. The selenoenzyme family of deiodinase isozymes controls local thyroid hormone availability. Rev Endocr Metab Disord. 2000;1:49–58.
8. Wolff J, Chaikoff IL. Plasma inorganic iodide as a homeostatic regulator of thyroid function. J Biol Chem. 1948;174:555–64.
9. Lechan RM, Fekete C. The TRH neuron: a hypothalamic integrator of energy metabolism. Prog Brain Res. 2006;153:209–35.
10. Kádár A, Sánchez E, Wittmann G, et al. Distribution of hypophysiotropic thyrotropin releasing hormone (TRH) synthesizing neurons in the hypothalamic paraventricular nucleus of the mouse. J Comp Neurol. 2010;518:3948–61.
11. Amenta F, Caporuscio D, Ferrante F, et al. Cholinergic nerves in the thyroid gland. Cell Tissue Res. 1978;195:367–70.
12. Melander A, Sundler F, Westgren U. Sympathetic innervation of the thyroid: variation with species and with age. Endocrinology. 1975;96:102–6.
13. Schmitmeier S, Thole H, Bader A, et al. Purification and characterization of the thyrotropin releasing hormone (TRH) degrading serum enzyme and its identification as a product of liver origin. Eur J Biochem. 2002;269:1278–86.
14. Sugrue ML, Vella KR, Morales C, Lopez ME, Hollenberg AN. The thyrotropinreleasing hormone gene is regulated by thyroid hormone at the level of transcription in vivo. Endocrinology. 2010;151:793–801.
15. Segerson TP, Kauer J, Wolfe HC, et al. Thyroid hormone regulates TRH biosynthesis in the paraventricular nucleus of the rat hypothalamus. Science. 1987;238:78–80.
16. Kakucska I, Rand W, Lechan RM. Thyrotropin releasing hormone gene expression in the hypothalamic paraventricular nucleus is dependent upon feedback regulation by both triiodothyronine and thyroxine. Endocrinology. 1992;130:2845–50.
17. Fekete C, Mihály E, Herscovici S, et al. DARPP32 and CREB are present in type 2 iodothyronine deiodinase producing tanycytes: implications for the regulation of type 2 deiodinase activity. Brain Res. 2000;862:154–61.
18. Jansen J, Friesema EC, Milici C, Visser TJ. Thyroid hormone transporters in health and disease. Thyroid. 2005;15:757–68.
19. Pascual A, Aranda A. Thyroid hormone receptors, cell growth and differentiation. Biochim Biophys Acta. 2013;1830:3908–16.

20. Tata JR. The road to nuclear receptors of thyroid hormone. Biochim Biophys Acta. 1830;2013:3860–6.
21. DelViscovo A, Secondo A, Esposito A, et al. Intracellular and plasma membrane-initiated pathways involved in the [Ca2C]i elevations induced by iodothyronines (T3 and T2) in pituitary GH3 cells. American Journal of Physiology. Endocrinol Metab. 2011;302:E1419–30.
22. Cheng SY, Leonard JL, Davis PJ. Molecular aspects of thyroid hormone actions. Endocr Rev. 2010;31: 139–70.
23. Senese R, Cioffi F, de Lange P. Thyroid: biological actions of 'nonclassical' thyroid hormones. J Endocrinol. 2014;221:R1–12.
24. Remaud S, Gothié JD, Morvan-Dubois G, et al. Thyroid hormone signaling and adult neurogenesis in mammals. Front Endocrinol (Lausanne). 2014;5:62.
25. Oppenheimer JH, Schwartz HL. Molecular basis of thyroid hormone-dependent brain development. Endocr Rev. 1997;18:462–75.
26. Pop VJ, Kuijpens JL, van Baar AL, et al. Low maternal free thyroxine concentrations during early pregnancy are associated with impaired psychomotor development in infancy. Clin Endocrinol (Ofx). 1999;50:149–55.
27. Chan S, Kilby MD. Thyroid hormone and central nervous system development. J Endocrinol. 2000;165: 1–8.
28. Novitzky D, Cooper DK. Thyroid hormone and the stunned myocardium. J Endocrinol. 2014;223:R1–8.
29. Ririe DG, Butterworth JF, Royster RL, et al. Triiodothyronine increases contractility independent of b-adrenergic receptors or stimulation of cyclic-30,50-adenosine monophosphate. Anesthesiology. 1995;82:1004–12.
30. Klein I. Clinical, metabolic, and organ-specific indices of thyroid function. Endocrinol Metab Clin North Am. 2001;30:415–27.
31. Warner MH, Beckett GJ. Mechanisms behind the non-thyroidal illness syndrome: an update. J Endocrinol. 2010;205:1–13.
32. Luo Y, Cha DG, Liu YL, Zhou SF. Coronary microcirculation changes during myocardial stunning in dogs. Cardiology. 2010;117:68–74.
33. Heusch G. The regional myocardial flow-function relationship: a framework for an understanding of acute ischemia, hibernation, stunning and coronary microembolization. Circ Res. 1980;112:1535–7.
34. Allain TJ, McGregor AM. Thyroid hormones and bone. J Endocrinol. 1993;139:9–18.
35. Mosekilde L, Eriksen EF, Charles P. Effects of thyroid hormones on bone and mineral metabolism. Endocrinol Metab Clin North Am. 1990;19:35–63.
36. Huang BK, Golden LA, Tarjan G, et al. Insulin-like growth factor I production is essential for anabolic effects of thyroid hormone in osteoblasts. J Bone Miner Res. 2000;15:188–97.
37. Glautchnig H, Varga F, Klaushofer K. Thyroid hormone and retinoic acid induce the synthesis of insulin-like growth factor-binding protein 4 in mouse osteoblastic cells. Endocrinology. 1996;137:281–6.
38. Ailhaud G, Grimaldi P, Negrel R. Cellular and molecular aspects of adipose tissue development. Annu Rev Nutr. 1992;12:207–33.
39. Flores-Delgado G, Marsch-Moreno M, Kuri-Harcuch W. Thyroid hormone stimulates adipocyte differentiation of 3 T3 cells. Mol Cell Biochem. 1987;76: 35–43.
40. Oppenheimer JH, Schwartz HL, Lane JT, et al. Functional relationship of thyroid hormone-induced lipogenesis, lipolysis, and thermogenesis in the rat. J Clin Invest. 1991;87:125–32.
41. Kinlaw WB, Church JL, Harmon J, et al. Direct evidence for a role of the "spot 14" protein in the regulation of lipid synthesis. J Biol Chem. 1995;270: 16615–8.
42. Tuca A, Giralt M, Villarroya F, et al. Ontogeny of thyroid hormone receptors and c-erbA expression during brown adipose tissue development: evidence of fetal acquisition of the mature thyroid status. Endocrinology. 1993;132:1913–20.
43. Silva JE, Larsen PR. Adrenergic activation of triiodothyronine production in brown adipose tissue. Nature. 1983;305:712–3.
44. Lowell BB, Susulic VS, Hamann A, et al. Development of obesity in transgenic mice after genetic ablation of brown adipose tissue. Nature. 1993;366:740–2.
45. Leonhardt U, Gerdes E, Ritzel U, et al. Immunoreactive leptin and leptin mRNA expression are increased in rat hypo- but not hyperthyroidism. J Endocrinol. 1999;163:115–21.
46. Oppenheimer JH, Schwartz HL, Mariash CN, et al. Advances in our understanding of thyroid hormone action at the cellular level. Endocr Rev. 1987;8: 288–308.
47. Oppenheimer JH, Schwartz HL, Strait KA. An integrated view of thyroid hormone actions in vivo. In: Weintraub B, editor. Molecular endocrinology: basic concepts and clinical correlations. New York: Raven; 1995. p. 249–68.
48. Petty KJ, Desvergne B, Mitsuhashi T, et al. Identification of a thyroid hormone response element in the malic enzyme gene. J Biol Chem. 1990;265: 7395–400.
49. Brent GA. The molecular basis of thyroid hormone action. N Engl J Med. 1994;331:847–53.
50. Tan KC, Shiu SW, Kung AW. Effect of thyroid dysfunction on high-density lipoprotein subfraction metabolism: roles of hepatic lipase and cholesteryl ester transfer protein. J Clin Endocrinol Metab. 1998;83:2921–4.
51. Underwood AH, Emmett JC, Ellis D, et al. A thyromimetic that decreases plasma cholesterol levels without increasing cardiac activity. Nature. 1986;324:425–9.
52. Falcone M, Miyamoto T, Fierro-Renoy F, et al. Antipeptide polyclonal antibodies specifically recognize each human thyroid hormone receptor isoform. Endocrinology. 1992;131:2419–29.

53. Feng X, Jiang Y, Meltzer P, Yen PM. Thyroid hormone regulation of hepatic genes in vivo detected by complementary DNA microarray. Mol Endocrinol. 2000;14:947–55.
54. Samuels HH, Forman BM, Horowitz ZD, et al. Regulation of gene expression by thyroid hormone. J Clin Invest. 1988;81:957–67.
55. Wood DF, Docherty K, Ramsden DB, et al. Thyroid status affects the regulation of prolactin mRNA accumulation by tri-iodothyronine and thyrotrophin-releasing hormone in cultured rat anterior pituitary cells. J Endocrinol. 1987;115:497–503.
56. Sugawara A, Yen PM, Qi YP, et al. Isoform-specific retinoid X receptor (RXR) antibodies detect differential expression of RXR proteins in the pituitary gland. Endocrinology. 1995;136:1766–74.
57. Chung HR. Adrenal and thyroid function in the fetus and preterm infant. Korean J Pediatr. 2014;57: 425–33.
58. Ng PC. The fetal and neonatal hypothalamic-pituitary-adrenal axis. Arch Dis Child Fetal Neonatal Ed. 2000;82:F250–4.
59. Kester MH, Martinez de Mena R. Iodothyronine levels in the human developing brain: major regulatory roles of iodothyronine deiodinases in different areas. J Clin Endocrinol Metab. 2004;89:3117–28.
60. Thorpe-Beeston JG, Nicolaides KH, et al. Maturation of the secretion of thyroid hormone and thyroid-stimulating hormone in the fetus. N Engl J Med. 1991;324:532–6.
61. Feingold SB, Brown RS. Neonatal thyroid function. NeoReviews. 2010;11:e640–6.
62. Biswas S, Buffery J, Enoch H, et al. Pulmonary effects of triiodothyronine (T3) and hydrocortisone (HC) supplementation in preterm infants less than 30 weeks gestation: results of the THORN trial: thyroid hormone replacement in neonates. Pediatr Res. 2003;53:48–56.
63. Seri I, Tan R, Evans J. Cardiovascular effects of hydrocortisone in preterm infants with pressor-resistant hypotension. Pediatrics. 2001;107: 1070–4.
64. Yen PM. Physiological and molecular basis of thyroid hormone action. Physiol Rev. 2001;81:1097–142.

3 Iodine and the Thyroid

Hernando Vargas-Uricoechea,
Anilza Bonelo-Perdomo,
and Carlos Hernán Sierra-Torres

Abstract

Iodine Deficiency Disorders (IDD) are among the most significant public health problems in the world at the present time, especially among children and pregnant women, considered the highest risk population. These disorders hinder socio-economic development in the affected areas. IDD are a permanent natural occurrence that affects the entire planet, which means that the people living in iodine-deficient areas will always be exposed to the consequences of that deficiency, in particular increased perinatal mortality, mental retardation and brain developmental delay. Consequently, it is the major cause of preventable brain damage in childhood, and its elimination is one of the biggest challenges in public health. Iodine is present in small amounts in the body and its main role is to act as the substrate for thyroid hormone synthesis. When dietary requirements are not met, the frequency of IDD increases. In general, these disorders are underdiagnosed and, in many countries, there is no awareness of the associated problems or of the iodine status in the population.

Introduction

Iodine deficiency is a public health problem in 54 countries, occurring equally in marginal economies as well as in industrialized regions of the world. Close to 2 billion people are at risk globally as a result of the low intake of this halogenated trace element, including one third of school-age children. A minor iodine deficiency still prevails approximately in 50 % of continental Europe, and the problem has reappeared in industrialized countries like the United States (US) and Australia. In the US, although the general population is

H. Vargas-Uricoechea, MD, MSc, Ph.Dc (✉)
Division of Endocrinology and Metabolism, Internal Medicine Department, University of Cauca, Popayán-Cauca, Colombia
e-mail: hernandovargasu10@yahoo.com

A. Bonelo-Perdomo, BSc, MSc, Ph.D
Division of Basic Immunology and Biomedical Sciences, University of Valle, Cali-Valle, Colombia

C.H. Sierra-Torres, Ph.D
Division of Genetic and Molecular Epidemiology, University of Cauca, Popayán-Cauca, Colombia

S.K. Imam, S.I. Ahmad (eds.), *Thyroid Disorders: Basic Science and Clinical Practice*,
DOI 10.1007/978-3-319-25871-3_3

iodine-"sufficient", it is not clear whether iodine intake during pregnancy is appropriate; and in other geographical areas such as Australia, deficiency has increased as a result of a decreased use of iodophors in the food industry (an iodophor is defined as an iodine complex with non-ionic tensioactive agents that act as iodine transporters and solubilizers in water). This lower industrial use of iodophors may also explain – at least in part – minor iodine deficiencies in the United Kingdom and the Republic of Ireland. In marginal economies such as southern Asia and Sub-Saharan Africa, the problem is greater [1, 2]. The lowest frequency is found in the Americas. The most vulnerable groups are pregnant mothers and children, and the consequences of the lack of iodine during brain development in utero were the trigger that led the International Public Health Community, with the support from United Nations (UN) agencies, particularly the World Health Organization (WHO) and the United Nations Children's Fund (UNICEF), to adopt sustainable iodine deficiency elimination as a goal. Food iodine content depends on the amount of iodine in the soil, and soil degradation as a result of erosion, excess cattle grazing and cutting of trees is associated with significant losses of this trace element. Consequently, food grown in degraded soils has low iodine content. The term Iodine Deficiency Disorders (IDD) is used to define a group of diseases resulting from a relative loss of iodine in the diet, including multiple defects. The definition also encompasses the concept that those disorders are preventable by means of an adequate iodine intake. However, iodine-induced hyperthyroidism is a metabolic disorder that is relatively frequent in areas with very high iodine intake; in fact, in those areas where iodine intake is marginal – although not iodine-deficient – moderate increases in iodine intake may induce hyperthyroidism in individuals with autonomous thyroid nodules [3–5].

Epidemiology

In an analysis of data collected in 2003, the WHO estimated that the Americas and Western Pacific had the lowest proportion of people with insufficient iodine intake (9.8 % and 24 %, respectively). In the other WHO regions, the figures were 56.9 % for Europe; 54.1 % for Eastern Mediterranean; 42.6 % for Africa; and 39.8 % for Southeast Asia [3, 4]. Between 1990 and 2003, the proportion of households using iodized salt increased from 10 to 66 %. As a result, the WHO estimated that the number of countries where iodine deficiency disorders were a public health problem had dropped from 110 to 54; and later it dropped from 54 to 30. On the other hand, the number of "iodine-sufficient" countries increased from 67 to 112. In 2006, 15 countries had reached the goal of sustainable elimination of iodine deficiency disorders. The prevalence of iodine deficiency was published in 2008 on the basis of the world population estimated for 2006 – without including data from countries such as the US and Western Europe. The highest prevalence was found in Europe (52 %), followed by Eastern Mediterranean (47.2 %) and Africa (41.5 %), taking into consideration that iodine deficiency in school-age children in countries like Ethiopia is unacceptably high. The lowest prevalence was found in Southeast Asia, Western Pacific and the Americas –30 %, 21.2 % and 11 %, respectively – [5, 6]. Despite efforts to achieve universal salt iodization, there are still areas where results are conflicting – Table 3.1 [7–9].

Moreover, iodine intake is more than adequate and even too high in at least 34 countries globally. Over the past decade, the number of countries with excess iodine intake increased from 5 to 10 as a result of very high levels of salt iodization or poor monitoring and follow-up of the iodization programs. This is important to note that even minor changes in iodine intake (above or below the normal population reference range) in the different geographical regions are associated with marked differences in the frequency of thyroid disorders. It has even been found that primary elimination of IDD achieved in some regions may be accompanied by "overiodization" of salt, resulting in a substantial increase in ioduria, and highlighting the need for permanent monitoring of all IDD prevention programs. Currently, 111 countries have adequate iodine dietary intake; of these, 30 remain iodine-deficient, nine are moderately deficient, 21 are

Table 3.1 Prevalence of iodine deficiency in numbers (millions) and percentages, in the general population (all age groups) and in school children (6–12 years) for 2007. The percentage of households with access to iodized salt is also shown

WHO regions (193 member states)	General population	School age children	Households with access to iodized salt (%) not including Western Europe or the UN
Africa	312.9 (41.5 %)	57.7 (40.8 %)	66.6 %
Americans	98.6 (11 %)	11.6 (10.6 %)	86.8 %
Eastern Mediterranean	259.3 (47.2 %)	43.3 (48.8 %)	47.3 %
Europe	459.7 (52 %)	38.7 (52.4 %)	49.2 %
Southeast Asia	503.6 (30 %)	73.1 (30.3 %)	61 %
Western Pacific	374.7 (21.2 %)	41.6 (22.7 %)	89.5 %
Total	**2000 (30.6 %)**	**263.7 (31.5 %)**	**70 %**

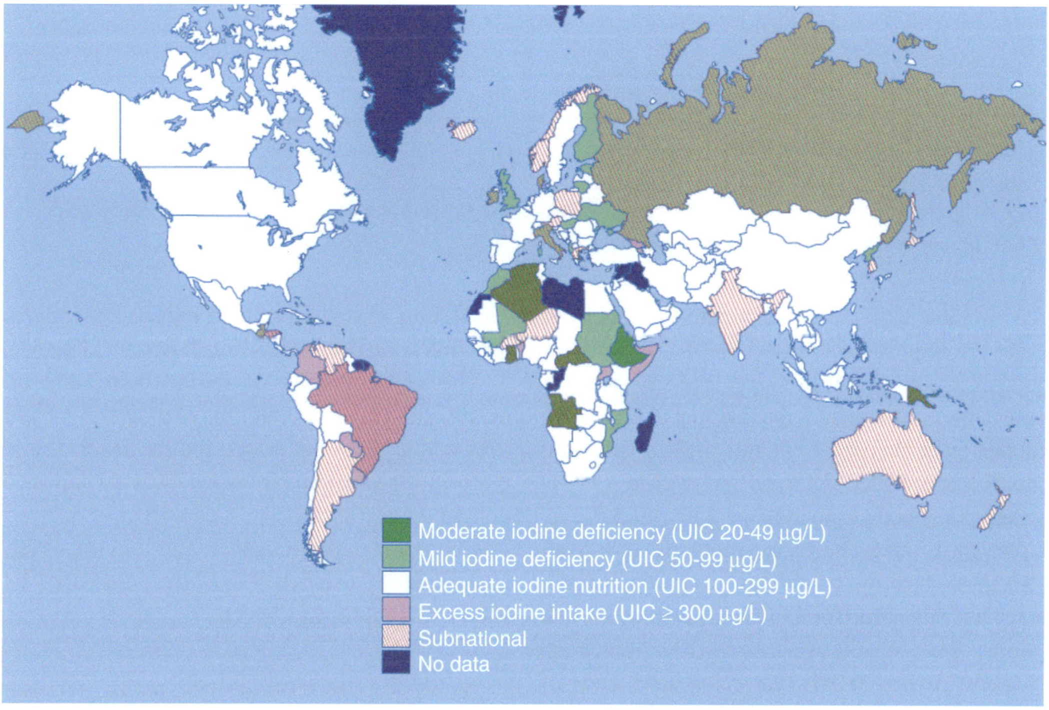

Fig. 3.1 Iodine status worldwide in 2014; based on the median urinary iodine concentration

mildly deficient, and none are currently considered severely iodine-deficient. Ten countries have excess iodine intake – Fig. 3.1 – [10–13].

Definition of IDD and Its Impact on Health and on the Population

Iodine deficiency emerges when iodine intake is below the recommended levels. The term IDD refers to the consequences of iodine deficiency in a population, and which may be prevented by ensuring adequate intake [14, 15]. WHO, UNICEF, and International Council for Control of Iodine Deficiency Disorders (ICCIDD) recommends an adequate daily intake of iodine aimed at reducing IDD in the population to the largest extent (Table 3.2). For the USA and Canada, the Institute of Medicine established Dietary Reference Intakes (DRI) for iodine, and specifically an Adequate Intake (AI) for infants, which is defined as a recommended daily intake level that is expected to meet or exceed the requirement in essentially all individuals of a specific life-stage and sex group; and an Estimated Average Requirement (EAR) which is defined as

Table 3.2 Recommendations for iodine intake by age or life-stage group and tolerable upper intake levels for iodine

WHO-UNICEF-ICCIDD (RNI) (μg/day)		USA Institute of Medicine			Tolerable upper intake Levels for iodine (μg/day)		
Children 0–59 months	90	Life Stage Group	EAR (μg/day)	AI or RDA (μg/day)	Age Group[a]	USA Institute of Medicine	ECSC[b]
Children 6–12 years	120	Infants aged 0–12 months	–	110–130	1–3	200	200
>12 years and adults	150	Children Aged 1–8 years	65	90	4–6	300	250
Pregnancy and location	250	Children aged 9–13 years	73	120	7–10	600	300
		Adults aged ≥14 years	95	150	11–14	–	450
		Pregnancy	160	220	15–17 and (14–18) years	900	500
		Location	200	290	Adults pregnant and lactating women	1100	600

[a]Age categories in parenthesis are for the Tolerable Upper Intake Level defined by the US Institute of Medicine
[b]*ECSC* European Commission/Scientific Committee on Food

the average daily level of intake estimated to meet the requirements of 50 % of healthy individuals in a particular life-stage and sex group; It is usually used to assess the adequacy of nutrient intakes in populations but not individuals. And the Recommended Dietary Allowance (RDA) which is defined as the average daily intake level sufficient to meet the requirements of nearly all (97–98 %) healthy individuals in a particular life-stage and sex group for children, adolescents, and adults. The WHO established Recommended Nutrient Intakes (RNI) that cover the needs of nearly all healthy individuals in a specific life-stage group. On the other hand, programs focusing on universal salt iodization have increased the risk of overiodized salt. This has led to the recommendation of the "Tolerable Upper Intake Levels for iodine", bearing in mind that some populations with profound iodine deficiencies may respond adversely to intakes far below recommended levels [15, 16].

Disorders caused either by iodine deficiency or excess intake (measured using median ioduria or ioduria concentrations) occur in ranges between <100 μg/L (insufficiency) and more than 300 μg/L (excess). The epidemiological criteria for the evaluation of iodine nutrition in a population –based on median ioduria and ioduria concentration (or both) – are shown in Table 3.3.

The consequences of iodine deficiency on health and the community may be disastrous and irreversible. For the WHO, iodine deficiency is the primary preventable cause of brain injury – both in fetuses and infants – as well as of delayed psychomotor development in children; however, consequences reach beyond brain disorders, as shown in Table 3.4 [17–19].

Iodine Chemistry

The discovery of iodine, like most discoveries, was a fortuitous accident. In 1811, Bernard Courtois serendipitously discovered iodine while extracting saltpeter (ammonium nitrate) from seaweed to produce gunpowder for Napoleon's army. He mistakenly added excess sulfuric acid, which caused a violet-colored vapor to exude and recrystallize. Iodine derives its name from the Greek word iodes, which means violet.

Iodine is included in the element list of the lesser 1/3 in abundance and is therefore classified as a rare element. It is classified as a nonmetallic element, showing that it has little of the

Table 3.3 Epidemiological criteria for dietary iodine contribution in a population

	Iodine intake	Dietary iodine contribution
School-age children		
<20 μg/L	Insufficient	Severe deficiency
20–49 μg/L	Insufficient	Moderate deficiency
50–99 μg/L	Insufficient	Mild deficiency
100–199 μg/L	Adequate	Optimal
200–299 μg/L	More than adequate	Risk of iodine-induced hyperthyroidism in susceptible groups
>300 μg/L	Excess	Risk of harmful consequences for health (hyperthyroidism, autoimmune thyroid disease)
Pregnant women		
L150 μg/L	Insufficient	–
150–249 μg/L	Adequate	–
250–499 μg/L	More than adequate	–
≥500 μg/L	Excess[a]	–
Breastfeeding women[b]		
<100 μg/L	Insufficient	–
≥100 μg/L	Adequate	–
Children <2 years of age		
<100 μg/L	Insufficient	–
≥100 μg/L	Adequate	–

There is no information on dietary iodine contribution in pregnant and breastfeeding women in the UN evaluation table

[a]The term excess means that it exceeds the amount required to prevent and control iodine deficiency

[b]In breastfeeding women, median ioduria numbers are lower than iodine requirements due to iodine excretion in breast milk

characteristics of metallic elements. It is a solid, not a liquid or gas like the halogens above it in the periodic table. It is however volatile and therefore when heated it sublimes to a purple vapor. It is included in the seventh column of the periodic table, fourth in this halogen column. It has a characteristic odor and a sharp acrid taste [20, 21]. Like the other halogen elements it is diatomic, meaning that in its atomic state there are two atoms bound together to give one entity referred to as I2. Iodine is present on the surface of the earth in a very small amounts and it is known as a trace element. As a non-metallic element, its atomic number is 53, it belongs under group 17 in the periodic table with a relative mass of 126.904, and it is considered the heaviest among halogens found in nature. Under normal conditions, it is found in the form of a black, volatile, shiny solid. The chemistry of iodine, as that of other halogens, is dominated by the ease with which the atom acquires an electron to form the iodide ion (I^-) or a single covalent bond, and the formation, with more electronegative elements, of compounds in which the formal iodine oxidation state is +1, +3, +5 or +7; however, like the rest of halogens, it may form a large number of compounds with other elements although it is in fact the least reactive of the whole group. Despite the low concentration of iodine in seawater, some algae species may extract and accumulate this element. In the form of calcium iodate, iodine is found in saltpeter beds in Chile, and it is also found as iodide ion in some oil well brines in California, Michigan and Japan. Iodine may be obtained from iodides found in seawater and some algae, or in the form of iodates from niter. Iodine exists in the form of diatomic molecules (I_2) in solid, liquid and vapor phases,

Table 3.4 Consequences of iodine deficiency for health

Age	Consequence
All ages	Goiter (even nodular hyperthyroid disease); hypothyroidism in areas with moderate-to-severe deficiency; lower presence of hyperthyroidism in areas with mild-to-moderate deficiency; hyperavidity of the thyroid for iodine (which increases the risk of thyroid irradiation in the event of a nuclear accident).
In-utero and perinatal state:	Miscarriages, increased risk of fetal death, congenital abnormalities, increased perinatal mortality
Neonates:	Endemic cretinism, increased risk of infant mortality
Children and adolescents:	Growth delay, reduced intellectual and mental abilities
Adults:	Diminished intellectual and mental abilities, hypothyroidism, apathy, significant reduction of working capacity and productivity leading to poor social and economic development

although dissociation for atom formation is quite significant at high temperatures (>200 °C). Although it is less strong in its reactions with other halogens (halogenides), iodine combines directly with most of the elements, important exceptions being noble gases, carbon, nitrogen and some noble metals [22, 23].

Iodine has several valence states and exists naturally in inorganic and organic forms including iodide (I^-), iodate (IO_3^-), elemental iodine (I_2), methylated forms and iodine-substituted humic substances. The chemical form of iodine depends on pH and the redox status of the surrounding environment. Iodide and organic iodine forms were reported as the most prevalent species of iodine in river water while iodate is believed to be the most common iodine form in oceans. In soil, iodide was reported to be the dominant inorganic iodine species in humid acidic soils whereas iodate prevails in the arid oxidizing conditions [20, 24].

Iodine Ecology and Cycle

Close to 95 % of the crust of the earth is made of igneous rocks that form when magma (molten rock) cools and solidifies. Those rocks contain a definite amount of iodine – approximately 500 μg per kilogram of dry material (considering that these rocks consist mainly of silicates and are covered by a fine layer of sedimentary and metamorphic rocks) – Soils derived from igneous rocks contain substantial amounts of iodine, as is to be expected. Once the rocks have formed from molten magma that rises to the surface, they may go through different transformation processes. Moreover, they may be turned to dust by erosion, or their fragments may give rise to sedimentary rocks. On the other hand, they may sink or never rise to the surface, and become transformed by heat and pressure, giving rise to metamorphic rocks. The two types of rocks and the soils they give rise to contain varying amounts of iodine. From among the magmatic and metamorphic rocks, metasedimentary gneisses, mica schists and granulites have as little as 12–25 μg/kg iodine, and have lost from 75 to >95 % of their iodine content at metamorphic temperatures. Granites, granodiorites, tonalites, and basalts are even lower in iodine and contain 4–9 μg/kg Iodine, almost independent of the class of magmatic rock.

The planet that we know today looks very different from what it was like shortly after its birth. At that time, it was a huge clump of molten rock; eventually, the crust cooled and turned solid. Water pooled in the lower areas and a layer of gas began to form above the surface. In the meantime, lava leaked abundantly though multiple cracks in the crust and this volcanic activity released a huge amount of gas that ended up forming a layer above the surface. Oxygen and hydrogen produced water vapor during the eruptions; as water vapor rose through the atmosphere, it condensed, giving rise to the primordial rainfall. As the first rains fell on the planet, they pushed iodine into the sea, hence its substantial concentration in seawater [25–27]. Certain marine plants and animals have developed mechanisms that enable them to concentrate large amounts of iodine in their tissues and when they die and fall to the bottom of the sea, iodine becomes part of the sediment and the sedimentary rocks that may form later on. Part of the iodine contained in seawater evaporates and rises to the atmosphere, probably attached to dust particles (Fig. 3.2).

When water vapor forms clouds and then falls in the form of rain or snow, the latter also contain iodine, completing the entire circulation cycle [20, 24]. Seawater has the highest iodine concentration – close to 58 μg/L, iodate being the most stable form which is reduced to iodide in the water surface through the biological activity mediated by algae and phytoplankton, both of which release iodine-containing organic gases (especially methyl iodide [CH3I] and diiodomethane [CH2I2]) that rise to the atmosphere and undergo chemical changes under the action of sunlight. About 400.000 ton of iodine escapes from the oceans every year as iodide in sea spray or as iodide, hydrochloric acid and methyl iodide, produced by marine organisms. Much of it is deposited on land where it may become part of the bio cycle. In the atmosphere, iodine migrates

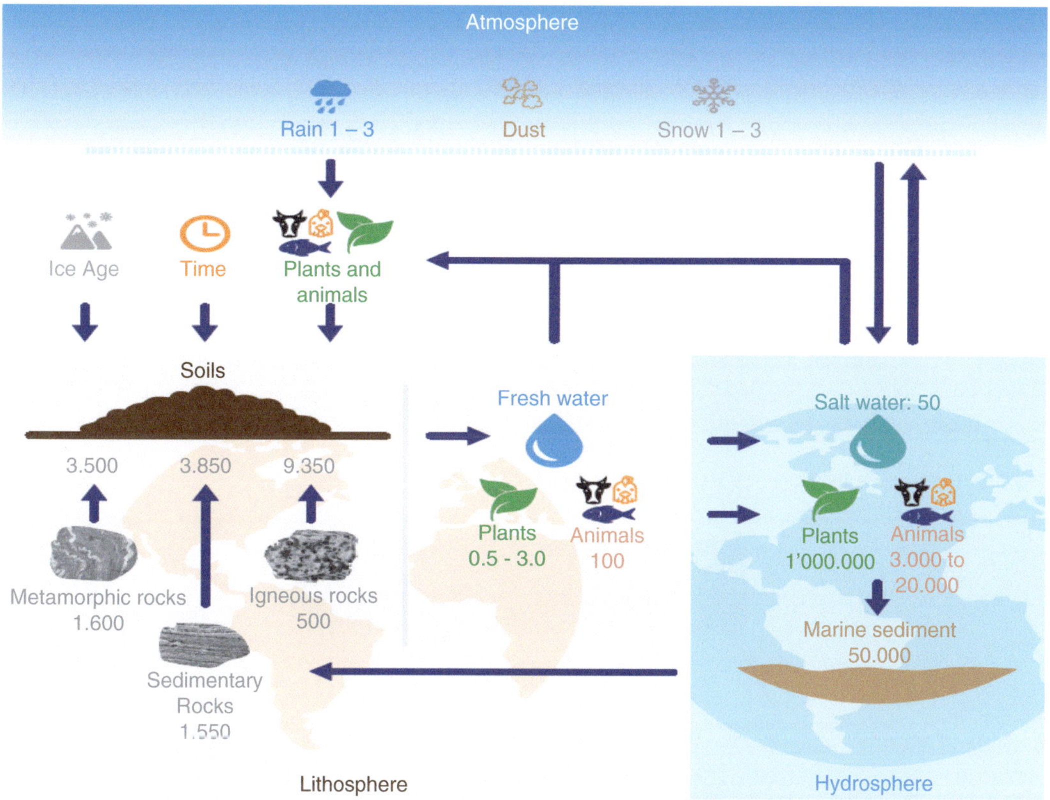

Fig. 3.2 Iodine ecology in nature: Certain marine plants and animals have developed mechanisms that enable them to concentrate large amounts of iodine in their tissues and when they die and fall to the bottom of the sea, iodine becomes part of the sediment and the sedimentary rocks that may form later on. Part of the iodine contained in seawater evaporates and rises to the atmosphere, probably attached to dust particles (See text for more details)

to other parts of the earth and is deposited by wet or dry precipitation, depending on climatic and topographic conditions; as a result, areas near coastal regions tend to have a more iodine-rich environment. For example, soils within 0–50 km from the sea have a higher – though variable – level of iodine when compared with those found far from the sea. Iodine may become "revolatilized" from the soil and the plants, probably due to biological conversion to organic forms, allowing it to travel far from the coasts until it precipitates down to the earth again (Fig. 3.3). Although organic matter plays an important role in fixing iodine in the soil, in areas known to be rich in organic matter soils with high iodine content is not a good source of this trace element for the food chain because of strong binding of iodine to the soil, precluding its bioavailability. From a medical geology point of view, the iodine status of soils is most important. The amount of soil and its ability to retain it are two factors that need consideration in the study of the geochemical pathways of iodine. There are three main forms of iodine in the soil: *mobile iodine*; *insoluble iodides* and *fixed iodine*. The property of the soil which fixes the iodine was termed Iodine Fixation Potential (IFP). The IFP is particularly important for tropical soils since iron, manganese and aluminum oxides are abundant in such soils and these have the ability to fix iodine strongly. The organic matter in the soil also absorbs iodine strongly and the bioavailability of iodine may therefore be relatively small (Fig. 3.4).

The iodine status of a soil is a combination of the supply of iodine and the soil's ability to retain it. A soil from a coastal zone may have a high input of iodine but if it cannot hold on to the iodine then it will remain deficient. The iodine

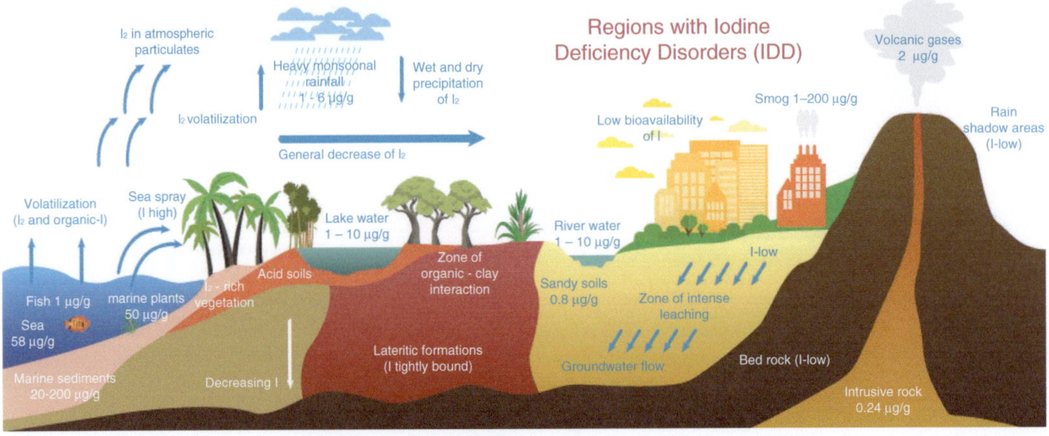

Fig. 3.3 Iodine cycle in nature (see text for more details)

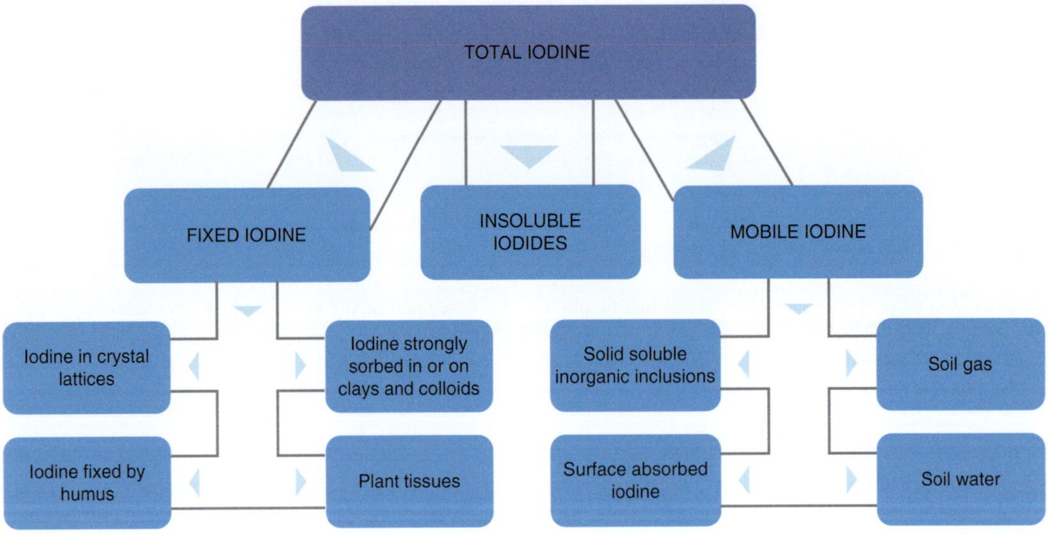

Fig. 3.4 Main forms of iodine in the soil: There are three main forms of iodine in the soil: mobile iodine, insoluble iodides and fixed iodine. The property of the soil which fixes the iodine is called Iodine Fixation Potential (IFP). The IFP is particularly important for tropical soils since iron, manganese and aluminum oxides are abundant in such soils and these have the ability to fix iodine strongly (See text for more details)

fixation potential of a soil is a complex mixture of many factors that include the soil's organic content, the soil texture, the chemical form of the iodine, and the prevailing oxidation and acidity conditions [28, 29].

This means that any consideration regarding iodine status in the population and its relationship with the environment must be evaluated in accordance with the bioavailability and not on the basis of the total iodine content. Water surfaces may be the best indicator of iodine status in the environment, considering that they represent its bioavailability. It is suggested that a level below 3 µg/L defines iodine deficiency. Finally, Iodine is primarily obtained as a by-product with nitrate minerals that are associated with caliche deposits in places such as the Atacama Desert of Chile. It is present in seawater, which contains about 0.05 parts per million (ppm) iodine, meaning that there is approximately 35 million metric tons of iodine in the world's oceans. Iodine was first isolated from seaweed, and dried seaweeds (particularly those of the Liminaria family) contain as much as 0.45 % iodine. Prior to 1959, seaweed was a major source of iodine and it remains a significant source for iodine in the diets of many people around the world. Iodine is also retrieved from underground brines (formation waters containing many dissolved salts and ions) which are associated with natural gas and oil deposits as in Japan and the US [30, 31].

Food Sources of Iodine

Seaweed (such as kelp, nori, kombu, and wakame) is one of the best food sources of iodine, but it is highly variable in its content. Other good sources include seafood, dairy products (partly due to the use of iodine feed supplements and iodophors sanitizing agents in the dairy industry), grain products, and eggs. Dairy products, especially milk, and grain products are the major contributors of iodine to the American diet. Iodine is also present in human breast milk and infant formulas. Fruits and vegetables contain iodine, but the amount varies depending on the iodine content of the soil, fertilizer use and irrigation practices. Both leaf vegetables and fruit vegetables can absorb exogenous iodine from soil. The uptake amounts increases with the application intensity of algal organic iodized fertilizer. However, uptake capacity is different for different vegetable. The leaf vegetables have a greater absorbing capacity than the fruit vegetables, although there are variations in uptake capacity, usually less significant, between different species within the same type vegetables. Iodine concentrations in plant foods can range from as little as 10 mcg/kg to 1 mg/kg dry weight. This variability in turn affects the iodine content of meat and animal products because it affects the iodine content of foods that the animals consume. Certain food sources are associated with various effects on iodine metabolism in the population [32, 33]. Universal restrictions regarding salt intake, as a way to prevent and manage diseases like hypertension, have been associated with iodine deficiency, particularly in women; and the growing consumption of soy products that may contain isoflavones (genistein and daidzein) may be associated with iodine deficiency and hypothyroidism. The goitrogenic effects of genistein -the major soy isoflavone- seem to derive from a direct interaction of this isoflavone with key pathways involved in thyroid hormones synthesis, metabolism, and thyroid hormone transport proteins. In vitro and in vivo studies showed that genistein is a potent inhibitor of Thyroid Peroxidase (TPO). Indeed, TPO catalyzes the iodination of thyroglobulin (Tg) and oxidative coupling of diiodothyronine resulting in the thyroid hormone formation. Thus, inhibition of TPO leads to a reduction of thyroid hormones levels, with a subsequent increment of TSH release that, in turn, provides a strong growth stimulus to the thyroid gland. Moreover, genistein also affects the metabolism of thyroid hormones and iodide re-utilization by inhibition of sulfotransferase enzymes.

On the other hand, perchlorate content in food and its intake may affect the *Symporter* Na/I (SNI) in the thyroid gland and reduce active intra-thyroid iodine transport, leading to hypothyroidism [34, 35]. Thiocyanates are mainly the result of the reaction of free cyanide with sulfur. Like perchlorate, these compounds may reduce active intrathyroid iodine transport through SNI involvement. Thiocyanate is the main product that forms when cyanide enters the body, and it is the way the body gets rid of cyanide. Thiocyanates are found in water, mainly due to discharges from coal processing, gold and silver extraction, and mining. Thiocyanates in the soil come from the direct application of herbicides, pesticides and rodenticides, and the disposal of industrial by-products. Some vegetables like cabbage, cauliflower and Brussels sprouts are part of a large genus called *Brassica* which, apart from their high content of diet fiber and vitamins, also contain detectable levels of thiocyanates. In individuals that eat large amounts of these vegetables may get an increased vulnerability to iodine deficiency and hypothyroidism. Most foods and beverages for human consumption have a low iodine concentration. Foods of marine origin have the highest iodine content. In

Table 3.5 Iodine content in some foods, in μg for every 100 g of the product (content may vary according to the geographical area and the content of iodine in the soil

Foods	Iodine content
Red mullet (150 g)	150
Calms, cockles and bi-valve mollusks in general	120
Allioids (garlic)	94
Crustaceans such as shrimp, prawns and scampi	90
Salmon (150 g)	60
Perciform fish (grouper)	52
Fresh fish (150 g)	45
Pineapple (150 g)	45
Lobsters and decapode crustaceans like king crabs	40
Tuna, bonito, sardines in oil (100 g)	37
Green beans, chards	35
Eggs	20
Herbaceous plants like onions	20
Edible mushrooms	18
Whole rice (80 g)	18
Pleuronectiform or flat fish (sole)	17
Fabaceous plants like dry faba beans and peanuts	14
Cow's milk	9
Carrot-type vegetables	9
Solanaceous plants (tomatoes)	7
Prunes	7
Lean pork	5.2
Lettuce	5
Yogurt	3.8
Potatoes	3
Lime	3
Spanish ham (20 g)	2.2

general, iodine concentrations in frequently consumed foods are highly variable (3–80 μg per serving). In the mid 90s in the US, mean iodine intake was estimated at 190–210 μg/day for women, the most abundant sources being milk and bread. The situation is similar in other countries like Switzerland where the mean iodine intake measured directly from food is 140 μg/day. Other food sources of iodine are shown in Table 3.5. It is important to bear in mind that some iodophors and fertilizers may modify iodine content in food. In countries like Japan, iodine intake from food is among the highest in the world, most probably because of the high consumption of algae in the diet. It is estimated that the daily iodine intake in this population ranges between 5280 and 13,800 μg, 5–14 times higher than the upper safety limit of 1 mg for the United States. In Japanese women, this high iodine intake is associated with low rates of goiter, autoimmune thyroid disease, breast cystic disease, or breast cancer [36, 37]. Some additional sources of iodine are iodized contrast media, water purification tablets and medications such as multivitamins, anti-arrhythmics like amiodarone (that contains close to 75 mg in each 200 mg tablet), topical disinfectants like povidone (10 mg/mL), and Lugol's solution, with a content of 6 mg of iodine for every drop, and saturated potassium iodide solution which contains 38 mg of iodine per drop [36].

Iodine Metabolism

Biosynthesis and secretion of thyroid hormones require several steps, including the following: *iodide absorption* from the gastrointestinal tract into the blood stream; *iodide uptake* in the thyroid by the NIS and its *transport* into the follicular lumen, which is partly mediated by Pendrin (PDS); *oxidation of iodide*, which involves TPO and H_2O_2 generated by dual oxidases (DUOXs); *iodination of Tg*; *storage of thyroid hormones* in a Tg-bound form; and *reabsorption and hydrolysis* of follicular Tg and *secretion* of thyroid hormones (Fig. 3.5).

Iodine, as a component of thyroid hormones, accounts for 65 % and 58 % of the weight of thyroxin (T4) and triiodothyronine (T3), respectively. When ingested, iodine is absorbed through the small intestine and transported in plasma to the thyroid where it is concentrated, oxidized and incorporated into Tg to form monoiodotyronine (MIT) and diiodotyronine (DIT), and then gives rise to T3 and T4 formation. Of the total iodine used by the body, 96–99 % is metabolized in the thyroid gland, while the rest is used by other organs or systems like the retina and the choroid plexus. The thyroid and the kidneys remove most of the iodine from plasma, regardless of the

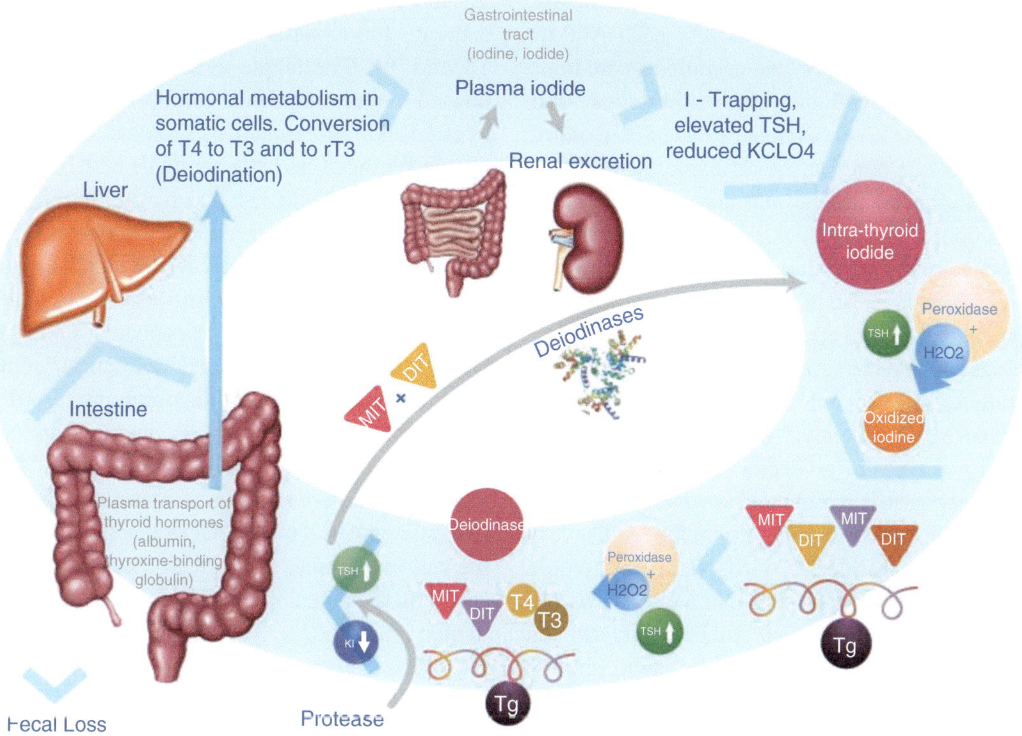

Fig. 3.5 Iodine metabolism: When ingested, iodide is trapped and oxidized in the thyroid gland and binds to tyrosine to form iodotyrosines; the coupling of iodotyrosyl residues forms T4 and T3; the hormone secreted by the gland is transported in the serum, and a fraction of the T4 is deiodinated to T3. The hormone plays out its metabolic effects in the cell and is finally deiodinated; iodide is reutilized or excreted in the kidneys. A second cycle occurs inside the thyroid through deiodination of iodotyrosines

amount of iodine or other anions present [37, 38]. Renal clearance of iodine depends mainly on the glomerular filtration rate, with no evidence of a tubular secretion mechanism or phenomenon, or of active transport. Reuptake is partial and passive and hypothyroidism may decrease renal clearance while as hyperthyroid states may increase it. Using a mean value of iodine intake in the diet of 150 μg/day, the thyroid clears serum iodine at an average rate of approximately 17 mL per minute, but rates could be as high as 100 mL/min in iodine deficient areas. A normal thyroid gland maintains a free iodine concentration 20–50 times higher than plasma levels – depending on the amount of iodine available and gland activity – the concentration gradient may be greater than 100:1 in primary hyperthyroidism. SNI is the plasma membrane glycoprotein that mediates active iodine transport in the thyroid and other tissues, such as salivary glands, stomach, lactating breast, and small intestine mediates iodine transport to the inside of follicular cells in what is considered the first step in thyroid hormone biosynthesis. In the thyroid, the transport of iodide from the extracellular space to the follicular lumen requires two steps: the transport in the cell at the basal side and in the lumen at the apical side. The first step is mediated by the NIS and the second step by PDS. The NIS is located at the basolateral plasma membrane of the thyroid follicular cells actively transports iodide into the thyroid using the electrochemical gradient generated by the Na,K-ATPase pump (a member of the P-type class of ATPases, is a critical protein found in the membranes of all animal cells. It functions in the active transport of sodium and potassium ions across the cell membrane against their concentration gradients. For each ATP the pump breaks down, two potassium ions are transported into the cell and three sodium ions out of the cell. Ion (K+) channels provide a K+–selective aqueous pore for the diffusion of K+ across the plasma membrane and are essential for the function of most, if not all, mammalian cell types. Voltage-gated potassium (Kv) channels are gated (opened and closed) by changes in membrane potential. They are opened by membrane depolarization and are essential for the timely repolarization of excitable cells. KCNQ1-KCNE2 channels are essential for the physiology of at least two types of no excitable, polarized epithelial cells: gastric parietal cells, which secrete gastric acid, and thyroid epithelial cells. The requirement for KCNQ1-KCNE2 for thyroidal iodine uptake may indicate that KCNQ1-KCNE2 is necessary for adequate function of NIS, the primary thyrocyte iodine uptake conduit (the first step in thyroid hormone biosynthesis requires a constitutive active potassium channel promoting potassium efflux). Iodide efflux into the follicular lumen is mediated in part by PDS, in conjunction with an as of yet unidentified channel. PDS is a highly hydrophobic membrane protein located at the apical membrane of thyrocytes. In addition to the thyroid, PDS is also expressed in the kidney and in the inner ear. In the kidney, PDS plays an important role in acid–base metabolism as an exchanger of chloride and bicarbonate in β-intercalated cells. In the inner ear, PDS is important for generation of the endocochlear potential. PDS belongs to the SLC26A family, which includes several anion transporters, as well as the motor protein prestin that is expressed in outer hair cells. PDS is encoded by the SLC26A4 gene, which is located on chromosome 7q21-31 and contains 21 exons with an open reading frame of 2343 bp. At the intraluminal side, iodide is oxidized, a reaction that requires H_2O_2 (which is the final electron acceptor for the biosynthesis of the thyroid hormone catalyzed by TPO at the apical surface of thyrocytes). The oxidation of iodide is mediated by TPO. Human TPO is a 110 kDa membrane-bound, glycosylated, heme-containing protein that catalyzes the iodination of Tg and the coupling of iodotyrosyl residues to generate functionally active thyroid hormones, T3 and T4. The single gene encoding TPO is located on chromosome 2p25 which spans at least 150 kb and contains 17 exons. The matrix for the synthesis and storage of T4 and T3 is Tg, a large glycoprotein secreted by the thyroid follicular cells. H_2O_2 is produced by two isoform enzymes, DUOX1 and DUOX2 –which were initially identified in the thyroid as Nicotinamide Adenine Dinucleotide Phosphate Oxidases (NOX) that produce H_2O_2. DUOX1 and DUOX2 are a calcium dependent flavoproteins NADPH oxidase, which requires a maturationfactor known as DUOXA1 and DUOXA2. DUOXA1 and DUOXA2 are required as maturation factors to localize DUOX1 and DUOX2, respectively, to the cell membrane. Both DUOX and TPO colocalize on the apical membrane of the thyroid follicular epithelium. The H2O2 produced by DUOXs is used by TPO to oxidize iodide, to iodinate tyrosyl residues of Tg to form MIT and DIT; then, they subsequently couple to the iodotyrosines to form T3 and T4. Finally, Monocarboxylate Transporter 8 (MCT8, SLC16A2) is a thyroid hormone transmembrane transport; MCT8 belongs to the major facilitator superfamily of 12 transmembrane-spanning proteins and mediates energy-independent bidirectional transport of iodothyronines across the plasma membrane [37–39].

In order to ensure the necessary supply of iodide for thyroid hormonogenesis the iodotyrosine deiodinase enzyme (DEHAL1) deiodinates MIT and DIT, molecules that are formed in excess within the Tg pre-hormonal matrix and become again free after hydrolysis of Tg by cathepsines, leading to the liberation and secretion of T3 and T4. DEHAL1 then "Recovers" one or two iodide molecules contained in MIT and DIT for further synthesis of thyroid hormones, and this function represents an intrathyroidal mechanism of iodide recycling and efficient hormonogenesis (Fig. 3.6). This allows the re-utilization of iodide within the thyroid cell. When dietary iodine is sufficient, the major product of the thyroid gland is T4 which is secreted at a rate of 10-fold that of T3. Thus, a rate-limiting step in

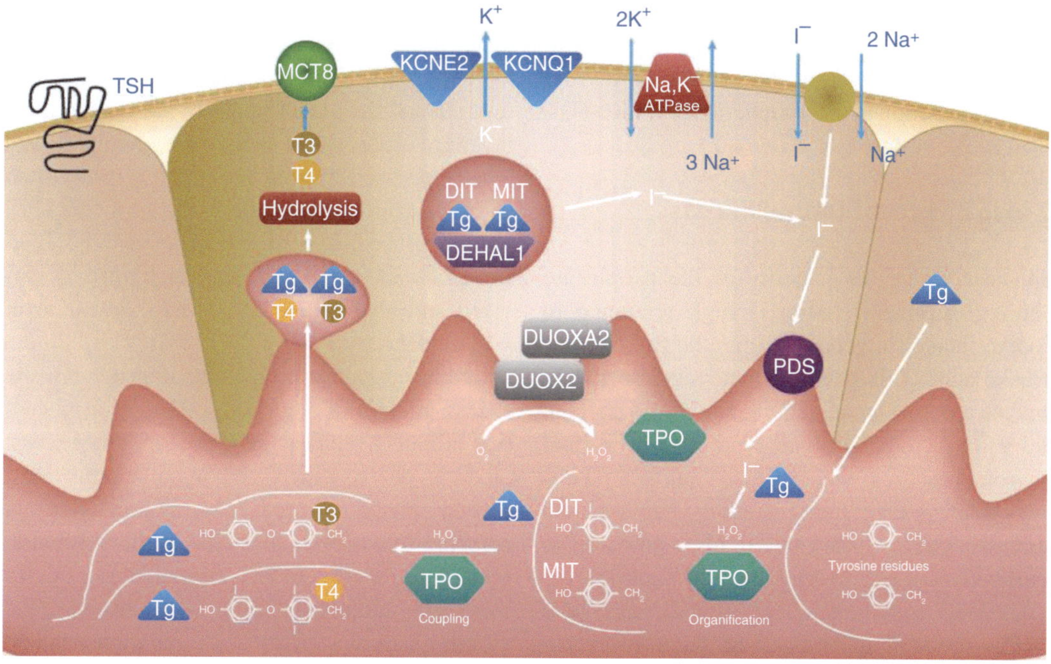

Fig. 3.6 Iodine transport mechanism: The fine balance between each of the components present in the figure, involves the proper metabolism and transport of iodine in the thyroid follicular cell, see text for more details

thyroid hormone action is the conversion of the prohormone T4 to T3. This is the major role of two enzymes –type 1 and 2 iodothyronine deiodinases. Deiodinases exert a major metabolic control of intracellular thyroid hormones concentrations leading to a tissue-specific thyroid hormones bioavailability. All deiodinases are membrane-anchored proteins of 29–33 kDa that share substantial sequence homology. They catalyze and sequentially remove stereo-specific iodine atoms from T4, generating active and inactive isomers of both T3 and DIT. The deiodination of T4, T3, and other iodothyronines is an integral component of thyroid hormones homeostasis. There are three deiodinases: Type 1 (D1), localized to the plasma membrane and catalyzes removal of inner or outer ring iodine atoms in equimolar proportions to generate T3, reverse T3 (rT3), or DIT, depending on the substrate. Most of the circulating T3 is derived from conversion of T4 to T3 by the actions of D1. Type 2 (D2), which is considerably more efficient than D1, catalyzes only the removal of an outer ring iodine atom from T4, generating the active product T3. DIT is considered the main T4 activating enzyme, given its high substrate affinity. DIT-mediated T3 production happens intracellularly. Subsequently, T3 leaves the cells and enters the plasma compartment, being responsible for 70 % of all extrathyroidal T3 production in healthy humans. The major role of DIT is to control the intracellular T3 concentration, its availability to the nucleus, and the saturation of the nuclear T3 receptor in target tissues. It is mainly active in brain, pituitary, and skeletal muscle. Type 3 (D3) is expressed in the brain and other tissues. It irreversibly inactivates T3 or prevents activation of T4 by catalyzing removal of an inner ring iodine atom to generate DIT or rT3, respectively. D3 is an integral membrane protein that exerts its role as a homodimer. It is recycled through a system of endosomal clathrin-coated vesicles, this might suggest a possible mechanism for D3 reactivation, and furthermore the possibility that this enzyme acts on both extracellular and intracellular pools of T3 and T4. Moreover, the inactivation of D3 prevents thyroid hormones access to specific tissues at critical times and reduces thyroid hormones receptors saturation. Given these functions, D3 is considered the major physiological inactivator and terminator of thyroid hormones action at the peripheral level [40, 41].

Toxic Effects of Iodine Excess

In areas where the majority of the people are iodine "sufficient", there is high tolerance to iodine intake. In general terms, the thyroid carries a pool of iodine and may regulate iodine uptake within a broad margin, allowing a specific level of thyroid hormone synthesis (in normal thyroids). In areas where dietary iodine intake is very high – e.g., Japan – adults may tolerate amounts greater than 1,000 μg/day; however, in children, amounts greater than 500 μg/day are associated with goiter [42]. If iodization programs are not appropriate or there is excess dietary salt consumption, the population will have a given risk of disorders due to excess iodine intake. The main consequence is iodine-induced hyperthyroidism, which usually occurs in people with endemic goiter due to iodine deficiencies supplemented with the trace element. This response is known as the "Jod-Basedow effect' and occurs only in a small proportion of the patients at risk [43]. The best documented experience was described in Tasmania, where a temporary increase in the diagnosis of thyrotoxicosis occurred shortly after the addition of small amounts of iodine to bread as the selected method selected for addressing iodine deficiency. The analysis of that population revealed two patterns of underlying thyroid dysfunction. The first pattern was the presence of nodular goiter with autonomous function areas, especially in elderly individuals, with no finding of TSH receptor antibodies. The second pattern occurred in the younger population in the form of diffuse goiter and the presence of TSH receptor antibodies, suggesting that the Jod-Basedow effect occurred only in thyroid glands where function was independent from TSH-mediated stimulation. However, iodine-induced hyperthyroidism is a metabolic disorder that is relatively frequent in areas with very high iodine intake. In fact, in those areas where iodine intake is marginal, moderate increases in iodine intake may induce hyperthyroidism in individuals with autonomous thyroid nodules. Consequently, clinicians must be aware of the risk of inducing hyperthyroidism when prescribing iodine-containing drugs such as amiodarone and iodinated contrast media [44]. Iodine-induced hyperthyroidism may be confirmed by means of ioduria which appears elevated and also by means of thyroid scan with I-131 uptake.

Iodine organification will depend on the excess amount of iodine provided in a process that exhibits a biphasic response to iodine excess: an initial phase of increased organification, and a second phase of reduced organification in response to a relative blockade of this phenomenon. This reduced iodine organification due to increased supplementation is known as the "Wolff-Chaikoff effect", a TSH-independent self-regulated blockade based on an intracellular iodine molar concentration ≥10-3. Susceptibility to this phenomenon may be due either to iodine "trapping" mechanisms, as is the case in Graves-Basedow disease, or to the inability to form organic iodine, as is the case after giving radioactive iodine therapy or during thionamide treatment, or in patients with Hashimoto's disease. Goiter or hypothyroidism may develop in those situations if iodine supply is maintained for long periods of time. The exact biochemical mechanism underlying the Wolff-Chaikoff effect is still unclear, but it could be explained – at least partially- by the generation of several inhibitory substances (such as intrathyroidal iodolactones, iodoaldehydes and/or iodolipids) on thyroid peroxidase activity, or also on the basis of triiodide reaction: $I^- + I_2 \leftrightarrow I_3^-$

At high iodide concentrations, this reaction is displaced to the right due to mass action, trapping I_2, considered to be an intermediary in iodine organification [40]. When moderate or high iodine doses are given repeatedly, organification and thyroid hormone formation inhibition is partially corrected. This "escape" or "adaptation" mechanism occurs because iodine transport diminishes and thyroid iodine concentration is insufficient to maintain the complete

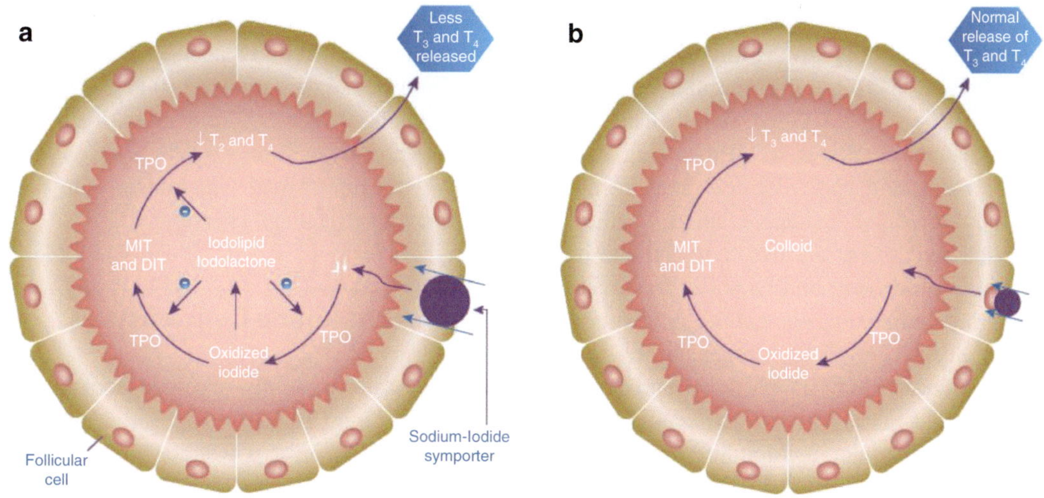

Fig. 3.7 (**a**, **b**) The Wolff–Chaikoff effect and escape mechanism: Is a reduction in thyroid hormone levels caused by ingestion of a large amount of iodine; is an auto-regulatory phenomenon that inhibits organification in the thyroid gland, the formation of thyroid hormones inside the thyroid follicle, and the release of thyroid hormones into the bloodstream. This becomes evident secondary to elevated levels of circulating iodide. When moderate or high iodine doses are given repeatedly, organification and thyroid hormone formation inhibition is partially corrected; this "escape" or "adaptation" mechanism occurs because iodine transport diminishes and thyroid iodine concentration is insufficient to maintain the complete Wolff-Chaikoff effect (See text for more details)

Wolff-Chaikoff effect (Fig. 3.7). This response is a manifestation of the thyroid self-regulated inhibition of iodine transport, preventing the development of hypothyroid goiter in the normal population [45, 46]. On occasions, the "escape" or "adaptation" phenomenon does not occur, giving rise to the persistent inhibition of thyroid hormone formation, leading to hypothyroidism and goiter (myxedema). The Wolff-Chaikoff effect is short-lived because SNI biosynthesis comes quickly to a halt, intracellular iodine drops below the molar concentration of ≥10(−3), and iodine organification resumes. This marked drop in SNI activity occurs through TSH-independent self-Toxic effects of iodine excess. In areas where the majority of the people are iodine "sufficient", there is high tolerance to iodine intake. In general terms, the thyroid carries a pool of iodine and may regulate iodine uptake within a broad margin, allowing a specific level of thyroid hormone synthesis (in normal thyroids).

In summary, excessive iodine intake can cause "thyroid dysfunction", especially in patients with underlying autoimmune thyroiditis – due to a failure to escape from the Wolff-Chaikoff effect-Iodine excess can cause hypothyroidism and/or goiter, but if autonomously functioning nodules or a subclinical form of Graves' disease are present, it can also induce hyperthyroidism (Jod-Basedow effect). Both phenomena are thought to lead to some thyroid destruction and hence presentation of the most important antigens involved in thyroid autoimmunity, such as Tg and TPO.

Although the mechanisms are not fully elucidated, excess iodine is a well-recognized environmental factor for Autoimmune Thyroid Disease (ATD) in autoimmune-prone individuals, particularly Autoimmune Thyroiditis (AIT), which is characterized by lymphocytic infiltration of the thyroid gland with the development of thyroid autoantibodies and primary hypothyroidism [47–49].

Thyroid autoimmunity in the context of an iodine excess state could be induced by: (a) Excess iodine induces the production of cytokines and chemokines that can recruit immunocompetent cells to the thyroid – has been reported that high concentrations of iodine induced thyroid cell injury and subsequent inflammation with production of reactive oxygen species, which may contribute to the initiation of thyroid autoimmunity: (b) It seems that iodide preferentially induces chemokines rather than other inflammatory cytokines: (c) Processing excess iodine in thyroid epithelial cells may result in elevated levels of oxidative stress leading to harmful lipid oxidation and thyroid tissue injuries: (d) Iodine incorporation in the protein chain of thyroglobulin may augment the antigenicity of this molecule: (e) The mechanism of iodine excess-induced ATD is partly regarded as T helper type 1 (Th1) cell and/or T helper type 17 (Th17) cell dominant autoimmune disease. Both the hyperactivation of Th17 cells and the suppression of Th1 (and T helper type 2), and regulatory T cells may be involved in the pathogenesis of ATD [50, 51].

On the other hand, amiodarone is a potent class III anti-arrhythmic drug used in clinical practice for the prophylaxis and treatment of many cardiac rhythm disturbances, ranging from paroxysmal atrial fibrillation to life-threatening ventricular tachyarrhythmias. Amiodarone often causes changes in thyroid function tests mainly related to the inhibition of 5′-deiodinase activity resulting in a decrease in the generation of T3 from T4, with a resulting increase in reverse T3 (rT3) production and a decrease in its clearance.

Amiodarone is a benzofuran derivative containing two atoms of iodine per molecule. This amount to 37.5 % of organic iodine by molecular weight, and 10 % of the drug's iodine content is released daily as free iodide. Drug doses range from 200 to 600 mg daily and treatment releases about 7–20 mg of iodide daily, which is about 50–100 fold the optimal daily iodine intake.

Although the majority of the adverse effects of amiodarone on several organs are due to deposition of the drug in the parenchyma, its effects on the thyroid gland can be divided into two groups: intrinsic effects resulting from the inherent properties of the compound, and iodine-induced effects due solely to the pharmacologic effects of a large iodine load – it has the potential to cause thyroid dysfunction because of its iodine-rich chemical structure.

Amiodarone can lead to both hypothyroidism (Amiodarone-Induced Hypothyroidism (AIH) with a prevalence ranging from 10 to 20 %) and, less commonly to hyperthyroidism with a prevalence ranging from 2 to 9.6 %). Most patients treated with amiodarone will remain euthyroid throughout the treatment course.

Diagnosis of Iodine Deficiency

There are four generally accepted and recommended methods for assessing the nutritional aspects of iodine in a population: *urine iodine concentration, goiter rates, Tg levels, and thyroid stimulating hormone (THS) levels.* These measurements are not exclusive but complementary since ioduria is a sensitive indicator of recent iodine intake (days), while Tg levels show iodine status in the population (over weeks to months), and changes in goiter rates show long-term iodine nutritional status in a population (over months and years).

Ioduria: Essentially 90 % of the total iodine content absorbed is cleared through the urine. This is why measuring this trace element in urine is considered a way to assess recent intake, although concentrations may vary from day to day and even throughout the same day. Iodine urine concentration may be expressed in μg/L, or in relation with creatinine (μg/g creatinine), or also as 24 h urine concentration (μg/day). Considering that 24-h urine is impractical in population studies, it is usually recommended to measure ioduria in a urine sample taken either in the morning or at random (0.5–1 mL) in a specific group, and it is expressed as median ioduria in μg/L. Although median ioduria does not reflect thyroid function, it is clear that a low urine concentration points to an increased risk of suffering thyroid disorders. Creatinine and creatinuria are not taken into consideration in the vast majority of studies designed to determine iodine status in a population, given that creatinine concentration is low in those regions with a significant frequency of malnutrition [52, 53]. Ioduria may be used to extrapolate daily iodine intake in the population using the estimated 24-h mean urinary volume and assuming an average iodine bioavailability of 92 % on the basis of the following formula:

$$\textit{Daily iodine intake} = \text{urinary iodine}(\mu g / L) \times 0.0235 \times \text{body weight } (kg)$$

Using this formula, a median ioduria of 100 μg/L would correlate with an average mean intake of 150 μg. Several methods for measuring ioduria have been described; however, these methods are not universally available. The method most widely available is "Method A" which uses ammonium persulfate and requires the use of spectrophotometry. The second is "Method B" which uses chloric acid, although it has the drawback of explosion risk during the test. There are other tests, but Method A is preferred in population studies, followed by Method B [52].

Thyroid volume: There are two methods for assessing thyroid volume: physical inspection and palpation, and thyroid ultrasound. On palpation, goiter is considered to be present when each lateral lobe is longer that the distal phalanx of the examiner's thumb. According to the WHO classification system, grade 0 is non-palpable or visible thyroid gland; grade I is palpable but non-visible goiter with the neck in normal position; and grade II is evidently visible goiter with the neck in a the normal position. This is perhaps the most widely accepted classification because it is easy to use and interpret even in the hands of an inexperienced examiner. Goiter prevalence may be determined also with the use of thyroid ultrasound. In those areas with mild IDD, goiter prevalence may be low, hence the low diagnostic sensitivity and specificity of palpation alone. Moreover, classification error may be as high as 40 %, and in those situations ultrasound may be more reliable than palpation. However, there are few data comparing ultrasound with palpation in areas where IDD is more prevalent. In fact, thyroid ultrasound is considered to have lower accuracy in areas with severe IDD and, consequently, palpation is a better way to estimate goiter prevalence. In areas with moderate-to-severe IDD, goiter screening using palpation must be the option of choice because of ease of application, reproducibility and low cost. Goiter rate in school children is an indicator of IDD severity in a specific population. A rate ≥5 % in this age group is an indicator of a public health problem. Thyroid volume interpretation requires validated reference ranges in children living in iodine "sufficient" areas. In 1997, the WHO together with International Council for the Control of Iodine Deficiency Disorders (ICCIDD) proposed reference values for thyroid volume based on data of European children, but those reference values were much higher than they actually are. Thyroid volumes in other areas of the world (Switzerland, the United States, Malaysia) were shown to be much lower than those referenced in the European school population, although this could be explained on the basis of the residual effect from iodine deficiency prevailing in Europe in the early 1990s. Later, thyroid volumes were measured in children between 6 and 12 years of age in areas that had been "sufficient" for a long time in North and South America, Central Europe, Eastern Mediterranean, Western Pacific Africa, and children from most ethnic majorities in the world. The sample consisted of 3529 children, divided by age and gender; the median ioduria range was 118–288 μg/L. Significant differences were found in mean thyroid volume adjusted by age and body surface, suggesting that reference values for a specific population in countries with long standing iodine "sufficiency" may be more accurate than an international reference standard. These reference values are recommended for goiter screening during IDD monitoring, and they are more conservative than those previously used, although it is clear that inter-observer variability with this method is high – up to 26 % – [52, 54, 55]. In order to improve thyroid volume data reliability and comparability on ultrasound when monitoring for IDD, a standardized approach has to be adopted worldwide [32, 40]. Thyroid volume is calculated by adding the volume of each lobe, and it does not include thyroid isthmus volume. The following formula is used to calculate the volume of each lobe:

$$\text{Volume (mL)} = 0.479 \times D \times w \times 1\,(\text{cm})$$

Where D is depth and W is width.

For classification purposes, body surface calculation in IDD screening programs uses the Dubois and Dubois formula:

$$\text{Body surface area } (m^2) = W^{0.425} \times H^{0.725} \times 71.84 \times 10^{-4}$$

Where W is weight and H is height.

In accordance with the ultrasound criteria, goiter is considered to be present when thyroid volume is above the 97th percentile of the volume found in an area where the population is iodine "replete" [56]. Table 3.6 shows the reference values for the 97th percentile of the thyroid volume as a function of age and body surface area.

TSH: TSH is not a sensitive indicator for IDD either in school-age populations or in adults. However, in neonates, where iodine concentration is very low, iodine turnover is very high and this increased iodine turnover is exaggerated in iodine deficient areas. When it is present, an increase in TSH levels is required, explaining why in iodine deficient areas TSH rises far above normal in the first weeks of life, creating a state called "transient hyperthyrotropinemia" [52].

Table 3.6 Specific 97th percentile for thyroid volume (mL) by age and body surface area, measured by ultrasound in iodine "sufficient" school children 6–12 years of age

Age	Boys 97th P	Girls 97th P	Body surface area (m^2)	Boys 97th P	Girls 97th P
6	2.91	2.84	0.7	2.62	2.56
7	3.29	3.26	0.8	2.95	2.91
8	3.71	3.76	0.9	3.32	3.32
9	4.19	4.32	1.0	3.73	3.79
10	4.73	4.98	1.1	4.2	4.32
11	5.34	5.73	1.2	4.73	4.92
12	6.03	6.59	1.3	5.32	5.61
			1.4	5.98	6.4
			1.5	6.73	7.29
			1.6	7.57	8.32

Therefore, TSH elevation in this age group is of great value for determining the severity of iodine deficiency in a given population.

Thyroglobulin: Tg is the most abundant thyroid protein. In areas with endemic goiter, the major determinants of serum Tg are thyroid cell mass and TSH stimulation. Studies that have examined Tg as a potential indicator of the effects of iodine supplementation in populations with IDD show that this protein drops rapidly with iodine supplementation and, consequently, it is considered a more sensitive indicator of iodine repletion than TSH itself. The international Tg range in whole blood samples of school-age populations is between 4 and 40 μg/L. Tg correlates very well with iodine deficiency severity determined by ioduria and, for this reason, Tg is now considered a promising biochemical indicator of thyroid function in school-age populations after the introduction and implementation of universal salt iodization programs. However, it must be complemented with the use of ioduria and thyroid volume, although it has not yet been adopted as a universal indicator for IDD [38, 52].

IDD Prevention and Treatment

The most effective way to control IDD is universal salt iodization, which refers to iodization of all salt used for human consumption (industrial and household use) and for cattle. This strategy is recommended because salt is used essentially in all foods and its intake is consistent throughout the year. Iodization is a simple, inexpensive technique, and does not affect salt color or flavor. The WHO/UNICEF/ICCIDD recommendation is to add iodine to the salt at a concentration of 20–40 mg of iodine per kilogram of salt. Iodine may be added in the form of potassium iodide or iodate. However, considering that potassium iodate is more stable than iodide when in contact with moisture and impurities, it is the recommended iodization form in tropical countries. Iodine is usually added once the salt has gone through a "drying" process. Bread may be a good vehicle for adjusting salt intake by introducing iodine-enriched salt in the baking process. Iodization of water and irrigation systems may also be useful, but this requires costly methods that limit its application. Countries like Switzerland and US have additional iodine sources through milk in the diet, more because of the use of iodophors in the food industry than the deliberate addition of iodine. In countries affected by IDD, it is considered that iodine must be added routinely to complementary foods in order to increase iodine content derived from daily intake. In remote areas or areas of difficult access, or where small-scale salt producers exist, salt iodization programs may not work or create the expected social impact. In those situations, the recommendation is to replace iodine by means of iodized oils administered orally or intramuscularly. The oral route is easier, but the intramuscular route is more effective and has longer lasting effects. The oral dose ranges between 200 and 400 mg of iodine per year and it is usually administered to the most vulnerable population (pregnant women, children and women in childbearing age). Iodine may also be given in the form of potassium iodide or iodate drops or tablets; the monthly (30 mg) or biweekly (8 mg) dose of potassium iodide may be sufficient to provide the adequate amount of iodine, in particular to the population at risk [52, 56].

Impact of Iodine Supplementation in Deficient Populations

A review of the evidence of the health consequences of mild iodine deficiency reveals that:

- There is a limited number of published studies investigating the health consequences of mild iodine deficiency.
- There is reasonable evidence of an association between mild iodine deficiency and suboptimal neurological development, specially reduced Intelligence Quotient (IQ).
- Of the studies that have attempted to investigate the effects of mild iodine deficiency, many have limitations. Consequently, the current literature does not provide unequivocal evidence for significant health effects for populations with urinary iodine in the upper range of mild iodine deficiency.
- There is sufficient evidence to suggest that the known association between neurological outcomes and moderate and severe iodine deficiency is likely to extend to mild iodine deficiency. However, there is a suggestion of a dose response relationship with increasing effects on neurological development with higher iodine deficiency levels. Neurological effects associated with mild iodine deficiency include reduced IQ, increased auditory threshold and increased rates of attention-deficit hyperactivity disorder. Although the relation between iodine intake during pregnancy, thyroid function, and child neurodevelopment needs further evaluation, the evidence on the safety and effectiveness of iodine supplementation during pregnancy is needed before it is systematically recommended in iodine-sufficient or mildly deficient areas.
- In constructing a reasonable health-based standard using the precautionary approach, it is clear that urinary iodine levels below 100 μg/L, which are in the mild iodine deficiency range, warrant intervention [1, 57, 58].

Iodine requirements are increased ≥50 % during pregnancy, and iodine deficiency can cause maternal and fetal hypothyroidism and impair neurological development of the fetus. The consequences depend upon the timing and severity of the hypothyroidism. The most severe manifestation is cretinism. In moderate-to-severely iodine-deficient areas, controlled studies have demonstrated that iodine supplementation before or during early pregnancy eliminates new cases of cretinism, increases birth weight, reduces rates of perinatal and infant mortality and generally increases developmental scores in young children by 10–20 %. Mild maternal iodine deficiency can cause thyroid dysfunction but whether it impairs cognitive and/or neurologic function in the offspring remains uncertain. To date, measures to address iodine deficiency in populations with mild-to-moderate deficiencies have been shown to prevent (during gestation) increases in maternal thyroid volume and in Tg levels. On the other hand, the impact of iodine supplementation for the mother on the neurological development of the new-born is yet to be ascertained given the absence of clinical trials designed to evaluate those outcomes appropriately. In school-age children, iodine supplementation has been associated with modest benefits in terms of cognitive development. Iodine supplementation has proven to be an effective method for reducing goiter rates and improving iodine status in this age group. Moreover, there is some indication of positive effects on the physical and mental development and on mortality, although the results of the studies have not always been statistically significant [52, 56]. Recently, WHO proposed a guideline aims to help member states and their partners in their efforts to make informed decisions on the appropriate nutrition actions to achieve the Millennium Development Goals, in particular, reduction of child mortality and improvement of maternal health. This guideline provides global, evidence-informed recommendations on fortification of food-grade salt with iodine, for the prevention and control of iodine deficiency disorders, with the purpose of improving iodine nutrition and preventing iodine deficiency disorders in populations [57–59].

Conclusion

Although substantial progress has been made, iodine deficiency remains a significant public health problem worldwide, even in developed countries. Consequently, good quality population data on iodine status are required to assess population status and design strategies to correct deficiencies without introducing excessive intakes. If programs of iodine prophylaxis are carefully monitored for both iodine deficiency and excess, the relatively small risks of iodine excess are far outweighed by the substantial risks of iodine deficiency. In addition to monitoring iodine nutrition, effective surveillance systems should also include monitoring of iodized salt quality at all levels (industrial, retail, and household) to ensure that salt iodization programs are safe and effective in their control of iodine deficiency.

References

1. Zimmerman MB, Boelaert K. Iodine deficiency and thyroid disorders. Lancet Diabetes Endocrinol. 2015. Published Online 13 Jan 2015. http://dx.doi.org/10.1016/S2213-8587(14)70225-6.
2. Lazarus JH. The importance of iodine in public health. Environ Geochem Health. 2015;37(4):605–18.
3. Nyenwe EA, Dagogo-Jack S. Iodine deficiency disorders in the iodine-replete environment. Am J Med Sci. 2009;337(1):37–40.
4. Zimmermann MB, Andersson M. Assessment of iodine nutrition in populations: past, present, and future. Nutr Rev. 2012;70:553–70.
5. de Benoist B, McLean E, Andersson M. Iodine deficiency in 2007: global progress since 2003. Food Nutr Bull. 2008;29:195–202.
6. Bath SC, Rayman MP. A review of the iodine status of UK pregnant women and its implications for the offspring. Environ Geochem Health. 2015;37(4):619–29.
7. Masoodi SR, Ali A, Wani AI, Bashir MI, Bhat JA, Mudassar S, Zargar AH. Goitre and urinary iodine excretion survey in schoolchildren of Kashmir Valley. Clin Endocrinol. 2014;80:141–7.
8. Ahmed M, Zama SY, Nagarajarao V, Khan MA. Iodine deficiency in children: a comparative study in two districts of south-interior Karnataka. India J Family Community Med. 2014;21(1):48–52.
9. Zou Y, Lou X, Ding G, Mo Z, Zhu W, Mao G, Zhou J. An assessment of iodine nutritional status and thyroid hormone levels in children aged 8–10 years living in Zhejiang Province, China: a cross-sectional study. Eur J Pediatr. 2014;173(7):929–34.
10. Zimmermann MB. Iodine deficiency and excess in children: worldwide status in 2013. Endocr Pract. 2013;19(5):839–46.
11. Pearce EN, Andersson M, Zimmermann MB. Global iodine nutrition: where do we stand in 2013? Thyroid. 2013;23(5):523–8.
12. Chung HR. Iodine and thyroid function. Ann Pediatr Endocrinol Metab. 2014;19(1):8–12.
13. Huang W, Peng C, Huang H, Zhang J, Liu J, Mao L, Luo R, Xiao Y. Control of iodine-deficiency disorders following universal salt iodization in Shenzhen, China, 1997–2011. Food Nutr Bull. 2013;34(3):331–7.
14. WHO/UNICEF/ICCIDD. Assessment of iodine deficiency disorders and monitoring their elimination: a guide for programme managers [updated 1st September 2008]. 3rd ed. Geneva: World Health Organization; 2007.
15. Rohner F, Zimmermann M, Jooste P, Pandav C, Caldwell K, Raghavan R, Raiten DJ. Biomarkers of nutrition for development-Iodine review. J Nutr. 2014. pii:jn.113.181974.
16. Doggui R, El Atia J. Iodine deficiency: Physiological, clinical and epidemiological features, and pre-analytical considerations. Ann Endocrinol (Paris). 2015;76(1):59–66.

17. Girma K, Nibret E, Gedefaw M. The status of iodine nutrition and iodine deficiency disorders among school children in Metekel Zone. Northwest Ethiopia Ethiop J Health Sci. 2014;24(2):109–16.
18. Bath SC, Rayman MP. Iodine deficiency in the U.K.: an overlooked cause of impaired neurodevelopment? Proc Nutr Soc. 2013;72(2):226–35.
19. Andersson M, de Benoist B, Rogers L. Epidemiology of iodine deficiency: salt iodisation and iodine status. Best Pract Res Clin Endocrinol Metab. 2010; 24(1):1–11.
20. Fuge R, Johnson CC. The geochemistry of iodine – a review. Environ Geochem Health. 1986;8(2): 31–54.
21. Johnson CC. The geochemistry of iodine and its application to environmental strategies for reducing the risks from iodine deficiency disorders. British Geological Survey, CR/03/057N; 2003.
22. Leung AM, Braverman LE, Pearce EN. History of U.S. iodine fortification and supplementation. Nutrients. 2012;4:1740–6.
23. Gong T, Zhang X. Determination of iodide, iodate and organo-iodine in waters with a new total organic iodine measurement approach. Water Res. 2013; 47(17):6660–9.
24. Kaplan DI, Denham ME, Zhang S, Yeager C, Xu C, Schwehr KA, Li HP, Ho YF, Wellman D, Santschi PH. Radioiodine biogeochemistry and prevalence in groundwater. Crit Rev Environ Sci Technol. 2014;44(20):2287–335.
25. Amachi S. Microbial contribution to global iodine cycling: volatilization, accumulation, reduction, oxidation, and sorption of iodine. Microbes Environ. 2008;23(4):269–76.
26. Chameides W, Davis D. Iodine: its possible role in tropospheric geochemistry. J Geophys Res. 1980;85: 7383–98.
27. Fuge R. The role of volatility in the distribution of iodine in the secondary environment. Appl Geochem. 1990;5:357–60.
28. Fuge R. Sources of halogens in the environment, influences on human and animal health. Environ Geochem Health. 1988;10(2):51–61.
29. Hong C, Weng H, Jilani G, Yan A, Liu H, Xue Z. Evaluation of iodide and iodate for adsorption-desorption characteristics and bioavailability in three types of soil. Biol Trace Elem Res. 2012; 146(2):262–71.
30. Hu Q, Zhao P, Moran JE, Seaman JC. Sorption and transport of iodine species in sediments from the Savannah River and Hanford Sites. J Contam Hydrol. 2005;78(3):185–205.
31. Kolb CE. Atmospheric chemistry: Iodine's air of importance. Nature. 2002;417:597–8.
32. Gahche JJ, Bailey RL, Mirel LB, Dwyer JT. The prevalence of using iodine-containing supplements is low among reproductive-age women, NHANES 1999–2006. J Nutr. 2013;143(6):872–7.
33. Wolka E, Shiferaw S, Biadgilign S. Epidemiological study of risk factors for goiter among primary school-children in southern Ethiopia. Food Nutr Bull. 2014;35(1):20–7.
34. Zimmerman MB, Jooste PL, Pandav CS. Iodine-deficiency disorders. Lancet. 2008;372:1251–62.
35. Kuriti M, Pearce EN, Braverman LE, He X, Leung AM. Iodine content of U.S. weight-loss food. Endocr Pract. 2014;20(3):232–5.
36. Pearce EN. National trends in iodine nutrition: is everyone getting enough? Thyroid. 2007;17(9): 823–7.
37. Pesce L, Kopp P. Iodide transport: implications for health and disease. Int J Pediatr Endocrinol. 2014;1:8. doi:10.1186/1687-9856-2014-8.
38. Sellitti DF, Suzuki K. Intrinsic regulation of thyroid function by thyroglobulin. Thyroid. 2014; 24(4):625–38.
39. Nicola JP, Reyna-Neyra A, Carrasco N, Masini-Repiso AM. Dietary iodide controls its own absorption through post-transcriptional regulation of the intestinal Na+/I-symporter. J Physiol. 2012;590(Pt 23):6013–26.
40. Portulano C, Paroder-Belenitsky M, Carrasco N. The Na+/I- Symporter (NIS): mechanism and medical impact. Endocr Rev. 2014;35(1):106–49.
41. Schweizer U, Johannes J, Bayer D, Braun D. Structure and function of thyroid hormone plasma membrane transporters. Eur Thyroid J. 2014;3(3):143–53.
42. Bürgi H. Iodine excess. Best Pract Res Clin Endocrinol Metab. 2010;24:107–15.
43. Vargas-Uricoechea H, Sierra-Torres CH. Thyroid hormones and the heart. Horm Mol Biol Clin Investig. 2014;18(1):15–26.
44. Leung AM, Braverman LE. Consequences of excess iodine. Nat Rev Endocrinol. 2014;10(3):136–42.
45. Bizhanova A, Kopp P. Minireview: the sodium-iodide symporter NIS and PDS in iodide homeostasis of the thyroid. Endocrinology. 2009;150:1084–90.
46. Sun X, Shan Z, Teng W. Effects of increased iodine intake on thyroid disorders. Endocrinol Metab (Seoul). 2014;29(3):240–7.
47. Vargas-Uricoechea H, Bonelo-Perdomo A, Sierra-Torres CH. Effects of thyroid hormones on the heart. Clin Invest Arterioscl. 2014;26(6):296–309.
48. Roti E, Uberti ED. Iodine excess and hyperthyroidism. Thyroid. 2001;11(5):493–500.
49. Mansourian ARA. review on the metabolic disorders of iodine deficiency. Pak J Biol Sci. 2011; 14(7):412–24.
50. Kawicka A, Regulska-Ilow B, Regulska-Ilow B. Metabolic disorders and nutritional status in autoimmune thyroid diseases. Postepy Hig Med Dosw (Online). 2015;69:80–90.
51. Yang X, Gao T, Shi R, Zhou X, Qu J, Xu J, Shan Z, Teng W. Effect of iodine excess on Th1, Th2, Th17, and Treg cell subpopulations in the thyroid of NOD.H-2 h4 mice. Biol Trace Elem Res. 2014;159(1–3):288–96.
52. World Health Organization, United Nations Children's Fund, International Council for the Control of Iodine Deficiency Disorders. Assessment of iodine deficiency disorders and monitoring their elimination: a

guide for programme managers. 3rd ed. Geneva: World Health Organization; 2007.
53. Zhou SJ, Anderson AJ, Gibson RA, Makrides M. Effect of iodine. supplementation in pregnancy on child development and other clinical outcomes: a systematic review of randomized controlled trials. Am J Clin Nutr. 2013;98(5):1241–54.
54. Zimmerman MB. Assessing iodine status and monitoring progress of iodized salt programs. J Nutr. 2004;134:1673–7.
55. Zimmermann MB, Hess SY, Molinari L, De Benoist B, Delange F, Braverman LE, Fujieda K, Ito Y, Jooste PL, Moosa K, Pearce EN, Pretell EA, Shishiba Y. New reference values for thyroid volume by ultrasound in iodine-sufficient schoolchildren: a World Health Organization/Nutrition for Health and Development Iodine Deficiency Study Group Report. Am J Clin Nutr. 2004;79(2):231–7.
56. Vargas-Uricoechea H, Sierra-Torres CH, Holguín-Betancourt CM, Cristancho-Torres L. Iodine-deficiency disorders. Permanent surveillance of vulnerable zones is poor. MEDICINA. (Bogotá). 2012;34, No. 2(97):119–44.
57. Taylor PN, Okosieme OE, Dayan CM, Lazarus JH. Therapy of endocrine disease: impact of iodine supplementation in mild-to-moderate iodine deficiency: systematic review and meta-analysis. Eur J Endocrinol. 2014;170:R1–15.
58. WHO. Guideline: fortification of food-grade salt with iodine for the prevention and control of iodine deficiency disorders. Geneva: World Health Organization; 2014.
59. Aburto N, Abudou M, Candeias V, Wu T. Effect and safety of salt iodization to prevent iodinedeficiency disorders: a systematic review with meta-analyses. WHO eLibrary of EvidenceforNutrition Actions (eLENA). Geneva: World Health Organization; 2014.

4 The Role of Thyroid Hormones in Neural Development

Alan J. Hargreaves

Abstract

A key aim of this chapter was to review the molecular events associated with the regulation of neural development by thyroid hormones. These molecules are produced in the thyroid gland, and secreted into the bloodstream, where they interact with a number of carrier proteins to facilitate distribution to target tissues. A range of transporter proteins are also present to facilitate uptake in tissues that require TH for their normal development. Research over several decades has shown that TH can regulate neural gene expression both at the transcriptional and post-transcriptional levels. This review focuses partly on the ability of TH to modulate genes encoding cytoskeletal proteins involved in the regulation neural cell proliferation and differentiation, and how dysregulation of TH is associated with cytoskeletal disruption. It also discusses selected non-genomic mechanisms by which TH can influence cytoskeletal involvement in development and other important cell functions.

Introduction

Thyroid hormones (THs) regulate a range of metabolic and developmental processes. Of particular interest to this review is the essential role of THs and their receptors in neural development, which is underlined by evidence that irreversible brain damage and mental retardation can occur as a result of thyroid deficiency during foetal or perinatal development [1–5]. THs may also continue to be important in the regulation of certain neural cell activities throughout adult life [6, 7]. This chapter discusses the factors influencing the delivery of TH to nerve tissue, reviews evidence for the involvement of THs in neural development, and examines the cellular and molecular pathways modulated by TH with a particular emphasis on the cytoskeleton.

A.J. Hargreaves
Interdisciplinary Biomedical Research Centre,
School of Science & Technology,
Nottingham Trent University, Nottingham, UK
e-mail: alan.hargreaves@ntu.ac.uk

S.K. Imam, S.I. Ahmad (eds.), *Thyroid Disorders: Basic Science and Clinical Practice*,
DOI 10.1007/978-3-319-25871-3_4

Fig. 4.1 Chemical structures of thyroid hormones. Shown are planar diagrams of the structures of the two principal thyroid hormones, namely triiodothyronine (*T3*) and L-thyroxine (*T4*). These molecules account for approximately 99 % of circulating hormone

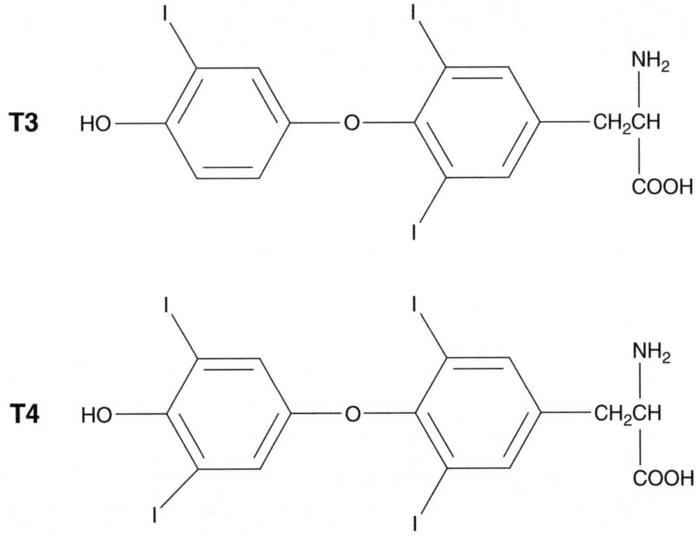

Thyroid Hormone Synthesis and Secretion

The two main forms of TH are the active hormone tri-iodothyronine (T3) and the pro-hormone thyroxine (T4), the chemical structures of which are illustrated in Fig. 4.1. The neurodevelopmental effects of TH are believed to occur largely as a result of the binding of T3 to specific nuclear receptors in nerve cells, to which T4 binds with much lower affinity, resulting in the regulation of a variety of genes that encode proteins involved in neural development, although relatively rapid non-genomic effects have also been described. TH is synthesised in the thyroid gland in a process involving iodination of the amino acid tyrosine in a specific domain of the protein thyroglobulin, which is first synthesised as a glycoprotein in the lumen of the endoplasmic reticulum of thyroid follicular cells and then secreted by exocytosis into the thyroid follicle colloid region [8, 9]. The thyroid gland accumulates and concentrates iodine from the circulation with the aid of a plasma membrane associated Na^+/I^- symporter, whereas iodine efflux into the intrafollicular compartment (colloid) is regulated by the action of the Cl^-/I^- exchanger pendrin in conjunction with one or more Cl^- transporters that also have the ability to transport I^- across membranes [10–12].

In a series of reactions catalysed by thyroperoxidase, the accumulated iodine is oxidised, coupled to thyroglobulin-bound tyrosines producing monoiodo- and diiodo-tyrosine, which are then conjugated to form thyroglobulin-bound T3 and T4 [13, 14]. The thyroglobulin bound hormone can be stored in the colloid and released when required, whereupon it is taken up into the follicular cells by endocytosis, proteolytically degraded by lysosomal proteases, and the liberated T3 and T4 released into the circulation by exocytosis [8, 15].

The thyroid gland is under the control of hormones secreted via the hypothalamo-pituitary axis. The overall process of TH synthesis and release is regulated by thyroid stimulating hormone (TSH) under a feedback loop modulated by the levels of circulating TH, which acts to reduce the response of pituitary cells that produce TSH to the hormones that stimulate this process [8, 16]. The production and secretion of TSH is stimulated by the tripeptide thyrotrophin-releasing hormone (TRH), which is derived by cleavage of a pro-hormone released from hypothalamic neurosecretory cells into the bloodstream for transport to the pituitary thyrotroph cells that synthesise and secrete TSH [8]. TSH secretion is down-regulated by agents such as somatostatin, dopamine and certain cytokines (e.g. TNF-α).

Thyroid Hormone Transport, Uptake and Metabolism

Due to their hydrophobic nature, after being secreted from the thyroid gland, THs utilise a number of proteins in the circulation and within target cells that can facilitate their movements to their target tissues (e.g. brain), maternal-foetal transfer during early development, transfer across the blood brain barrier in children and adults, and their metabolism [8, 17–20]. Major TH-binding proteins in serum include albumin, transthyretin, thyroxine-binding globulin and apolipoprotein B-100 [17, 20, 21]. Collectively these proteins help to maintain an equilibrium between protein-bound and free (i.e. non protein-bound) TH, such that the necessary amount of free hormone is available in the circulation of healthy individuals [8].

While this system effectively maintains a supply of free TH to target cells and tissues in healthy adults, during embryonic and foetal development there are other barriers to TH reaching its target tissue, namely the placental barrier. For example, during early development as foetal thyroid gland dose not secrete TH in the first 4 months of gestation, the foetus is dependent on the maternal supply of TH during this period [22]. Its transport across the placental barrier involves TH binding proteins, such as albumin and transthyretin, which are actually synthesised in the placental trophoblast cells and are also secreted and taken up by them, the latter involving an LDL-mediated receptor mediated endocytosis pathway [18, 23]. Transplacental transfer is further dependent on the action of a number of TH transporters, which are expressed by trophobasts from 6 weeks of gestation [24]. On entry into the placental cells T4 can be converted to T3 by deiodination mediated by type III deiodinase (D3) [18]. Thus, the delivery of T3 to the foetus is dependent on the coordinated action of TH binding proteins, TH transporters and deiodinase activities in trophoplasts [4, 18].

The delivery of TH to the brain requires its transfer across the blood brain barrier, which is the main route of entry for T4, or the brain-cerebrospinal fluid barrier. The four serum proteins mentioned above transport bound T4 to the blood brain barrier but, of these, only transthyretin has been detected in large amounts in cerebrospinal fluid, as a result of its synthesis and secretion by the choroid plexus epithelial cells [20, 25, 26]. On arrival at the blood brain barrier, TH requires the assistance of a number of transmembrane transporter proteins, which facilitate uptake and release in a variety of cell types and brain regions, to enable it to reach the appropriate tissue [20]. Several brain TH transporter proteins have been described, including Mct8, Mct10, Lat1, Lat2 and Oatp14, which exhibit both similarities and differences in their regional distribution and developmentally regulated expression patterns [20, 27]. It has been suggested that coordinated expression of TH transporters occurs in alignment with the expression and activities of deiodinases D2 and D3, in order to enable timely maturation of brain cells during development [28, 29].

Having crossed the blood brain barrier, T4 can then be bioactivated (i.e. converted to T3) by the deiodinase D2; alternatively T4 and T3 can be converted to an inactive from of TH termed reverse T3 [20]. Deiodinases exhibit distinct distribution patterns in neural cells and tissues [30, 31], D2 being more prevalent in glial cells [32, 33], while D3 may be more abundant in certain neurons [30], although developmental fluctuations can occur.

On entering the cytoplasm of target cells, T3 interacts with a thyroid hormone receptors (TRs) present in the nucleus [34–36]. Members of the steroid-retinoic acid-thyroid hormone superfamily, TRs exist in two main forms termed TRα and TRβ, each of which has at least 2 isoforms, showing regional variation within the brain and differential patterns of expression during early and late development which may reflect distinct functions at key developmental stages [35]. Like other members of the nuclear receptor superfamily, TRs contain an amino terminal domain, a central DNA binding domain with two zinc fingers, a hinge region containing the nuclear localisation signal and a carboxy terminal ligand binding domain which is essential for TH attachment [36]. The TRs are effectively T3-inducible transcription factors that, once activated, induce changes in the expression of a variety of neural genes of importance during development and in later life, whereas the unliganded receptors act as repressors. However, TH may interact with other proteins in the cell membrane or the cytoplasm to induce a range of rapid non-genomic effects, as discussed later.

Disruption of Brain Development by Thyroid Hormone Depletion

The development of all organ systems is disrupted by the lack of active TH, leading to a range of developmental abnormalities [37]. However, the brain is so severely affected that mental retardation and other neurological effects can result from deficiencies during foetal or perinatal development [4, 5, 8, 36–39].

Studies in humans have shown that TH deficiency disrupts the normal patterns of brain development and is associated with neurological lesions such as attention deficit and hyperactivity disorders, and impaired cognitive function [40–43]. A study performed on rats transiently treated with 2-mercapto-1-methylimidazole to induce hypothyroxinemia resulted in a statistically significant impairment of spatial learning in the offspring in adulthood, as determined by the water maze test, in conjunction with impairment of long term potentiation (LTP) in the hippocampus, a process which is known to be important in cognitive processes such as spatial learning [44]. The same study showed that these physiological changes were associated with reduced phosphorylation of c-fos, an immediate early gene-encoded protein which is phosphorylated at specific sites to support its role in spatial learning. Increased levels of the post synaptic density protein PSD-95, the NMDA receptor NR1 with which it normally co-localises, and the neurotrophin receptor TrkB were found, although no significant change was observed in the levels of brain derived neurotrophic factor (BDNF), which binds to the latter. These observations, together with the inability of NR1 to colocalise with PSD-95 in offspring from treated dams, suggest that there is disruption of the action of neurotrophins, molecular organisation and signalling at glutamatergic synapses in the hippocampus of adults born from thyroxinemic mothers [44].

A study by Chakraborty et al. [45] on neonatal rats from mothers that were treated prenatally with propylthiouracil (PTU) to induce mild hypothyroidism, detected a significant reduction in the levels of the BDNF in the hippocampus. These findings suggested that mild hypothyroidism during pregnancy could contribute to the adverse neurodevelopmental effects observed in later life by causing reduced levels of BDNF in the hippocampus during early postnatal development.

In a study by Berbel et al. [46], pregnant female rats were thyroidectomised at embryonic day 18 and infused with calcitonin and parathormone until giving birth as a model of late maternal hypothyroidism (LMH). Analysis of LMH pups revealed major disruption of the same hippocampal region as that affected by chemically-induced hypothyroidism [44], as well as disruption of signalling pathways known to be important in neural cell differentiation and learning deficits. The fact that maternal administration of T4 ablated the effects of thyroidectomy suggests that, although foetal thyroid function is up and running by this stage of pregnancy, there is still a dependence on maternal TH for normal brain development in the offspring and that its depletion can have serious developmental consequences.

Effects of Thyroid Hormones on Neural Cell Proliferation and Differentiation

One interpretation of the above findings is that TH plays a key role in the differentiation of specific groups of neural cells. To address this question, a range of studies have been performed on cellular models of neural cell differentiation to determine the role of TH in the morphological development of neurons and glial cells. An early study found that T3 stimulated the outgrowth of neurites from cultured cells of neuronal (N2a neuroblastoma) but not glial (C6 glioma) origin, suggesting that T3 was able to induce neuronal cell differentiation [47]. The presence of elevated levels of the microtubule associated protein MAP 1B on western blots of N2a cell lysates and in axon-like neurites of immunofluorescently stained cell monolayers confirmed that this effect was associated with increased levels of cytoskeletal proteins known to be important in axon development. Interestingly, the levels of other cytoskeletal components such as neurofilament proteins, which are linked to axon stabilisation, have also been shown to be dependent on TH during development [48, 49]. Indeed, regulation of cytoskeletal proteins during peripheral nerve regeneration, which mirrors many of the cytoskeletal events of axon growth during nerve development, was also found to be regulated by T3 [50, 51], supporting the notion that TH plays a key role in the regulation of nerve repair [52].

Enhanced outgrowth of axon-like neurites, which were visualised by indirect immunofluorescence staining with antibodies to the axon-enriched microtubule stabilising protein tau, increased expression of mRNA for the synaptic vesicle protein synaptophysin, and enhanced cell survival were reported in primary cultures of rat cerebellar neurons [53] while enhanced synthesis of synapsin I and synaptogenesis were observed in primary cultures of foetal rat cortical neurons [54, 55]. Garza et al. [56] found increased neurite outgrowth in acetylcholinesterase (AChE) positive cells cultured from rat cerebral hemisphere cultures from 15 day embryos. These morphological changes were associated significant dose dependent stimulation of choline acetyl transferase and AChE activities from 2 to 15 days of treatment, respectively, suggesting T3 mediated stimulation of cholinergic neuron differentiation. TH has also been shown to modulate the outgrowth and arborisation of dendrites by differentiating neurones [57, 58]. Furthermore, developmental TH deficiency leads to disruption in dendrites of Ca^{2+}/calmodulin-dependent protein kinase II and the expression and/or phosphorylation-dependent activity of MAP2 and stathmin, which play opposing roles in the stabilisation and destabilisation of MTs, respectively, and are important in the regulation of dendrite arborisation [59, 60]. Taken together, the above studies provide strong evidence that T3 can regulate the expression of cytoskeletal and other proteins that play critical roles in the maturation of specific groups of neurons in the brain cortex and cerebellum.

It is well established that, as well as neurons, glial cells contain TRs and that T3 can regulate the development of some glial cell types particularly in brain cortex [2, 34, 35, 61–64]. A study using oligodendrocyte progenitor cells derived from neonatal rat brain indicated that T3 participates in the regulation of oligodendrocyte proliferation and differentiation, as well as in the regulation of cell maturation and that the two are not causally linked [64]. Such differences in the responses to T3 are likely to be due to the reported developmental changes in the patterns of expression of TRs [35, 65].

Other studies, using primary cultures of glial cells from developing rat brain, suggested that T3 could induce astroglial differentiation as determined by the outgrowth of neurites and increased levels of glial fibrillary acidic protein (GFAP) [66–68]. Further work showed that T3 induced proliferation in cerebellar astrocytes but stimulated differentiation in cerebral hemisphere derived astrocytes, effects that may be at least partly due to T3-induced synthesis of glial derived neurotrophic factors [69]. Thus, T3 can directly regulate multiple key events in both astrocyte and neuronal cell development. The different responses of astrocytes from these two brain regions may be due to a number of factors including differences between their cellular and tissue environments and variations in the regional and developmental patterns of TR receptor expression [35].

As factors secreted by glial cells can exert trophic effects on neuronal cells, it is interesting to note that conditioned medium derived from primary cultures of T3-treated cerebellar astrocytes stimulates proliferation of cultured cerebellar neurons, particularly when the two cell types were grown in co-culture, an effect that involves altered extracellular matrix deposition and activation of the EGF receptor-protein kinase A signalling pathway [70, 71]. Thus, as well as having a direct effect on neuronal cells, T3 can mediate neuronal development indirectly through its influence on glial cell activities.

The above mentioned studies suggest that THs regulate important developmental changes in neural cells at least in part by regulating the synthesis and/or distribution of cytoskeletal proteins. This notion is further supported by the observation of rapid T3-stimulated tubulin and/or actin synthesis in cultured brain explants from late foetal and neonatal rat brain, in primary cultures of neurons and glial cells from neonatal rat brain and fetal human brain [72–74]. It has also been shown that T3 regulates the expression of immature (early) and mature (late) tau isoforms during rat brain development [75]. The fact that T3 deprivation in development was shown to down-regulate the synthesis of proteins of the neuronal axon stabilising IF proteins α-internexin and neurofilament light chain (in addition to the GFAP in astrocytes) shows that the activities of all 3 cytoskeletal networks are under the influence of TH [48, 49]. Given the well-established importance of the cytoskeleton in neural form and function, it is clear that a range of genes encoding cytoskeletal proteins are modulated by TH and that such regulation plays a central role in neural development and function.

While the classical interpretation of the effects of THs on mammalian brain development has been that they are largely due to the interaction of T3 with nuclear receptors, not all genes modulated by thyroid hormone contain TR-responsive elements, suggesting that many are indirectly regulated by TH at the post-transcriptional level. Indeed, in terms of cytoskeletal genes, the up-regulation of tubulin synthesis was suggested to be post-transcriptionally controlled via an effect on mRNA stability whereas the regulation of actin was thought to be at the level of transcription [72–74, 76, 77]. T3 was also shown to regulate the process of differential splicing of tau isoforms that enables the replacement of juvenile forms of tau by mature tau variants in post natal rat brain, an effect that is modulated by the RNA binding protein Musashi-1 [75, 78]. It has also been found that the regulation of genes for other MAPs linked to dendrite outgrowth is not under the direct control of TH but involves specific transcription factors or such as RORα and basic transcription element-binding protein [57, 58, 79]. Furthermore, the stability of the mRNA encoded by a number of genes including that of acetylcholinesterase is repressed by T3, indicating that THs are capable of regulating neural gene expression patterns via a range of both direct and indirect mechanisms.

Non-genomic and Mitochondrial Effects of Thyroid Hormones

A number of studies have indicated that THs can exert non-genomic neuroprotective or neurodevelopmental effects on the nervous system via protein interactions at the cell surface [80–82]. For example the state of polymerisation of microfilaments in astrocytes is regulated by thyroid hormone and this, in turn, modulates the TH mediated inactivation of [83, 84]. Thyroxine treatment was found to cause a rapid loss of microfilaments but had no effect on total cellular levels of actin in cultured astrocytes, suggesting a direct influence on the equilibrium between monomer and polymer [83, 84]. The T4 induced depolymerisation of microfilaments was associated with reduced internalisation and hence reduced turnover of type II iodothyronine 5′-deiodinase [83]. The ability to have rapid effects on microfilament dynamics may contribute to the influence of THs on neurite branching, axonal transport and cell-cell contact in developing brain dendrite arborisation. Such a rapid influence may be under the direct or indirect regulation of signalling events shown to be triggered by TH. For example, rapid signalling at the plasma membrane in cultured rat pituitary cells, associated with modulation of the KCNH2 potassium channel by phosphatidylinositol 3-kinase, has been shown to involve the interaction of T3 with TRβ2 in the nucleus via a mechanism that is independent of DNA binding [85]. The activity of mitogen-activated protein kinase, which plays a key role in the regulation of neurite outgrowth, is also up-regulated [86, 87]. Furthermore, protein kinase C is an important

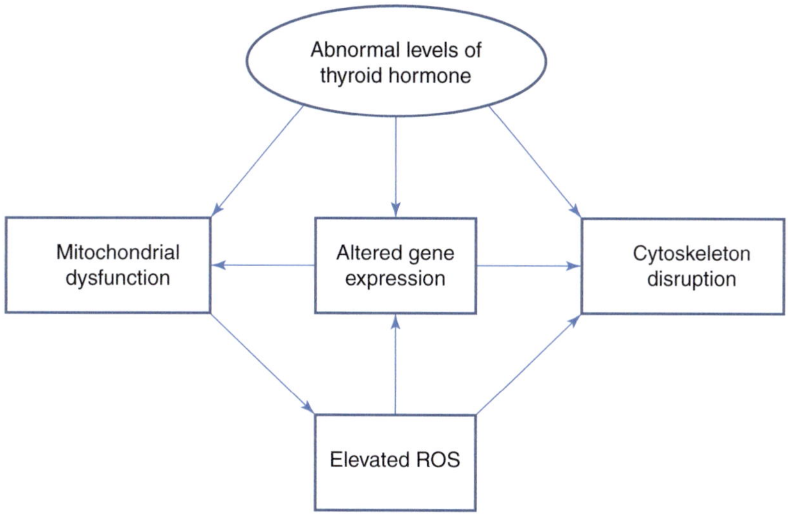

Fig. 4.2 Key events involved in the disruption of cell proliferation and differentiation in thyroid deficient brain. Shown is a schematic representation of key events that contribute to the disruption of neural development as a result of thyroid hormone imbalance. T3 induces direct or indirect changes in gene expression during normal development, leading to coordinated modulation of the levels of many neural proteins and their activities. Disruption of gene expression occurs when the normal levels of hormone are not maintained. If genes encoding mitochondrial proteins are affected, mitochondrial dysfunction ensues, which can lead to energy deficit and elevated levels of reactive oxygen species (*ROS*) causing oxidative stress, and cytoskeletal protein dysfunction. Altered levels of cytoskeletal proteins disrupt microtubule, microfilament and intermediate filament networks that support neural cell proliferation, differentiation and function. Thyroid hormones may also induce direct effects on cytoskeleton proteins forming the microfilaments networks and other cellular events via disruption of cell signalling pathways

modulator of the developmental events triggered by THs; it has been found that production of downstream messengers of this kinase such as diacyl glycerol, which regulates cytoskeletal dynamics, are up-regulated in tissue slices and cultured cells exposed to T4 [88].

Thyroid hormones can also affect mitochondrial activity either by short or long term effects, with higher rates of O_2 consumption in mitochondria from hyperthyroid rats while the converse is found for hypothyroid rats [87, 89]. The mitochondrial antioxidant defence system is severely disrupted in hypothyroid rats and restored on treatment with T3, suggesting that oxidative stress is a major contributor to abnormal development when thyroid levels are sub-optimal [90, 91]. The consequence of elevated levels of reactive oxygen species would be oxidative damage to proteins, lipids and DNA, which could contribute to a range of cytoskeletal effects, such as the neurofilament accumulations, altered gene expression and other activities observed in developing hypothyroid rats [49, 92, 93].

Conclusion

THs play a key role in neural development, abnormal TH levels being associated with a number of neurodevelopmental abnormalities. A schematic representation of key events is illustrated in Fig. 4.2. Disruption of key developmental molecular events by TH deficiency occurs by both genomic and non-genomic pathways and may, for example, be associated with down-regulation of the production of neurotrophins by glial cells. Not all genes exhibiting altered expression patterns are directly affected at the transcriptional level by T3, which can induce changes in gene expression or protein synthesis via other intermediary pathways such as the regulation of RNA stability. A complex combination of changes at the gene and protein levels leads to impaired proliferation and/or differentiation of both neuronal and glial cells in specific brain regions. A major consequence TH deficiency at the protein level is the disruption of the expression levels, distribution and/or dynamics of microtubules, microfilaments and intermediate filaments, all of which play important roles in the development and maintenance of neurites during nerve development and peripheral nerve regeneration. Some of these cytoskeletal changes may be the result of altered gene expression or alternatively may arise as a consequence of impaired mitochondrial function and/or disruption of cell signalling pathways that regulate cytoskeletal proteins of importance in the regulation of neural cell differentiation and function.

References

1. Bernal J. Thyroid hormones and brain development. Vitam Horm. 2005;71:95–122.
2. Bernal J. Thyroid hormone receptors in brain development and function. Nat Clin Prac Endocrinol Metab. 2007;3:249–59.
3. Ahmed OM, El-Gareib AW, El-Bakry AM, El-Tawab SMA, Ahmed RG. Thyroid hormones states and brain development interactions. Int J Dev Neurosci. 2008;26:147–209.
4. Patel J, Landers K, Li H, Mortimer RH, Richard K. Delivery of maternal thyroid hormone to the fetus. Trends Endocrinol Metab. 2011;22:164–70.
5. Patel J, Landers K, Mortimer RH, Richard K. Thyroid hormones and foetal neurological development. J Endocrinol. 2011;209:1–8.
6. Bauer M, Heinz A, Whybrow PC. Thyroid hormones serotonin and mood: of synergy and significance in the adult brain. Mol Psychiatry. 2002;7:140–56.
7. Diez D, Gritoja-Martinez C, Agretti P, De Marco G, Tonacchera M, Pinchera A, Morreale de Escobar G, Bernal J, Morte B. Thyroid hormone action in the adult brain: Gene expression profiling of the effects of single and multiple doses of triiodo-L-thyronine in the rat striatum. Endocrinology. 2008;149:3989–4000.
8. Nussey S, Whitehead S. Endocrinology: an integrated approach. Oxford: BIOS Scientific Publishers; 2001.
9. Zimmermann MB. Iodine deficiency. Endocr Rev. 2009;30:376–408.
10. Bizhanova A, Kopp P. Minireview: the sodium-iodide symporter and pendrin in iodide homeostasis of the thyroid. Endocrinology. 2009;150:1084–90.
11. Fong P. Thyroid iodide efflux: a team effort? J Physiol. 2011;589:5929–39.
12. Twyffels L, Massart C, Goldstein PE, Raspe E, Van Sande J, Dumont JE, Beauwens R, Kruys V. Pendrin: the thryocyte apical membrane iodide transporter? Cell Physiol Biochem. 2011;28:491–6.
13. Pommier J, Deme D, Nunez J. Effect of iodide concentration on thyroxine synthesis catalysed by thyroid peroxidase. Eur J Biochem. 1973;37:406–14.
14. Ruf J, Carayon P. Structural and functional aspects of thyroid peroxidase. Arch Biochem Biophys. 2006;445:269–77.
15. Marinò M, McCluskey RT. Role of thyroglobin endocytic pathways in the control of thyroid hormone release. Am J Physiol Cell Physiol. 2000;279:C1295–306.
16. Chatterjee KK, Lee JK, Rentoumis A, Jameson JL. Negative regulation of the thyroid-stimulating hormone α gene by thyroid hormone: receptor interaction adjacent to the TATA box. Proc Natl Acad Sci U S A. 1989;86:9114–8.
17. Larsson M, Petterson T, Carlström A. Thyroid hormone binding in serum of 15 vertebrate species. Isolation of thyroxine binding globulin and prealbumin analogs. Gen Comp Endocrinol. 1985;58:360–5.
18. McKinnon B, Li H, Richard K, Mortimer R. Synthesis of thyroid binding proteins transthyretin and albumin by human trophoblast. J Clin Endocrinol Metab. 2005;90:6714–20.
19. Kassem NA, Deane R, Segal MB, Preston JE. Role of transthyretin in thyroxine transfer from cerebrospinal fluid to brain and choroid plexus. Am J Physiol Regul Integr Comp Physiol. 2006;291:R1310–5.
20. Wirth EK, Schweizer U, Köhrle J. Transport of thyroid hormone in brain. Front Endocrinol. 2014;5:98.
21. Benvenga S, Cahnmann HJ, Robbins J. Localization of the thyroxine binding sites in apolipoprotein B-100 of human low density lipoproteins. Endocrinology. 1990;127:2241–6.
22. Morreale de Escobar G, Obregon MJ, Escobar del Rey F. Maternal thyroid hormones early in pregnancy and foetal brain development. Best Prac Res Clin Endocrinol Metab. 2004;18:225–48.
23. Landers KA, Li H, Subramaniam VN, Mortimer RH, Richard K. Transerythretin-thyroid hormone internalisation by trophoblasts. Placenta. 2013;34:716–8.
24. Loubière LS, Vasilopoulou E, Bulmer JN, Taylor PM, Steiger B, Verrey F, McCabe CJ, Franklyn JA, Kilby MD, Chan SY. Expression of thyroid hormone transporters in the human placenta and changes associated with intrauterine growth restriction. Placenta. 2010;31:295–304.
25. Larsen PD, DeLallo L. Cerebrospinal fluid transthyretin in the neonate and blood cerebrospinal fluid permeability barrier. Ann Neurol. 1985;25:628–30.
26. Zheng W, Lu YM, Lu GY, Zhao Q, Cheung O, Blaner WS. Transthyretin, thyroxine and retinol-binding protein in human cerebrospinal fluid: Effect of lead exposure. Toxicol Sci. 2001;61:107–14.

27. Wirth E, Roth S, Blechschmidt C, Hölter SM, Becker L, Racz I, Zimmer A, Klopstock T, Gailus-Durner V, Fuchs H, Wurst W, Naumann T, Bräuer A, Hrabé de Angelis M, Köhrle J, Grüters A, Schweizer U. Neuronal 3',3,5-triiodothyronine (T3) uptake and behavioural phenotype of mice deficient in Mct8, the neuronal T3 transporter mutated in Allan-Herndon-Dudley Syndrome. J Neurosci. 2009;29:9439–49.
28. Freisema ECH, Visser TJ, Borgers AJ, Kalsbeek A, Swaab DF, Fliers E, Alkemade A. Thyroid hormone transporters and deiodinases in the developing human hypothalamus. Eur J Endocrinol. 2012;167:379–86.
29. Braun D, Wirth EK, Schweizer U. Thyroid hormone transporters in the brain. Rev Neurosci. 2010;21: 173–86.
30. Verhoelst CH, Roelens SA, Darras VM. Role of spatiotemporal expression of iodothyronine deiodinase proteins in cerebellar cell organisation. Brain Res Bull. 2005;67:196–202.
31. Dentice M, Salvatore D. Deiodinases: the balance of thyroid hormone local impact. Local impact of thyroid hormone inactivation. J Endocrinol. 2011;209: 273–82.
32. Farwell AP, Leonard JL. Identification of a 27 kDa protein with the properties of type II iodothyronine 5'-deiodinase in dibutyryl cAMP-stimulated glial cells. J Biol Chem. 1989;264:20561–7.
33. Guadaño-Ferraz A, Obregón MJ, St Germain DL, Bernal J. The type 2 iodothyronine deiodinase is expressed primarily in glial cells in the neonatal rat brain. Proc Natl Acad Sci U S A. 1997;94:10391–6.
34. Ruel J, Faure R, Dussault JH. Regional distribution of nuclear T3 receptors in rat brain and evidence for preferential localization in neurons. J Endocrinol Invest. 1985;8:343–8.
35. Forrest D, Hallbook F, Persson H, Vennström B. Distinct functions for thyroid hormone receptors α and β in brain development as indicated by differential expression of receptor genes. EMBO J. 1991;10:269–75.
36. Yen PM. Physiological and molecular basis of thyroid hormone action. Physiol Rev. 2001;81:1097–142.
37. Thompson CP, Potter GB. Thyroid hormone action in neural development. Cereb Cortex. 2000;10:939–45.
38. DeLong GR. The neuromuscular system and brain in hypothyroidism. In: Braverman LE, Utiger RD, editors. The thyroid. New York: JP Lippincott; 1996. p. 826–35.
39. Gong J, Liu W, Dong J, Wang Y, Xu H, Wei W, Zhong J, Xi Q, Chen J. Developmental iodine deficiency and hypothyroidism impair neural development in rat hippocampus: Involvement of doublecortin and NCAM-180. BMC Neurosci. 2010;11:50.
40. Glinoer D, Delange F. The potential repercussions of maternal, fetal and neonatal hypothyroxinemia on the progeny. Thyroid. 2000;10:871–87.
41. Vermiglio F, Lo Presti VP, Moleti M, Sidoti M, Tortorella G, Scaffidi G, Castagna MG, Mattina F, Violi MA, Crisa A, Atremisia A, Trimarchi F. Attention deficit and hyperactivity disorders in the offspring of mothers exposed to mild-moderate iodine deficiency: a possible novel iodine deficiency disorder in developed countries. J Clin Endocrinol Metab. 2004;89:6054–60.
42. Kasatkina EP, Samsonova LN, Ivakhnenko VN, Ibragimova GV, Ryabykh AV, Naumenko LL, Evodkimova YA. Gestational hypothyroxinemia and cognitive function in offspring. Neurosci Behav Physiol. 2006;36:619–24.
43. Kooistra L, Crawford S, van Baar AL, Brouwers EP, Pop VJ. (2006) Neonatal effects of maternal hypothyroxinemia during early pregnancy. Pediatrics. 2006;117:161–7.
44. Opazo MC, Gianini A, Pancetti F, Azkcona G, Alarcón L, Lizana R, Noches V, Gonzalez PA, Porto M, Mora S, Rosenthal D, Eugenin E, Naranjo D, Bueno SM, Kalergis AM, Riedel CA. Maternal hypothyroxinemia impairs spatial learning and synaptic nature and function in the offspring. Endocrinology. 2008;149:5097–106.
45. Chakraborty G, Magagna-Poveda A, Parratt C, Umans JG, MacLuskey NJ, Scharfman HE. Reduced hippocampal brain-derived neurotrophic factor (BDNF) in neonatal rats after prenatal exposure to propylthiouracyl (PTU). Endocrinology. 2012;153: 1311–6.
46. Berbel P, Navarro D, Ausó E, Varea E, Rodríguez AE, Ballesta JJ, Salina M, Flores E, Faura CC, Morreale de Escobar G. Role of late maternal thyroid hormones in cerebral cortex development: an experimental model for human prematurity. Cereb Cortex. 2010;20:1462–75.
47. Hargreaves A, Yusta B, Aranda A, Avila J, Pascual A. Triiodothyronine (T3) induces neurite formation and increases synthesis of a protein related to MAP 1B in cultured cells of neuronal origin. Brain Res. 1988;38:141–8.
48. Sampson D, Pickard MR, Sinha AK, Evans IM, Leonard AJ, Ekins RP. Maternal thyroid status regulates the expression of neuronal and astrocytic cytoskeletal proteins in the fetal brain. J Endocrinol. 2000;167:439–45.
49. Rahaman SO, Ghosh S, Mohanakumar KP, Das S, Sarkar PK. Hypothyroidism in the developing rat brain is associated with marked oxidative stress and aberrant intraneuronal accumulation of neurofilaments. Neurosci Res. 2001;40:273–9.
50. Volnesco F, Glauser L, Kraftsik R, Barakat-Walter I. Local administration of thyroid hormones in silicone chamber increases regeneration of transacted rat sciatic nerve. Exp Neurol. 1998;150:69–81.
51. Schenker M, Riederer BM, Kuntzer T, Barakat-Walter I. Thyroid hormones stimulate expression and modification of cytoskeletal protein during rat sciatic nerve regeneration. Brain Res. 2002;957:259–70.
52. Barakat-Walter I. Role of thyroid hormones and their receptors in peripheral nerve regeneration. J Neurobiol. 1999;40:541–59.

53. Salemi G, Ferraro D, Savettieri G. Triiodothyronine accelerates the synthesis of synapsin I in developing neurons from rat brain cultured in a synthetic medium. Neurochem Res. 1990;15:827–31.
54. Heisenberg CP, Thoenen H, Lindholm D. Triiodothyronine regulates survival and differentiation of rat cerebellar granule neurons. Neuroreport. 1992;3:685–8.
55. Hosoda R, Nakayama K, Kato-Negishi M, Kawahara M, Muramoto K, Kuroda Y. Thyroid hormone enhances the formation of synapses between cultured neurons of rat cerebral cortex. Cell Mol Neurobiol. 2003;23:895–906.
56. Garza R, Dussault JH, Puymirat J. Influence of triiodothyronine (L-T3) on the morphological and biochemical development of fetal brain acetylcholinesterase-positive neurons cultured in a chemically defined medium. Brain Res. 1988;43:287–97.
57. Cayrou C, Denver RJ, Puymirat J. Suppression of the basic transcription element-binding protein in brain neuronal cultures inhibits thyroid hormone induced neurite branching. Endocinology. 2002;143:2242–9.
58. Boukhtouche F, Brugg B, Wehrlé R, Bois-Joyeux B, Danan JL, Dusart I, Mariani J. Induction of early Purkinje cell dendritic differentiation by thyroid hormone requires RORα. Neural Dev. 2010;5:18.
59. Ohkawa N, Fujitani K, Tokunaga E, Furuya S, Inokuchi K. The microtubule destabilizer stathmin mediates the development of dendritic arbors in neuronal cells. J Cell Sci. 2007;120:1447–56.
60. Wang Y, Wang Y, Dong J, Wei W, Song B, Min H, Teng W, Chen J. Developmental hypothyroxinaemia and hypothyroidism limit dendritic growth of cerebellar Purkinje cells in rat offspring: involvement of microtubule-associated protein 2 (MAP2) and stathmin. Neuropathol Appl Neurobiol. 2014;40:398–415.
61. Ortiz-Caro J, Yusta B, Montiel F, Villa A, Aranda A, Pascual A. Identification and characterization of L-triiodothyronine receptors in cells of glial and neuronal origin. Endocrinology. 1986;119:2163–7.
62. Luo M, Puymirat J, Dussault JH. Immunocytochemical localization of nuclear 3,5,3'-triiodothyronine ($_{L}$-T3) receptors in astrocyte cultures. Brain Res. 1989;46:131–6.
63. Hubank M, Sinha AK, Gullo D, Ekins RP. Nuclear triiodothyronine (T3) binding in neonatal rat brain suggests a direct glial requirement for T3 during development. J Endocrinol. 1990;126:409–15.
64. Baas D, Bourbeau D, Sarliève LL, Ittel ME, Dussault JH, Puymirat J. Oligodendrocyte maturation and progenitor cell proliferation are independently regulated by thyroid hormone. Glia. 1997;19:324–32.
65. Carré JL, Demerens C, Rodríguez-Peña A, Floch HH, Vincendron G, Sarliève LL. Thyroid hormone receptor isoforms are sequentially expressed in oligodendrocyte lineage cells during rat cerebral development. J Neurosci Res. 1998;54:584–94.
66. Trentin AG, Moura Neto V. T3 affects astrocyte proliferation, GFAP and fibronectin organization. Neuroreport. 1995;6:293–6.
67. Paul S, Das S, Poddar R, Sarkar PK. Role of thyroid hormone in the morphological differentiation and maturation of astrocytes: temporal correlation with synthesis and organisation of actin. Eur J Neurosci. 1996;8:2361–70.
68. Lima FRS, Trentin AG, Rosenthal D, Chaga C, Moura Neto V. Thyroid hormone induces protein secretion and morphological changes in astroglial cells with an increase in expression of glial fibrillary acidic protein. J Endocrinol. 1997;154:167–75.
69. Trentin AG, Rosenthal D, Moura Neto V. Thyroid hormone and conditioned medium effects on astroglial cells from hypothyroid and normal rat brain: factor secretion, cell differentiation and proliferation. J Neurosci Res. 1995;41:409–17.
70. Trentin AG, Nedel Mendes de Aguiar CB, Castilho Garcez R, Alvarez-Silva M. Thyroid hormone modulates the extracellular matrix organization and expression in cerebellar astrocytes: Effects on astrocyte adhesion. Glia. 2003;42:359–69.
71. Martinez R, Carvalho Alcantara Gomes F. Proliferation of cerebellar neurons induced by astrocytes treated with thyroid hormone is mediated by a co-operation between cell contact and soluble factors and involves the epidermal growth factor-protein kinase A pathway. J Neurosci Res. 2005;80:341–9.
72. Chaudhury S, Sarkar PK. Stimulation of tubulin synthesis by thyroid hormone in the developing rat brain. Biochim Biophys Acta. 1983;763:93–8.
73. De A, Chaudhury S, Sarkar PK. Thyroidal stimulation of tubulin and actin in primary cultures of neuronal and glial cells of rat brain. Int J Dev Neurosci. 1991;9:381–90.
74. Pal U, Biswas SC, Sarkar PK. Regulation of actin and its mRNA by thyroid hormones in cultures of fetal human brain during second trimester of gestation. J Neurochem. 2002;69:1170–6.
75. Aniello F, Couchie D, Bridoux AM, Gripois D, Nunez J. Splicing of juvenile and adult tau mRNA variants is regulated by thyroid hormone. Proc Natl Acad Sci U S A. 1991;88:4035–9.
76. Poddar R, Paul S, Chaudhury S, Sarkar PK. Regulation of actin and tubulin gene expression by thyroid hormone during rat brain development. Mol Brain Res. 1996;35:111–8.
77. Lorenzo PI, Ménard C, Miller FD, Bernal J. Thyroid hormone-dependent regulation of Tα1 α-tubulin during brain development. Mol Cell Neurosci. 2002;19:333–43.
78. Cuadrado A, García-Fernández LF, Imai T, Okano H, Muñoz A. Regulation of tau RNA maturation by thyroid hormone is mediated by the neural RNA-binding protein Musashi-1. Mol Cell Neurosci. 2002;20:198–210.

79. Cuadrado A, Navarro-Yubero C, Furneaux H, Muñoz A. Neuronal HuD gene encoding a mRNA stability regulator is transcriptionally repressed by thyroid hormone. J Neurochem. 2003;86:763–73.
80. Davis PJ, Davis FB. Nongenomic actions of thyroid hormone. Thyroid. 1996;6:497–594.
81. Davis PJ, Davis FB, Lin HY. L-thyroxine acts as a hormone as well as a prohormone at the cell membrane. Immunol Endocr Metab Agents Med Chem. 2006;6:2235–40.
82. Lin HY, Davis FB, Luidens MK, Mousa SA, Cao JH, Zhou M, Davis PJ. Molecular basis for certain neuroprotective effects of thyroid hormone. Front Mol Neurosci. 2011;4:29.
83. Farwell AP, Lynch RM, Okulicz WC, Comi AM, Leonard JL. The actin cytoskeleton mediates the hormonally regulated translocation of type II iodothyronine 5'-deiodinase in astrocytes. J Biol Chem. 1990;265:18546–53.
84. Siegrist-Kaiser CA, Juge-Aubry C, Tranter MP, Ekenbarger DM, Leonard JL. Thyroxine dependent modulation of actin polymerisation in cultured astrocytes. J Biol Chem. 1990;265:5296–302.
85. Storey NM, Gentile S, Ullah H, Russo A, Muessel M, Erxleben C, Armstrong DL. Rapid signalling at the plasma membrane by a nuclear receptor for thyroid hormone. Proc Natl Acad Sci U S A. 2006;103:5197–201.
86. Lin HY, Davis FB, Gordinier JK, Martino LJ, Davis PJ. Thyroid hormone induces activation of mitogen-activated protein kinase in cultured cells. Am J Physiol. 1999;276:1014–24.
87. Bassett JHD, Harvey CB, Williams GR. Mechanisms of thyroid hormone receptor-specific nuclear and extra nuclear actions. Mol Cell Endocrinol. 2003;213:1–11.
88. Kavok NS, Krasilnikova OA, Babenko NA. Thyroxine signal transduction in liver cells involves phospholipase C and phospholipase D activation. Genomic independent action of thyroid hormone. BMC Cell Biol. 2001;2:5.
89. Wrutniak-Cabello C, Casas F, Cabello G. Thyroid hormone action in mitocondria. J Mol Endocrinol. 2001;26:67–77.
90. Das K, Chainy GBN. Modulation of rat liver mitochondrial antioxidant defence system by thyroid hormone. Biochim Biophys Acta. 2003;1537:1–13.
91. Messarah M, Boumendgel A, Chouabia A, Klibet F, Abdennour C, Boulakoud MS, El Feki A. Influence of thyroid dysfunction on liver lipid peroxidation and antioxidant status in experimental rats. Exp Toxicol Pathol. 2010;62:301–10.
92. Ghosh S, Rahaman SO, Sarkar PK. Regulation of neurofilament gene expression by thyroid hormone in the developing rat brain. Neuroreport. 1999;10:2361–5.
93. Brent GA. Mechanism of thyroid hormone action. J Clin Invest. 2012;122:3035–43.

Autoimmune Thyroid Disease (Flajani-Parry-Graves-von Basedow Disease): Etiopathogenesis, Clinical Manifestations and Diagnosis

5

Hernando Vargas-Uricoechea, Anilza Bonelo-Perdomo, Carlos Hernán Sierra-Torres, and Ivonne Meza-Cabrera

Abstract

Autoimmune thyroid disease is the most common organ-specific autoimmune disorder affecting 2–5 % of the population in Western countries. Graves-Basedow disease is the most frequent form of hyperthyroidism in iodine sufficient countries; while the exact etiology of thyroid autoimmunity is not known, interaction between genetic susceptibility and environmental factors appears to be of fundamental importance to initiate the process of thyroid autoimmunity. The identified autoimmune thyroid disease susceptibility genes include immune-modulating genes, such as the Major Histocompatibility Complex, Cytotoxic T Lymphocyte Antigen-4, CD40 molecule, Protein Tyrosine Phosphatase-22, TSH receptor and Thyroglobulin. The exact nature of the role environmental factors play in Graves-Basedow disease is still not well known, but the involvement of several factors such as: iodine diet, drugs, stress, and infections has been reported. In Graves-Basedow disease the lymphocytic infiltration of the thyroid leads to activation of TSH Receptor (TSHR)-reactive B-cells that secrete TSHR stimulating antibodies causing hyperthyroidism. These antibodies bind to TSH receptors on the surface of thyroid follicular cells, leading to continuous and uncontrolled thyroid stimulation, associated with excess synthesis of the thyroid hormones T4 and T3, and thyroid

H. Vargas-Uricoechea, MD, MSc, Ph.Dc (✉)
Division of Endocrinology and Metabolism, Internal Medicine Department, University of Cauca, Popayán-Cauca, Colombia
e-mail: hernandovargasu10@yahoo.com

A. Bonelo-Perdomo, BSc, MSc, Ph.D
Division of Basic Immunology and Biomedical Sciences, University of Valle, Cali-Valle, Colombia

C.H. Sierra-Torres, Ph.D
Division of Genetic and Molecular Epidemiology, University of Cauca, Popayán-Cauca, Colombia

I. Meza-Cabrera, MD
Laboratory of Pathology, Hospital Universitario San José, Popayán-Cauca, Colombia

S.K. Imam, S.I. Ahmad (eds.), *Thyroid Disorders: Basic Science and Clinical Practice*,
DOI 10.1007/978-3-319-25871-3_5

hypertrophy. Graves-Basedow disease includes thyrotoxicosis, goiter, exophthalmos, and pretibial myxedema when fully expressed, but can occur with one or more of these features.

Introduction

Graves-Basedow Disease (GD) affects approximately 0.5 % of the population and is the underlying cause of 50–80 % of the total number of cases of hyperthyroidism. The disease originates from the presence of circulating IgG antibodies that come together and activate the Thyrotropin (TSH) G-protein coupled receptor. Such activation leads to follicular hyperplasia and hypertrophy that in the long run is clinically translated into goiter, with increased production of the final elements of thyroid metabolism –Triiodothyronine (T3) and Thyroxin (T4)- The clinical spectrum of the disease is broad and although the triad of exophthalmos, goiter and dermopathy has traditionally defined GD, a considerable number of patients may express isolated symptoms and signs (tachycardia, diarrhea and unexplained weight loss). Biochemically, GD is expressed with suppressed TSH levels and usually elevated levels of T3 and T4 in the context of classic primary hyperthyroidism, or may be expressed with suppressed TSH and normal T3 and T4 (as part of subclinical hyperthyroidism). Thyroid ophthalmopathy in GD is evidenced in 30–50 % of the patients and its frequency is higher when intentionally screened for using specific orbital images, whereby ophthalmopathy is detected in up to 80 % of the patients. Thyroid Dermopathy (TD) is a rare extra-thyroid manifestation of the disease that consists in a localized thickening of the skin, usually in the pretibial area; it is often called "pretibial myxedema", though other sites may be involved. The treatment of the disease is based on three main aspects: thionamide management, radioactive iodine therapy (I-131), and surgery.

Background and History

The oldest bibliographical reference known about this condition dates back to Egyptian culture. The Ebers papyrus written around 1550 B.C. –a 22 lines and 108 columns manuscript- described what is currently termed goiter (from the Latin word *Guttur:* throat) or Struma (from the Latin word *Struma:* a term used to describe the inflammation of the "neck gland"). The manuscript even recommended surgical excision as potential treatment, or the intake of some particular salts from a specific place in Lower Egypt.

Ibn Sina, also called Abu Ali al-Husayn ibn Abd Allah ibn Sina (980–1037) was a Persian philosopher physician and scientist, commonly referred to in the Western world as "Avicenna", is accepted and acknowledged as the father of modern medicine. Some of his extensive literary work includes "The book of healing" and "The Canon of Medicine", also known as the "Canon of Avicenna". The latter, his most famous book, describes in great detail exophthalmos and goiter, symptoms that today we accept as evidence of thyroid hyperactivity. Another historical document describing the disease was the work by André Du Laurens [Laurentius] (1558–1609) entitled: "De Mirabili Strumas Sanadi" published in Paris in 1609, followed by other works during the XVII and XVIII Centuries and the first quarter of the nineteenth Century, until the Italians Giuseppe Flajani in 1802 and Antonio Giuseppe Testa in 1810 described patients with palpitations, apprehension, tremor, nervousness, and psychotic disorders [1, 2]. In 1825, Caleb Hillier Parry wrote what is considered the most comprehensive review on exophthalmic goiter. About 10 years later, Robert James Graves published what according to many people is the first accurate description of the disease, and in 1840 Carl Adolph von Basedow published an extensive article about the results of his research about treatment approaches [3–5]. Although von Basedow described many of the key characteristics we currently know, his publication took place 5 years after Robert Graves's description, despite he had followed his patients' evolution for several years. The transcendental importance of the last three authors above mentioned, had established that exophthalmic goiter was indistinctively identified as Parry, Graves or von Basedow disease. Though it is well known that in English-speaking countries the term Graves Disease is commonly used, in most European countries the condition is referred to as von Basedow's disease. In Germany for instance, the description of the clinical characteristics of the disease is attributed to von Basedow; so much so, that the description of the so called Merseburg's triad –exophthalmos, goiter, and tachycardia, similar to the triad described by Robert Graves is attributed to von Basedow- [5, 6]. Currently there is little controversy about the fact that Parry was the first to describe the disease, though historically modestly acknowledged. According to some of Robert Graves's biographers, this could be due to the fact that Graves very astutely hired the services of Armand Trousseau, a very influential advertiser in France at that time, in addition to the fact that he was the head of Medicine at the Hotel-Dieu hospital in Paris. Trousseau was a strong admirer of Graves, and often quoted his work in his clinical lectures and in his multiple publications. When Grave's book was translated into French, Trousseau praised the author and in fact, used the term Graves-Basedow Disease for the first time. It should also be noted that most publications about this condition are in English, thus perpetuating the term "Graves' Disease". However, the autoimmune hyperthyroid diffuse goiter should in all fairness, and from the historical and descriptive point of view, be called *"Flajani-Parry-Graves-von Basedow Disease"*. Other names used in the medical literature to describe GD are March disease, Parsons disease, Flajani disease and Begbie disease [6, 7].

Epidemiology

According to the National Health Institutes (NIH) of the United States of America, autoimmune diseases affect approximately 23.5 million people in the country, although the American Autoimmune Related Disease Association (AARDA) estimates that there are about 50 million people affected by the disease, of which 75 % are women. It is currently stated that there are about 100 types of autoimmune diseases identified, affecting a larger population than the number affected by cancer and heart disease. The numerical differences based on the figures identified by the various associations responsible for studying autoimmune diseases are due to definitions adopted for each particular disease; for instance, the NIH only involve 24 autoimmune diseases (based on trials with specific epidemiological designs); it has been estimated however, that the number of diseases with some autoimmune background is close to 150. Autoimmune diseases have a variable rate of presentation and ethnic and geographical differences have been documented to impact the incidence of particular autoimmune diseases. Some specific groups may be at higher risk than others for certain diseases with even some variation among the same populations. Autoimmune disease is highly prevalent in the pediatric population and adolescents (representing one of the ten most frequent causes of death among children 1–14 years old). Likewise, autoimmune disease is one of the ten most important causes of death among women over 65 years of age, and is the fifth cause of death among women less than 65. The incidence and prevalence of autoimmune diseases has been rising in the last two decades worldwide, with diseases such as Diabetes Mellitus Type 1 (DM1), Celiac Disease (CD), Multiple Sclerosis (MS) and Systemic Lupus Erythematous (SLE) being some of the most frequent. Such a rapid rise in frequency strongly suggests that environmental factors play a key role in such increase, since genes do not change so fast, in such short periods of time. The frequency of autoimmune asymptomatic thyroid syndrome indicates an association between the levels of thyroid autoantibodies [Thyroid Peroxidase (TPO) Autoantibodies and anti-Thyroglobulin (Tg) Autoantibodies] and the presence of focal thyroid inflammation in biopsy specimens and biopsies of individuals that never showed any evidence of hypothyroidism in their life. Post-mortem analyses show histopathological evidence of autoimmune thyroiditis in over one fourth of adult women; diffuse changes were identified in 5 % of females and in 1 % of males;

furthermore, the prevalence of thyroid antibodies among the healthy population ranges between 10 and 12 %. With regards to hypothyroidism, its frequency may vary depending on whether the diagnosis is considered as subclinical or overt hypothyroidism. The former shows a TSH value above the upper reference limit, with a normal Free T4 (FT4) level (assuming that the hypothalamic-pituitary-thyroid axis is normal, and in the absence of current or recent severe critical disease). The variation in prevalence of subclinical hypothyroidism is consistent with the TSH values; for instance, The National Health and Nutrition Examination Survey (NHANES III) used an upper normal TSH level above 4.5 mIU/L; at this cut point, the prevalence of subclinical hypothyroidism was 4.3 % and the prevalence of overt hypothyroidism was 0.3 %. The Colorado thyroid disease prevalence survey used an upper normal TSH level of 5.0 mIU/L, and a prevalence of 8.5 % was reported for subclinical hypothyroidism while the reported prevalence for overt hypothyroidism was 0.4 %. In the Framingham trial, 5.9 % of females and 2.3 % of males over 60 years of age had TSH values over 10 mIU/L, while in the British Whickham survey, 9.3 % of females and 1.2 % of males had TSH values exceeding 10 mIU/L. The frequency of hypothyroidism in people 85–89 years old in the Netherlands was 7 % among 558 people evaluated. Furthermore, the incidence of hypothyroidism in females is established at 3.5 per 1000 individuals per year, and in males at 0.6 per 1000 individuals per year. The risk to develop hypothyroidism in females with positive thyroid Autoantibodies and elevated TSH is 4 % per year, in contrast with those women that only have one of the two conditions with a risk of 2–3 % per year. For males the risk is higher in either condition, but the rate of development of overt hypothyroidism is still lower than the rate for women. According to the 20-year follow-up Whickham cohort, the annual average incidence of spontaneous hypothyroidism (in the 20 years of follow-up), was 3.5 per 1000 in females, and of 0.6 per 1000 in males; the presence of elevated TSH and/or positive thyroid antibodies was associated with an increase risk of developing hypothyroidism. In females, the annual risk of spontaneous overt hypothyroidism was 4 % (in women with elevated TSH and positive thyroid antibodies); 3 % if only the TSH was elevated and 2 % when only the thyroid antibodies were positive. The likelihood of developing hypothyroidism was higher in women with TSH >2.0 mIU/L and elevated anti-TPO values [8–10].

Although GD may present at any age, the incidence peak is found between the fifth and the seventh decade of life; the female:male ratio is 5–10:1. The incidence of the disease varies depending on the series reviewed, the geographical area studied, the intake of dietary iodine and gender. Most series report an incidence rate from 15 to 50 per 100,000 people/year of follow-up; however, trials based on the British population report an incidence rate of 80 per 100,000 women/year and of 10 per 100,000 males/year. The prevalence of the disease among the general population is of 0.5–1.0 %. The National Health and Nutrition Survey (NHANES III) showed that in individuals older than 12, the general prevalence of hypothyroidism was 1.3 %, with a lower prevalence in Hispanics (0.7 %) and a higher prevalence among whites (1.4 %). In "The Nurses' Health Study" the overall incidence of GD hypothyroidism was 4.6 per 1000 women in 12 years of follow-up. There are limited comparative incidence data for males. In the "Rochester Epidemiology Project" trial, the age-adjusted incidence of ophthalmopathy due to GD was 5 times higher in white females than in males –16 per 100,000 patients/year and 2.9 per 100,000 patients/year, respectively- In a cohort trial in Stockholm between 2003 and 2005, the total incidence of hypothyroidism among the population over 18 years of age was 32.7/100,000 patients/year, of which 75 % had GD [10, 11]. Changes in incidence may reflect improved diagnostic methods, rather than an actual change in the incidence rates. The higher iodine intake has been considered a factor that impacts the incidence of GD among the population in places such as Japan, where the dietary iodine intake may be much higher than in most other countries, with an incidence of 200 per 100,000. Moreover, dietary iodine supplementation in mild to moderately deficient populations may increase the number of GD cases. Moreover, it has been shown that in some areas with some iodine deficiency, supplementation is associated with a drop in up to 33 % in the incidence of GD [12].

Genetics and Etiopathogenesis

GD is defined as an antibody-mediated autoimmune process that affects the thyroid gland and the extra-thyroid tissues in about 90 % of the cases. The production of Autoantibodies targeted against the TSH receptor (anti-TSHR) leads to excessive synthesis of thyroid hormones; however, the underlying inflammation and remodeling mechanisms in the extra-thyroid tissues are still ambiguous. Family occurrence of autoimmune thyroid disorders are frequently identified in GD patients; for instance, in individuals with GD ophthalmopathy 36 % have a first or second degree relative affected either with GD or another Autoimmune Thyroid Disease (AITD). While in monogenic diseases Monozygotic (MZ) twins show complete concordance, in complex inherited disorders the concordance is incomplete, but is comparatively higher in Dizygotic twins (DZ). Cohort studies in twins have identified a concordance rate of 0.36 and 0.03 for MZ and DZ respectively; moreover, the analysis of these data shows that 79 % of the predisposition to develop GD is attributable to genetics, while the specific individual environmental factors that are not shared by the twins may account for the remaining 21 % [13]. The estimated concordance for GD may be different for the populations studied; for example, la concordance for American twins is 0.17–0.02 in MZ and DZ siblings, respectively, suggesting a small contribution of genes for GD in the American population versus Europeans. Studies in families and twins have clearly shown that GD is not the result of a single gene defect, but rather that it has a complex inheritance pattern; consequently, the predisposition results from multiple genes with individual and very modest effects. Most of the loci identified represent a low risk of disease (between 1.2 and 1.5).

From the genetic perspective, the studies are aimed at identifying an association between two or more genetic polymorphisms and a characteristic genetic trait. Association studies differ from binding trials where the same allele (or alleles) are associated with that trait in a similar manner to the population as a whole; in contrast, binding studies allow for different alleles to be associated with that trait in different families. These associated studies may be done among unrelated patients (cases) and healthy controls to identify markers that significantly differ between the two groups or in family groups usually comprised of a sick individual and his/her parents. The association analysis is a very sensitive method to identify weak genetic risk factors and is currently the preferred method to study diseases with this type of pattern. Association analyses are based on a comparison between a group of patients with a particular outcome and ethnical "matched" controls; if a statistically significant difference in the frequency of a variable is observed between the cases and the controls, the conclusion is that such variable is associated with the disease or the outcome [14–16]. The most frequent type of genetic variability in humans occurs at specific sites in the genome where individual nucleotide variations develop from one member of the population to another. These sites are called Single Nucleotide Polymorphisms (SNPs). Most SNPs exist as alternate alleles; i.e., A or G; in average, two randomly selected human genomes have approximately three million differences in individual nucleotides between them; in other words, one per one thousand base pairs. Generally speaking, the SNPs are single nucleotide mutations giving rise to changes in one amino acid in the protein – the frequency of the minor allele shall be more than 1 % of the population- [17]. The identification of complex disease genes involves four phases: ***Phase 1:*** Analysis of candidate genes; ***Phase 2:*** Genome-wide association studies; ***Phase 3:*** Extended genome association studies; and ***Phase 4:*** Whole genome sequencing.

The implementation of these technologies has led to further developments in this area, identifying at least seven genes whose variants have been associated with AITD, including: HLA-DR gene, immunoregulatory genes (CTLA-4, CD 40, PTPN-22 y CD 25) and thyroid-specific genes: Tg gene and TSHR gene [16–18].

***HLA-DR* Gene** The available evidence suggests that the HLA (6p21) region predisposes to AITD; the alleles within the HLA class II region (genes *DRB1* and *DQA1* are the ones with the strongest association to GD). An important association has also been identified in the HLA Class I region, *HLA-C* and *HLA-B*. GD Caucasian patients have an increased prevalence of the *DRB1**03 *DQA1**05 and *DQB1**02 haplotype, though these are not always present in other ethnic groups. In fact, it has been found that the HLA-*DPB1**05:01 is the major gene that predisposes to GD among the Asian population, in a sub-population of Chinese patients with an OR = 2.3 and a population attributable risk of 48 %. Other susceptibility variables with independent effects include the *B**46:01, *DRB1**15:02 and 16:02, whilst *DRB1**12:02 and *DQB1**03:02 are protective. Arginine in the position 74 of the HLA-DRb1 (Deb-Arg74) has been recently identified as the critical DR amino acid that causes GD susceptibility. Furthermore, the presence of the glutamine amino acid at the position 74 of the DRb1 chain is protective against GD [15, 18].

CTLA-4 (Cytotoxic T Lymphocyte Antigen-4) The CTLA-4 attenuates T-cell activity. Its structural resemblance to CD28, both in terms of the chromosomal localization as in terms of the exon-intron organization, suggests that both genes share the same origin. CD28 is a 44 KD membrane glycoprotein with a 202 amino acid sequence, whose gene is localized in the long arm of chromosome 2. It is the principal co-stimulating molecule in the activation of T cells, where it plays a broad range of roles. One of the most important effects identified is the dramatic increase in the production of IL-2, 4, 5 & 13, in addition to other cytokines such as TNFα-, inter alia. These cytokines act as growth factors, with an autocrine and paracrine action, in addition to reducing the T-cell response threshold and preventing apoptosis. CTLA-4 is expressed in activated T-cells, CD4 and CD8, at levels 10 and 100 times lower than those of CD28, but binds to CD80 and CD86 with a dissociation constant 20–50 times higher. Although a similar role was initially attributed to CD28 in the activation of T-cells, the most recent experimental findings indicate that CTLA-4 has a negative regulatory action. Some trials have established that CTLA-4 is a GD-susceptible gene; in the Chinese population, for instance, the A49G and CT60 polymorphisms are associated with increased susceptibility for GD. The Odds Ratio (OR) for A49G was 1.49, whilst for CT60 was 1.45 [18, 19].

CD 40 Among the identified susceptibility genes in Graves' Disease, CD40 is the only one involved with regulating the B cells response; the physiological ligand for CD40 is the CD154 (CD40L) molecule, that is expressed on the surface of the T helper cells. Binding of CD40 by CD40L helps to drive the resting B cell from G_0 into the cell cycle, playing an essential role in the activation and proliferation of B-lymphocytes. The CD40 gene has been associated with GD and a plausible explanation is the a C allele may induce an overexpression of the CD40 molecule, leading to the activation of B-lymphocytes with a prevalence of the Th2-type immune response. Bases on extended genome studies, CD40 is one of the candidates for GE. These studies have involved the 20q11 chromosome region – called GD-2 – as a susceptibility locus. The C allele in the rs 1883832 has been found to generate an OR = 1.6 for Graves' Disease among Caucasians, though the same association has been identified among the Japanese population [19, 20].

The PTPN22 Gene (Protein Tyrosine Phosphatase Nonreceptor-22) PTPN22 is involved in the antigen adaptive response via the dephosphorylation and inactivation of the T-cells receptor. The PTPN22 gene has been associated with the presence of AITD and other autoimmune diseases; it is localized at the 1p13 chromosome and codes for the so-called signaling protein Lymphoid Tyrosine Phosphatase (PTP), which is a potent t-cell activation regulator. This protein inhibits T-cell activation through binding to signal transduction molecules such as Csk kinase that mediates T-cell activation. The best association documented of the PTPN22 variants with autoimmune diseases, including GD is with rs2476601 (C1858T). This polymorphism has been studied and considered as a candidate susceptibility gene for AITD in several ethnic groups (particularly Caucasians). The PTPN22 C1858T polymorphism triggers a change in the 620 position from an Arginine to Tryptophan, resulting in a less efficient binding to Csk kinase. Hence, T-cells express T alleles that may be hypersensitive and lead to autoimmune disorders. However, the association of these polymorphisms with increased susceptibility in AITD has been variable, with both negative and positive associations due in part to the genetic heterogeneity among the populations studied and to other potential confounders [19, 20].

Interleukin-2 Receptor α Gene (IL-2RA) This gene codes for the α chain of the IL-2 receptor (IL-2R) complex, also known as CD25, which plays a key immunoregulatory role as an important auto-tolerance and immunity modulator. The IL-2RA gene has been associated with Graves' disease [15, 19].

Thyroglobulin (Tg) Tg represents one of the major auto-antigens involved in AITD; however, the anti-Tg are not specific and occur in 80–90 % of the patients with Hashimoto's disease and in 50–70 % of the patients with Graves' disease (usually at low concentrations). The association of Tg polymorphisms with GD has been identified with relapse of the disease following antithyroid treatment; nonetheless, these conclusions are based on studies with a small sample size that have not been homogenously replicated [14, 18].

Fc Receptor-Like Gene (FCRL) This gene codes for products that play a key role in the control of B cell signals and it has been shown to be associated with autoimmune diseases. The FCRL3 is one of the five genes preferentially expressed in B-lymphocytes and are structurally similar to the Fc receptors. The FCRL3 plays an inhibitory role in the B cells signaling process, resulting in B-cells disrupted tolerance and activity. The association of SNP rs7528684 was replicated in Japanese subjects with GD and Systemic Lupus Erythematosus (SLE). The 1p21-23 cytoband in which the FCRL resides has been identified as a candidate locus for several autoimmune disorders with a strong association identified for SNPs in that region, and increased susceptibility to GD in the Japanese population. This suggests that the origin of the association is a regulatory SNP in the FCRL3 promoter region. The rs7522061 SNP in the FCRL3 gene has also been associated with AITD in Caucasians, and more recently the SNP rs3761959 and the rs7522061 has also been associated with GD [13, 19, 20].

TSH Receptor (TSHR) TSHR and its ligand -TSH- are critical thyroid activity regulators. The TSHR stimulating antibodies simulate the TSH action, resulting in the characteristic hyperthyroid status. The TSHR is considered to exacerbate the autoimmune process, as a key component for the onset of GD. The TSHR is made up of 10 exons that code for 764 amino acids of approximately 95 kDa. The genetic variants of the TSHR probably stimulate autoimmunity in GD, particularly in individuals that exhibit other loci or general autoimmune risk; it is then possible for the TSHR genetic variants to influence the post-translational changes in the TSHR and/or the gene expression, thus increasing the risk for the TSHR to be an immune target; anti-TSHR can be found in 95–96 % of GD patients [15, 18].

GD has a strong genetic component, and hence is influenced by family history. The interaction between genetic susceptibility and environmental factors is extremely complex and poorly understood. Many of the genes associated with the onset of the disease are involved in other autoimmune diseases, including Type 1 Diabetes Mellitus, Rheumatoid Arthritis, and Multiple Sclerosis. This apparent genetic susceptibility convergence raises the risk for autoimmunity and when combined with specific risk factors triggers autoimmune diseases [21]. Several factors have been suggested to increase the risk of developing GD, including gender (the disease is more frequent in females than in males), prior infections

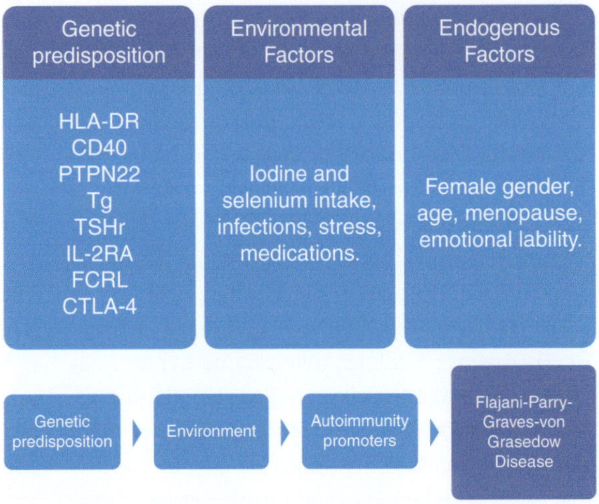

Fig. 5.1 Etiopathogenic considerations about GD. Genetic predisposition, together with environmental and endogenous factors trigger a cascade of events, with an increased expression of autoimmunity promotors, resulting in GD

due to germs such as *Yersinia enterocolítica*, *Yersinia pseudotuberculosis* and *Mycoplasma arthritidis,* iter alia. The way in which these infectious agents may trigger a specific auto-antigenic response is controversial, though a large number of mechanisms may be argued. One of these mechanisms is the induction of an inflammatory response leading to the production of pro-inflammatory cytokines that may cause the aberrant over-expression of Class III MHC, resulting from the presentation of auto-peptides through the MHC molecules that lead to antigen-specific T-cell activation. The production of cytokines and their imbalance is caused by infection that may trigger the immune response. The post-partum period is a potential "predisposing" factor, though clearly the pregnant woman regulates some genetic and autoimmune expressions that tend to activate after the end of the post-partum period. Consequently, while the likelihood of GD expressing during the post-partum period is higher as compared to gestation, the most plausible explanation may be the "attenuation" of autoimmune manifestations typical of pregnancy, rather than an increased risk during the post-partum period. Furthermore, during pregnancy fetal cells may reach the maternal circulation and may somehow infiltrate various tissues – a process called "fetal microchimerism". The infiltration of fetal cells into the maternal tissues influences the maternal immune response, though at a level that is difficult to quantify; these fetal cells are valid candidates to explain the autoimmune modulation of thyroid disease, both during pregnancy as during the post-partum period. The use of drugs such as amiodarone, lithium derivatives, α-interferon, anti-retrovirals, and monoclonal antibodies, increase the risk of developing GD. Smoking is another factor associated with the presence of GD and is considered a predictor of GD-related risk of hyperthyroidism. Most likely the existing relationship depends on the exposure time; active smokers have a higher risk than patients who smoked in the past or those that never smoked. These effect is also dose-dependent; i.e., the larger the number of cigarette packs smoked per year, the higher the frequency of Graves' Disease, particularly in women that are heavy smokers [22, 23].

In summary, the combination of genetic, environmental and endogenous factors is the etiopathological foundation for GD (Fig. 5.1).

Clinical Manifestations

The GD patient may focus on the context of a "*Hyperthyroidism Syndrome*" covering the basic signs of morphological-structural manifestations of the thyroid gland (particularly goiter), alterations triggered by excessive circulating thyroid hormones (more frequently the *hyperadrenegic status*) and the tissue manifestations of the circulating TSHR expression (*exophtalmos and dermopathy*).

The clinical spectrum may be divided into general and tissue manifestations. The most frequent general manifestations include the paradoxical weight loss (meaning that despite the accompanying hyperphagia, the patient experiences accelerated and considerable weight loss), heat intolerance, diaphoresis, hyperkinesia, and emotional lability with a feeling of sadness, anxiety, and apprehension. Asthenia and adynamia may prevail and can be associated with difficulty to fall asleep and frequent awakenings, with physical and intellectual performance decline as the condition progresses. The libido is preserved early on, but as time goes by, patients express some sexual apathy and seek medical advice [24].

At the ***cardiovascular*** level, palpitations, exertion dyspnea and dyspnea at rest are overt. Arterial hypertension may be the first sign of the disease and it divergence may be suggestive of hyperthyroidism. The cardiovascular manifestations are the result of two intervening factors: the direct and indirect effect of thyroid hormones on the cardiovascular system and the interaction with the autonomous sympathetic system leading to a hyperdynamic status called "thyrotoxic cardiomyopathy", chest pain at rest and with minimal exertion, may be suggestive of coronary disease. Since cardiac manifestations may be the first to be expressed, with no evidence of other systemic – and even less thyroid- alterations, the condition is referred to as "masked thyrotoxicosis that mimics heart disease". Tachycardia with atrial fibrillation may be the only clinical manifestation in the elderly; in these patients, the presence of diarrhea and tachycardia may be the key expressions of GD. So the term "apathetic hyperthyroidism" has been coined and in fact, atrial fibrillation is the most frequent rhythm disorder in GD that may be present in over one third of patients over 60 years of age. The heart rate is usually high, the arterial pulse is jerky and broad, the first heart sound is accentuated and the second sound is often split; in patients with a classical high-output heart failure, S3 or S4 may be identified. Occasionally there is scratch murmur in the apex, called "Means-Lerman murmur" that is attributed to the friction of the hyperdynamic precordium against the pleura [25]. It is common knowledge that the cardiac contractile function, as well as the blood volume are significantly altered in patients with thyroid disease, because of the decreased vascular resistance that results in Renin-Angiotensin-Aldosterone system stimulation. Consequently, there is a significant increase in sodium and water reabsorption, with the corresponding increase in volume and preload, resulting in dilatation and increased cardiac output. Additionally, as a direct short-term effect, there are changes in the various sodium, potassium, and calcium channels configuration and of their respective intracellular levels in the heart, hence raising both inotropism and chronotropism, in addition to ventricular hypertrophy due to increased protein synthesis. Failure to properly control these processes may lead to contractile function and ejection fraction impairment, and finally to heart failure. Furthermore, experimental studies have shown a shorter duration of the action potential and increased spontaneous activity (automaticity), similar to the effect of the sinus node and in the cardiomyocytes around the pulmonary veins, which may facilitate the genesis of re-entry and atrial fibrillation circuits. The advent of Echocardiogram (EKG) has led to the identification of images inherent to GD. Among the most extensively described and characterized using EKG are the closing time of the mitral valve until the opening of the aortic valve (the so-called Isovolumetric Contraction Time –ICT-), the time from the opening of the aortic valve until the end of ventricular systole (the left ventricular ejection fraction time –LVEFT-) and the time from the closing of the aortic valve until the opening of the mitral valve (known as the Isovolumetric Relaxation Time –IRT-). GD patients exhibit increased values for these three parameters: ICT, LVEFT, and IRT, indicating systolic and/or diastolic dysfunction [25, 26].

At the ***Gastrointestinal*** level, the acceleration of the intestinal rhythm prevails, with hyperdefecation or diarrhea. The frequency and the severity of bowel movements predisposes to hydro-electrolytic imbalances that may impact mortality, particularly in the elderly. Flatulence and borborigmi are frequent manifestation. The autoimmune characteristic of GD favors the association with other equally relevant conditions, including CD, that has a growing frequency among patients with autoimmune thyroid disease –with a prevalence ranging from 5 to 10 %- Anorexia, abdominal pain, and vomiting are less frequent manifestation; jaundice and hepato/splenomegaly are manifestations of severe hyperthyroidism, although splenomegaly may occur in the initial forms of the disease. Just as in the case of CD, GD may be associated with severe forms of autoimmune hepatitis, ulcerative colitis, and primary biliary cirrhosis. Paradoxical weight loss is a frequent manifestation and is a specific sign of GD, that may be explained by increased thermogenesis and by the presence of hyperadrenergic factor-mediated lipolysis; though rare, weigh gain may present in the hyperadrenergic status; in fact, up to 10 % of the patients with hyperadrenergic Graves' Disease experience a relative weight gain [27, 28].

Skin manifestations are very conspicuous; the skin looks moist and hot as a result of cutaneous vasodilatation and diaphoresis; patients with GD often present with intertrigo, facial and palmar erythema, fine and brittle hair with excessive turnover resulting in a marked tendency to early baldness, with sparse fine hair, particularly on the forehead, giving rise to the expression "ash on the forehead under flaring gaze". Gray hair on one or both temples has been called "hyperthyroid Sainton tuft". Hair loss is frequent and alopecia areata are part of the capillary spectrum in GD patients. Spoon-shaped nails or koilonyquia (concave contour with distal onycholysis) with longitudinal striae are found in 5 % of patients with hyperthyroidism and are called "Plummer nails". Onycholysis, platonychia and onicorrhexis may be present. The elbow and knee skin tends to be soft and pink; itching is very common and may be associated with atopic dermatitis; skin hyperpigmentation is infrequent and similar to Addison's disease, but does not affect the mucosae. The hyperpigmentation is apparently mediated by accelerated cortisol metabolism in GD, that stimulates an excessive Adrenocorticotropic Hormone (ACTH), resulting in an elevation of the Melanocyte Stimulating Hormone (MSH), particularly its alpha fraction (α-MSH). The pretibial myxedema is an induration of the pretibial skin and develops as a result of hyaluronic acid and chondroitin sulfate deposits at this level. While in normal skin the percentage of hyaluronic acid is close to 5 %, it raises to 90 % in GD. Myxedema is a rare extra-thyroid manifestation in GD; its frequency increases in patients with ophthalmopathy, is more frequent in females and usually manifests over the third and fourth decade of life. The underlying mechanism of myxedema is unclear, though animal studies suggest that thyroid hormones affect the synthesis and catabolism of mucopolysaccharides and collagen from dermal fibroblasts [29, 30]. The myxedema usually presents at sites previously injured and manifests mostly as infiltrated plaques or asymmetrically distributed nodules over the pretibial region, either of a color similar to that of the normal skin or brownish, purple or erythematous occurring in 0.5–4.5 % of patients of GD. Diffuse myxedema presents in 43 % of the patients with dermopathy and the nodular variety occurs in 18 % of the patients with myxedema. The lesions have a hard consistency, with dilatation of the follicular orifices giving the affected surface an "orange peel" aspect; pressure on the lesions does not result in pitting. Whilst the classical localization is on the pretibial skin area, lesions may also be found on the foot dorsum, the face, the forearms, the abdominal wall and the chest. Hyperhidrosis may also be present on the affected surface, with itching, burning sensation, and pain. The combination of exophthalmos, pretibial myxedema, and hypertrophic osteoarthopathy is referred to as "EMO syndrome, or Diamond Syndrome" [30, 31].

At the level of the ***Nervous System***, the manifestations triggered by the activation of the sympathetic nervous system; restlessness and anxiety, emotional lability, hyperkinesia, psychotic status and panic attacks are usual and may be the initial manifestations of the disease. Hypokalemic Thyrotoxic Periodic Paralysis (HTPP) is a rare disease that may coexist with some hyperthyroidism conditions and is frequently described in GD patients. When HTPP occurs, patients develop some degree of hypokalemia attributed to transcellular potassium turnover, and a subsequent reduction of extracellular potassium. High thyroid hormone levels result in an over-regulation of the ATPase activity in the muscle, the kidney, the liver, and platelets. Furthermore, there is an increased trans-cellular potassium flow due to a yet undetermined mechanism that interferes with the actual ability of potassium to promote muscle contraction. The level of hypokalemia is directly related to the amount of muscle weakness, paraparesis and varying degrees of hemiplegia or quadriplegia present in patients with HTPP. Fine distal tremor is one of the most prevalent signs of GD; tongue tremor is also frequent when purposefully screened. Proximal muscle weakness may be present, as well as lid ptosis, which may be suspicious for Myasthenia Gravis (MG). This neurological presentation is not unusual and between 2 and 17.5 % of patients with MG express GD associated hyperthyroidism. Some epidemiological studies have shown the co-existence of GD and ocular MG in 41 % of cases and in 28 % generalized MG. The underlying reasons for this strong association, particularly for ocular MG, are not yet well established, but immune cross-reactivity against epitopes or auto-antigens that are shared by the thyroid and the eye muscles is suspected. The strong association between GD and generalized MG may be due to the fact that both share a common genetic history, and also because the HLA-B8 and DR3 expression are present in a large number of patients with both entities. Other neurological manifestations include the carpal tunnel syndrome, the cerebellar and pyramidal syndrome, chorea, and nonspecific myopathies [32–34]. Overall, patients respond very well to treatment (based on potassium electrolyte replacement and non-selective beta blockers). Total remission is achieved when the underlying hyperthyroidism is finally controlled.

The ***Ocular*** manifestations of GD are quite striking, ranging from almost imperceptible manifestations that can only be detected through imaging techniques, up to edematous and infiltrative manifestation with considerable orbital disfiguration. Periorbital edema, lid retraction, exophthalmos and diplopia are frequent signs and symptoms. It has been estimated that 50 % of GD patients will express ocular manifestations of the disease, though it is clinically relevant in 20–30 % of the cases, and between 3 and 5 % of the patients may have severe ocular disease. The clinical findings in patients with ophthalmopathy due to GD may be segregated into two groups: thickening of the retro-lobular space due to the Glucose-Aminoglycans (GAG) deposit or to the restriction of extra-ocular motility that is due to initial tumefaction and further fibrosis. The initial manifestations are particularly related to foreign body sensation, tearing, photophobia, and retroocular pain. Usually patients are diagnosed during the initial stages of the disease with "allergic Conjunctivitis" and transiently respond to the use of topical steroids. Then upper lid retraction develops which is considered the most common clinical orbital characteristic in GD; this leads to eyeball protrusion, bilateral eye protrusion together with upper eyelid retraction (caused by increased sympathetic activity of Müller's muscle and hyper function of the "superior rectus-elevator muscle", secondary to fibrosis-related hypophoria and contraction of the inferior rectus muscle), which is pathognomonic of GD. Most GD eye expression signs and symptoms are the result of orbital soft tissue expansion, resulting in increased pressures of the orbital cavity. Diplopia may be the initial symptom and results from the inflammation and tumefaction of the muscles involved, mainly the inferior rectus muscle; overall, this sign has a restrictive pattern, and does not cause ocular paralysis [35–37]. Diplopia is one of the most poorly tolerated signs because it is a major hindrance for the patient's performance and everyday tasks. Diplopia may even be more disruptive than the typical hyperadrenergic manifestations. Periorbital edema is very frequent at the onset of the disease and mainly affects the upper lids (particularly in young patients, where there is the above described increase in periorbital fat). The presence of orbital edema in GD is the reflection of delayed venous drainage due to compression at the orbital space. Lid edema in GD differs from hyperthyroidism edema because the latter is usually localized in the lower lid. The conjunctivas frequently present edema or chemosis; severe cases of conjuntival prolapse at the level of the lower lid are less frequent. Conjunctiva hyperemia is particularly visible near the horizontal rectus tendon and is indicative of the significant underlying autoimmune disease. In the event of severe proptosis, the elevator aponeurosis may be detached, resulting in lid ptosis that may be undistinguishable from the condition expressed in MG patients. GD ophthalmopathy occurs unilaterally in 5–15 % of the cases and is probably the most frequent cause of unilateral ocular protrusion. The reason for this presentation is yet unknown, but it may be the reflection of an early but still incomplete expression of orbital antibodies. These patients often do not show any signs or symptoms of hyperthyroidism (except proptosis), though the orbital imaging findings, in addition to the high level of antibodies against the TSH receptor, enables the identification of this group of patients. Exophthalmos, reduced blinking, and lid retraction give rise to exposure keratopathy of variable presentation, ranging from mild forms with just a fine punctiform de-epithelialization on the lower hemicornea –which is more exposed due to the nocturnal lagophthalmos- to corneal-conjuntival de-epithelialization resulting in stromal ulcerations and eventually corneal perforation [38]. The optical neuropathy derived from GD ophthalmopathy is compressive in nature, and occurs in 3–5 % of the patients with ocular manifestations. Optical neuropathy develops mainly in cases of major involvement of the orbital apex. In addition to the direct compression of the nerve in its apical segment, other factors that contribute to nerve damage are disruptions in venous return and stretching of the nerve in the orbit, losing the meandering trajectory and the hypertony of the aqueous humor. When the apical compression of the nerve is the rule, the disk may look normal, edematous, or slightly ischemic [37, 38]. The earlier disruptions develop around color perception, since the axons from the macula are more prone to injury. The progression of the neuropathy to absolute scotoma, the atrophy-cupping and stasis are dependent on the ophthalmopathy due to GD proper, and on the previous nerve circulatory status (increased sensitivity to compressive ischemia in patients with a history of vascular pathology). The hypertension at the orbital apex due to increased muscle and soft tissue volume, gives rise to a compressive syndrome of the orbital apex called "Crowded Orbital Apex Syndrome" and occurs in around 5–6 % of the patients with GD ophthalmopathy who had good eyesight in the past but experienced progressive or even fast eyesight impairment. Horner's syndrome (miosis, enophthalmos, and ptosis) is rarely present but when it occurs it is accompanied by loss of hemi facial sweating. Horner's syndrome in GD patients indicates compression of the cervical sympathetic chain due to the presence of goiter. From the ocular semiology point of view, the most relevant signs sings described throughout history are: [6, 36, 38].

- **Abadie's sign:** Spasm of the elevator palpebrae superioris muscle
- **Ballet's sign:** External ophthalmoplegia with loss of voluntary eye movements and preservation of the pupillary and reflex eye movements
- **Becker's Phenomenon:** Pulsation of retinal arteries visible in the eye fundus
- **Boston's Sign:** Abrupt closure of the upper eyelid when the eyeball looks downward
- **Cowen's Sign:** Jerky consensual pupillary light reflex
- **Dalrymple's Sign:** Retraction of the upper eyelids with abnormally wide palpebral opening
- **Dieulafoy's Sign:** Patients with GD develop a horror gaze (tragic eye) that sometimes is so marked that the eye develops a subluxation (Dieulafoy's subluxation)
- **Dunphy's Sign:** The injection of the conjunctiva in front of the lateral rectus muscle insertion
- **Enroth's Sign:** Eyelid edema, specially the upper lid close to the supraorbital rim
- **Griffith's Sign:** Lower lid lag on upward gaze
- **Gifford's Sign:** Evident difficulty in averting the upper eyelid
- **Grove's Sign:** Resistance of the upper eyelid to do downward traction
- **Jellinek-Rasin Sign:** Increased eyelid pigmentation, particularly of the upper lid.
- **Jendrassk-Brain Sign:** Paralysis of the extraocular muscles in GD
- **Joffroy's Sign:** Absence of wrinkles when the gaze is forced upwards, resulting from poor contraction of the frontal muscle
- **Knie's sign:** Unequal pupillary dilatation

- **Kocher's Reflex:** Fixed and frightening gaze
- **Lagophthalmos:** Incomplete eyelid closure due to exophthalmos
- **Loewi's Sign:** Pupil dilation following adrenalin stimulation
- **Mann's Sign:** The two eyes appear not to be on the same level due to decreased scalp resistance.
- **Means-Griffith-Von Koller Sign:** Lower lid lag on upward gaze
- **Möbius Sign:** Inability to keep the eyeballs converged due to insufficiency of the internal rectus muscles
- **Rosembach's Sign:** Fine upper lid tremor when closing the eyes softly
- **Rusell-Fraser Sign:** The fold between the upper eyelid and eyeball is narrowed when closing the eyes
- **Sainton's Sign:** Frontal muscle contraction on upward gaze
- **Snellen-Riesman Sign:** Is the murmur heard over the stethoscope gently placed over the eye closed
- **Stellwag's Sign:** Apparent widening of the palpebral opening
- **Sucker's Sign:** Deficient complementary fixation in lateral eye rotation
- **Tellais Sign:** Eyelid pigmentation, particularly of the lower lids.
- **Topolanski's Sign:** Pericorneal eye congestion
- **Von Graefe's Sign (Graefe's):** Lack of synergy between the eyelid and eyeball movements, particularly on downward gaze
- **Wilder's Sign:** Slight twitch of the eyeball when it changes its movement from adduction to abduction or vice versa.

Enophthalmos is rare and sometimes presents with orbit swelling and paresis or paralysis of the extrinsic muscles and is sometimes called "Brain ophthalmopathy". Orbital dull pain is considered a severe symptom indicative of orbital swelling with subsequent distension of the tissues around the eyeball [36–38].

The ***Respiratory*** manifestations are quite frequent with a relative weakness of the respiratory muscles, in addition to poor ventilation control due to alterations in the chemoreceptor expression and the center of respiration. All of this results in poor gaseous exchange that, in the presence of higher oxygen consumption typical of thyrotoxicosis, expresses clinically as the initial manifestation of the disease. Patients with pulmonary hypertension have also been identified as the initial manifestation of GD [39, 40].

Renal alterations reflect a condition of generalized vasodilatation present in these patients. The renal plasma flow and glomerular filtration are increased and polyuria –usually accompanied by polydipsia- seem to be mediated by increased levels of Angiotensin II, which causes sodium and water retention by mediating aldosterone release, worsening the palpebral, facial and pedal edema typical of GD. Thyrotoxicosis results in increased renal plasma flow and glomerular filtration, that gives rise to a decline in creatinine levels. Furthermore, hyperthyroidism is associated with a decrease in the total body water content and potassium turnover. Though sodium turnover is increased, sodium and potassium serum levels are normal and those imbalances normalize once the thyroid function is controlled if adequately managed [41].

At the ***Bone*** level, the manifestations are the result of faster bone turnover with hypercalciuria present in many cases; hypercalcemia however is rare and is also accompanied by an increased N-telopeptide urinary excretion rate, in addition to elevated osteocalcin and alkaline phosphatase. Intolerance to heat in these patients leads to decreased sun exposure that together with increased vitamin D catabolism translates into a progressive vitamin D deficiency. Such low vitamin D levels eventually result in reduced calcium absorption and patients may develop mild hypocalcemia. Although initially the Parathormone (PTH) level is below the normal range, some cases may present mild hypocalcemia and minor PTH elevations. All of this results in a marked loss of bone mass, osteopenia or osteoporosis, with a known risk of fractures, even higher than in patients with prior vitamin D deficit [42, 43].

Other ***systemic*** manifestations include: Hypoalbuminemia, oligomenorrhea, polymenorrhea, menorrhagia, hypermenorrhea and galactorrhea. Fertility may be compromised but pregnancy is possible, though there is a higher rate of abortions and a considerable increase in

Table. 5.1 Common, less common and atypical clinical manifestations in GD

Common manifestations	Less common manifestations	Atypical manifestations
Tremor	Depression	Vomiting
Goiter	Apathy	Jaundice
Tachyarrhythmia	Muscle weakness	Leucopenia
Fatigue	Paraparesis, quadriparesis	Thrombocytopenia
Left ventricular dysfunction	Altered liver tests	Chronic disease anemia
Increased peristalsis	Agitation	Pulmonary hypertension
Heat intolerance	Psychosis	Right heart failure
Exophthalmos	Erectile dysfunction	Angioedema
Weight loss	Gynecomasty	Acute coronary syndrome
Dyspnea	Alopecia	Venous thromboembolism
Anxiety	Cachexia	Vasculitis
Nervousness	koilonyquia	Angioedema
Palmar erythema (Lane's Palm)	Polydipsia	Chorea
Hyperreflexia	Weight gain	Pruritus
Diaphoresis	Polymenorrhea/oligomenorrhea	Sialorrhea
Insomnia	galactorrhea	Polyuria

peripartum morbidity. Erectile dysfunction and loss of libido are frequent in males; anemia may be present with an increased mean corpuscular volume (macrocytic) resulting from enhanced vitamin B12 and folic acid metabolism, and from the presence of anti-intrinsic factor antibodies and anti-parietal cells. This anemia is usually asymptomatic. The presence of splenomegaly with leukopenia-neutropenia and lymphocytosis has been called "Kocher Syndrome" [6, 44].

At the ***thyroid*** level, a lobulated, soft, usually smooth gland may be found and sometimes it can be nodular. In the classical GD, the gland is asymmetrical and variable in size. Thyroid gland growth is conspicuous in some cases, even at a distance and seldom imperceptible to palpation (in 1 % of the cases the gland is not palpable, either because of its small size or because it is localized under the sternal manubrium). Size is somehow associated with the severity of the disease, but is not infallible as a parameter since clinically the patient may present a severe GD with barely palpable goiter. In contrast, there are patients with mild signs and symptoms of the disease, with remarkable gland sizes. Murmur or "fremitus" are important findings, but are usually absent; their presence is indicative of gland hyperfunction [36, 45].

GD presents some ***rare*** manifestations that affect several organs and systems including cases compatible with cerebral vasculitis, venous thromboembolism, vomiting, jaundice, pulmonary hypertension and elevated alkaline phosphatase [46] (Table 5.1).

Clinical Diagnosis

In 1959 Crooks et al. described a statistical method to assist in the diagnosis of thyrotoxicosis, using a weighted score based on 19 different signs and symptoms. The score discriminated between individuals with and without thyrotoxicosis with a relatively high sensitivity. The strength of this scoring system was that it relied on the classical symptoms of hyperthyroidism, and its weakness was the fact that most of the findings were just based on the presence or absence of the factor studied. The authors also used their scoring system to assess treatment and were able to contrast the efficacy of various therapeutic modalities [47, 48]. With a view to improving the clinical evaluation of patients with hyperthyroidism, the authors themselves suggested and validated the hyperthyroidism symptoms scale that was used for the diagnosis and treatment of Graves' disease patients (Table 5.2). When newly diagnosed and untreated GD patients are administered the above symptoms scale; the mean score reported was

Table 5.2 Hyperthyroid symptoms scale proposed by Crooks et al. (Refs. [47, 48])

Characteristics	Score
Nervousness:	
0. None	
1. Anxious, only under stress	——
2. Anxious at rest, occasionally	
3. Frequently anxious, difficulty to complete tasks or to concentrate	
4. Very nervous most of the time	
Sweating:	
0. Only when active	
1. At rest, but under hot temperature	
2. At rest in temperate climates, mainly involving the hands and intertriginous areas	——
3. At rest, involving large body areas	
4. Profuse, almost constant diaphoresis	
Heat Tolerance:	
0. Normal tolerance	
1. Periods of time when heat perception is higher than the perception by other people in the same room	
2. Extremely difficult to manage heat sensation in warm environments, constantly requiring air conditioning during summer time	——
3. Extremely difficult to manage heat sensation, even in temperate climates	
4. Extremely difficult to manage heat sensation; feels uncomfortable even in cold weather, evidenced by the fact that no coats of blankets are needed for protection against cold.	
Hyperactivity:	
0. Normal level of activity	
1. Increased level of activity and productivity	
2. Increased productivity and less sleep hours	——
3. Performs some kind of senseless or purposeless activity	
4. Frequent episodes of senseless activity unable to stay still during the examination	
Tremor: Examined while the patient keeps his/her hands extended	
0. Absent	
1. Barely noticeable	
2. Tremor easily identified during the examination	——
3. Marked tremor, but able to properly perform fine motor activities	
4. Exaggerated handshake; difficulty to perform fine motor skills	
Weakness:	
0. Normal strength	
1. Subjective weakness, but with tolerance to normal exercising	
2. Reduced exercise tolerance at a near maximal activity	——
3. Reduce exercise tolerance when climbing up the stairs or standing up from a chair	
4. Extreme weakness – patients are barely able to raise any objects or climb the stairs	
Hyperdynamic Precordium:	
0. Normal precordial activity and apical impulse	
1. Tachycardia, 90 beats per minute with normal apical impulse	——
2. Tachycardia, 90 beats per minute with increased apical impulse	
3. Tachycardia, 110 beats per minute with increased apical impulse	
4. Tachycardia, 110 beats per minute, apical impulse and increased carotid pulse; systolic murmur present	

(continued)

Table 5.2 (continued)

Characteristics		Score
Diarrhea:		
0.	A bowel movement per day, formed stools	
1.	Two to four bowel movements per day, formed stools	
2.	One to four bowel movements per day, watery stools	——
3.	Four bowel movements per day; solid feces	
4.	Four watery bowel movements per day	
Appetite:		
0.	Normal appetite, no weight loss	
1.	Normal appetite, with weight loss	
2.	Increased appetite with no weight loss	——
3.	Increased appetite with weight loss	
4.	Decreased appetite with weight loss	
Evaluation of daily function (level of disability):		
0.	Normal (none)	
1.	Minimal disruption (10 %)	
2.	Mild disruption (30 %)	——
3.	Moderate disruption (60 %)	
4.	Severe disruption (90 %)	
Total score:		——

24.3 ± 4.6, which was significantly higher than the reported score for the same patients under beta blockers (14.3 ± 5.9) and at the same time was significantly higher than the score for patients that remained euthyroid (4.7 ± 2.2). When the scale was applied to a large group of newly diagnosed GD individuals, there was no correlation between the hyperparathyroidism scale and the total T3, T4 levels and the free thyroxine index [48]. The scale was directly correlated against other parameters such as goiter size, and inversely proportional to age –probably due to the lower prevalence of adrenergic symptoms in people over 50 years old-.

Sir Edward Wayne also described a scale called the Wayne's Index; the purpose of this index was to help in the diagnosis of hyperthyroidism and to limit the need to do any other diagnostic tests. The score ranges from +45 to −25; a score of less than 11 defines "euthyroidism", while a score above 19 implies "toxic hyperthyroidism" [47–49]. Values between 11 and 19 are classified as "questionable"; Wayne's index provides an 85 % diagnostic accuracy (Table 5.3).

Laboratory Diagnosis

Any patient that presents in a hyper-adrenergic status, with exophthalmos, goiter and dermopathy virtually has GD; however, the manifestations are not always florid. The diagnosis of GD is based on sound clinical judgment and on the biochemical manifestations of the disease. From the laboratory point of view, TSH measurements (ideally together with free fraction T3 and T4 because "total" titration may vary depending on the intake of certain medications and thyroid-binding hormones that give rise to falsely elevated TSH) allow for the identification of hyperthyroidism, TSH suppression and increased levels of free T3 and T4 are pathognomonic for primary hyperthyroidism. The presence of suppressed TSH with normal free T3 and T4 levels identifies the patient with subclinical hyperthyroidism. The TSH measurement through different forms and trials has been identified in "Generations" based on the functional sensitivity of the trial. The National Academy of Clinical Biochemistry (NACB) recommends the various laboratories to use third generation functional

Table 5.3 Wayne index (Refs. [47, 49])

Recent onset symptoms and/or increased severity	Score	Signs	Present	Absent
Dyspnea on exertion	+1	Palpable thyroid	+3	−3
Palpitations	+2	Thyroid murmur	+2	−2
Fatigue	+2	Exophthalmus	+2	
Heat preference	−5	Lid retraction	+2	–
Cold preference	+5	Lazy lid (lid lag)	+1	–
Excessive sweating	+3	Hyperkinetics	+4	−2
Nervousness	+2	Hot hands	+2	−2
Appetite: Increased	+3	Sweaty hands	+1	−1
Appetite: Decreased	−3	Casual pulse rate:		
		<80/min	0	
		80–90/min	+3	−3
		>90/min		
Weight changes (increase)	−3	Atrial fibrillation	+4	–
Weight changes (decrease)	+3			

sensitivity essays (0.02 mIU/L) or greater. The lower normal population level for TSH values ranges between 0.4 and 4.0 mIU/L (based on 95 % of the values identified in apparently healthy individuals). Overall, this lower range of values for TSH is not as debated as the upper normal range [50–52]. Other laboratory parameters such as the titration of the antibody against the TSH receptor (Anti-TSHr) may be useful in some cases, but is not a prerequisite for making the diagnosis of GD [53].

Some recommendations to measure anti-TSHr are [53, 54]:

A. Since practically every GD patient expresses such antibodies, its detection is useful for the serological diagnosis of autoimmune hyperthyroidism.
B. The detection of such antibodies allows for the differentiation of autoimmune hyperthyroidism from the non-autoimmune type.
C. The antibody expression, particularly when present at elevated titers, may be predictive of GD ophthalmopathy.
D. The presence of these antibodies may predict relapses in patients treated with tionamides, though this is a debatable argument.
E. Early titration of the antibody is recommended in women with a history of GD, previously managed with I-131 or with surgery, since the antibody expression, regardless of the functional thyroid status of the mother, is a predictor for neonatal hyperthyroidism.
F. During pregnancy, in patients treated with anti-thyroid medication or a history of prior children with neonatal hyperthyroidism. Anti-TSHr titration is recommended in these patients during the first trimester and at week 22–26 of gestation.
G. In patients with multinodular hyperthyroidism goiter, with findings of ophthalmopathy and/or dermopathy, the measurement and the expression of the antibody helps in identifying those patients with GD expressed with a multinodular goiter.
H. In individuals with thyrotoxicosis within the framework of Immune Reconstitution Syndrome, patients treated with lymphocyte-depleting agents such as Alemtuzumab (AMPCATH) and in patients undergoing anti-retroviral therapy due to HIV infection (HAART). Thyroid dysfunction, hyperthyroidism and positive Anti-TSHr titers may result in both cases.
I. Presence of unilateral orbital pathology or with euthyroidism.
J. Presence of orbital pathology with hyperthyroidism.

Imaging Diagnosis

Ultrasound in GD patients usually shows an enlarged gland with low thyroid echogenicity. Color Doppler blood flow evaluation shows increased intra-thyroid and diffuse blood flow; such increase is well correlated with iodine uptake –in the gammagraphy- and with the thyroid hormone values. The ultrasound evaluation takes several imaging variables into consideration, including in particular the thyroid gland size, the vascularity, and the Systolic Peak Velocity (SPV) of the Inferior Thyroid Artery (ITA); overall, untreated patients with active GD show enlarged gland and increased vascularity and thyroid blood flow (determined based on the increased SPV of the ITA). It has been further suggested that the gland vascularity may be predictive of the long-term course of the disease under medical therapy. From the pathophysiological point of view, it is clear that hyperthyroidism induces increased arterial flow with a rise in heart output; however, the increased intra-thyroid blood flow is not exclusive of GD, since it may also occur in Hashimoto's disease –with hypothyroidism- hence, some authors recommend that in addition to the SPV measurement of the ITA, the SPV of the common carotid arteries should be assessed [55, 56]. One additional benefit of thyroid ultrasound is the diagnostic performance offered to identify the presence of nodules (that may not even be detected with the gammagraphy or at physical examination, but may be part of the spectrum of GD presentation). It may be probable that in the future glandular echogenicity may allow for improved accuracy in the determination of the I-131 dose that is estimated for the treatment of GD in patients who are amenable to this therapeutic modality. It may then be concluded that ultrasound as a diagnostic support method for GD is safe, avoids patient exposure to ionizing radiation, and is usually available and affordable to a large segment of the population; furthermore, it enables the evaluation of other neck structures and allows for targeted procedures such as Fine Needle Aspiration Biopsy (FNAB) and does not require the use of contrast medium. The disadvantage is that it is an operator-dependent method, though this hurdle is significantly reduced with extensive experience and a growing number of scans performed by the operator. The thyroid scan (Scintigraphy Technique) –within the context of nuclear imaging techniques of the thyroid gland is done using a gamma Scintigraphy. Camera that renders images from various views: oblique, anterior, and posterior. The morphological details of the gland are obtained using certain radionuclides such as Technetium 99 Pertechnetate (Tc99m), the I-123 and the I-131. When using Tc99m the images are obtained 20 min following its administration (dose of 10 mCi –370 MBq-); when I-123 is used, the images are obtained 4–24 h after intake and when using I-131, the images are obtained 24–72 after intake. The use of these imaging techniques allows for the determination of the gland's functional status, in addition to establishing the presence of nodules with malignant characteristics ("hypo and hyper-uptake"). In a way, Tc99m evaluates functionality, but mostly morphology, since the thyroid gland captures the Tc99m but does not result in organification. In contrast, in the case of I-123 and I-131, the thyroid gland captures and organifies the radionuclides. Hence, for instance, I-131 is used to determine the thyroid iodine uptake in 24 h and the thyroid uptake reflects the percentage of the dose given to the patient, which is then accumulated in the thyroid. The range of normal uptake in 24 h is from 10 to 30 % (following a dose of 5 μCi –0.19 MBq- of I-131). The same applies for I-123 (using a dose of 300 μCi –11.11 MBq-). The amount of radiation released into the thyroid via the I-123 is 1 % of the radiation released by the same amount of I-131. Consequently, I-123 is preferred over I-131, although the cost and the relatively low availability of the former, limits its routine administration. Generally speaking, since GD expresses with an increase in the production and turnover of thyroid hormones, the evaluation of the gland function with I-131 or I-123 shows increased tracer uptake (usually homogeneous); however, there are some cases when the uptake at 4–6 h is elevated and normalizes at 24 h. This is the result of an accelerated radioactive iodine clearance [57–59]. Certain agents such as iodine contrast, anti-thyroid agents, thyroid hormone, some antibiotics and antihistaminic agents, may lower the uptake range. Occasionally, nodular thyroid disease may be present together with GD; its presence is variable, but may escalate up to 25–30 %. A high percentage of these patients exhibit "hyperactive or autonomous" nodules. These subjects with GD-associated thyrotoxicosis and toxic nodular goiter are called "Marine-Lenhart Syndrome". These cases may exhibit a gland with increased diffuse uptake, "enhancement" areas in one or several areas that are consistent with the findings of nodules in the scan (autonomous functional nodules in GD individuals). This characteristic is present in 0.8–2.7 % of GD patients [60, 61]. When the diagnosis of hyperthyroidism is clear (both clinical and biochemical) in the presence of diffuse goiter, but when the evolution as described upon questioning the patient indicates that signs and symptoms have only been present for some weeks or a few months, the presence of non-GD hypothyroidism should be entertained. In these cases, the differential diagnosis should mainly be based on sub-acute or chronic thyroiditis in the hyperthyroid phase. Under such circumstances, I-131 or I-123 uptake is extremely helpful. Uptake increases in the presence of GD, whilst it declines or will be suppressed in the case of thyroiditis.

Histopathological Diagnosis

From the macroscopic point of view, GD presents a gland that may be mild to moderately enlarge and is symmetrical, involves both lobules and the isthmus, with a vascularized surface and it is usually smooth, though mild nodularity is occasionally visible. The section surface is soft and reddish due to marked vascularization of the gland. Mild fibrosis may be observed, usually when previous tionamide treatment has been received. Microscopically, thyroid follicles in different sizes may be appreciated, either hyperplastic or too small; some follicles have a prominent papillary shape occasionally misperceived for thyroid papillary carcinoma. The nucleus is rounded or oval in shape, with smooth margins and localized towards the base; chromatin is finely granular without atypia. The nuclei in the aspirate may exhibit a clear, marginal cytoplasmic vacuole adjacent to the nucleus; these are called flame cells that show small nucleoli without a nuclear bar or intranuclear vacuole. These findings are also characteristic of papillary carcinoma. The cytoplasm of thyrocytes in GD may adopt a pink or anophillic color, with a granular or micro-vacuolated appearance. The colloid is paler than usual, vacuolated and with a scalloped shape adjacent to the epithelium, indicating follicular cell activity. In long-standing cases, mild Hürthle cells metaplasia has been described, in contrast to what is usually appreciated in Hashimoto's thyroiditis. A mild increase in the lymphocytic infiltrate at the stroma is observed, though occasionally this infiltrate may be more significant and even develop into lymphoid follicles [62–64]. Frequently marked edema of the papillary and reticular dermis can be seen on the skin, with nuclear fibroblast activity. This edema turns blue under alcian blue stain, showing the positivity of mucopolysaccharides produced by active fibroblasts secreted into the extracellular matrix (Figs. 5.2, 5.3, 5.4, 5.5, and 5.6).

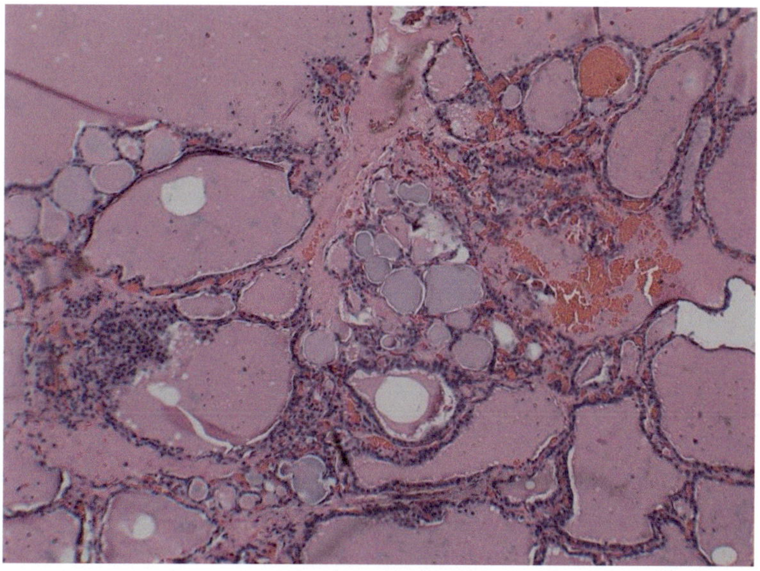

Fig. 5.2 4× image. Varying thyroid follicular size. Hematoxylin-Eosin staining (Author´s files)

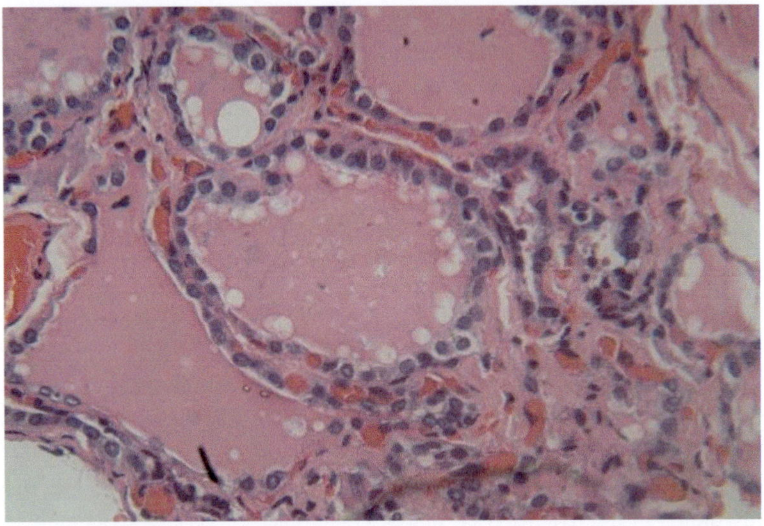

Fig. 5.3 10× image. Small follicles with mild fibrosis are observed in the middle of the follicle with the characteristic colloid scallop. Hematoxylin–eosin staining (Author's files)

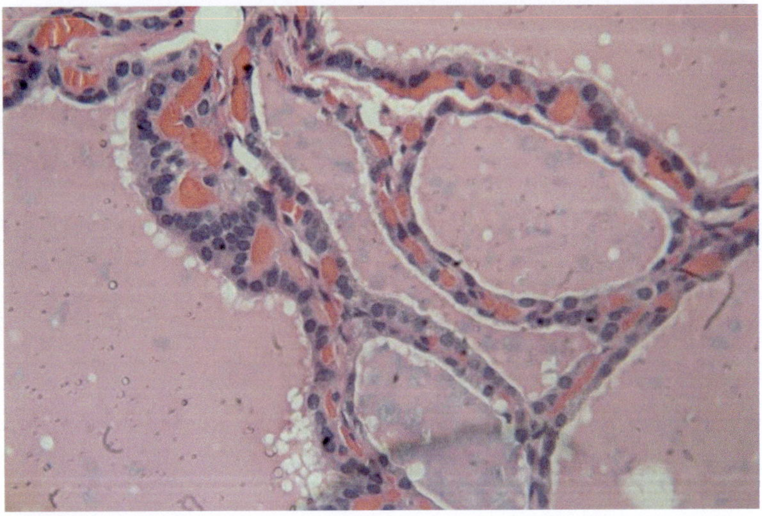

Fig. 5.4 40× image. The follicle is observed on the left side of the image, covered with columnar cells. Every follicle has the colloid scallop on the epithelium. A marked increase in the stromal vessels is also appreciated (Author's files)

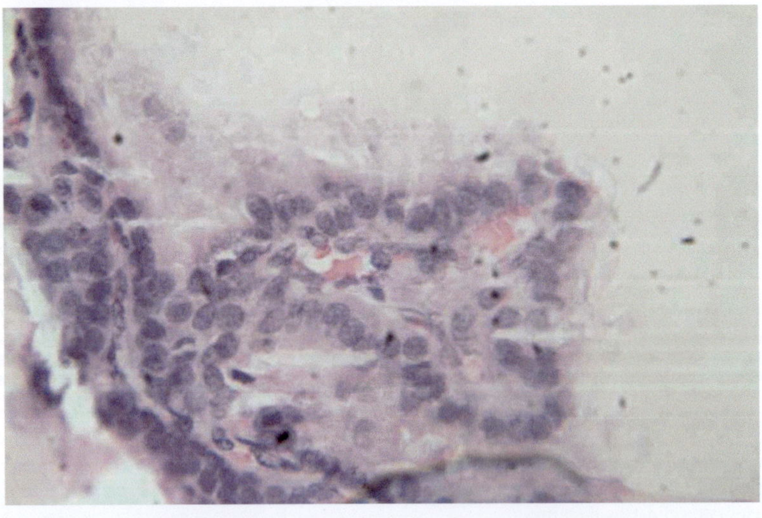

Fig. 5.5 10× image. Observe the formation of papillae with fibro vascular stem, covered with columnar cells. Hematoxylin-eosin staining (Author's files)

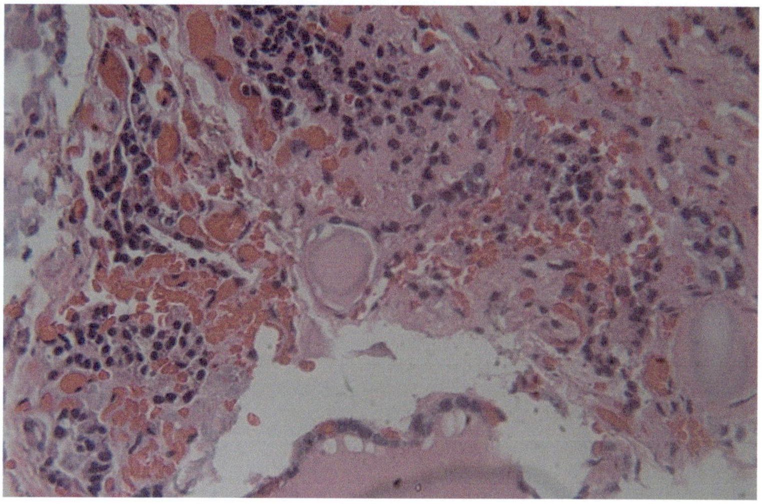

Fig. 5.6 10× image. This microphotograph shows a mild stromal fibrosis with vascular proliferation and moderate lymphocytic infiltrate. There is no formation of lymphoid formation. A scalloped colloid follicle can be appreciated on the lower segment (Author's files)

Conclusions

Graves-Basedow disease is an example of organ specific autoimmune disorder in which both humoral and cell mediated immunity directed against differentthyroid antigens areinvolved; the disease is an autoimmune disorder characterized by hyperthyroidism, diffuse goiter, ophthalmopathy and, rarely, dermopathy. When thyrotoxicosis, goiter and ocular signs and symptoms coexist, the diagnosis is evident.

Bibliography

1. Testa AG. Delle malattie del cuore, loro cagioni, specie, segni e cura. 2nd ed, vol. 3. Bologna; 1810.
2. Flajani G. Sopra un tumor freddo nell'anterior parte del collo broncocele (Osservazione LXVII). Collezione d'osservazioni e reflessioni di chirurgia, Rome, Milano, A Ripa Presso Lino Contedini. 1802;3:270–3.
3. Basedow CA. Exophthalmos durch Hypertrophie des Zellgewebes in der Augenhöhle. Wochenschrift fur die gesammte Heilkunde Berlin. 1840;6:197–220.
4. Graves RJ. New observed affection of the thyroid gland in females. London Med Surg J. 1835;7:516–7.
5. Parry CH. Enlargement of the thyroid gland in connection with enlargement or palpitations of the heart. In: Parry CH, editor. Collections from the unpublished medical writings of H. Parry. London: Underwoods; 1825. p. 111–29.
6. Young P, Finn BC, Bruetman JE. La enfermedad de Graves, signos y síntomas. An Med Interna (Madrid). 2007;24:505–8.
7. McKenna TJ. Graves' disease. Eponym Lancet. 2001; 357:1793–6.
8. McLeod Donald SA, Cooper DS. The incidence and prevalence of thyroid autoimmunity. Endocrine. 2012;42:252–65.
9. Vargas-Uricoechea H, Sierra-Torres CH, Meza-Cabrera IA. Enfermedad de Graves-Basedow. Fisiopatología y diagnóstico. Medicina (Bogotá). 2013;35,1(100):41–66.
10. Golden SH, Robinson KA, Saldanha I, Anton B, Ladenson PW. Prevalence and incidence of endocrine and metabolic disorders in the United States: a comprehensive review. J Clin Endocrinol Metab. 2009; 94:1853–78.
11. Abraham-Nordling M, Torring O, Lantz M, Hallengren B, Ohrling H, Lundell GJ, et al. Incidence of hyperthyroidism in Stockholm, Sweden, 2003–2005. Eur J Endocrinol. 2008;158(6):823–7.
12. Manji N, Carr-Smith JD, Boelaert K, Allahabadia A, Armitage M, Chatterjee VK, et al. Influences of age, gender, smoking, and family history on autoimmune thyroid disease phenotype. J Clin Endocrinol Metab. 2006;91:4873–80.
13. Ploski R, Szymanski K, Bednarczuk T. The genetic basis of Graves' disease. Curr Genomics. 2011;12: 542–63.
14. Ban Y. Genetic factors of autoimmune thyroid diseases in Japanese. Autoimmune Dis. 2012;2012:9. doi:10.1155/2012/236981. Article ID 236981.
15. Davies TF, Latif R, Yin X. New genetic insights from autoimmune thyroid disease. J Thyroid Res. 2012;2012:6. doi:10.1155/2012/623852. Article ID 623852.
16. Clayton DG, McKeigue PM. Epidemiological methods for studying genes and environmental factors in complex diseases. Lancet. 2001;358:1357–60.
17. Lohmueller KE, Pearce CL, Pike M, Lander ES, Hirschhorn JN. Meta-analysis of genetic association studies supports a contribution of common variants to susceptibility to common disease. Nat Genet. 2003;33: 177–82.

18. Płoski R, Szymański K, Bednarczuk T. The genetic basis of Graves' disease. Curr Genomics. 2011;12: 542–63.
19. Gu LQ, Zhu W, Zhao SX, Zhao L, Zhang MJ, Cui B, Song HD, Ning G, Zhao YJ. Clinical associations of the genetic variants of CTLA-4, Tg, TSHR, PTPN22, PTPN12 and FCRL3 in patients with Graves' disease. Clin Endocrinol (Oxf). 2010;72(2):248–55.
20. Sibarani RP. Genetics of Graves' disease: the lost concept. Acta Med Indones. 2009;41(1):37–40.
21. Brand OJ, Gough SCL. Immunogenetic mechanisms leading to thyroid autoimmunity: recent advances in identifying susceptibility genes and regions. Curr Genomics. 2011;12(8):526–41.
22. Nagayama Y, Nakahara M, Abiru N. Animal models of Graves' disease and Graves' orbitopathy. Curr Opin Endocrinol Diabetes Obes. 2015;22(5):381–6.
23. Nagayama Y, Nakahara M, Abiru N, Manson JE, Michels K, et al. Smoking and other lifestyle factors and the risk of Graves' hyperthyroidism. Arch Intern Med. 2005;165:1606–11.
24. Ando T, Imaizumi M, Graves PN, Unger P, Davies TF. Intrathyroidal fetal microchimerism in Graves' disease. J Clin Endocrinol Metab. 2002;87:3315–20.
25. Brent GA. Clinical practice. Graves' disease. N Engl J Med. 2008;358(24):2594–605.
26. Fadel BM, Ellahham S, Ringel MD, Lindsay J, Wartofsky L, Burman KD. Hyperthyroid heart disease. Clin Cardiol. 2000;23:402–8.
27. Mansourian AR. A review of literature on the adverse effects of hyperthyroidism on the heart functional behavior. Pak J Biol Sci. 2012;15:164–76.
28. Ebert EC. The thyroid and the gut. J Clin Gastroenterol. 2010;44(6):402–6.
29. Maser C, Toset A, Roman S. Gastrointestinal manifestations of endocrine disease. World J Gastroenterol. 2006;12(20):3174–9.
30. Burman KD, McKinley-Grant L. Dermatologic aspects of thyroid disease. Clin Dermatol. 2006;24(4):247–55.
31. Doshi DN, Blyumin ML, Kimball AB. Cutaneous manifestations of thyroid disease. Clin Dermatol. 2008;26(3):283–7.
32. Niepomniszcze H, Amad RH. Skin disorders and thyroid diseases. J Endocrinol Invest. 2001;24(8):628–38.
33. Yudiarto FL, Muliadi L, Moeljanto D, Hartono B. Neuropsychological findings in hyperthyroid patients. Acta Med Indones. 2006;38(1):6–10.
34. Canton A, de Fabregas O, Tintore M, Mesa J, Codina A, Simo R. Encephalopathy associated to autoimmune thyroid disease: a more appropriate term for an underestimated condition? J Neurol Sci. 2000;176:65–9.
35. Doherty C. Neurologic manifestations of thyroid disease. Neurologist. 2001;7:147–57.
36. Wiersinga WM, Smit T, van der Gaag R, Mourits M, Koornneef L. Clinical presentation of Graves' ophthalmopathy. Ophthalmic Res. 1989;21:73–82.
37. Pérez Moreiras JV, Prada Sánchez MC, Coloma J, et al. Oftalmopatía distiroidea. En: Pérez Moreiras JV, Prada Sánchez C. Patología orbitaria. Exploración, diagnóstico y cirugía. Barcelona: Edika Med 2002;2:940–90.
38. Gaddipati RV, Meyer DR. Eyelid retraction, lid lag, lagophthalmos, and von Graefe's sign. Quantifying the eyelid features of Graves' ophthalmopathy. Ophthalmology. 2008;115:1083–8.
39. Fernández-Hermida RV, Pinar S, Muruzábal N. Manifestaciones clínicas de la oftalmopatía tiroidea. An Sist Sanit Navar. 2008;31(Supl. 3):45–56.
40. Li JH, Safford RE, Aduen JF, Heckman MG, Crook JE, Burger CD. Pulmonary hypertension and thyroid disease. Chest. 2007;132(3):793–7.
41. Armigliato M, Paolini R, Aggio S, Zamboni S, Galasso MP, Zonzin P, Cella G. Hyperthyroidism as a cause of pulmonary arterial hypertension: a prospective study. Angiology. 2006;57(5):600–6.
42. Mariani LH, Berns JS. The renal manifestations of thyroid disease. J Am Soc Nephrol. 2012;23(1):22–6.
43. Dhanwal DK. Thyroid disorders and bone mineral metabolism. Indian J Endocrinol Metab. 2011;15:S107–12.
44. Mosekilde L, Eriksen EF, Charles P. Effects of thyroid hormones on bone and mineral metabolism. Endocrinol Metab Clin North Am. 1990;19:35–63.
45. Kendall-Taylor P. Thyrotoxicosis. In: Grossman A, editor. Clinical endocrinology. Oxford: Blackwell Science; 1998. p. 328–58.
46. Trzepacz PT, Klein I, Roberts M, Greenhouse J, Levey GS. Graves' disease: an analysis of thyroid hormone levels and hyperthyroid signs and symptoms. Am J Med. 1989;87:558–61.
47. Hegazi MO, Ahmed S. Atypical clinical manifestations of Graves' disease: an analysis in depth. J Thyroid Res. 2012;2012:8. doi:10.1155/2012/768019. Article ID 768019.
48. Kalra S, Khandewal SK, Goyal A. Clinical scoring scales in thyroidology: a compendium. Indian J Endocrinol Metab. 2011;15 Suppl 2:S89–94.
49. Klein I. Clinical, metabolic and organ-specific indices of thyroid function. Endocrinol Metab Clin North Am. 2001;30(2):415–27.
50. Klein I, Trzepacz PT, Roberts M, Levey GS. Symptom rating scale for assessing hyperthyroidism. Arch Intern Med. 1988;148:387–90.
51. Nayak B, Hodak SP. Hyperthyroidism. Endocrinol Metab Clin North Am. 2007;36(3):617–56.
52. Ross DS. Serum thyroid-stimulating hormone measurement for assessment of thyroid function and disease. Endocrinol Metab Clin North Am. 2001; 30(2):245–64.
53. Dufour RD. Laboratory tests of thyroid function: uses and limitations. Endocrinol Metab Clin North Am. 2007;36:579–94.
54. Kamath C, Adlan MA, Premawardhana LD. The role of thyrotrophin receptor antibody assays in Graves' disease.

J Thyroid Res. Vol. 2012;2012:8. doi:10.1155/2012/525936. Article ID 525936.
55. Lytton SD, Kahaly GJ. Bioassays for TSH-receptor autoantibodies: an update. Autoimmun Rev. 2010;10(2):116–22.
56. Soto GD, Halperin I, Squarcia M, Lomeña F, Domingo MP. Update in thyroid imaging. The expanding world of thyroid imaging and its translation to clinical practice. Hormones (Athens). 2010;9(4):287–98.
57. Chaudhary V, Bano S. Imaging of the thyroid: recent advances. Indian J Endocrinol Metab. 2012;16:371–6.
58. Meller J, Becker W. The continuing importance of thyroid scintigraphy in the era of high-resolution ultrasound. Eur J Nucl Med. 2002;29 Suppl 2:425–38.
59. Piga M, Cocco MC, Serra A, Boi F, Loy M, Mariotti S. The usefulness of 99mTc-sestaMIBI thyroid scan in the differential diagnosis and management of amiodarone-induced thyrotoxicosis. Eur J Endocrinol. 2008;159(4):423–9.
60. Avci E, Narci H. Coexistence of Graves' disease and toxic adenoma: a rare presentation of Marine-Lenhart syndrome. J Ayub Med Coll Abbottabad. 2015;27(1):248–50.
61. Lagaru A, McDougall IR. Treatment of thyrotoxicosis. J Nucl Med. 2007;48:379–89.
62. Intenzo C, Jabbour S, Miller JL, Ahmed I, Furlong K, Kushen M, Kim SM, Capuzzi DM. Subclinical hyperthyroidism: current concepts and scintigraphic imaging. Clin Nucl Med. 2011;36(9):e107–13.
63. Brahma A, Beadsmoore C, Dhatariya K. The oldest case of Marine-Lenhart syndrome? JRSM Short Rep. 2012;3:21. doi:10.1258/shorts.2011.011164.
64. LiVolsi VA. The pathology of autoimmune thyroid disease: a review. Thyroid. 1994;4:333–9.

Part II

Thyroid Dysfunction and Clinical Application

Thyroiditis

6

Henrique Vara Luiz, Isabel Manita,
and Jorge Portugal

Abstract

Thyroiditis is defined by the occurrence of thyroid inflammation and involves a diverse group of conditions. It is usually classified by the presence or absence of pain and tenderness. The most important forms include Hashimoto's thyroiditis, painless and postpartum thyroiditis, drug-induced thyroiditis, Riedel's thyroiditis, subacute and suppurative thyroiditis. Each type has particular characteristics, such as specific epidemiological data, etiopathogenesis, clinical features, laboratory and image results, pathology findings, differential diagnosis and therapeutic options. It is crucial that physicians and other health professionals be aware of the differences between the main forms of thyroiditis, so they can make a correct and prompt diagnosis and start the appropriate treatment.

Introduction

The term thyroiditis indicates the presence of thyroid inflammation and comprises a diverse group of conditions [1]. A universal classification of thyroiditis has not been established and it can be categorized based on etiology, pathology or clinical features. We agree with some authors who classify thyroiditis according to whether it is associated with thyroid pain and tenderness, because that distinction is important in the differential diagnosis of the disease [2] (Table 6.1).

In this chapter the authors perform a review of the literature and attempt to systematize the characteristics of the most important forms of thyroiditis. For each form, we discuss the following topics: epidemiology, etiology and pathogenesis, clinical features, diagnostic evaluation, differential diagnosis and treatment.

H.V. Luiz, MD (✉) • I. Manita, MD
J. Portugal, MD
Department of Endocrinology and Diabetology,
Hospital Garcia de Orta, Avenida Torrado da Silva,
2801-951 Almada, Portugal
e-mail: hvaraluiz@gmail.com; isabelmanita@sapo.pt;
jportugal@hgo.min-saude.pt

S.K. Imam, S.I. Ahmad (eds.), *Thyroid Disorders: Basic Science and Clinical Practice*,
DOI 10.1007/978-3-319-25871-3_6

Table 6.1 Classification of thyroiditis based on the presence or absence of pain and tenderness

No thyroid pain and tenderness
Hashimoto's thyroiditis
Painless thyroiditis
Postpartum thyroiditis
Amiodarone-associated thyroiditis
Thyroiditis induced by other drugs (lithium, interferon-alpha, interleukin-2, tyrosine kinase inhibitors)
Riedel's thyroiditis
Infiltrative thyroid disorders (amyloidosis, sarcoidosis)
Thyroid pain and tenderness
Subacute thyroiditis
Suppurative thyroiditis
Radiation-induced thyroiditis
Palpation or trauma-induced thyroiditis

Thyroiditis Without Thyroid Pain and Tenderness

Hashimoto's Thyroiditis

Epidemiology

Hashimoto's thyroiditis (HT) was first reported in 1912 by Hakaru Hashimoto, who described four patients with a chronic disorder of the thyroid gland, termed struma lymphomatosa [3]. This entity was rarely identified for many years, but an increase in its incidence was noticed since 1940 [4]. The diagnosis was usually made after surgery. Furthermore, the routine use of the fine needle aspiration biopsy (FNAB) and measurement of thyroid autoantibodies have contributed to a significant rise in its frequency.

The annual incidence of HT for women and men is approximately 3.5 and 0.6 cases per 1000 population, respectively [5] and its estimated prevalence is about 8 cases per 1000 [6]. Women are at least six to eight times more likely to develop the disease. It occurs especially between 40 and 60 years of age, but it may be seen in any age group, including children [5, 6].

HT is now considered the most common cause of hypothyroidism in areas of the world where dietary iodine is sufficient [7], the most frequent autoimmune disease [8] and one of the main endocrine disorders [9].

It is also reported in the literature as chronic lymphocytic thyroiditis or chronic autoimmune thyroiditis.

Etiology and Pathogenesis

HT is an autoimmune disorder, thought to be caused by a combination of genetic susceptibility and environmental factors.

It seems that there is no dominant gene conferring major susceptibility to the disease. However, an association was described with human leukocyte antigen (HLA) alleles and with other genes, namely CTLA-4, thyroglobulin (Tg), PTPN22, FCRL3 and IL2RA [10, 11].

Some precipitating factors have been identified, but their role remains unknown. They include infection (e.g. hepatitis C virus, human T lymphotrophic virus-I, rubella virus, herpes simplex virus, parvovirus and Epstein-Barr virus), stress, postpartum period, iodine intake, selenium and vitamin D deficiency, drugs such as interleukin-2 (IL-2) and interferon-alpha (IFN-α), environment pollutants and radiation exposure. More women than men have HT, which can be explained by skewed X chromosome inactivation, the role of sex steroids and fetal microchimerism. The prevalence of the disease increases with age, which may reflect an increasing loss of tolerance to self. Smoking has a surprisingly beneficial effect on HT, in contrast to its detrimental role on Graves' disease (GD) [11, 12].

Several mechanisms have been proposed to be related to HT, namely: molecular mimicry, bystander activation, thyroid-cell expression of HLA antigens with subsequent activation of T cells, and thyroid expression of functional Fas and Fas ligand contributing to thyroid cell apoptosis [13].

Thyroid inflammation is typically characterized by both T and B lymphocytes. T cells are thought to play the main role in the disease and can act by inducing antibody production, activating cytotoxic T cells with apoptotic destruction of thyroid cells and regulating the local immune response. Type 1 and type 2 T helper cells are present in patients with HT, with a predominance of the former [14]. In addition, patients may have dysfunctional regulatory T cells [15]. B cells can produce antibodies and nearly all individuals have high serum concentrations of Tg antibodies (TgAb) and thyroid peroxidase antibodies (TPOAb), which are polyclonal and have the potential to fix complement. As a result, complement-mediated cytotoxicity may contribute to thyroid damage, but this is thought to be a second line effect [16]. Thyroid-stimulating hormone receptor antibodies (TRAb) can also be identified in the serum of patients with HT. However, these antibodies block the action of thyroid-stimulating hormone (TSH) rather than activating thyroid tissue as seen in GD [17].

Clinical Features

The disease usually occurs as a painless, diffuse and gradual enlargement of the thyroid gland [18]. The goiter is often firm and symmetrical with pyramidal lobe enlargement. The presence of well-defined nodules is unusual. Rare patients have pain and tenderness [19] or symptoms related to neck pressure such as dyspnea or dysphagia, particularly if there is a rapid thyroid swelling. The thyroid gland may also remain unchanged for several years and some patients do not develop goiter or have an atrophic gland. In fact, two forms of HT, goitrous and atrophic, were described representing extremes within the distribution rather than separate disorders [20].

The patient is usually euthyroid but symptoms and signs of mild hypothyroidism may be present [18]. Occasionally, clinical features of mild thyrotoxicosis can occur, especially during the early phase of the disease [21].

One uncommon and controversial finding of HT is Hashimoto's encephalopathy. A review published in 2006 identified only 121 cases in the literature [22]. Its mechanism is unknown and it does not appear to be related to thyroid dysfunction, as the majority of reported patients are euthyroid at the time of presentation. Evidence suggests an autoimmune vasculitis, but the role of thyroid antibodies is not clear [23]. Patient most often have an acute to subacute onset of confusion with alteration of consciousness and other neurologic signs, such as seizures, myoclonus, tremor, hyperreflexia and psychosis [22, 24]. The diagnosis is usually performed by the presence of clinical manifestations in patients with elevated thyroid antibodies. A response to corticosteroids can also favor the diagnosis [25]. Other exams may be performed and are important in the differential diagnosis. Most patients respond to steroid therapy and prognosis is usually good [22, 24].

Diagnostic Evaluation

Patients with HT usually undergo a gradual loss of thyroid function. Approximately 75 % have normal thyroid function at diagnosis but they can develop subclinical or overt hypothyroidism [18], which is permanent in most cases. However, some patients may recover and reach euthyroidism, possibly explained by the decrease over time of TSH receptor blocking antibodies [26]. Rarely, the inflammatory process in the early course of the disease may cause severe apoptosis and thyroid damage, with subsequent thyroid hormone release and transient hyperthyroidism; this condition is termed Hashitoxicosis and usually evolves into permanent hypothyroidism [18, 21].

Serum concentrations of thyroid antibodies are almost always elevated. TPOAb and TgAb are positive in about 95 % and 60–80 % of patients, respectively [18].

A cervical ultrasound (US) may display an enlarged gland with very low echogenicity, or a suggestion of multiple ill-defined nodules. Most commonly the gland is two to four times the normal size.

Radioactive iodine uptake (RAIU) test, although rarely required, is variable and ranges from below normal to elevated values. Thyroid scan is not necessary in most cases and the typical finding is a diffuse or mottled uptake in an enlarged gland.

FNAB can be useful in patients with nodular disease. It usually reveals lymphocytes, macrophages, scant colloid and epithelial cells which may show Hurthle cell features. However, some aspirates lack inflammatory cells and consist almost exclusively of Hurthle cells, leading to a misleading result of Hurthle cell tumor [27].

Histological examination often reveals lymphoplasmacytic infiltration, lymphoid follicles with germinal center formation, epithelial cell destruction, the presence of large follicular cells with abundant granular eosinophilic cytoplasm, known as oxyphilic, Hurthle or Askanazy cells, and various degrees of fibrosis [18].

HT is often associated with type 1 diabetes mellitus (T1DM), celiac disease, Addison's disease, Sjögren syndrome and other autoimmune disorders in the context of polyglandular autoimmune syndromes. The link between HT and thyroid cancer remains controversial. This association was first described by Dailey et al. in 1955 [28]. Some authors reported that patients with HT have a threefold increased risk of papillary thyroid carcinoma (PTC) as compared to non-HT patients [29], but others stated that there is inconsistent evidence favoring a causal relationship between these entities [30]. Thyroid cancer may be associated with a less aggressive disease and a better prognosis in patients with coexisting HT [31].

The diagnosis of HT is usually performed in a patient with a diffuse goiter and one other biochemical or histological feature, such as positive TPOAb, positive TgAb or lymphocytic infiltration of the thyroid gland [32]. However, goiter can be absent and the presence of serum thyroid autoantibodies may be sufficient evidence of the diagnosis. For many years, HT has been characterized as a well-defined clinicopathologic entity. However, it is now considered a heterogeneous disease, with several subtypes: classic form, fibrous variant, IgG4-related variant, juvenile form (presented before 18 years of age), Hashitoxicosis and painless thyroiditis, the latter occurring either sporadically or in the postpartum period. They share the diagnostic characteristics of HT but have some interesting particularities [18].

The fibrous variant accounts for 10–13 % of HT cases and usually affects older patients. Its diagnostic criteria were defined by Katz and Vickery in 1974 and included a marked fibrous replacement of more than one-third of the thyroid parenchyma and changes typical of HT in the remaining tissue [33]. Most patients are hypothyroid at presentation.

The IgG4-related variant of HT is a new subtype, first recognized by Li et al. in 2009 [34]. It may be part of the systemic IgG4-related disease. The diagnosis of this systemic disorder includes, independently of the affected organ, histological features such as a dense lymphoplasmacytic infiltrate, storiform-type fibrosis and obliterative phlebitis, along with the demonstration of an increased population of IgG4-positive plasma cells [35, 36]. Cheuk and Chan considered that it requires an increase in the absolute number of IgG4-positive cells of > 50 per high power field and a raised IgG4-positive/IgG-positive ratio of > 40 % [37]. Deshpande et al. stated that histological data are the mainstay for diagnosis, since both elevated numbers of IgG4-positive plasma cells and IgG4/IgG ratios have been described in other inflammatory conditions and malignancies [38]. A high serum IgG4 concentration is often present but approximately 20–30 % of patients with classic histopathological and immunochemical findings of the disease have normal serum levels [39].

Therefore, the IgG4 variant of HT is characterized by thyroid inflammation rich in IgG4-positive plasma cells and marked fibrosis (Fig. 6.1). It is usually associated with male gender, rapid progress requiring surgery, more subclinical hypothyroidism, higher levels of thyroid autoantibodies and more diffuse low echogenicity on US, when compared with the non-IgG4 variant [40]. In 2012, Kakudo et al. studied 105 patients with HT and classified 28 cases (27 %) as IgG4 thyroiditis based on immunohistochemistry [41]. We recently presented the first case of IgG4-related HT in a non-Asian patient [42] (Fig. 6.2). Since this condition seems to be more common than previously thought, we suggest performing the immunostaining in a patient who presents with these typical clinical features and with lymphoplasmacytic infiltration and marked fibrosis of the thyroid gland.

Differential Diagnosis

HT has to be distinguished from nontoxic multinodular goiter, thyroid cancer and GD.

In multinodular goiter, thyroid function tests are usually normal and thyroid autoantibodies are absent or identified at low titers. Cervical US shows well-defined nodules and the thyroid scan can also be helpful. FNAB can distinguish these entities but is usually not performed.

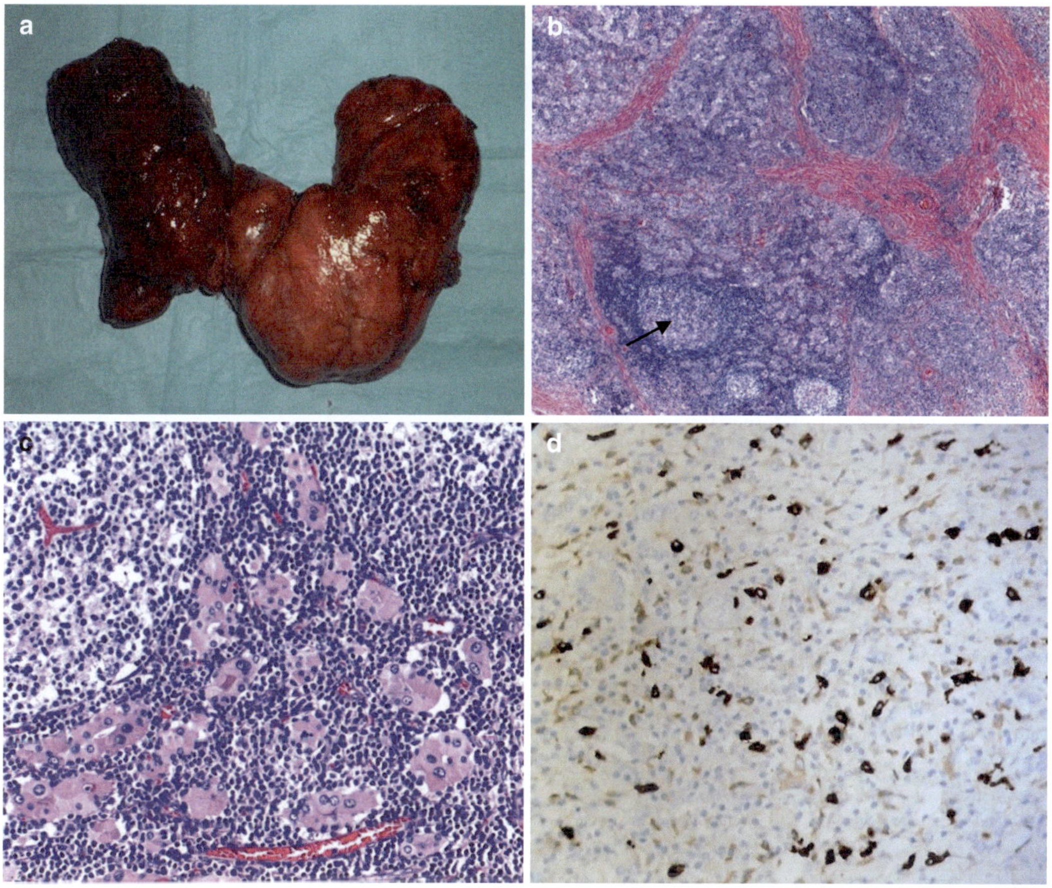

Fig. 6.1 Typical histopathological findings of a patient with the diagnosis of IgG4-related Hashimoto's thyroiditis. (**a**) Large thyroid gland with a hard consistency. (**b**) An inflammatory infiltrate is seen, along with lymphoid follicles with germinal centers (*black arrow*) and marked fibrosis (hematoxylin and eosin, 40×). (**c**) Lymphoplasmacytic infiltration is found and atrophic follicles with oxyphilic cells predominate (hematoxylin and eosin, 200×). (**d**) Increased number of IgG4-positive plasma cells are seen, with > 50 cells per high-power field (IgG4 immunostaining, 400×). (From Luiz et al. [42], with permission)

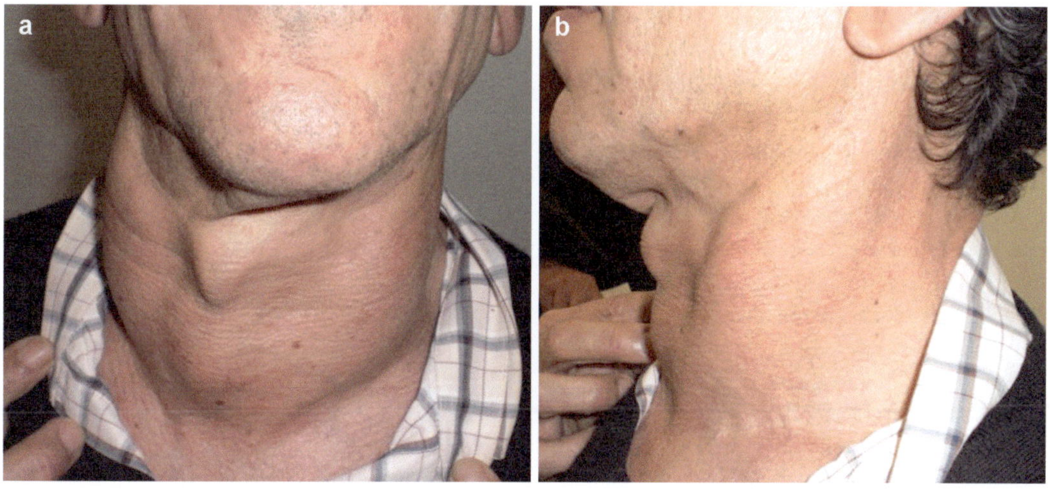

Fig. 6.2 A male patient with IgG4-related Hashimoto's thyroiditis, presenting with a diffuse neck swelling of rapid growing. (**a**) anterior view. (**b**) lateral view

Thyroid carcinoma must also be considered, especially if there is rapid growth of the gland or evidence of pain. Clinical findings, cervical US, thyroid scan and FNAB can be useful in the differential diagnosis. Thyroid lymphoma may also be considered in a patient with progressive and asymmetric enlargement of the thyroid gland, or if pain and tenderness appear. HT is a known risk factor for primary thyroid lymphoma [43].

The differentiation between HT and GD relies on clinical, biochemical and image exams, but the distinction of these entities is sometimes difficult because findings may overlap.

Treatment

Patients with HT should have regular follow-up. Treatment options are dependent on the thyroid function and the presence of symptoms. Asymptomatic and euthyroid patients do not require treatment. When hypothyroidism develops, it is usually permanent and replacement treatment with levothyroxine (L-T4) is required indefinitely in these patients. We suggest starting L-T4 in those with overt hypothyroidism or subclinical hypothyroidism with a TSH level above 10 mIU/L. Treatment can also be considered in patients with a TSH level between 4.5 and 10 mIU/L and positive thyroid antibodies. Ideal body weight is used for dose calculations, usually 1.6–1.8 μg/Kg of ideal body weight daily in adults. It is recommended to start with the full calculated dose in healthy young and middle-aged patients. A low starting dose should be given to older patients and those with coronary heart disease, with gradual dose increase. Some authors also recommend L-T4 therapy if a large goiter causing local pressure symptoms is present [1, 2]. The size of the thyroid gland decreases at least 30 % in about half of treated cases. The results are better in younger patients possibly because of the presence of fibrosis in those with a long-standing goiter.

Glucocorticoids are not usually recommended but can be used in cases presenting with pain.

Surgery is not indicated, unless significant pain, cosmetic and pressure symptoms occur, or in the presence of a nodule with a cytology suspicious for malignancy [44].

When a preoperative suspicion of IgG4-related HT is high, glucocorticoid therapy may improve local symptoms and clinical outcomes. However, as these patients usually present with a rapidly progressing neck swelling, surgery is often the first choice for treatment.

Painless Thyroiditis

Epidemiology

Painless thyroiditis is considered a subtype of HT [1].

It accounts for 1–23 % of hyperthyroidism cases [45] and usually presents between 20 and 40 years of age. When compared to other forms of thyroiditis, it has a lower female to male ratio of 2:1 to 3:1 [46].

Synonyms for this disorder include silent thyroiditis, subacute lymphocytic thyroiditis, and lymphocytic thyroiditis with spontaneously resolving hyperthyroidism.

Postpartum thyroiditis is considered a similar condition but, because of the particular features of the postpartum period, it will be discussed separately.

Etiology and Pathogenesis

Painless thyroiditis is an autoimmune disorder [1]. It seems to be associated with specific HLA haplotypes, suggesting a genetic susceptibility [47].

The inflammatory process damages thyroid follicles with a release of stored thyroid hormones into the circulation. The resulting hyperthyroidism is transient and occurs only until the stores are exhausted. New hormone synthesis is absent due to thyroid inflammation and destruction of follicular cells, and also because of the low levels of TSH during the hyperthyroid state. Thereafter, a transient period of hypothyroidism may ensue. As inflammation subsides, thyroid follicles recover and normal thyroid function occurs in most cases (Fig. 6.3).

Clinical Features

This disorder is classically characterized by a triphasic course of hyperthyroidism followed by hypothyroidism, and then recovery, similar to the

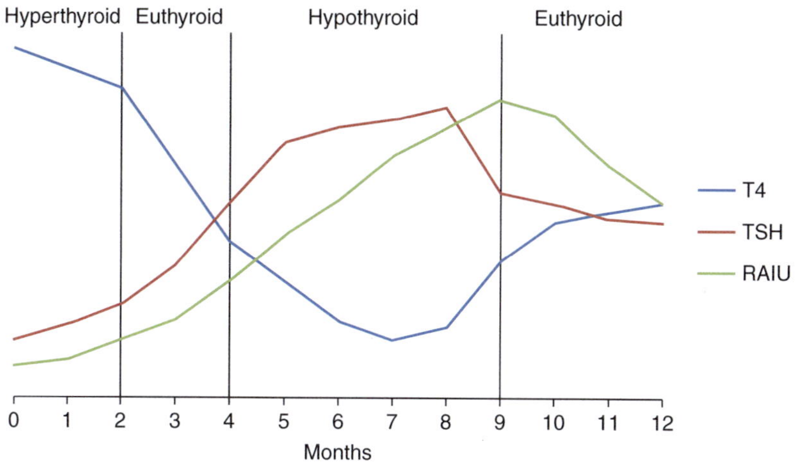

Fig. 6.3 Characteristic triphasic course of painless, postpartum and subacute thyroiditis. Abbreviations: *RAIU* radioactive iodine uptake, *T4* thyroxine, *TSH* thyroid-stimulating hormone

pattern found in postpartum and subacute thyroiditis [1, 2]. However, some patients only have a transient hyperthyroid or hypothyroid phase.

Hyperthyroid symptoms have an abrupt onset over 1–2 weeks but are usually mild, lasting from 4 to 8 weeks. Hypothyroidism is also mild or even asymptomatic, and may be present for 2–9 months [48, 49]. Some patients have no symptoms or signs related to thyroid dysfunction and are diagnosed incidentally by routine exams.

The thyroid gland is not painful or tender and has a normal or slightly increased size [49, 50].

Diagnostic Evaluation

The diagnosis of painless thyroiditis relies on clinical manifestations, laboratory findings and thyroid scan images.

If clinical suspicion is high, measurement of serum thyroid function is recommended. The results vary over the course of the disease, and changes in free thyroxine (T4) and triiodothyronine (T3) usually precede those of TSH. During the early period, overt or subclinical hyperthyroidism may be present and an increase of free T4 over T3 is typically found. Thyroid function tests should be monitored on a regular basis (e.g. every 4–8 weeks). Some patients may recover and others develop overt or subclinical hypothyroidism. When inflammation subsides, euthyroidism is almost always achieved, but some may remain hypothyroid. Chronic thyroid disease can also appear in almost 50 % of patients during subsequent follow-up, usually related to the development of goiter but permanent hypothyroidism may occur in 6 % of patients [45, 51].

Positive serum TPOAb and TgAb are present in about 57 and 38 % of patients, respectively, with lower titers when compared to HT [46, 49]. The white blood cell (WBC) count is often normal, and the erythrocyte sedimentation rate (ESR) and C-reactive protein (CRP) are also normal or slightly increased [46, 49].

The RAIU test can be performed in the hyperthyroid phase if the diagnosis is uncertain, yielding a low result of about 1 % [46, 48, 49]. Similarly, thyroid scan shows a very low radiotracer accumulation in the thyroid gland.

Cervical US may be helpful in some patients, showing a normal-sized or slightly enlarged, heterogeneous and hypoechogenic thyroid gland. Color flow Doppler sonography (CFDS) is normal or low during the hyperthyroid period.

FNAB is not typically performed. It can reveal lymphocytes and macrophages, thyroid epithelial cells and masses of colloid.

Histological features are similar to those found in HT, but patients with painless thyroiditis often show fewer lymphoid follicles and germinal centers, less fibrosis and lack Hurthle cells [46, 52].

Differential Diagnosis

During the hyperthyroid period, painless thyroiditis must be distinguished from the more common GD. The former is usually self-limited, lacks ophthalmopathy, presents with mild thyroid enlargement and has a low thyroid RAIU, which contrast to the findings found in the latter. Laboratory data suggesting painless thyroiditis include a predominance of T4 over T3 and absence of TRAb, while in GD the rise in T3 prevails and antibodies are typically elevated. In addition, thyroid CFDS is normal or decreased in patients with painless thyroiditis and increased in Graves' hyperthyroidism [2, 53]. During the hypothyroid phase, the differential diagnosis between painless and HT may be difficult. Clues that suggest the former include the presence of self-limited symptoms of hyperthyroidism preceding hypothyroidism and spontaneous normalization of thyroid function over weeks.

Treatment

Some patients do not need treatment during either the hyperthyroid or the hypothyroid periods, because thyroid dysfunction is often mild and transient.

Patients with biochemical confirmation of hyperthyroidism who develop symptoms or those with an increased risk for atrial fibrillation should be treated with a beta-blocker. Glucocorticoid therapy is rarely used and should be reserved for more severe cases [49, 51]. Antithyroid drugs or radioactive iodine are not indicated, because thyrotoxicosis is not caused by excess thyroid hormone synthesis and the RAIU is low. During the hypothyroidism phase, treatment with L-T4 should be started in patients with symptoms. It may also be considered when the TSH exceeds 10 mIU/L, even if symptoms of hypothyroidism are absent. Hormone replacement can be progressively discontinued after 3–6 months, with subsequent regular monitoring of thyroid function.

After recovery, the follow-up should be continued due to the risk of permanent hypothyroidism. Furthermore, additional episodes of thyroiditis can occur in approximately 10 % of patients [51, 54].

Postpartum Thyroiditis

Epidemiology

Postpartum thyroiditis is characterized by the occurrence of painless thyroiditis within 1 year after a delivery in women who were euthyroid prior to pregnancy [55, 56]. It can also appear after an abortion [57].

The general prevalence of the disease varies widely, ranging from 1 to 17 % of pregnancies, with a mean value of approximately 8 % [58, 59]. An increased prevalence is found in some groups of women, such as in those with T1DM (25 %), chronic viral hepatitis (25 %), prior history of GD (44 %), previous episode of postpartum thyroiditis (42–70 %) and positive TPOAb early in pregnancy (40–60 %) [55, 56, 59].

Etiology and Pathogenesis

Postpartum thyroiditis is an autoimmune disorder and it reflects the immune suppression that occurs during pregnancy followed by the rebound in the postpartum period [56].

It is also associated with particular HLA haplotypes [60], suggesting that genetic susceptibility is important. As previously noted, several factors increase the risk of developing the disease.

The inflammatory process results in damage of thyroid follicles with the same thyroid function abnormalities described for painless thyroiditis (Fig. 6.3).

Clinical Features

The presentation can be identical to painless thyroiditis, but the course of postpartum thyroiditis may be more variable. Approximately 20–30 % have the triphasic course of hyperthyroidism, which usually occurs within 3 months after delivery and lasts 1–3 months, followed by a period of hypothyroidism, often lasting 4–6 months, and then recovery. However, 20–40 % present only with transient hyperthyroidism, and the remaining 40–50 % have only a transient period of hypothyroidism [55, 61, 62].

During the thyrotoxic phase, most women are asymptomatic or develop mild symptoms. Clinical findings related to hypothyroidism are more common but also usually not severe [56, 61, 62]. Some authors suggest a relationship between the hypothyroid phase of postpartum thyroiditis and postpartum depression [63, 64], but others did not find any association [65]. There is insufficient data to conclude if these entities are related [62]. Most women have a slightly enlarged, diffuse, painless and nontender thyroid gland.

Diagnostic Evaluation

The diagnosis is based upon clinical manifestations and thyroid function tests.

There is insufficient data to recommend screening for postpartum thyroiditis in all cases. However, measuring of TSH levels at 3 and 6 months postpartum is recommended for women at highest risk for developing the disease, namely those with positive TPOAb, T1DM, chronic viral hepatitis, GD in remission and previous episode of postpartum thyroiditis [55]. A recent article suggests gestational diabetes as an additional risk factor and recommends screening for thyroid disorders in this group of women [66].

If clinical suspicion of postpartum thyroiditis is high, measurement of serum thyroid function is recommended. Given the potential association with postpartum depression and since hypothyroidism is a reversible cause of depression, thyroid function tests should also be performed in women with postpartum depression [55, 56]. The biochemical findings are similar to those found in patients with painless thyroiditis with variable results during the course of the disease. Overt or subclinical hyperthyroidism may be present during the early period. Thyroid function tests should be monitored every 4–8 weeks until 1 year postpartum to confirm resolution or to detect the development of hypothyroidism. When inflammation subsides, most patients achieve euthyroidism. However, some women with reversible hypothyroidism can develop permanent hypothyroidism in approximately 38–64 % of cases during long-term follow-up [62, 67, 68], especially those who have high TPOAb [69].

Positive TPOAb are present in about 60 % of patients [70].

The WBC count, ESR and CRP levels are typically normal, but may be slightly elevated.

Cervical US findings can be similar to those described in painless thyroiditis.

Thyroid scan is usually not necessary and special care should be taken in women who are breastfeeding. During the hyperthyroid phase, RAIU is typically low.

FNAB and histological findings are also similar to those reported for painless thyroiditis.

Recently, the first association between postpartum thyroiditis and thyroid hormone resistance was described [71].

Differential Diagnosis

During the hyperthyroid phase, postpartum thyroiditis has to be distinguished from GD, which can also present during the postpartum period. The former usually occurs within 3 months after delivery and the latter often develops after 4–6 months. CFDS and serum TRAb can be useful [72]. Other clues to distinguish these entities are discussed in the differential diagnosis of painless thyroiditis.

During the hypothyroid phase, HT should be considered. Normalization of thyroid function within weeks without the need of thyroid hormone replacement suggests the diagnosis of postpartum thyroiditis.

Treatment

There is no recommended treatment to prevent the disease. Administration of L-T4 or iodine in the postpartum period to women with high serum levels of TPOAb did not decrease the incidence of postpartum thyroiditis [73]. Selenium supplementation administered during and after pregnancy may reduce the incidence of this disorder in women with positive TPOAb [74]. However, the routine use of this supplementation needs further study [56, 62].

Most women with postpartum thyroiditis do not require any treatment during either the hyperthyroid or the hypothyroid phases. If needed, the therapeutic options are the same as were discussed for painless thyroiditis.

Women who have bothersome symptoms of hyperthyroidism can be treated with beta-blockers. Propranolol is usually the preferred and safest drug for those who are breastfeeding because, compared to other beta-blockers, it has high protein binding resulting in low diffusion into breast milk [75]. Antithyroid drugs or radioactive iodine are not indicated.

Women with symptomatic hypothyroidism, TSH levels exceeding 10 mIU/L or considering another pregnancy should be treated with L-T4. Patients not treated have to be monitored with thyroid function tests and treatment may be considered if hypothyroidism persists [55, 56]. The decision to discontinue L-T4 should be individualized. Many experts favor weaning L-T4 after 6–12 months, unless the woman is pregnant, attempting pregnancy, or breastfeeding. Thyroid function should be regularly monitored. A rise in the TSH level suggests permanent hypothyroidism. If normal thyroid function is achieved after thyroid hormone withdrawal, lifelong follow-up for persistent hypothyroidism is required, initially more frequently and then on an annual basis [56].

Amiodarone-Associated Thyroiditis

Epidemiology

Amiodarone is associated with thyroid dysfunction, including both hypothyroidism and thyrotoxicosis [76–78].

The prevalence of amiodarone-induced thyrotoxicosis (AIT) ranges between 5 and 12 % of treated patients [79, 80] and is more common in men [78]. It can be related to an increased synthesis of thyroid hormone (type I) in iodine-deficient regions or to a destructive thyroiditis (type II) in iodine-sufficient areas [76]. Only the latter will be discussed in this chapter.

Type II AIT usually presents in patients without prior thyroid disease [81]. It is the main type in the United States due to normal dietary iodine intake.

Etiology and Pathogenesis

The type II form is not related to iodine and results from a direct toxic effect of the drug on thyroid follicular cells [76, 81, 82]. This results in a destructive thyroiditis with excess release of preformed thyroid hormones into the bloodstream. It may be followed by a transient period of hypothyroidism with recovery of normal thyroid function in most cases [77].

Clinical Features

Manifestations of hyperthyroidism are sometimes masked due to the beta-blocking activity of the drug. Patients may be asymptomatic or have weight loss along with other nonspecific symptoms. However, atrial fibrillation, exacerbation of ischemic heart disease or heart failure may also occur.

The thyroid gland is usually normal or mildly enlarged and is usually painless and nontender [77].

Diagnostic Evaluation

Thyroid function should be ordered before amiodarone is started and monitored every 3–6 months during treatment. The drug has a half-life of 50–100 days and remains available for a long period after its discontinuation. For that reason, thyrotoxicosis may occur after amiodarone withdrawal and therefore assessment of thyroid function after treatment should be considered [83].

Type II AIT is characterized by thyroid function tests consistent with hyperthyroidism, sometimes followed by transient hypothyroidism and recovery [77].

Thyroid US usually shows a hypoechoic gland with absent vascularity on CFDS. RAIU is low or absent.

Differential Diagnosis

The distinction between type I and type II AIT is crucial, because the therapeutic approach varies depending on the type. However, the differential diagnosis may be difficult and some patients may have a mixture of both mechanisms [78]. Some features help in distinguishing the two types. If the RAIU is detectable, it suggests type I AIT. Patients with type I often have a goiter, whereas those with type II usually present with a normal thyroid gland. CFDS shows increased vascularity in type I and absent vascularity in type II hyperthyroidism (Table 6.2) [76, 84–86].

Table 6.2 Differential diagnosis between type I and type II amiodarone-induced thyrotoxicosis (AIT)

Feature	Type I AIT	Type II AIT
Epidemiology	Iodine-deficient areas	Iodine-sufficient areas
Underlying thyroid disease	Present	Absent
Pathogenesis	Iodine-induced hyperthyroidism	Destructive thyroiditis
Hypothyroid phase	Absent	Sometimes present
Thyroid antibodies	Often present	Usually absent
Thyroid ultrasound	Goiter	Normal-sized and hypoechoic thyroid gland or small goiter
Color flow Doppler sonography	Increased vascularity	Reduced or absent vascularity
Radioactive iodine uptake	Low, normal or increased	Low or absent
Spontaneous remission	No	Possible
Treatment	Thionamides (e.g. methimazole)	Glucocorticoids (e.g. prednisone)

Treatment

There is no consensus if amiodarone should be discontinued after the development of thyrotoxicosis but most authors consider that, if possible, the drug should be suspended [76, 87]. However, the decision should be determined on an individual basis and often shared with a cardiologist [78, 88].

AIT is associated with increased mortality and treatment should be promptly started. The type II form is treated with glucocorticoids (e.g. prednisone 40–60 mg/day), usually for 1–3 months and then slowly discontinued [77, 78]. Patients usually respond well and achieve euthyroidism. A delayed improvement can be related to a large goiter or to severe initial thyrotoxicosis [89].

In patients with a "mixed" form, a therapeutic combination for both type I and type II thyrotoxicosis may be started using prednisone and methimazole [78]. Combination therapy should also be considered for those who fail to respond to glucocorticoids [88]. Total thyroidectomy may be necessary in individuals who are refractory to other treatment options and if a rapid restoration of euthyroidism is needed [76, 90]. Surgery is usually performed after a short course of iopanoic acid to restore euthyroidism [91]. Radioiodine is not indicated.

Patients can develop transient or permanent hypothyroidism when the hyperthyroidism resolves and may benefit from L-T4 replacement.

In those who recover from thyroiditis and that have suspended amiodarone, reintroducing the drug may be considered and most patients remain euthyroid [92].

Thyroiditis Induced by Other Drugs

In addition to amiodarone, several drugs are associated with the development of thyroiditis, including lithium, IFN-α, IL-2 and tyrosine kinase inhibitors (TKI) [93].

Lithium

Epidemiology

Lithium can cause goiter, thyroid autoimmunity, hypothyroidism and hyperthyroidism [93, 94].

The incidence of hyperthyroidism in patients treated with the drug may be more than three times greater than that predicted for the general population [95].

Etiology and Pathogenesis

Hyperthyroidism can be related to GD, toxic nodular goiter and destructive thyroiditis [95]. In fact, lithium might directly damage thyroid cells, with consequent release of Tg and thyroid hormones into the circulation [94].

Clinical Features, Diagnostic Evaluation and Differential Diagnosis

These characteristics depend on the etiology of the thyroid disorder.

Patients treated with this drug should have a thyroid physical examination and be checked for thyroid dysfunction before it is started. Thyroid function has to be monitored during treatment on a regular basis (e.g. every 6–12 months).

Treatment

The occurrence of thyroid dysfunction does not typically require discontinuation of the drug. Therapeutic options are variable regarding the form of thyroiditis. The development of symptomatic destructive thyroiditis can be treated with beta-blockers [93].

Interferon-alpha

Epidemiology

IFN-α is indicated in the treatment of chronic hepatitis C, in combination with ribavirin [96].

Interferon-induced thyroiditis (IIT) is a common adverse effect of the drug, accounting for up to 40 % of treated patients [97–99].

Etiology and Pathogenesis

IIT can be classified as autoimmune and non-autoimmune [100], and each category represents 50 % of cases. It is thought to occur in genetically predisposed individuals. The autoimmune form can manifest as HT in patients who have positive thyroid antibodies before treatment and, less frequently, as GD. A subclinical disease characterized by positive thyroid autoantibodies and normal thyroid function is also commonly found.

Non-autoimmune IIT can occur as destructive thyroiditis due to a direct effect of the drug on the thyroid gland. It usually starts with an early thyrotoxic phase, caused by the release of preformed thyroid hormones, and then progresses to a late hypothyroid period, with recovery in most cases. The non-autoimmune form can also present as clinical hypothyroidism with no detectable thyroid antibodies, also suggesting a direct effect of the drug [100, 101].

Clinical Features, Diagnostic Evaluation and Differential Diagnosis

Features are variable, depending on the thyroid disorder.

Patients should undergo routine thyroid screening before starting IFN-α therapy, during treatment (usually every 3–6 months) and at least 6 months after withdrawal because thyroid disease can develop later [98, 99, 102].

Treatment

IFN-α can usually be continued but in some cases reduction in the dose or even cessation of the drug may be needed, especially when thyrotoxicosis is present [97]. Patients should be treated according to the type of thyroid disease. In most cases thyroid dysfunction is reversible on completion of antiviral treatment [99].

Interleukin-2

Epidemiology

The incidence of hypothyroidism in patients treated with IL-2 alone or in combination with lymphokine-activated killer cells is about 20–50 % [103–105]. The occurrence of hyperthyroidism is less frequently found [106, 107].

Etiology and Pathogenesis

Hypothyroidism is caused by an autoimmune process.

Hyperthyroidism also seems to be induced by autoimmunity and usually presents with an early phase of thyrotoxicosis followed by a period of hypothyroidism and then resolution, similar to the pattern found in painless thyroiditis [93, 107].

Clinical Features, Diagnostic Evaluation and Differential Diagnosis

These characteristics vary depending on the pathogenesis.

Thyroid function should be monitored in patients receiving IL-2 [107].

Treatment

Those who develop symptoms of hypothyroidism can be treated with L-T4 [106]. Symptoms related to thyrotoxicosis may be controlled with beta-blockers [93].

Tyrosine Kinase Inhibitors

Epidemiology

TKI have a role in some specific types of cancer.

Common adverse effects include the development of hypothyroidism or hyperthyroidism [108].

Sunitinib can induce hypothyroidism in 53–85 % of patients [109, 110]. The incidence of thyroid dysfunction with sorafenib and other drugs from this therapeutic class is lower [108].

Etiology and Pathogenesis

The pathogenesis is unknown, but it seems that hypothyroidism can be related to the drug induction of autoimmunity and that hyperthyroidism results from destructive thyroiditis as a direct effect of treatment. Other hypotheses include drug inhibition of vascular endothelial growth factor receptor with subsequent reduction of thyroid vasculature and tissue damage, or the reduction of iodine uptake induced by the drug [108].

Clinical Features, Diagnostic Evaluation, Differential Diagnosis

Different findings may be present, depending on the thyroid disorder.

Monitoring thyroid function during treatment is advisable.

Treatment

Management of thyroid dysfunction should be considered, namely using L-T4 for patients with symptomatic hypothyroidism [108, 110].

Riedel's Thyroiditis

Epidemiology

Riedel's thyroiditis (RT) is a rare condition, first recognized in 1896 by Bernhard Riedel [111].

At the Mayo Clinic, 37 cases of RT were diagnosed in a series of 56,700 thyroidectomies performed between 1920 and 1984, giving an incidence of 0.06 %. The same authors reported an outpatient incidence of 1.06/100,000 [112]. Women are four to five times more likely to be affected, and the mean age at diagnosis is about 42–48 years [113, 114].

Etiology and Pathogenesis

The true etiology of this disorder is unclear. It has been described as a characteristic of end-stage subacute thyroiditis or as a primary inflammatory disorder of the thyroid gland [115, 116].

However, the most accepted mechanism considers RT as a thyroid manifestation of a systemic fibrosclerosis disorder triggered by autoimmunity. The antigen initiating the disorder is not localized within the thyroid gland, which is affected secondarily by a systemic fibroinflammatory process. This probably occurs because thyroid cells express molecules that contribute to local activation of the disease. B and T lymphocytes along with other inflammatory cells are recruited. The role of eosinophils appears to be crucial and some of their products can induce fibrosis [115].

Some authors proposed an association between RT and systemic IgG4-related disease. Therefore, IgG4-related disease of the thyroid gland may also include RT, but this is still to be confirmed [40, 117, 118].

Clinical Features

Patients usually present with a slowly growing and painless goiter. It is frequently associated with compressive symptoms including dysphagia, hoarseness and dyspnea resulting from the extension of the fibroinflammatory process beyond the thyroid capsule. In fact, the diagnosis can be suggested by the presence of local restrictive or infiltrative symptoms out of proportion to the size or extent of the thyroid lesion [116]. Features related to hypoparathyroidism may occur in 14 % of cases and are related to parathyroid gland involvement [114]. Some patients may develop mild hypothyroidism due to the extensive replacement of the thyroid gland by fibrosis, whereas hyperthyroidism is rare [113, 115].

On physical examination, the goiter is typically nontender, firm, rock-hard, and adherent to the adjacent structures [2]. It is usually symmetric and often moves poorly with swallowing.

Symptoms and signs related to the involvement of other organs in the context of systemic fibrosclerotic disease may be present [115].

Diagnostic Evaluation

Most patients have normal thyroid function tests at presentation. Hypothyroidism can develop during the course of the disease in up to 85 % of patients, and hyperthyroidism is rarely found [113, 114].

Approximately two-thirds of patients have elevated serum thyroid autoantibody concentrations [113].

The WBC count and the ESR may be normal or mildly elevated. Measurement of serum calcium and phosphorus should be performed to screen for coexistent hypoparathyroidism.

US usually reveals a diffuse hypoechoic appearance with absence of vascular flow on CFDS, due to the extensive fibrosis [119].

In patients with significant obstructive symptomatology a neck computed tomography (CT) may be ordered to establish the extent of fibrosis. It often shows a hypodense area and extrathyroidal invasion. Magnetic resonance imaging typically identifies a homogenous hypointensity on both T1 and T2 images [115, 120].

Thyroid radionuclide imaging is not routinely performed and frequently shows a low uptake [116].

FNAB usually yields non-diagnostic results. It may reveal inflammatory cells and fibrous tissue, but thyroid epithelial cells are often absent [114].

Pathologic data show an intense infiltration of lymphocytes, plasma cells and eosinophils in a dense hyalinized fibrous tissue [116, 121]. The fibrosis extends beyond the thyroid into adjacent tissues. Occlusive phlebitis is present and results from a diffuse infiltration of the walls of small and medium-sized veins by lymphocytes and plasma cells [115, 122].

The diagnostic criteria of RT were established by Woolner et al. in 1957, based on histological data [123]. They have been modified to include a fibroinflammatory process involving all or a portion of the thyroid gland, the presence of fibrous extension beyond the thyroid capsule into adjacent anatomic structures, infiltration of inflammatory cells without giant cells, lymphoid follicles, oncocytes or granulomas, evidence of occlusive phlebitis and absence of a neoplasm.

Once the diagnosis of RT is performed, a search for related fibrotic conditions should be considered. In fact, about one-third of patients with RT may develop fibrosclerosis of other tissues, namely the retroperitoneal space, mediastinum, retroorbital space or the biliary tract [112].

RT can be also associated with other autoimmune and non-autoimmune thyroid disorders [115], such as HT [124], GD [125], subacute thyroiditis [126] and thyroid cancer [127].

Differential Diagnosis

RT should be distinguished clinically and histologically from several entities, namely the fibrosing variant of HT, PTC, the paucicellular variant of anaplastic cancer, thyroid lymphoma and sarcoma [115, 116].

In addition, recent data suggest that some characteristics can help to distinguish IgG4-related HT and RT. The absence of extensive fibrosis beyond the thyroid capsule is still the most reliable evidence to confirm a diagnosis of IgG4-related HT. Furthermore, when IgG4-related disease occurs in a systemic pattern, the thyroid involvement may present as RT, since IgG4-related HT is organ-specific. In addition, obliterative phlebitis is not present in any subtype of HT [128].

Treatment

In the setting of clinical suspicion of RT, patients commonly undergo surgery to improve obstructive symptoms, establish a definitive diagnosis and rule out malignancy [115, 116]. Total thyroidectomy is often not possible because of the lack of resection planes and the high risk of complications. For that reason most authors prefer to perform a less aggressive surgery, usually an isthmusectomy to relieve constrictive pressure. Despite limited surgical intervention, approximately 39 % of patients can develop complications involving the vocal cords and the parathyroid glands [114].

After establishing the diagnosis, medical treatment should be started. Glucocorticoids are used as first-line therapy, usually prednisone at an empiric dose of 100 mg daily given for long-term. It can provide a dramatic improvement in compressive symptoms, especially when initiated early in the course of the disease [129]. In patients who fail to respond to steroids or relapse after withdrawal, tamoxifen therapy can be tried [130, 131].

Hypothyroidism, if present, should be treated with L-T4. Patients with hypoparathyroidism require treatment with calcium and calcitriol.

Infiltrative Thyroid Disorders

Several systemic infiltrative disorders can cause thyroiditis without evidence of pain or tenderness, namely amyloidosis [132, 133] and sarcoidosis [134–136].

Thyroiditis with Thyroid Pain and Tenderness

Subacute Thyroiditis

Epidemiology

The reported overall incidence of subacute thyroiditis is 4.9 cases per 100,000/year [137]. Females are four to seven times more affected than men. The disease is rare in children and usually occurs between 30 and 50 years of age [137–139].

Subacute thyroiditis is used as a synonym of subacute granulomatous thyroiditis. Other terms found in the literature are subacute nonsuppurative thyroiditis, giant cell thyroiditis, painful thyroiditis and de Quervain's thyroiditis.

Etiology and Pathogenesis

It is probably caused by a viral infection of the thyroid gland [50]. In fact, several patients have a history of an upper respiratory infection a few weeks prior to the onset of thyroiditis. Some authors suggested that the disease may have a higher incidence in summer, possibly related to the seasonal variations of viral infections [140], but others did not identify significant differences throughout the year [137].

In patients with subacute thyroiditis diagnosed during a mumps epidemic, circulating anti-mumps antibodies were identified and the virus was isolated from the thyroid gland, suggesting the mumps virus as a cause of thyroiditis [141]. Direct evidence of infection was also found for human foamy virus [142], but its implication in subacute thyroiditis has not been confirmed [143]. Numerous attempts to culture other viruses in the thyroid gland have failed. However, viral antibody titers were identified in these patients, suggesting a possible association. Some examples include measles, chicken pox, influenza, rubella, adenovirus, coxsackievirus, Epstein-Barr virus and cytomegalovirus [143].

Approximately 70 % of patients with subacute thyroiditis manifest HLA-B35 [144]. Therefore, it appears that the disease might occur through viral infections in genetically predisposed individuals. Autoimmunity does not seem to have an important role in this disorder.

Inflammation and damage to thyroid follicles occur, with development of the same thyroid dysfunction pattern described for painless and postpartum thyroiditis (Fig. 6.3).

Clinical Features

Subacute thyroiditis is characterized by neck pain in more than 95 % of cases [137, 138]. Rare patients have minimal or absent pain [145]. The onset can be sudden or gradual and it is usually bilateral but may be located in one lobe and then spreads rapidly to involve the other lobe, a process known as creeping thyroiditis. Pain may radiate to the jaw, ears or occiput and some patients also complaint of dysphagia, mimicking disorders arising in these areas [48]. Sometimes the clinical presentation is preceded by an upper respiratory infection.

The thyroid gland is typically enlarged two or three times the normal size and nearly always tender. Myalgia, arthralgia, tremor, sweating and weight loss may be present along with mild to moderate fever [137].

A triphasic course is often identified, characterized by hyperthyroidism followed by hypothyroidism and then recovery. At least one-half of patients have mild and transient symptoms and signs of hyperthyroidism [139], usually subsiding in 3–6 weeks [50]. However, rare patients can develop severe side effects such as adverse cardiac outcomes and thyroid storm [146]. The hypothyroid phase occurs in about one-third of cases and is usually asymptomatic lasting from 2 weeks to 6 months [50].

Diagnostic Evaluation

The diagnosis relies mostly on clinical findings.

If a patient presents with the typical symptoms and signs, thyroid function tests should be performed, showing variable results over the course of the disease. Almost all patients have biochemical evidence of hyperthyroidism in the early stage of the inflammatory process. Thyroid function tests should be monitored on a regular basis to confirm recovery or to identify the occurrence of overt or subclinical hypothyroidism. Most patients achieve euthyroidism but permanent hypothyroidism can occur in approximately 5–15 % during follow-up [137, 147].

A high ESR and/or CRP measurement may help in confirming the diagnosis [148]. Liver function test abnormalities are also frequently found [149].

About 25 % of patients have positive serum thyroid antibodies, often present at low titers [138, 150].

In some cases a thyroid scan can be useful. It often shows low uptake during the thyrotoxic period [151], returning to normal or even becoming elevated in a late phase of the disease.

Thyroid US with CFDS may help in the differential diagnosis. The thyroid gland is normal or enlarged and typically hypoechogenic, showing absent vascularization during the hyperthyroid period [152, 153].

Rarely, FNAB is necessary to exclude infection or thyroid cancer. It usually reveals neutrophils, lymphocytes, histiocytes and giant cells, along with follicular cells and masses of colloid.

Histological examination shows an inflammatory process and destruction of follicles in the early phase of the disease. The most distinctive feature is the presence of granulomas, comprising clusters of giant cells within the degenerating thyroid follicles. Progressive destruction of the thyroid parenchyma with the development of fibrosis is found later in the course of this disorder [154].

Differential Diagnosis

Subacute thyroiditis is the most common cause of thyroid pain. However, another important condition to be considered is suppurative thyroiditis. Some characteristics help in distinguishing these two disorders (Table 6.3) [155, 156].

Hemorrhage into a thyroid nodule can also cause severe thyroid pain and tenderness, but it is often more sudden and transient, and the thyroid abnormalities are predominantly unilateral.

Other causes of hyperthyroidism with a low RAIU, including administration of exogenous iodine, should be excluded based on clinical findings and laboratory evaluation.

Rare patients with HT or GD can present with neck pain and tenderness and these entities should also be considered.

Painless and postpartum thyroiditis are characterized by the same triphasic pattern of thyroid dysfunction and also have a low RAIU. However, they do not usually present with thyroid pain, and their ESR is often normal.

Rarely, patients with thyroid carcinoma or lymphoma may have thyroid pain and tenderness [157]. Thyroid US and FNAB are useful in ruling out a malignancy.

Some authors reported the coexistence of subacute thyroiditis and thyroid carcinoma, and noticed that US changes related to thyroiditis may obscure the diagnosis of a PTC. Therefore, it is important to repeat US after recovery of the inflammatory process and to perform a FNAB in

Table 6.3 Differential diagnosis between subacute and suppurative thyroiditis

Characteristics	Suppurative thyroiditis	Subacute thyroiditis
History		
Preceding upper respiratory infection	88 %	17 %
Fever	100 %	54 %
Symptoms of thyrotoxicosis	Uncommon	47 %
Sore throat	90 %	36 %
Physical examination of the thyroid gland		
Painful thyroid swelling	100 %	77 %
Left side affected	85 %	Not specific
Migrating thyroid tenderness	Possible	27 %
Erythema of overlying skin	83 %	Not usually
Laboratory		
Elevated white blood cell count	57 %	25–50 %
Erythrocyte sedimentation rate (>30 mm/h)	100 %	85 %
Abnormal thyroid hormone levels (elevated or depressed)	5–10 %	60 %
Alkaline phosphatase, transaminases increased	Rare	Common
Needle aspiration		
Purulent, bacteria or fungi present	100 %	0
Lymphocytes, macrophages, some polys, giant cells	0	100 %
Radiological		
123I uptake low	Common	100 %
Abnormal thyroid scan	92 %	Non-visualized
Thyroid scan or ultrasound helpful in diagnosis	75 %	Non-specific
Gallium scan positive	100 %	100 %
18 F-fluorodeoxyglucose positron emission tomography	Positive	Positive
Barium swallow showing fistula	Common	0
Computed tomography scan useful	Varies	Not indicated
Clinical course		
Clinical response to glucocorticoid treatment	Transient	100 %
Incision and drainage required	85 %	No
Recurrence following operative drainage	16 %	No
Pyriform sinus fistula discovered	96 %	No

Republished from Lazarus J, Hennessey J. Acute and Subacute, and Riedel's Thyroiditis. In: www.thyroidmanager.org, the free on-line *Endocrinology Textbook*, version 30 March 2015, with permission

cases of hypoechoic regions measuring more than 1 cm [158, 159].

Treatment

In some patients no treatment is required, because symptoms can be mild and transient. Pain can be managed with nonsteroidal antiinflammatory drugs (NSAIDs). Glucocorticoids are typically reserved for severe cases or if NSAIDs are not effective, usually starting with prednisone 40 mg daily, with a gradual dose reduction thereafter over approximately 6 weeks [88, 160]. If pain reoccurs the dose must be increased again and tapered some weeks after. Patients treated with corticosteroids have a rapid resolution of pain in about 4 days, whereas NSAIDs provide a relief of pain in 3 weeks [137].

Patients with bothersome symptoms of hyperthyroidism may be treated with a beta-blocker. Thionamides and radioactive iodine should not be used.

Therapy for hypothyroidism is also often not needed. However, L-T4 treatment should be introduced in patients with symptoms or a TSH level above 10 mIU/L, and is usually discontinued after 3–12 months [50, 88]. Regular monitoring of thyroid function should be performed to confirm that the hypothyroidism is not permanent.

Recurrence of the inflammatory process can occur during subsequent follow-up in 1–4 % of patients with a prior episode of subacute thyroiditis [137, 161].

Suppurative Thyroiditis

Epidemiology

Suppurative thyroiditis is a rare but potentially life-threatening condition, accounting for 0.1–0.7 % of thyroid diseases [162]. Its incidence is increasing due to the higher number of immunocompromised patients.

It occurs especially in children because of the association with pyriform sinus fistula, whereas about 8 % of cases are diagnosed in adults [163].

Etiology and Pathogenesis

Suppurative thyroiditis is caused by an infection. The thyroid gland is usually resistant to infection because of its encapsulation, high iodide content, rich blood supply, and extensive lymphatic drainage [1]. However, several factors may overcome these mechanisms and predispose patients to this disorder. In children, an anomaly in the third or fourth branchial arch can be related to the development of a fistula extending from the pyriform sinus to the thyroid capsule. It is almost always left-sided, explained by the fact that the right ultimobranchial body is often atrophic. Pyriform sinus fistula is associated with a high risk of recurrent suppurative thyroiditis [164, 165]. Patients with a thyroglossal duct remnant, and immunocompromised patients such as those infected by the human immunodeficiency virus (HIV) or harboring a malignancy are predisposed to this condition [166]. It is also most likely to occur in individuals with preexisting thyroid disease [1]. FNAB can also contribute to the occurrence of suppurative thyroiditis by direct spread of pathogenic organisms, although this is a very rare complication of the procedure [167, 168].

Several organisms may reach the thyroid gland by hematogenous route or direct spread from an adjacent organ. Aerobic Gram-positive bacteria are the most common pathogens, especially *Staphylococcus aureus*, *Streptococcus pyogenes* and other Staphylococcus and Streptococcus species [166, 169, 170]. In 2013, three cases of suppurative thyroiditis caused by *Streptococcus milleri* were published [171, 172]. This organism is associated with head and neck abscess formation. Recently, in our hospital, we treated two patients with thyroid infection caused by this agent, one of them presenting with extensive involvement of cervical structures [173] and later developing recurrent disease.

Aerobic Gram-negative bacteria can also be associated with this disorder and include Klebsiella species, *Eschericia coli*, *Haemophilus influenzae*, *Eikenella corrodens* and Salmonella species. Anaerobic bacteria such as Peptostreptococcus, Bacteroides, Actinomyces and Fusobacterium species were also identified [166, 170].

Polymicrobial infection involving these agents is present in about 37 % of patients [173]. Organisms that are more rarely identified include *Mycobacterium tuberculosis*, atypical mycobacteria, fungal infections such as Aspergillus species, *Coccidioides immitis*, *Cryptococcus neoformans*, *Histoplasma capsulatum*, Candida species and *Pneumocystis jiroveci* (previously classified as *Pneumocystis carinii*) and some parasites, namely Echinococcus species and *Strongyloides stercoralis* [166, 170].

Clinical Features

Most cases present with a sudden onset of pain, often after an upper respiratory tract infection. Pain is typically unilateral and may radiate to the jaw, ears or occiput. It is reduced by neck flexion and worsened by neck hyperextension. Associated features include fever, hoarseness, dysphagia, dysphonia, local warmth and dermal erythema [169, 174]. In general, there are no signs or symptoms of hyper or hypothyroidism.

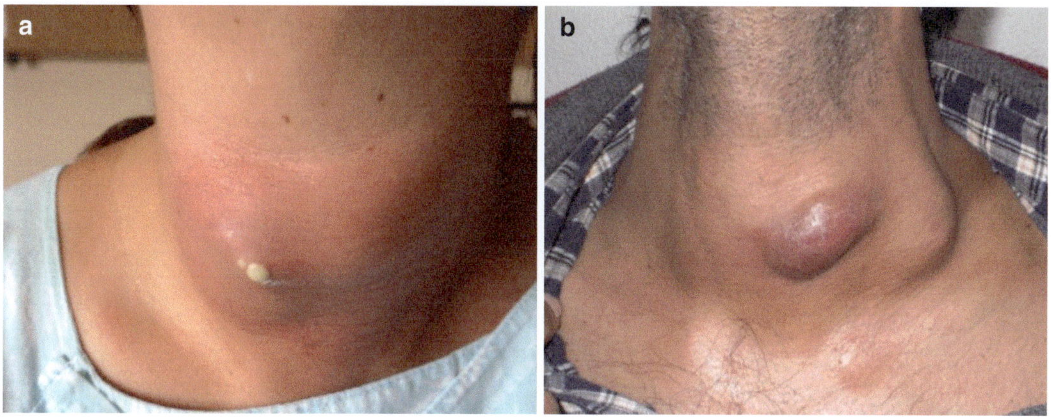

Fig. 6.4 Clinical features of two patients with suppurative thyroiditis presented to our hospital. (**a**) *Streptococcus milleri*. (**b**) *Mycobacterium tuberculosis*

On examination, a firm, tender, red and warm swelling is noticed in the anterior region of the neck (Fig. 6.4). In children the left lobe is involved in 90 % of cases due to the predominance of a left-side pyriform sinus fistula [174]. A thyroid abscess can be identified on physical exam.

The course of the disease is usually more indolent in patients with tuberculous and fungal thyroiditis, when compared to those presenting with an acute bacterial infection [175, 176].

Diagnostic Evaluation

Thyroid function tests are normal in about 90 % of patients [174]. However, this depends on the causative agent. Euthyroidism is the rule in bacterial thyroiditis, but fungal infections are often associated with hypothyroidism [171]. Patients with thyroid tuberculosis are usually euthyroid but are most likely to develop hyperthyroidism, whereas hypothyroidism is very rare [171, 175].

Leukocytosis, high ESR and elevated CRP are typical [156, 174]. Screening for HIV is recommended.

Cervical US often reveals a unifocal hypoechoic region and/or abscess formation, along with effacement of the plane between the thyroid and perithyroid tissues. Thyroid atrophy can be identified in the late inflammatory stage [177].

CT of the neck can be performed if the US is unclear or if there is extension of a thyroid abscess to other locations.

A radionuclide thyroid scan shows absent or decreased uptake in the affected lobe, but is often not needed [174].

Evaluation for pyriform sinus fistula is usually indicated, especially in children. A barium swallow study or direct laryngoscopy of the hypopharynx can be used, and the latter may be more sensitive [178, 179]. Thyroid US and CT may also suggest the presence of a fistula [180, 181].

Aspiration of the lesion by FNAB or surgical drainage should be performed to identify the causative organism, and the specimen has to be analyzed for Gram stain, culture of possible involved organisms and cytology. For patients presenting acutely, some authors choose to order blood cultures and then start empiric antibiotic treatment prior to thyroid aspiration. However, for hemodynamically stable patients, this procedure can be performed before starting antibiotic treatment [170].

In those presenting with bacterial infections, pathological examination reveals a polymorphonuclear and lymphocytic infiltrate, often with necrosis and abscess formation.

Differential Diagnosis

This entity should be differentiated from thyroid adenoma, goiter or subacute thyroiditis. The differences between suppurative and subacute thyroiditis are described in Table 6.3 [155, 156]. In summary, systemic manifestations are less severe in subacute thyroiditis and the inflammation process is usually transient, whereas untreated suppurative thyroiditis typically results in severe complications.

Intracystic hemorrhage, painful HT and malignancy should also be considered. The latter is usually distinguished by US and FNAB. Thyroid malignancy and suppurative thyroiditis may coexist, and the inflammatory condition can be the presenting manifestation disclosing the diagnosis of a carcinoma [182].

Treatment

Traditional therapy has been surgery, either thyroidectomy or surgical drainage, combined with targeted antibiotic therapy. However, antibiotic therapy without invasive surgery is now considered the mainstay of treatment in most cases [170].

Suppurative thyroiditis requires immediate parenteral antibiotics which are started empirically. Given the wide range of potentially involved organisms, broad spectrum antibiotics are indicated and the regimen is usually individualized. In an immunocompetent patient, initial empiric therapy can include a penicillin and a β-lactamase inhibitor (e.g. piperacillin/tazobactam). Options for patients with HIV infection require consideration of opportunistic organisms. Subsequent treatment should be adjusted to microbiology and antimicrobial susceptibility data. In addition, if an abscess is identified, surgical drainage should be performed. For mild infections or after clinical improvement, treatment with oral antibiotics may be an option [170, 178, 183, 184].

Cervical CT or US are used to monitor patients regarding the persistence or resolution of suppurative thyroiditis. If extensive disease is present or the infection persists despite treatment, thyroid lobectomy may be necessary [170]. Surgery is also important to repair the developmental abnormality that predisposed the patient to infection, most commonly a fistula from a pyriform sinus. This procedure can be performed surgically or by endoscopic cauterization, usually after resolution of the thyroid abscess and improvement of clinical symptoms [179, 185–187].

Antibiotic treatment should be administered for at least 14 days. In patients with pyriform sinus fistula, it is reasonable to continue antibiotic therapy until its elective correction [170].

The prognosis is usually excellent and clinical recovery is the rule after appropriate treatment [170]. Rare patients develop permanent hypothyroidism or extension of the infection into adjacent structures. However, local and systemic complications may be life-threatening if therapy is delayed or inadequate [1].

Radiation-Induced Thyroiditis

Epidemiology

Patients submitted to radioiodine may develop thyroiditis. The prevalence is about 1 % in those treated for hyperthyroidism and higher in those receiving radioiodine for postoperative thyroid remnant ablation in differentiated thyroid cancer [188, 189]. Radiation-induced thyroiditis may be most likely to occur after treatment of toxic multinodular goiter than GD [190] and when higher doses of 131I are administered [189].

Other individuals at higher risk include the elderly, those with severe thyrotoxicosis or significant weight loss, and those with cardiovascular or cerebrovascular disease [191].

Etiology and Pathogenesis

The most accepted mechanism is radiation-induced damage of the thyroid follicles with release of preformed thyroid hormones into the circulation, resulting in thyrotoxicosis and then recovery [188].

Clinical Features

Patients usually present with mild to severe neck pain, tenderness and neck swelling, starting within 2 weeks after 131I administration. Exacerbation of mild symptoms and signs of thyrotoxicosis are also common. Clinical findings are typically transient and disappear in days or weeks [192, 193].

However, severe hyperthyroidism may occur and thyroid storm as been very rarely described [191]. We recently evaluated a patient with GD that developed thyroid storm after radioiodine treatment; the hyperthyroidism was very difficult to control requiring plasmapheresis (unpublished work).

Diagnostic Evaluation

Thyroid function tests often reveal transient hyperthyroidism.

Other findings are similar to those identified in other forms of destructive thyroiditis.

Differential Diagnosis

After 131I therapy for hyperthyroidism, it can be difficult to differentiate between treatment failure and thyroiditis [194]. A retrospective study indicates that the former can be considered if thyrotoxicosis has not improved within 3 months [195].

Treatment

Some authors recommend pretreatment of hyperthyroid patients with antithyroid drugs, to prevent the occurrence of transient hyperthyroidism after radioiodine [191, 192]; but others did not find any beneficial effect [196].

NSAIDs are usually sufficient for analgesia, but prednisone may be required. Symptoms of hyperthyroidism may be managed with beta-blockers [188].

Palpation or Trauma-Induced Thyroiditis

Epidemiology

Vigorous palpation of the thyroid gland [197], manipulation during thyroid biopsy [198], neck surgery [199, 200] and trauma [201] can cause a particular form of thyroid inflammation, known as palpation or trauma-induced thyroiditis.

Carney et al. in 1975 identified specific pathological findings in dogs after vigorous squeezing of their thyroid glands. A similar disorder in humans was believed to result from traumatic injury or rupture of thyroid follicles caused by palpation. The authors also found the histological changes in at least 83 % of human thyroids removed surgically [197].

In addition, transient hyperthyroidism has been shown to occur postoperatively in 20–29 % of patients undergoing surgical treatment of primary hyperparathyroidism [199, 202].

Etiology and Pathogenesis

Manipulation and trauma of the thyroid gland is thought to induce leakage of thyroid hormones into the circulation, resulting in a transient period of thyrotoxicosis.

Clinical Features

It usually presents as neck pain, tenderness and symptoms of hyperthyroidism. New-onset atrial fibrillation due to thyrotoxicosis has been noticed following neck exploratory surgery [203].

Diagnostic Evaluation

Thyroid function tests often reveal transient hyperthyroidism with subsequent normalization of thyroid function [200].

As in other forms of destructive thyroiditis, ESR and CRP can be elevated, CFDS shows decreased vascularity and RAIU is usually low [2, 198, 203].

Histological changes typically found in these patents are described as multifocal granulomatous folliculitis [197, 204].

Differential Diagnosis

This entity should be distinguished from other causes of hyperthyroidism, including GD and subacute thyroiditis.

Treatment

Glucocorticoids can be used to induce symptoms relief [203].

Conclusion

Several types of thyroiditis were described, characterized by thyroid inflammation. However, each form has particular characteristics, such as specific incidence/prevalence, etiopathogenesis, clinical features, laboratory and image results, pathology findings, differential diagnosis and therapeutic options. Table 6.4 provides an overview of the main forms of thyroiditis.

It is crucial that physicians and other health professionals be aware of the classification

Table 6.4 Overview of the main forms of thyroiditis

	Epidemiology	Etiology and Pathogenesis	Clinical features	Diagnostic evaluation	Differential diagnosis	Treatment
Hashimoto's thyroiditis	Incidence: 3.5 (♀) and 0.6 (♂) /1000/year ♀:♂, 6:1–8:1 Peak age: 40–60 years	Autoimmune Genetic susceptibility Environmental factors	Painless goiter Mild hypothyroidism	Euthyroidism or hypothyroidism High thyroid antibodies US: low echogenicity Pathology: lymphocytic infiltration	Multinodular goiter Thyroid carcinoma Lymphoma Graves' disease	LT4
Painless thyroiditis	1–23 % of hyperthyroidism cases ♀:♂, 2:1–3:1 Peak age: 20–40 years	Autoimmune Genetic susceptibility	Variable symptoms of thyroid dysfunction Small painless goiter	Triphasic course (hyperthyroidism, hypothyroidism and recovery) US: hypoechogenicity CFDS: normal/low flow (hyperthyroid phase) RAIU: low (hyperthyroid phase) Pathology: lymphocytic infiltration	Hyperthyroid phase: Graves' disease Hypothyroid phase: Hashimoto's thyroiditis	No treatment Hyperthyroid phase: consider beta-blockers Hypothyroid phase: consider L-T4
Postpartum thyroiditis	8 % of pregnancies Within 1 year after a delivery	Autoimmune Genetic susceptibility Predisposing factors	Variable symptoms of thyroid dysfunction Small painless goiter	Triphasic pattern or only transient hyper or hypothyroidism US: hypoechogenicity RAIU: low (hyperthyroid phase) Pathology: lymphocytic infiltration	Hyperthyroid phase: Graves' disease Hypothyroid phase: Hashimoto's thyroiditis	No treatment Hyperthyroid phase: consider beta-blockers (propranolol) Hypothyroid phase: consider L-T4
Amiodarone -associated thyroiditis (type II AIT)	5–12 % of treated patients Iodine-sufficient areas	Direct toxic effect of the drug (destructive thyroiditis)	No symptoms or mild hyperthyroidism Small painless goiter	Transient hyperthyroidism US: hypoechoic gland CFDS: low flow RAIU: low or absent	Type I AIT	Consider amiodarone withdrawal Glucocorticoids
Riedel's Thyroiditis	Incidence: 1.06/100,000 ♀:♂, 4:1–5:1 Mean age: 42–48 years	Probably a manifestation of a systemic fibrosclerosis disorder triggered by autoimmunity	Painless, firm, rock-hard and adherent goiter Compressive symptoms Mild hypothyroidism	Euthyroidism or hypothyroidism US: diffuse hypoechogenicity CFDS: absent flow RAIU: low Pathology: extensive fibrosis	Fibrosing and IgG4 variants of Hashimoto's thyroiditis PTC, paucicellular variant of anaplastic cancer, lymphoma or sarcoma	Limited surgical intervention Glucocorticoids Hypothyroidism: L-T4

Subacute thyroiditis	Incidence: 4.9/100,000/ year ♀:♂, 4:1–7:1 Peak age: 30–50 years	Viral infection Genetic susceptibility	Painful/tender goiter Variable symptoms of thyroid dysfunction	Triphasic course (hyperthyroidism, hypothyroidism and recovery) High ESR and CRP US: hypoechogenicity CFDS: absent flow (hyperthyroid period) RAIU: low (thyrotoxic period) Pathology: granuloma, giant cells	Suppurative thyroiditis Intracystic hemorrhage Exogenous iodine Thyroid carcinoma or lymphoma	NSAIDs Glucocorticoids (severe cases) Hyperthyroidism: beta-blockers Hypothyroidism: L-T4
Suppurative thyroiditis	0.1–0.7 % of thyroid diseases Children >90 %	Infection Predisposing conditions	Painful/tender goiter Systemic symptoms	Euthyroidism Leukocytosis, high ESR and CRP US: unifocal hypoechogenicity and/or abscess RAIU: low in the affected lobe Barium swallow study or direct laryngoscopy: pyriform sinus fistula FNAB or surgical drainage: identify organism Pathology: abscess formation	Subacute thyroiditis Intracystic hemorrhage Painful Hashimoto's thyroiditis Malignancy	Antibiotic therapy Surgical drainage Surgery to repair a pyriform sinus fistula
Radiation-induced thyroiditis	1 % in patients treated for hyperthyroidism More frequent after thyroid remnant ablation	Destructive thyroiditis	Painful/tender goiter after radioiodine Symptoms of hyperthyroidism	Transient hyperthyroidism	Radioiodine failure	NSAIDs or glucocorticoids Hyperthyroidism: beta-blockers
Palpation or trauma-induced thyroiditis	Unknown incidence	Destructive thyroiditis	Painful/tender goiter Symptoms of hyperthyroidism	Transient hyperthyroidism CFDS: low flow RAIU: low Pathology: multifocal granulomatous folliculitis	Graves' disease Subacute thyroiditis	Glucocorticoids

Abbreviations: *AIT* amiodarone-induced thyrotoxicosis. *CFDS* color flow Doppler sonography, *CRP* C-reactive protein, *ESR* erythrocyte sedimentation rate, *FNAB* fine needle aspiration biopsy, *L-T4* levothyroxine, *NSAIDs* nonsteroidal antiinflammatory drugs, *PTC* papillary thyroid carcinoma, *RAIU* radioactive iodine uptake, *US* ultrasound and differences between the main forms of thyroiditis, so they can make a correct and prompt diagnosis and start the appropriate treatment.

Acknowledgement We thank Joan Kennedy for the assistance in preparing the chapter.

References

1. Pearce EN, Farwell AP, Braverman LE. Thyroiditis. N Engl J Med. 2003;348:2646–55.
2. Bindra A, Braunstein GD. Thyroiditis. Am Fam Physician. 2006;73:1769–76.
3. Hashimoto H. Zur kenntnis der lymphömatosen veränderung der schilddrüse (Struma lymphomatosa). Archiv für Klinische Chirurgie. 1912;97:219–48.
4. McConahey WM, Keating Jr FR, Beahrs OH, et al. On the increasing occurrence of Hashimoto's thyroiditis. J Clin Endocrinol Metab. 1962;22:542–4.
5. Vanderpump MP, Tunbridge WM, French JM, et al. The incidence of thyroid disorders in the community: a twenty-year follow-up of the Whickham Survey. Clin Endocrinol (Oxf). 1995;43:55–68.
6. Jacobson DL, Gange SJ, Rose NR, et al. Epidemiology and estimated population burden of selected autoimmune diseases in the United States. Clin Immunol Immunopathol. 1997;84:223–43.
7. Vanderpump MP. The epidemiology of thyroid disease. Br Med Bull. 2011;99:39–51.
8. McLeod DS, Cooper DS. The incidence and prevalence of thyroid autoimmunity. Endocrine. 2012;42: 252–65.
9. Golden SH, Robinson KA, Saldanha I, et al. Clinical review: prevalence and incidence of endocrine and metabolic disorders in the United States: a comprehensive review. J Clin Endocrinol Metab. 2009;94:1853–78.
10. Weetman AP. The genetics of autoimmune thyroid disease. Horm Metab Res. 2009;41:421–5.
11. Weetman AP. The immunopathogenesis of chronic autoimmune thyroiditis one century after hashimoto. Eur Thyroid J. 2013;1:243–50.
12. Brent GA. Environmental exposures and autoimmune thyroid disease. Thyroid. 2010;20:755–61.
13. Giordano C, Stassi G, De Maria R, et al. Potential involvement of Fas and its ligand in the pathogenesis of Hashimoto's thyroiditis. Science. 1997;275: 960–3.
14. Fisfalen ME, Palmer EM, Van Seventer GA, et al. Thyrotropin-receptor and thyroid peroxidase-specific T cell clones and their cytokine profile in autoimmune thyroid disease. J Clin Endocrinol Metab. 1997;82:3655–63.
15. Glick AB, Wodzinski A, Fu P, et al. Impairment of regulatory T-cell function in autoimmune thyroid disease. Thyroid. 2013;23:871–8.
16. Chiovato L, Bassi P, Santini F. Antibodies producing complement-mediated thyroid cytotoxicity in patients with atrophic or goitrous autoimmune thyroiditis. J Clin Endocrinol Metab. 1993;77:1700–5.
17. Tamaki H, Amino N, Kimura M. Low prevalence of thyrotropin receptor antibody in primary hypothyroidism in Japan. J Clin Endocrinol Metab. 1990;71:1382–6.
18. Caturegli P, De Remigis A, Rose NR. Hashimoto thyroiditis: clinical and diagnostic criteria. Autoimmun Rev. 2014;13:391–7.
19. Zimmerman RS, Brennan MD, McConahey WM, et al. Hashimoto's thyroiditis. An uncommon cause of painful thyroid unresponsive to corticosteroid therapy. Ann Intern Med. 1986;104:355–7.
20. Carlé A, Pedersen IB, Knudsen N, et al. Thyroid volume in hypothyroidism due to autoimmune disease follows a unimodal distribution: evidence against primary thyroid atrophy and autoimmne thyroiditis being distinct diseases. J Clin Endocrinol Metab. 2009;94:833–9.
21. Fatourechi V, McConahey WM, Woolner LB. Hyperthyroidism associated with histologic Hashimoto's thyroiditis. Mayo Clin Proc. 1971;46: 682–9.
22. Ferracci F, Carnevale A. The neurological disorder associated with thyroid autoimmunity. J Neurol. 2006;253:975–84.
23. Chaudhuri A, Behan PO. The clinical spectrum, diagnosis, pathogenesis and treatment of Hashimoto's encephalopathy (recurrent acute disseminated encephalomyelitis). Curr Med Chem. 2003;10:1945–53.
24. Kothbauer-Margreiter I, Sturzenegger M, Komor J, et al. Encephalopathy associated with Hashimoto thyroiditis: diagnosis and treatment. J Neurol. 1996;243:585–93.
25. Chong JY, Rowland LP, Utiger RD. Hashimoto encephalopathy: syndrome or myth? Arch Neurol. 2003;60:164–71.
26. Takasu N, Yamada T, Takasu M, et al. Disappearance of thyrotropin-blocking antibodies and spontaneous recovery from hypothyroidism in autoimmune thyroiditis. N Engl J Med. 1992;326:513–8.
27. Yang GC, Schreiner AM, Sun W. Can abundant colloid exclude oncocytic (Hürthle cell) carcinoma in thyroid fine needle aspiration? Cytohistological correlation of 127 oncocytic (Hürthle cell) lesions. Cytopathology. 2013;24:185–93.
28. Dailey ME, Lindsay S, Skahen R. Relation of thyroid neoplasms to Hashimoto disease of the thyroid gland. Arch Surg. 1955;70:291–7.
29. Konturek A, Barczynski M, Wierzchowski W, et al. Coexistence of papillary thyroid cancer with Hashimoto thyroiditis. Langenbecks Arch Surg. 2013;398:389–94.

30. Jankovic B, Le KT, Hershman JM. Clinical review: Hashimoto's thyroiditis and papillary thyroid carcinoma: is there a correlation? J Clin Endocrinol Metab. 2013;98:474–82.
31. Kwak HY, Chae BJ, Eom YH, et al. Does papillary thyroid carcinoma have a better prognosis with or without Hashimoto thyroiditis? Int J Clin Oncol. 2015;20:463–73.
32. Akamizu T, Amino N, De Groot LJ. Hashimoto's thyroiditis. In: Endotext. 2013. http://www.thyroidmanager.org.
33. Katz SM, Vickery Jr AL. The fibrous variant of Hashimoto's thyroiditis. Hum Pathol. 1974;5:161–70.
34. Li Y, Bai Y, Liu Z, et al. Immunohistochemistry of IgG4 can help subclassify Hashimoto's autoimmune thyroiditis. Pathol Int. 2009;59:636–41.
35. Umehara H, Okazaki K, Masaki Y, et al. A novel clinical entity, IgG4-related disease (IgG4RD): general concept and details. Mod Rheumatol. 2012;22:1–14.
36. Umehara H, Okazaki K, Masaki Y, et al. Comprehensive diagnostic criteria for IgG4-related disease (IgG4-RD), 2011. Mod Rheumatol. 2012;22:21–30.
37. Cheuk W, Chan JK. IgG4-related sclerosing disease: a critical appraisal of an evolving clinicopathologic entity. Adv Anat Pathol. 2010;17:303–32.
38. Deshpande V, Zen Y, Chan JK, et al. Consensus statement on the pathology of IgG4-related disease. Mod Pathol. 2012;25:1181–92.
39. Sah RP, Chari ST. Serologic issues in IgG4-related systemic disease and autoimmune pancreatitis. Curr Opin Rheumatol. 2011;23:108–13.
40. Li Y, Nishihara E, Hirokawa M, et al. Distinct clinical, serological, and sonographic characteristics of Hashimoto's thyroiditis based with and without IgG4-positive plasma cells. J Clin Endocrinol Metab. 2010;95:1309–17.
41. Kakudo K, Li Y, Taniguchi E, et al. IgG4-related disease of the thyroid glands. Endocr J. 2012;59:273–81.
42. Luiz HV, Gonçalves D, Silva TN, et al. IgG4-related Hashimoto's thyroiditis – a new variant of a well known disease. Arq Bras Endocrinol Metabol. 2014;58:862–8.
43. Ahmed R, Al-Shaikh S, Akhtar M. Hashimoto thyroiditis: a century later. Adv Anat Pathol. 2012;19:181–6.
44. Caturegli P, De Remigis A, Chuang K, et al. Hashimoto's thyroiditis: celebrating the centennial through the lens of the Johns Hopkins hospital surgical pathology records. Thyroid. 2013;23:142–50.
45. Ross DS. Syndromes of thyrotoxicosis with low radioactive iodine uptake. Endocrinol Metab Clin North Am. 1998;27:169–85.
46. Nikolai TF, Brosseau J, Kettrick MA, et al. Lymphocytic thyroiditis with spontaneously resolving hyperthyroidism (silent thyroiditis). Arch Intern Med. 1980;140:478–82.
47. Farid NR, Hawe BS, Walfish PG. Increased frequency of HLA-DR3 and 5 in the syndromes of painless thyroiditis with transient thyrotoxicosis: evidence for an autoimmune aetiology. Clin Endocrinol (Oxf). 1983;19:699–704.
48. Mandel SJ, Larsen PR, Davies TF. Thyrotoxicosis. In: Melmed S, editor. Williams textbook of endocrinology. 12th ed. Philadelphia: Elsevier Health Sciences; 2011. p. 362–405.
49. Woolf PD. Transient painless thyroiditis with hyperthyroidism: a variant of lymphocytic thyroiditis? Endocr Rev. 1980;1:411–20.
50. Samuels MH. Subacute, silent, and postpartum thyroiditis. Med Clin North Am. 2012;96:223–33.
51. Nikolai TF, Coombs GJ, McKenzie AK. Lymphocytic thyroiditis with spontaneously resolving hyperthyroidism and subacute thyroiditis. Long-term follow-up. Arch Intern Med. 1981;141:1455–8.
52. Volpe R. Is silent thyroiditis an autoimmune disease? Arch Intern Med. 1988;148:1907–8.
53. Kamijo K. Study on cutoff value setting for differential diagnosis between Graves' disease and painless thyroiditis using the TRAb (Elecsys TRAb) measurement via the fully automated electrochemiluminescence immunoassay system. Endocr J. 2010;57:895–902.
54. Mittra ES, McDougall IR. Recurrent silent thyroiditis: a report of four patients and review of the literature. Thyroid. 2007;17:671–5.
55. De Groot L, Abalovich M, Alexander EK, et al. Management of thyroid dysfunction during pregnancy and postpartum: an Endocrine Society clinical practice guideline. J Clin Endocrinol Metab. 2012;97:2543–65.
56. Stagnaro-Green A, Abalovich M, Alexander E, et al. Guidelines of the American Thyroid Association for the diagnosis and management of thyroid disease during pregnancy and postpartum. Thyroid. 2011;21:1081–125.
57. Marqusee E, Hill JA, Mandel SJ. Thyroiditis after pregnancy loss. J Clin Endocrinol Metab. 1997;82:2455–7.
58. Stagnaro-Green A. Postpartum thyroiditis. Best Pract Res Clin Endocrinol Metab. 2004;18:303–16.
59. Nicholson WK, Robinson KA, Smallridge RC, et al. Prevalence of postpartum thyroid dysfunction: a quantitative review. Thyroid. 2006;16:573–82.
60. Kologlu M, Fung H, Darke C. Postpartum thyroid dysfunction and HLA status. Eur J Clin Invest. 1990;20:56–60.
61. Stagnaro-Green A. Clinical review 152: postpartum thyroiditis. J Clin Endocrinol Metab. 2002;87:4042–7.
62. Stagnaro-Green A. Approach to the patient with postpartum thyroiditis. J Clin Endocrinol Metab. 2012;97:334–42.
63. Pop VJ, de Rooy HA, Vader HL, et al. Postpartum thyroid dysfunction and depression in an unselected population. N Engl J Med. 1991;324:1815–6.

64. Harris B, Othman S, Davies JA, et al. Association between postpartum thyroid dysfunction and thyroid antibodies and depression. BMJ. 1992;305:152–6.
65. Lucas A, Pizarro E, Granada ML, et al. Postpartum thyroid dysfunction and postpartum depression: are they two linked disorders? Clin Endocrinol (Oxf). 2001;55:809–14.
66. Maleki N, Tavosi Z. Evaluation of thyroid dysfunction and autoimmunity in gestational diabetes mellitus and its relationship with postpartum thyroiditis. Diabet Med. 2015;32:206–12.
67. Azizi F. The occurrence of permanent thyroid failure in patients with subclinical postpartum thyroiditis. Eur J Endocrinol. 2005;153:367–71.
68. Stuckey BG, Kent GN, Ward LC, et al. Postpartum thyroid dysfunction and the long-term risk of hypothyroidism: results from a 12-year follow-up study of women with and without postpartum thyroid dysfunction. Clin Endocrinol (Oxf). 2010;73:389–95.
69. Premawardhana LD, Parkes AB, Ammari F, et al. Postpartum thyroiditis and long-term thyroid status: prognostic influence of thyroid peroxidase antibodies and ultrasound echogenicity. J Clin Endocrinol Metab. 2000;85:71–5.
70. Nikolai TF, Turney SL, Roberts RC. Postpartum lymphocytic thyroiditis. Prevalence, clinical course, and long-term follow-up. Arch Intern Med. 1987;147:221–4.
71. Paragliola RM, Concolino P, De Rosa A, et al. The first case of association between postpartum thyroiditis and thyroid hormone resistance in an Italian patient showing a novel p.V283A THRB mutation. Thyroid. 2013;23:506–10.
72. Ide A, Amino N, Kang S, et al. Differentiation of postpartum Graves' thyrotoxicosis from postpartum destructive thyrotoxicosis using antithyrotropin receptor antibodies and thyroid blood flow. Thyroid. 2014;24:1027–31.
73. Kampe O, Jansson R, Karlsson FA. Effects of Lthyroxine and iodide on the development of autoimmune postpartum thyroiditis. J Clin Endocrinol Metab. 1990;70:1014–8.
74. Negro R, Greco G, Mangieri T, et al. The influence of selenium supplementation on postpartum thyroid status in pregnant women with thyroid peroxidase autoantibodies. J Clin Endocrinol Metab. 2007;92: 1263–8.
75. Beardmore KS, Morris JM, Gallery ED. Excretion of antihypertensive medication into human breast milk: a systematic review. Hypertens Pregnancy. 2002;21:85–95.
76. Bogazzi F, Bartalena L, Martino E. Approach to the patient with amiodarone-induced thyrotoxicosis. J Clin Endocrinol Metab. 2010;95:2529–35.
77. Basaria S, Cooper DS. Amiodarone and the thyroid. Am J Med. 2005;118:706–14.
78. Martino E, Bartalena L, Bogazzi F, et al. The effects of amiodarone on the thyroid. Endocr Rev. 2001;22:240–54.
79. Batcher EL, Tang XC, Singh BN, et al. Thyroid function abnormalities during amiodarone therapy for persistent atrial fibrillation. Am J Med. 2007;120:880–5.
80. Trip MD, Wiersinga W, Plomp TA. Incidence, predictability, and pathogenesis of amiodarone-induced thyrotoxicosis and hypothyroidism. Am J Med. 1991;91:507–11.
81. Roti E, Minelli R, Gardini E, et al. Thyrotoxicosis followed by hypothyroidism in patients treated with amiodarone. A possible consequence of a destructive process in the thyroid. Arch Intern Med. 1993;153:886–92.
82. Lambert M, Unger J, De Nayer P, et al. Amiodarone-induced thyrotoxicosis suggestive of thyroid damage. J Endocrinol Invest. 1990;13:527–30.
83. Yagishita A, Hachiya H, Kawabata M, et al. Amiodarone-induced thyrotoxicosis late after amiodarone withdrawal. Circ J. 2013;77:2898–903.
84. Bogazzi F, Bartalena L, Brogioni S, et al. Color flow Doppler sonography rapidly differentiates type I and type II amiodarone-induced thyrotoxicosis. Thyroid. 1997;7:541–5.
85. Bogazzi F, Martino E, Dell'Unto E, et al. Thyroid color flow doppler sonography and radioiodine uptake in 55 consecutive patients with amiodarone-induced thyrotoxicosis. J Endocrinol Invest. 2003;26:635–40.
86. Eaton SE, Euinton HA, Newman CM, et al. Clinical experience of amiodarone-induced thyrotoxicosis over a 3-year period: role of colour-flow Doppler sonography. Clin Endocrinol (Oxf). 2002;56:33–8.
87. Tanda ML, Piantanida E, Lai A, et al. Diagnosis and management of amiodarone-induced thyrotoxicosis: similarities and differences between North American and European thyroidologists. Clin Endocrinol (Oxf). 2008;69:812–8.
88. Bahn RS, Burch HB, Cooper DS, et al. Hyperthyroidism and other causes of thyrotoxicosis: management guidelines of the American Thyroid Association and American Association of Clinical Endocrinologists. Thyroid. 2011;21:593–646.
89. Bogazzi F, Bartalena L, Tomisti L, et al. Glucocorticoid response in amiodarone-induced thyrotoxicosis resulting from destructive thyroiditis is predicted by thyroid volume and serum free thyroid hormone concentrations. J Clin Endocrinol Metab. 2007;92:556–62.
90. Houghton SG, Farley DR, Brennan MD, et al. Surgical management of amiodarone-associated thyrotoxicosis: Mayo Clinic experience. World J Surg. 2004;28:1083–7.
91. Bogazzi F, Miccoli P, Berti P, et al. Preparation with iopanoic acid rapidly controls thyrotoxicosis in patients with amiodarone-induced thyrotoxicosis before thyroidectomy. Surgery. 2002;132:1114–7.
92. Ryan LE, Braverman LE, Cooper DS, et al. Can amiodarone be restarted after amiodarone-induced thyrotoxicosis? Thyroid. 2004;14:149–53.

93. Barbesino G. Drugs affecting thyroid function. Thyroid. 2010;20:763–70.
94. Lazarus JH. Lithium and thyroid. Best Pract Res Clin Endocrinol Metab. 2009;23:723–33.
95. Barclay ML, Brownlie BE, Turner JG, et al. Lithium associated thyrotoxicosis: a report of 14 cases, with statistical analysis of incidence. Clin Endocrinol (Oxf). 1994;40:759–64.
96. Fried MW, Shiffman ML, Reddy KR, et al. Peginterferon alfa-2a plus ribavirin for chronic hepatitis C virus infection. N Engl J Med. 2002;347:975–82.
97. Tomer Y, Blackard JT, Akeno N. Interferon alpha treatment and thyroid dysfunction. Endocrinol Metab Clin North Am. 2007;36:1051–66.
98. Tran HA, Jones TL, Ianna EA, et al. Thyroid disease in chronic hepatitis C infection treated with combination interferon-a and ribavirin: management strategies and future perspective. Endocr Pract. 2013;19:292–300.
99. Nadeem A, Hussain MM, Aslam M, et al. Interferon-alpha induced and ribavirin induced thyroid dysfunction in patients with chronic hepatitis C. Hepat Mon. 2010;10:132–40.
100. Mandac JC, Chaudhry S, Sherman KE, et al. The clinical and physiological spectrum of interferon-alpha induced thyroiditis: toward a new classification. Hepatology. 2006;43:661–72.
101. Tomer Y. Hepatitis C, and interferon induced thyroiditis. J Autoimmun. 2010;34:J322–6.
102. Bini EJ, Mehandru S. Incidence of thyroid dysfunction during interferon alfa-2b and ribavirin therapy in men with chronic hepatitis C: a prospective cohort study. Arch Intern Med. 2004;164:2371–6.
103. Weijl NI, Van der Harst D, Brand A, et al. Hypothyroidism during immunotherapy with interleukin-2 is associated with antithyroid antibodies and response to treatment. J Clin Oncol. 1993;11:1376–83.
104. Atkins MB, Mier JW, Parkinson DR, et al. Hypothyroidism after treatment with interleukin-2 and lymphokine-activated killer cells. N Engl J Med. 1988;318:1557–63.
105. Mattijssen VJ, De Mulder PH, Van Liessum PA, et al. Hypothyroidism and goiter in a patient during treatment with interleukin-2. Cancer. 1990;65:2686–8.
106. Schwartzentruber DJ, White DE, Zweig MH, et al. Thyroid dysfunction associated with immunotherapy for patients with cancer. Cancer. 1991;68:2384–90.
107. Vialettes B, Guillerand MA, Viens P, et al. Incidence rate and risk factors for thyroid dysfunction during recombinant interleukin-2 therapy in advanced malignancies. Acta Endocrinol (Copenh). 1993;129:31–8.
108. Ahmadieh H, Salti I. Tyrosine kinase inhibitors induced thyroid dusfunction: a review of its incidence, pathophysiology, clinical relevance, and treatment. Biomed Res Int. 2013;2013:725410.
109. Wong E, Rosen LS, Mulay M, et al. Sunitinib induces hypothyroidism in advanced cancer patients and may inhibit thyroid peroxidase activity. Thyroid. 2007;17:351–5.
110. Rini BI, Tamaskar I, Shaheen P, et al. Hypothyroidism in patients with metastatic renal cell carcinoma treated with sunitinib. J Natl Cancer Inst. 2007;99:81–3.
111. Riedel B. Die chronische, zur bildung eisenharter tumoren führende entzündung der schilddrüse. Ver Deutsch Ges Chirurg. 1896;25:101–5.
112. Hay ID. Thyroiditis: a clinical update. Mayo Clin Proc. 1985;60:836–43.
113. Schwaegerle SM, Bauer TW, Esselstyn Jr CB. Riedel's thyroiditis. Am J Clin Pathol. 1988;90:715–22.
114. Fatourechi MM, Hay ID, McIver B, et al. Invasive fibrous thyroiditis (Riedel thyroiditis): the Mayo Clinic experience, 1976–2008. Thyroid. 2011;21:765–72.
115. Papi G, LiVolsi VA. Current concepts on Riedel thyroiditis. Am J Clin Pathol. 2004;121:S50–63.
116. Hennessey JV. Clinical review: Riedel's thyroiditis: a clinical review. J Clin Endocrinol Metab. 2011;96:3031–41.
117. Dahlgren M, Khosroshahi A, Nielsen GP, et al. Riedel's thyroiditis and multifocal fibrosclerosis are part of the IgG4-related systemic disease spectrum. Arthritis Care Res (Hoboken). 2010;62:1312–8.
118. Pusztaszeri M, Triponez F, Pache JC, et al. Riedel's thyroiditis with increases IgG4 plasma cells: evidence for an underlying IgG4-related sclerosing disease? Thyroid. 2012;22:964–8.
119. Papi G, Corrado S, Cesinaro AM, et al. Riedel's thyroiditis: clinical, pathological and imaging features. Int J Clin Pract. 2002;56:65–7.
120. Ozgen A, Cila A. Riedel's thyroiditis in multifocal fibrosclerosis: CT and MR imaging findings. AJNR Am J Neuroradiol. 2000;21:320–1.
121. Heufelder AE, Goellner JR, Bahn RS, et al. Tissue eosinophilia and eosinophil degranulation in Riedel's invasive fibrous thyroiditis. J Clin Endocrinol Metab. 1996;81:977–84.
122. Meyer S, Hausman R. Occlusive phlebitis in multifocal fibrosclerosis. Am J Clin Pathol. 1976;65:274–83.
123. Woolner LB, McConahey WM, Beahrs OH. Invasive fibrous thyroiditis (Riedel's struma). J Clin Endocrinol Metab. 1957;17:201–20.
124. Baloch ZW, Saberi M, Livolsi VA. Simultaneous involvement of thyroid by Riedel's [correction of Reidel's] disease and fibrosing Hashimoto's thyroiditis: a case report. Thyroid. 1998;8:337–41.
125. Heufelder AE, Hay ID. Evidence for autoimmune mechanisms in the evolution of invasive fibrous thyroiditis (Riedel's struma). Clin Investig. 1994;72:788–93.
126. Kabalak T, Ozgen AG, Günel O, et al. Occurrence of Riedel's thyroiditis in the course of sub-acute thyroiditis. J Endocrinol Invest. 2000;23:399–401.

127. Hong JT, Lee JH, Kim SH, et al. Case of concurrent Riedel's thyroiditis, acute suppurative thyroiditis, and micropapillary carcinoma. Korean J Intern Med. 2013;28:236–41.
128. Li Y, Zhou G, Ozaki T, et al. Distinct histopathological features of Hashimoto's thyroiditis with respect to IgG4-related disease. Mod Pathol. 2012;25: 1086–97.
129. Vaidya B, Harris PE, Barrett P, et al. Corticosteroid therapy in Riedel's thyroiditis. Postgrad Med J. 1997;73:817–9.
130. Jung YJ, Schaub CR, Rhodes R, et al. A case of Riedel's thyroiditis treated with tamoxifen: another successful outcome. Endocr Pract. 2004;10:483–6.
131. De M, Jaap A, Dempster J. Tamoxifen therapy in steroid resistant Reidel's thyroiditis. Scott Med J. 2001;46:56–7.
132. Hamed G, Heffess CS, Shmookler BM. Amyloid goiter. A clinicopathologic study of 14 cases and review of the literature. Am J Clin Pathol. 1995;104: 306–12.
133. Villa F, Dionigi G, Tanda ML, et al. Amyloid goiter. Int J Surg. 2008;6:S16–8.
134. Manchanda A, Patel S, Jiang JJ, et al. Thyroid: an unusual hideout for sarcoidosis. Endocr Pract. 2013;19:e40–3.
135. Antonelli A, Fazzi P, Fallahi P, et al. Prevalence of hypothyroidism and Graves disease in sarcoidosis. Chest. 2006;130:526–32.
136. Ozkan Z, Oncel M, Kurt N, et al. Sarcoidosis presenting as cold thyroid nodules: report of two cases. Surg Today. 2005;35:770–3.
137. Fatourechi V, Aniszewski JP, Fatourechi GZ, et al. Clinical features and outcome of subacute thyroiditis in an incidence cohort: Olmsted County, Minnesota, study. J Clin Endocrinol Metab. 2003;88:2100–5.
138. Erdem N, Erdogan M, Ozbek M, et al. Demographic and clinical features of patients with subacute thyroiditis: results of 169 patients from a single university center in Turkey. J Endocrinol Invest. 2007;30: 546–50.
139. Nishihara E, Ohye H, Amino N, et al. Clinical characteristics of 852 patients with subacute thyroiditis before treatment. Intern Med. 2008;47:725–9.
140. Martino E, Buratti L, Bartalena L, et al. High prevalence of subacute thyroiditis during summer season in Italy. J Endocrinol Invest. 1987;10:321–3.
141. Eylan E, Zmucky R, Sheba C. Mumps virus and subacute thyroiditis; evidence of a causal association. Lancet. 1957;272:1062–3.
142. Werner J, Gelderblom H. Isolation of foamy virus from patients with de Quervain thyroiditis. Lancet. 1979;2:258–9.
143. Desailloud R, Hober D. Viruses and thyroiditis: an update. Virol J. 2009;6:5.
144. Ohsako N, Tamai H, Sudo T, et al. Clinical characteristics of subacute thyroiditis classified according to human leukocyte antigen typing. J Clin Endocrinol Metab. 1995;80:3653–6.
145. Daniels GH. Atypical subacute thyroiditis: preliminary observations. Thyroid. 2001;11:691–5.
146. Swinburne JL, Kreisman SH. A rare case of subacute thyroiditis causing thyroid storm. Thyroid. 2007;17:73–6.
147. Lio S, Pontecorvi A, Caruso M, et al. Transitory subclinical and permanent hypothyroidism in the course of subacute thyroiditis (de Quervain). Acta Endocrinol (Copenh). 1984;106:67–70.
148. Pearce EN, Bogazzi F, Martino E, et al. The prevalence of elevated serum C-reactive protein levels in inflammatory and noninflammatory thyroid disease. Thyroid. 2003;13:643–8.
149. Matsumoto Y, Amino N, Kubota S, et al. Serial changes in liver function tests in patients with subacute thyroiditis. Thyroid. 2008;18:815–6.
150. Benbassat CA, Olchovsky D, Tsvetov G, et al. Subacute thyroiditis: clinical characteristics and treatment outcome in fifty-six consecutive patients diagnosed between 1999 and 2005. J Endocrinol Invest. 2007;30:631–5.
151. Espinoza PG, Guendelman CL, Quevedo Limon LN, et al. A comparison between two imaging techniques for the diagnosis of subacute thyroiditis (de Quervain thyroiditis): brief communication. Clin Nucl Med. 2010;35:862–4.
152. Park SY, Kim EK, Kim MJ, et al. Ultrasonographic characteristics of subacute granulomatous thyroiditis. Korean J Radiol. 2006;7:229–34.
153. Hiromatsu Y, Ishibashi M, Miyake I, et al. Color Doppler ultrasonography in patients with subacute thyroiditis. Thyroid. 1999;9:1189–93.
154. Woolner LB, McConahey WM, Beahrs OH. Granulomatous thyroiditis (De Quervain's thyroiditis). J Clin Endocrinol Metab. 1957;17:1202–21.
155. DeGroot LJ, Larsen PR, Hennemann G. Acute and subacute thyroiditis. In: DeGroot LJ, editor. The thyroid and its diseases. 6th ed. New York: Churchill Livingstone; 1996. p. 700.
156. Szabo SM, Allen DB. Thyroiditis. Differentiation of acute suppurative and subacute. Case report and review of the literature. Clin Pediatr (Phila). 1989;28:171–4.
157. Yang YS, Wu MZ, Cheng AL, et al. Primary thyroid lymphoma mimicking subacute thyroiditis. Acta Cytol. 2006;50:710–2.
158. Nishihara E, Hirokawa M, Ohye H, et al. Papillary carcinoma obscured by complication with subacute thyroiditis: sequential ultrasonographic and histopathological findings in five cases. Thyroid. 2008;18:1221–5.
159. Ucan B, Delibasi T, Cakal E, et al. Papillary thyroid cancer case masked by subacute thyroiditis. Arq Bras Endocrinol Metabol. 2014;58:851–4.
160. Volpé R. The management of subacute (DeQuervain's) thyroiditis. Thyroid. 1993;3:253–5.
161. Iitaka M, Momotani N, Ishii J, et al. Incidence of subacute thyroiditis recurrences after a prolonged latency: 24-year survey. J Clin Endocrinol Metab. 1996;81:466–9.
162. Al-Dajani N, Wootton SH. Cervical lymphadenitis, suppurative parotiditis, thyroiditis, and infected cysts. Infect Dis Clin North Am. 2007;21:523–41.

163. Cases JA, Wenig BM, Silver CE, et al. Recurrent acute suppurative thyroiditis in an adult due to a fourth branchial pouch fistula. J Clin Endocrinol Metab. 2000;85:953–6.
164. Yolmo D, Madana J, Kalaiarasi R, et al. Retrospective case review of pyriform sinus fistulae of third branchial arch origin commonly presenting as acute suppurative thyroiditis in children. J Laryngol Otol. 2012;126:737–42.
165. Sai Prasad TR, Chong CL, Mani A, et al. Acute suppurative thyroiditis in children secondary to pyriform sinus fistula. Pediatr Surg Int. 2007;23: 779–83.
166. Yu EH, Ko WC, Chuang YC, et al. Suppurative Acinetobacter baumanii thyroiditis with bacteremic pneumonia: case report and review. Clin Infect Dis. 1998;27:1286–90.
167. Nishihara E, Miyauchi A, Matsuzuka F, et al. Acute suppurative thyroiditis after fine-needle aspiration causing thyrotoxicosis. Thyroid. 2005;15:1183–7.
168. Ünlütürk U, Ceyhan K, Çorapçioğlu D. Acute suppurative thyroiditis following fine-needle aspiration biopsy in an immunocompetent patient. J Clin Ultrasound. 2014;42:215–8.
169. Berger SA, Zonszein J, Villamena P, et al. Infectious diseases of the thyroid gland. Rev Infect Dis. 1983;5:108–22.
170. Paes JE, Burman KD, Cohen J, et al. Acute bacterial suppurative thyroiditis: a clinical review and expert opinion. Thyroid. 2010;20:247–55.
171. Wu C, Zhang Y, Gong Y, et al. Two cases of bacterial suppurative thyroiditis caused by Streptococcus anginosus. Endocr Pathol. 2013;24:49–53.
172. Dupret-Bories A, Caron P, Rouquette I, et al. Fatal neck necrotizing cellulitis in a patient with Riedel's thyroiditis. Thyroid. 2013;23:904–5.
173. Nunes da Silva TL, Vara Luiz H, Dias Pereira B, et al. Acute bacterial thyroiditis with no risk factors and a difficult treatment. In: Abstracts of the 16th international congress of endocrinology and 96th annual meeting & expo of The Endocrine Society, Chicago, 21–24 June 2014.
174. Rich EJ, Mendelman PM. Acute suppurative thyroiditis in pediatric patients. Pediatr Infect Dis J. 1987;6:936–40.
175. Luiz HV, Pereira BD, Silva TN, et al. Thyroid tuberculosis with abnormal thyroid function – case report and review of the literature. Endocr Pract. 2013;19:e44–9.
176. Guttler R, Singer PA, Axline SG, et al. Pneumocystis carinii thyroiditis. Report of three cases and review of the literature. Arch Intern Med. 1993;153:393–6.
177. Masuoka H, Miyauchi A, Tomoda C, et al. Imaging studies in sixty patients with acute suppurative thyroiditis. Thyroid. 2011;21:1075–80.
178. Smith SL, Pereira KD. Suppurative thyroiditis in children: a management algorithm. Pediatr Emerg Care. 2008;24:764–7.
179. Pereira KD, Davies JN. Piriform sinus tracts in children. Arch Otolaryngol Head Neck Surg. 2006;132: 1119–21.
180. Park NH, Park HJ, Park CS, et al. The emerging echogenic tract sign of pyriform sinus fistula: an early indicator in the recovery stage of acute suppurative thyroiditis. AJNR Am J Neuroradiol. 2011;32:E44–6.
181. Miyauchi A, Tomoda C, Uruno T, et al. Computed tomography scan under a trumpet maneuver to demonstrate piriform sinus fistulae in patients with acute suppurative thyroiditis. Thyroid. 2005;15:1409–13.
182. Crisafulli G, Wasniewska M, Ascenti G, et al. Acute suppurative thyroiditis disclosing diagnosis of thyroid cancer in a boy. J Endocrinol Invest. 2008;31: 1137–8.
183. Miyauchi A. Thyroid gland: a new management algorithm for acute suppurative thyroiditis? Nat Rev Endocrinol. 2010;6:424–6.
184. Shah SS, Baum SG. Diagnosis and management of infectious thyroiditis. Curr Infect Dis Rep. 2000;2:147–53.
185. Kim KH, Sung MW, Koh TY, et al. Pyriform sinus fistula: management with chemocauterization of the internal opening. Ann Otol Rhinol Laryngol. 2000;109:452–6.
186. Jordan JA, Graves JE, Manning SC, et al. Endoscopic cauterization for treatment of fourth branchial cleft sinuses. Arch Otolaryngol Head Neck Surg. 1998;124:1021–4.
187. Miyauchi A, Inoue H, Tomoda C, et al. Evaluation of chemocauterization treatment for obliteration of pyriform sinus fistula as a route of infection causing acute suppurative thyroiditis. Thyroid. 2009;19:789–93.
188. Ross D. Radioiodine therapy for hyperthyroidism. N Engl J Med. 2011;364:542–50.
189. Cherk MH, Kalff V, Yap KS, et al. Incidence of radiation thyroiditis and thyroid remnant ablation success rates following 1110 MBq (30 mCi) and 3700 MBq (100 mCi) post-surgical 131I ablation therapy for differentiated thyroid carcinoma. Clin Endocrinol (Oxf). 2008;69:957–62.
190. Koornstra JJ, Kerstens MN, Hoving J, et al. Clinical and biochemical changes following 131I therapy for hyperthyroidism in patients not pretreated with antithyroid drugs. Neth J Med. 1999;55:215–21.
191. McDermott MT, Kidd GS, Dodson Jr LE, et al. Radioiodine-induced thyroid storm: case report and literature review. Am J Med. 1983;75:353–9.
192. Hyer SL, Newbold K, Harmer CL. Early and late toxicity of radioiodine therapy: detection and management. Endocr Pract. 2010;16:1064–70.
193. Shah KK, Tarasova V, Davidian M, et al. Painful acute radiation thyroiditis induced by 131I treatment of Graves' disease. BMJ Case Rep. 2015.
194. Bonnema SJ, Hegedüs L. Radioiodine therapy in benign thyroid diseases: effects, side effects, and factors affecting therapeutic outcome. Endocr Rev. 2012;33:920–80.
195. Gayed I, Wendt J, Haynie T, et al. Timing for repeated treatment of hyperthyroid disease with radioactive iodine after initial treatment failure. Clin Nucl Med. 2001;26:1–5.

196. Burch HB, Solomon BL, Cooper DS, et al. The effect of antithyroid drug pretreatment on acute changes in thyroid hormone levels after 131I ablation for Graves' disease. J Clin Endocrinol Metab. 2001;86:3016–21.
197. Carney JA, Moore SB, Northcutt RC, et al. Palpation thyroiditis (multifocal granulomatous folliculitis). Am J Clin Pathol. 1975;64:639–47.
198. Kobayashi A, Kuma K, Matsuzuka F, et al. Thyrotoxicosis after needle aspiration of thyroid cyst. J Clin Endocrinol Metab. 1992;75:21–4.
199. Stang MT, Yim JH, Challinor SM, et al. Hyperthyroidism after parathyroid exploration. Surgery. 2005;138:1058–64.
200. Espiritu RP, Dean DS. Parathyroidectomy-induced thyroiditis. Endocr Pract. 2010;16:656–9.
201. Leckie RG, Buckner AB, Bornemann M. Seat belt-related thyroiditis documented with thyroid Tc-99 m pertechnetate scans. Clin Nucl Med. 1992;17:859–60.
202. Bergenfelz A, Ahrén B. Hyperthyroxinemia after surgery for primary hyperparathyroidism. Langenbecks Arch Chir. 1994;379:178–81.
203. Mai VQ, Glister BC, Clyde PW, et al. Palpation thyroiditis causing new-onset atrial fibrillation. Thyroid. 2008;18:571–3.
204. Hwang TS, Park SH. Histopathologic study of the so called "palpation thyroiditis". J Korean Med Sci. 1988;3:27–9.

Hypothyroidism

7

Henrique Vara Luiz, Isabel Manita,
and Jorge Portugal

Abstract

Hypothyroidism can be defined by a decrease in thyroid hormone production and/or by an impaired action of thyroid hormones on target tissues. It is a common condition with multiple etiologies and clinical manifestations. Currently, hypothyroidism is usually diagnosed at early stages which allow a timely treatment. Levothyroxine is still the modality of choice and other therapeutic options are not recommended. The administration of an appropriate hormone replacement dose leads to a normalization of thyroid function in virtually all cases. However, patients with severe long-standing hypothyroidism can develop life-threatening complications. Therefore, physicians must be aware of the typical clinical findings in order to promptly evaluate patients with suspected hypothyroidism. In addition, infants with congenital hypothyroidism should be properly managed.

Introduction

Hypothyroidism can be defined by a decrease in thyroid hormone production and/or by an impaired action of thyroid hormones on target tissues. It is a common condition with multiple etiologies and clinical manifestations. When hypothyroidism is suspected a prompt diagnosis and a proper treatment should be performed.

In this chapter the authors perform a review of the literature and attempt to systematize the relevant information about this topic. Primary and central types are discussed and we also focus on congenital hypothyroidism. The diagnosis and management of hypothyroidism during pregnancy, subclinical hypothyroidism and myxedema coma are reviewed in different chapters.

Historical

Curling in 1850 described the first case of hypothyroidism in children [1], whereas Gull in 1873 was the first to identify adult hypothyroidism [2].

H.V. Luiz, MD (✉) • I. Manita, MD • J. Portugal, MD
Department of Endocrinology and Diabetology,
Hospital Garcia de Orta, Avenida Torrado da Silva,
Almada 2801-951, Portugal
e-mail: hvaraluiz@gmail.com;
isabelmanita@sapo.pt; jportugal@hgo.min-saude.pt

S.K. Imam, S.I. Ahmad (eds.), *Thyroid Disorders: Basic Science and Clinical Practice*,
DOI 10.1007/978-3-319-25871-3_7

Ord in 1878 introduced the term myxedema to define the disease [3]. Kocher in 1883 noticed that the disorder occurs after thyroidectomy [4]. In the same year the Clinical Society of London appointed a committee to study the features of myxedema. An interesting report regarding its clinical and pathological findings was published by the committee in 1888 [5]. In 1891 Murray reported for the first time a successful treatment of a patient with myxedema using injections of sheep thyroid extract [6]. Hashimoto's thyroiditis (HT) was reported in 1912 by Hakaru Hashimoto, who described four patients with a chronic disorder of the thyroid gland, termed struma lymphomatosa [7]. In 1914, Kendall isolated thyroxine (T4) from the thyroid gland [8], and in 1927 Harington and Barger described its synthesis [9]. Gross and Pitt-Rivers in 1952 identified triiodothyronine (T3) in human plasma [10]. In 1956 Roitt et al. reported the presence of circulating thyroid autoantibodies in HT [11]. Purification of human thyroid-stimulating hormone (TSH) was performed by Condliffe in 1963 [12]. Braverman, Ingbar and Sterling in 1970 confirmed extrathyroidal conversion of T4 to T3 in humans [13]. Due to these findings, levothyroxine (L-T4) substituted desiccated thyroid extracts as the mainstay of treatment for hypothyroid patients in the latter half of the twentieth century.

Definitions

Hypothyroidism is usually defined as deficient production of thyroid hormone [14]. It can be classified in two main types: primary and central. Primary hypothyroidism is caused by a disorder of the thyroid gland which contributes to a decreased thyroid hormone secretion. It can be defined as overt if a high serum TSH concentration and a low serum free T4 (FT4) level are present or as subclinical if patients have a high serum TSH measurement along with a normal serum FT4. Central hypothyroidism is associated with decreased release of TSH from the pituitary gland (secondary hypothyroidism) or with reduced secretion of thyrotropin-releasing hormone (TRH) from the hypothalamus (tertiary hypothyroidism). In these cases decreased thyroid hormone production is caused by insufficient stimulation of the thyroid gland [14–16]. However, some patients with normal thyroid hormone production have reduced action of the thyroid hormones at the tissue level and present with symptoms and signs of hypothyroidism. Patients with resistance to thyroid hormone (RTH) and consumptive hypothyroidism are examples of this phenomenon. Thus, it seems more appropriate to define hypothyroidism as thyroid hormone deficiency on target tissues [14, 17].

Epidemiology

Primary hypothyroidism is a common disease. The National Health and Nutrition Examination Survey (NHANES III) studied patients from the US population. The prevalence of hypothyroid in this study was 4.6 % (0.3 % overt and 4.3 % subclinical), using a TSH upper limit of normal of 4.5 mIU/mL [18]. In the Colorado thyroid disease prevalence study an upper normal TSH value of 5.0 mIU/L was used. The authors reported a prevalence of subclinical and overt hypothyroidism of 8.5 % and 0.4 %, respectively, in people not taking medications for thyroid disease [19]. In the British Whickham survey the prevalence of overt hypothyroidism in people not treated for a thyroid disorder was 10/1000 in females and less than 1/1000 in males [20]. The incidence of hypothyroidism in women and men was 3.5 and 0.6 per 1000 survivors per year, respectively [21]. Females, the elderly and some racial groups (e.g. non-Hispanic whites and Mexican Americans) are thought to have a higher risk of developing hypothyroidism [18, 20–22]. A higher baseline TSH level and positive thyroid antibodies were also identified as predictors for this condition [21, 23].

Central hypothyroidism is a rare entity with an estimated prevalence of 1:20,000 to 1:80,000 in the general population [24].

In countries with neonatal screening the prevalence of congenital hypothyroidism is about 1:2000 to 1:4000 newborns, with a female to male ratio of 2:1 [25, 26].

Table 7.1 Causes of hypothyroidism

Primary hypothyroidism
Hashimoto's thyroiditis
Iodine deficiency
Iodine excess
Iatrogenic (thyroidectomy, radioiodine therapy, external irradiation)
Drugs (thionamides, amiodarone, lithium, interferon-alpha, interleukin-2, tyrosine kinase inhibitors)
Thyroid infiltration (Riedel's thyroiditis, amyloidosis, sarcoidosis, hemochromatosis, scleroderma, cystinosis)
Infections of the thyroid gland
Transient hypothyroidism (painless, postpartum and subacute thyroiditis)
Congenital (dysgenesis and dyshormonogenesis)
Central hypothyroidism
Acquired pituitary and hypothalamic disorders (tumors, Sheehan's syndrome, head trauma, surgery and irradiation, hypophysitis, infiltrative diseases, infections)
Congenital (structural lesions and genetic defects)
Drugs (dopamine, bexarotene, glucocorticoids, somatostatin analogues)
Other etiologies
Resistance to thyroid hormone
Consumptive hypothyroidism

Etiology

Hypothyroidism can be caused by several conditions (Table 7.1). Primary hypothyroidism accounts for about 99 % of patients. The remaining cases are related to central hypothyroidism and other rare etiologies namely RTH and consumptive hypothyroidism [14].

Primary Hypothyroidism

Hashimoto's Thyroiditis

HT is considered the most frequent cause of hypothyroidism in areas of the world where dietary iodine is sufficient [27]. It is an autoimmune disease, usually characterized by the presence of a diffuse goiter and positive thyroid antibodies. This disorder is discussed in the Chap. 6.

Iodine Deficiency

Iodine deficiency is the most common cause of hypothyroidism worldwide, affecting about two billion people [28]. It occurs in several countries especially in mountainous areas, and is commonly found in Africa, Asia, and in some European countries [28, 29]. Although iodine deficiency was present in many regions of the United States in the past, it is now rare in this country possibly explained by the introduction of iodized salt [28, 30]. Decreased iodine intake is associated with a deficient production of thyroid hormones, with subsequent increase in the TSH level. Continuous stimulation of the thyroid gland by TSH is responsible for the occurrence of a goiter (Fig. 7.1). The incidence and severity of endemic goiter is mainly dependent on the degree of iodine deficiency [14]. However, it seems to have a genetic component and to be related to some goitrogens such as thiocyanate that can be present in food [28, 31, 32]. Despite the presence of goiter, most patients do not have severe clinical features of hypothyroidism due to the preferential secretion of T3 and to the increased peripheral conversion of T4 to T3 [14, 33]. The diagnosis can be straightforward if a patient from a known iodine deficient region presents with a goiter. The differential diagnosis includes thyroiditis, thyrotoxicosis and thyroid carcinoma.

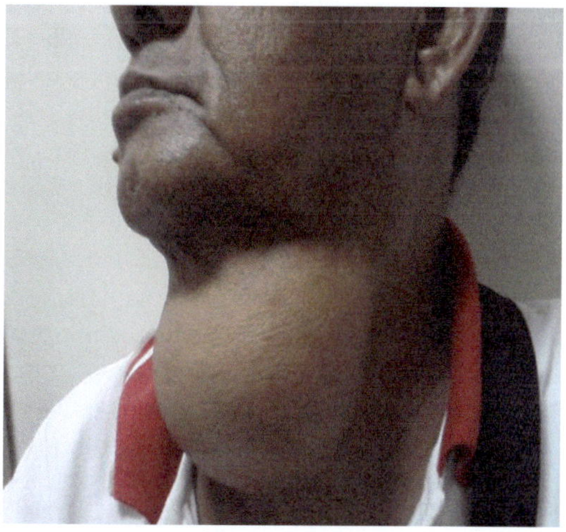

Fig. 7.1 Presence of a large goiter in a patient from an area of iodine deficiency (Courtesy of Dr. Ruby Guerrero and Dr. April Abcede)

Endemic cretinism refers to the presence of severe hypothyroidism in children occurring in regions of endemic goiter [14]. It is caused by severe iodine deficiency during pregnancy [28, 34, 35].

Iodine Excess

Iodine is present in the diet and in some drugs such as amiodarone, kelp tablets, vitamin preparations, topical antiseptics and radiographic contrast agents. Iodine excess can also cause hypothyroidism by inhibiting iodide organification and thyroid hormone synthesis, a phenomenon known as Wolff-Chaikoff effect [36]. Most subjects escape from this effect within a few weeks. However, failure to escape may occur especially in patients with an underlying thyroid disease such as HT, painless, postpartum or subacute thyroiditis and in those submitted to radioiodine therapy or partial thyroidectomy [14, 36]. Improvement is noticed after iodine withdrawal.

Iatrogenic

Iatrogenic hypothyroidism is common in adults and can be related to thyroidectomy, radioiodine therapy and external irradiation.

Hypothyroidism invariably occurs in patients submitted to total thyroidectomy. After partial thyroidectomy it develops in about 20–35 % of cases, especially within the first year [37, 38]. However, hypothyroidism can develop later or be transient. Some authors suggested an association between the development of hypothyroidism after surgery and both the presence of thyroid antibodies and higher preoperative TSH levels [37–39].

Radioiodine therapy is another iatrogenic cause of hypothyroidism. In patients with Graves' disease it is usually recommended to administer sufficient radiation in a single dose to render the patient hypothyroid [40], which occurs in about 70 % of cases within the first year [41]. Hypothyroidism can develop later at a rate of 2–3 % per year [42] and it may also be transient. The development of hypothyroidism in patients submitted to radioiodine therapy for toxic multinodular goiter or toxic adenoma is less common, occurring in 4 % of cases within the first year with an additional risk during long-term follow-up [43, 44]. It is also dependent on the administered dose.

External neck irradiation performed for several disorders can produce hypothyroidism. The estimated incidence in patients treated for Hodgkins' lymphoma is about 30 % [45], whereas those performing irradiation for larynx or pharynx cancer develop hypothyroidism in 13 % of cases [46]. The effect of radiation is dose-dependent and the onset of thyroid dysfunction is often gradual [47].

Drugs

Thionamides such as methimazole and propylthiouracil are used in the management of hyperthyroidism. Overtreatment can cause hypothyroidism.

Amiodarone is associated with thyroid dysfunction, including both hypothyroidism and thyrotoxicosis [48–50]. Overt and subclinical hypothyroidism develops in 5 and 26 % of treated patients, respectively [51] and is caused by iodine excess. It often affects patients living in iodine-sufficient regions [52], those with an underlying thyroid disorder who cannot escape from the Wolff-Chaikoff effect [36], and those with positive thyroid antibodies [53]. Thyroid function should be checked before amiodarone is started and monitored every 3–6 months during treatment. The drug has a half-life of 50–100 days and remains available for a long period after its discontinuation. For that reason, thyroid dysfunction may occur after amiodarone withdrawal and therefore assessment of thyroid function after treatment should be considered [54]. If hypothyroidism develops, amiodarone is usually not discontinued [50].

Lithium can cause goiter, hypo and hyperthyroidism [55, 56]. The prevalence of hypothyroidism ranges between 6 and 52 % of treated patients [56] and it can develop in those with or without an underlying thyroid disease. Risk factors include female gender, the elderly and patients with positive thyroid antibodies [56–59]. Lithium-associated hypothyroidism is related to the drug inhibition of thyroid hormone secretion and/or to the increasing of thyroid antibodies [55, 56, 60]. Patients treated with this drug should have a thyroid physical examination and be checked for thyroid dysfunction before it is started. Thyroid function needs to be monitored during treatment on a regular basis (e.g. every 6–12 months). The occurrence of hypothyroidism does not require discontinuation of the drug [56].

Interferon-alpha (IFN-α) is associated with the occurrence of both hypo and hyperthyroidism in about 5–10 % of treated patients [61–64]. Hypothyroidism can be autoimmune manifesting as HT, which especially affects patients with positive thyroid antibodies before treatment. Non-autoimmune hypothyroidism is due to a direct effect of the drug on the thyroid gland. Patients should undergo routine thyroid screening before starting IFN-α therapy, during treatment (usually every 3–6 months) and at least 6 months after withdrawal because thyroid disease can develop later [62, 63, 65]. IFN-α can usually be continued if thyroid dysfunction is identified. In most cases hypothyroidism is reversible on completion of antiviral treatment [63].

The incidence of hypothyroidism in patients treated with interleukin-2 alone or in combination with lymphokine-activated killer cells is about 20–50 % [66–68]. It is caused by an autoimmune process. Thyroid function should also be monitored in patients receiving this drug [69].

Tyrosine kinase inhibitors are associated with the development of hypo and hyperthyroidism [70]. Sunitinib can induce hypothyroidism in 53–85 % of patients [71, 72]. The incidence of thyroid dysfunction with sorafenib and other drugs from this therapeutic class is lower [70]. The pathogenesis is unknown, but it seems that hypothyroidism can be related to the drug induction of autoimmunity or to a destructive thyroiditis as a direct effect of treatment [70]. Monitoring thyroid function during treatment is advisable.

Thyroid Infiltration and Infections

Infiltrative disorders such as fibrous thyroiditis (Riedel's thyroiditis) [73, 74], amyloidosis [75], sarcoidosis [76], hemochromatosis [77], scleroderma [78] and cystinosis [79] are rare causes of hypothyroidism.

Infections of the thyroid gland are also uncommon and almost always present with normal thyroid function. We reported an interesting case of hypothyroidism due to thyroid tuberculosis [80].

Riedel's thyroiditis and infections are discussed in the Chap. 6.

Transient Hypothyroidism

Painless, postpartum and subacute thyroiditis are characterized by a triphasic course of hyperthyroidism followed by hypothyroidism, and then recovery to the euthyroid state. These entities are also discussed in the Chap. 6.

Primary Congenital Hypothyroidism

It is one of the most common preventable causes of mental retardation. About 90 % of permanent cases of congenital hypothyroidism are related to thyroid dysgenesis. This condition manifests in about two-thirds of cases as failure of the gland to descend properly during embryologic development (ectopy), whereas absence of the thyroid tissue (agenesis) is found in one-third of patients [81]. Thyroid dysgenesis is usually sporadic, but it can be rarely associated with genetic mutations in transcription factors predominantly expressed in the thyroid gland, namely PAX8, NKX2-1, FOXE1 and NKX2-5 [82]. The remaining 10 % of permanent cases are due to thyroid dyshormonogenesis, caused by mutations in genes encoding proteins involved in thyroid hormone synthesis, namely the sodium-iodine symporter, thyroid peroxidase (TPO), pendrin (Pendred's syndrome), thyroglobulin (TG) and iodotyrosine deiodinase [83]. Inheritance is autosomal recessive. Other patients present with resistance to TSH due to mutations in the TSH receptor gene [84].

Some infants may have transient congenital hypothyroidism, which is usually related to iodine deficiency or excess during pregnancy [85, 86], and to transplacental transfer of TSH receptor blocking antibodies or antithyroid drugs [87].

Central Hypothyroidism

Acquired Pituitary and Hypothalamic Disorders

Central hypothyroidism can be caused by any acquired disorder affecting the pituitary gland and producing TSH deficiency or any hypothalamic condition associated with TRH deficiency. Pituitary adenomas are the most common cause of central hypothyroidism in adults and these lesions can be functional and/or be associated with multiple pituitary hormone failure. Other tumors include craniopharyngiomas, meningiomas, gliomas or metastatic disease [24]. Intrasellar plasmacytomas are rare and usually present with intact anterior pituitary function. We recently evaluated a patient with panhypopituitarism due to a large plasmacytoma with intrasellar extension [88] (Fig. 7.2).

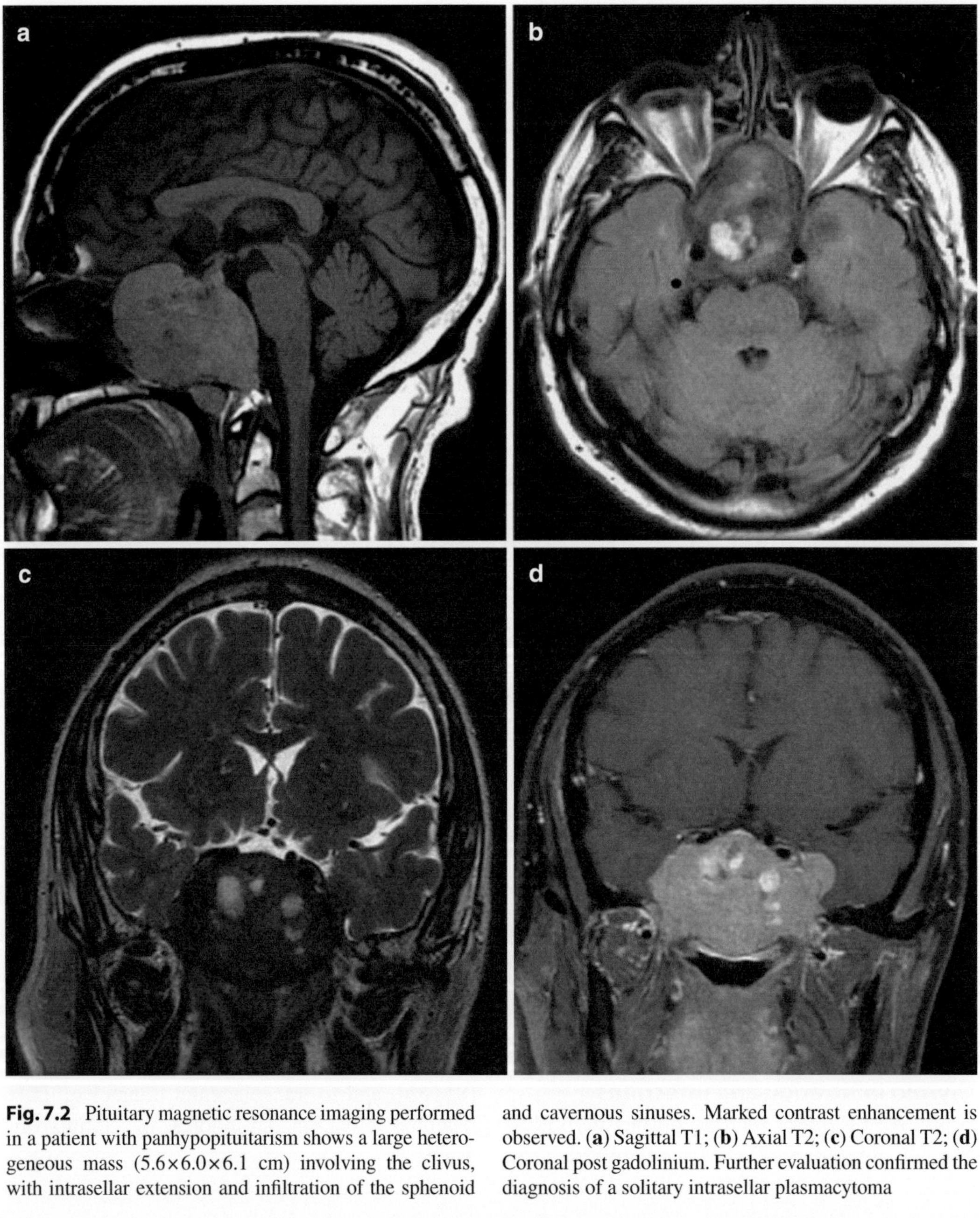

Fig. 7.2 Pituitary magnetic resonance imaging performed in a patient with panhypopituitarism shows a large heterogeneous mass (5.6×6.0×6.1 cm) involving the clivus, with intrasellar extension and infiltration of the sphenoid and cavernous sinuses. Marked contrast enhancement is observed. (**a**) Sagittal T1; (**b**) Axial T2; (**c**) Coronal T2; (**d**) Coronal post gadolinium. Further evaluation confirmed the diagnosis of a solitary intrasellar plasmacytoma

Mass lesions cause hypothyroidism by compression of pituitary thyrotrophs, interruption of the hypothalamic-pituitary portal blood flow thereby preventing delivery of TRH to the pituitary, or rarely by acute hemorrhage or infarction resulting in pituitary apoplexy [89]. Several other etiologies are associated with central hypothyroidism, namely postpartum pituitary necrosis (Sheehan's syndrome), head trauma, surgery and irradiation, autoimmune lymphocytic hypophysitis, infiltrative diseases (e.g. sarcoidosis, histiocytosis, hemochromatosis) and infections (e.g. tuberculosis, syphilis, toxoplasmosis) [24].

Central Congenital Hypothyroidism

The presence of hypothalamic and pituitary hypothyroidism in infants is very rare. It may be caused by structural lesions such as pituitary hypoplasia and septo-optic dysplasia. Some cases are associated with mutations in genes encoding proteins that are related to TSH synthesis and release, namely TRH receptor [90], TSH [91] and pituitary transcription factors such as POU1F1, PROP1, LHX3, LHX4, HESX1 and LEPR [24]. These genetic defects may produce hypothyroidism either isolated or combined with other pituitary hormone deficiencies.

Drugs

Dopamine, bexarotene (retinoid X receptor agonist used in the treatment of lymphoma), glucocorticoids and somatostatin analogues may suppress serum TSH and contribute to the development of central hypothyroidism [92].

Other Disorders

Resistance to Thyroid Hormone

It is characterized by reduced tissue response to thyroid hormone action and is caused in most cases by mutations in the thyroid hormone receptor β gene. RTH can be classified as generalized, pituitary or peripheral [93–95]. In generalized resistance, the most common form, all thyroid responsive tissues are affected and patients have a nonsupressed TSH, due to the reduced sensitivity in the pituitary gland, and elevated circulating concentrations of thyroid hormones. Due to the resistance in peripheral tissues they are usually euthyroid. Patients with pituitary resistance alone are hyperthyroid as the high levels of thyroid hormones have normal action peripherally. Those with predominantly peripheral resistance have normal TSH and thyroid hormone levels that are not sufficient to overcome tissue hyposensitivity and usually present with symptoms and signs of hypothyroidism. We recently identified a patient with an extremely rare association of RTH and papillary thyroid carcinoma [96]. Control of thyroid function after total thyroidectomy was only possible using supraphysiological dosages of L-T4 (500 μg/day; 6 μg/kg/day).

Consumptive Hypothyroidism

It is a very rare condition characterized by excessive degradation of thyroid hormones within tumors such as large hemangiomas [97]. These tumors express type 3 deiodinase (D3), which metabolizes T4 to reverse T3 and T3 to 3,3′-diiodothyronine. Consumptive hypothyroidism is especially found in infants but adult cases were also reported [98].

Clinical Features

Hypothyroidism can affect all organ systems. The presence and severity of clinical manifestations are usually dependent on the degree of hormone deficiency. Two mechanisms explain most of the symptoms and signs: the generalized slowing of metabolic processes and the accumulation of glycosaminoglycans in the interstitial space of many tissues [99]. To simplify the discussion the authors decided to group the clinical features in organ systems.

Skin and Appendages

A mucinous nonpitting edema known as myxedema can be found around the eyes given a puffy or moonlike appearance, on the dorsum of the hands and feet, and in the supraclavicular fossa. This is explained by the accumulation of hyaluronic acid and other glycosaminoglycans in the dermis. The secretions of the sweat and sebaceous glands are reduced, leading to dryness of the skin. The skin is pale and cool as a result of cutaneous vasoconstriction and/or anemia. Some patients may have hypercarotenemia, which gives the skin a yellow tint. Wounds heal slowly. Easy bruising can also occur due to an increase in capillary fragility [14, 100].

Head and body hair is dry and brittle, lacks shine, and tends to fall out. Hair may be lost from the lateral margins of the eyebrows (Queen Anne's sign), although this is not a specific feature. Eyebrows can totally disappear. The nails are thickened, brittle and grow slowly (Fig. 7.3).

Cardiovascular

The cardiac output is decreased due to a reduction in both stroke volume and heart rate, which can explain the symptoms of reduced exercise tolerance and dyspnea. Peripheral vascular resistance is increased. These hemodynamic alterations cause narrowing of pulse pressure, diastolic hypertension (10–25 % of patients) and a decrease in blood flow to organs [101, 102]. In most tissues, the reduction in blood flow is proportional to the decrease in oxygen consumption and therefore angina is an infrequent symptom [103]. When present it is usually explained by an underlying coronary heart disease (CHD). Serum levels of homocysteine [104, 105] and creatine kinase (CK) [106] may be increased in hypothyroidism. Dyslipidemia can be found in more than 90 % of patients, usually presenting as elevations of total and low-density lipoprotein (LDL) cholesterol [107]. These findings may contribute to an increased risk of atherosclerosis.

An electrocardiogram can show sinus bradycardia, low voltage, prolongation of the PR interval, alterations of the ST segment, prolonged QT interval and flattened or inverted T waves [14, 100]. Torsade de pointes can rarely occur [108]. Echocardiographic evaluation may reveal pericardial effusion [109], asymmetric septal hypertrophy or other abnormalities

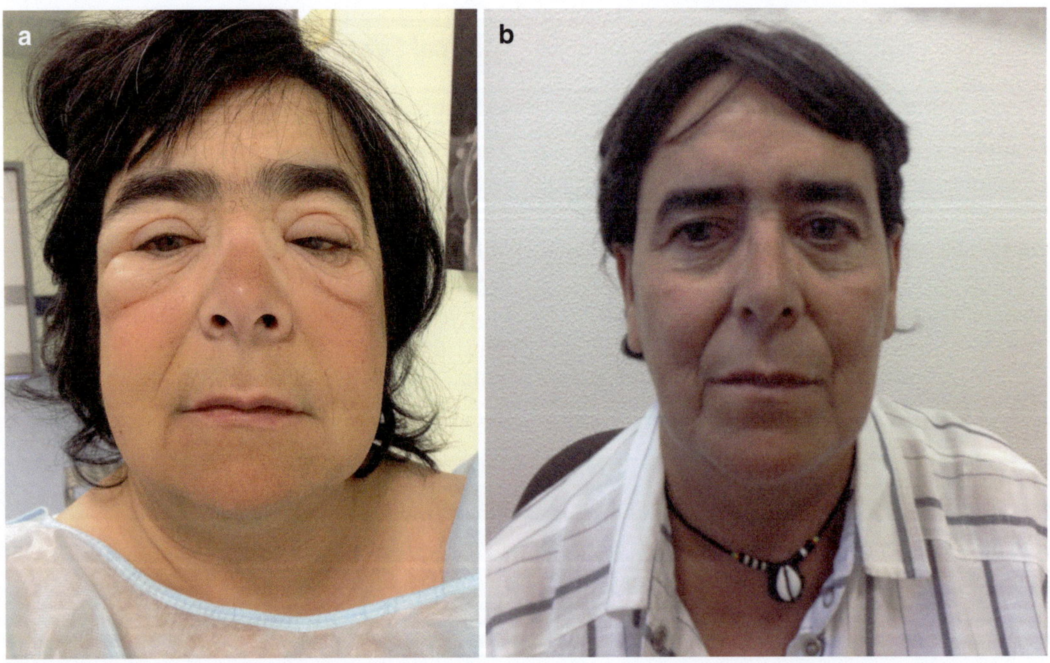

Fig. 7.3 Features of a patient with severe hypothyroidism. (**a**) Clinical presentation with marked periorbital myxedema, dry and cool skin and fatigue. (**b**) Significant improvement of signs and symptoms of hypothyroidism 3 months after the introduction of levothyroxine

[110]. Rarely, patients can develop congestive heart failure [111].

Respiratory

Pleural effusions can be present and may contribute to dyspnea [100]. In severe hypothyroidism, alveolar hypoventilation and carbon dioxide retention may occur, contributing to the development of myxedema coma [112, 113]. Obstructive sleep apnea is common as a result of macroglossia [114, 115].

Gastrointestinal

Appetite is usually reduced (anorexia). Modest weight gain can occur due to the decreased metabolic rate and retention of fluid in tissues. Contrary to popular belief, hypothyroidism is not related to an increase of fat and obesity [116]. Dysphagia or heartburn may be due to disordered esophageal motility, whereas dyspepsia, nausea or vomiting are related to delayed gastric emptying [117]. Decreased gut motility and decreased food intake result in constipation [118]. The latter may lead to fecal impaction, megacolon and ileus [119]. The rate of intestinal absorption is decreased and intestinal transit time is prolonged [120]. Ascites is rarely found [121]. Gallbladder motility is decreased in hypothyroid patients [122].

In addition, measurements of serum aspartate aminotransferase, lactate dehydrogenase [123] and carcinoembryonic antigen [124] may be elevated, and pernicious anemia can be present. Celiac disease is also associated with hypothyroidism [125].

Neurologic

Thyroid hormones are crucial for the development of the central nervous system. Congenital hypothyroidism is related to severe and irreversible neurologic abnormalities if left untreated. It can be associated with hypoplasia of cortical neurons, retarded myelination, and altered cell migration and differentiation [126, 127]. Manifestations include mental retardation, impaired motor development such as tremor, rigidity and spasticity of the trunk and proximal extremities, and also strabismus and sensorineural hearing loss [128].

Hypothyroidism occurring in adult life is characterized by less severe neurologic manifestations. Headaches can be identified in 30 % of hypothyroid patients [129]. Carpal tunnel syndrome is present in 29–38 % of cases due to compression of the median nerve by deposits of glycosaminoglycans [130, 131]. Body movements are slow and cerebellar ataxia may be identified [132]. The occurrence of delayed relaxation of deep tendon reflexes may be related to peripheral neuropathy [133]. Hearing loss, vertigo and tinnitus are frequent [134]. The voice is husky (hoarseness), low-pitched, and coarse.

The speech is slow and slurred [100]. These changes are caused by myxedematous infiltration of the tongue and larynx. Loss of initiative, memory and calculation defects, reduced attention span and poor concentration may be present. Irritability is decreased and apathy can occur. Psychiatric disorders are common and usually manifest as depression. However, some patients may present with psychosis and hallucinations (myxedema madness) [135]. An association between Alzheimer's disease and hypothyroidism was reported but an etiologic relationship has not been established [136, 137]. Lethargy and somnolence are sometimes found and epileptic seizures have been reported. The patient can evolve to myxedema coma. The pathogenesis of cognitive dysfunction in hypothyroidism is unknown. It may be related to a decrease in cerebral blood flow and a reduction in glucose metabolism [138].

Hashimoto's encephalopathy is a rare manifestation of HT [139]. Patients most often have an acute or subacute onset of confusion with alteration of consciousness and other neurologic signs, such as seizures, myoclonus, tremor, hyperreflexia and psychosis [139, 140]. The diagnosis is usually performed by the presence of these clinical manifestations in patients with elevated thyroid antibodies [141].

Musculoskeletal

Thyroid hormones are essential for normal growth and skeletal development. Thyroid hormone deficiency in infants results in growth failure and dwarfism in which the limbs are disproportionately short in relation to the trunk. Epiphyseal dysgenesis is a typical finding that can be identified in radiologic exams. Ossification centers appear late and bone age is retarded in relation to chronologic age [142]. Delayed closure of the fontanelles is also found. In older children hypothyroidism can cause short stature [143].

Adults may complain of arthralgias, joint stiffness and effusions [144]. Muscular symptoms can be identified in about 80 % of patients, namely muscle weakness and cramps [130]. Rarely, a combination of generalized muscular hypertrophy and weakness may be found, which is referred as Kocher-Debre-Semelaigne syndrome in children [145, 146] and Hofmann's syndrome in adults [147].

CK levels are sometimes high and patients may develop rhabdomyolysis [148]. Serum calcium levels are usually normal but may be elevated [149]. Serum phosphorus concentration is normal. Urinary excretion of calcium is decreased.

Renal

Renal blood flow is decreased due to the reduction of cardiac output and blood volume. The glomerular filtration rate is also low [150]. Other effects of hypothyroidism include impaired sodium reabsorption and renal ability to dilute urine. As a result, increased serum creatinine and hyponatremia can occur [151].

Hematopoietic

The red blood cell mass is decreased. Mild anemia may be found in one-third of patients [152], and it is usually normocytic and normochromic. Less commonly, a macrocytic form in the context of pernicious anemia or folate deficiency may occur [153]. Menorrhagia and the defective absorption of iron resulting from achlorhydria can contribute to a microcytic and hypochromic anemia.

White blood cell and platelet counts are usually normal. Hypothyroid patients have a higher risk of bleeding mainly due to acquired von Willebrand's syndrome [154, 155]. Some symptoms such as epistaxis, gum bleeding, menorrhagia and easy bruising may be present.

Endocrine

In primary hypothyroidism the increase in TSH levels stimulates the thyroid gland and results in the development of a goiter. Untreated primary hypothyroidism can also cause hyperplasia of the thyrotrophs and pituitary gland enlargement [156], which may result in hypopituitarism and visual field defects [157, 158]. About 39–63 % of patients have increased serum prolactin levels due to the increased TRH secretion. Galactorrhea may develop [159, 160]. Growth hormone secretion is decreased in hypothyroidism [161]. Serum aldosterone and cortisol levels are often normal in hypothyroid patients but the turnover rates are decreased. Plasma renin activity is also reduced [162]. Individuals may have an elevated plasma noradrenaline level, whereas the adrenaline concentration is usually normal [163]. A decreased adrenergic response is often found [164].

Reproductive

Thyroid hormones influence sexual development and reproductive function. Untreated infantile hypothyroidism results in sexual immaturity, whereas juvenile hypothyroidism causes a delay in the onset of puberty. However, it may also induce precocious puberty, which can be explained by the action of elevated levels of TSH on the follicle-stimulating hormone receptor [165].

In adult women, hypothyroidism may be associated with diminished libido and failure of ovulation [166]. Irregular menstrual cycles are present in more than 20 % of women, especially oligomenorrhea and menorrhagia [167]. Fertility may be reduced and both miscarriage and adverse neonatal outcomes can occur [168]. However, most women with untreated hypothyroidism have uneventful pregnancies and give birth to normal infants [169]. Hypothyroidism in adult men may cause decreased libido, erectile dysfunction, delayed ejaculation and defects in spermatogenesis [170, 171].

Energy Metabolism

Energy metabolism is decreased in hypothyroidism contributing to a lower energy expenditure, oxygen consumption and utilization of substrates. Both the synthesis and the degradation of protein are decreased, but nitrogen balance is usually positive. Permeability of capillaries to protein is increased, which explains the high levels of protein in effusions [14].

Hypothyroidism is usually associated with normal plasma glucose levels, whereas plasma insulin can be increased [172]. A lower glucose uptake in muscles and adipose tissue was reported [173]. In patients with preexisting diabetes mellitus who develop hypothyroidism, insulin requirements may be reduced possibly due to the decreased insulin degradation [174].

Both the synthesis and the degradation of lipid are reduced in hypothyroidism. As previously noted, hypothyroidism is associated with dyslipidemia usually presenting as elevations of total and LDL cholesterol [107].

Course of the Disease

Primary Hypothyroidism

In most cases a gradual loss of thyroid function occurs, resulting in an insidious onset of hypothyroidism that may go unnoticed by the patient and the family for several years. The presenting symptoms are highly variable. Dry skin, cold sensitivity, fatigue, muscle cramps, voice changes and constipation are among the most common features [16]. We frequently notice that older patients present with less clinical findings which can contribute to the delay in diagnosis. As hypothyroidism progresses, a slow intensification of all clinical manifestations occur. Progressive decrease in activity and responsiveness can finally evolve to coma. If left untreated, the length of time between the first symptoms and death may be as long as 15 years [17]. In contrast, symptoms are more abrupt if an acute loss of thyroid function occurs, such as when replacement therapy is discontinued or after thyroidectomy or radioiodine therapy. Thus, the clinical course may also be influenced by the etiology of the disorder. One interesting and recent study found that a diagnosis of hypothyroidism before the age of 60 is associated with loss of labor market income and a significantly increased risk of receiving a disability pension [175].

Central Hypothyroidism

The clinical manifestations are similar to those of primary hypothyroidism but the clinical picture is often milder [176]. Common symptoms of central hypothyroidism include fatigue and headaches [177]. Goiter is not a typical finding. Clinical features associated with deficiency or excess of other pituitary hormones are common and can mask those related to hypothyroidism [24]. For example, if hypogonadism is present patients may complaint of hot flashes and the cold intolerance typical of hypothyroidism is obscured. Acromegalic patients with central hypothyroidsm may present with sweating instead of dry skin.

Hypothyroidism in Infants and Children

Most infants with congenital hypothyroidism due to thyroid dysgenesis and dyshormonogenesis have no clinical features of thyroid dysfunction at birth, because maternal T4 is transferred to the fetus during late gestation [178]. Symptoms and signs can appear during the first months of life and include lethargy, hypotonia, poor feeding, hoarse cry, prolonged jaundice, large fontanelles, mottled and dry skin, distended abdomen, constipation and umbilical hernia [179]. This disorder can also be associated with additional congenital malformations especially affecting the heart [180]. If left untreated, prolonged hypothyroidism can be associated with dwarfism, sexual immaturity and severe neurological features, usually referred as cretinism. Other characteristic findings include disproportionately short limbs in relation to the trunk, broad and flat nose, widely set eyes, periorbital puffiness, and macroglossia [181] (Fig. 7.4).

Endemic cretinism in iodine deficient regions may manifest in a neurologic form characterized by goiter, mental retardation, strabismus, deaf-mutism, spasticity and other motor disorders, or present as a myxedematous form with thyroid atrophy, severe hypothyroidism, short stature, delayed sexual maturation and a less severe degree of mental retardation. However, these two clinical patterns may overlap [28, 34, 35]. Hypothyroidism in older children and adolescents is most commonly caused by HT. Common manifestations include declining growth velocity often resulting in short stature, delayed pubertal development and the presence of a goiter [143, 182, 183].

Screening

Congenital Hypothyroidism

Most developed countries perform newborn screening of congenital hypothyroidism, which is important for the early detection and treatment of affected infants and for the prevention of severe neurodevelopmental deficits associated with late diagnosis. Screening programs were proved to be successful and economically beneficial and are strongly recommended [184, 185]. Blood should be collected after heel prick and the best time for testing seems to be between 48 and 72 h of age [184]. Three screening strategies can be used including the measurement of

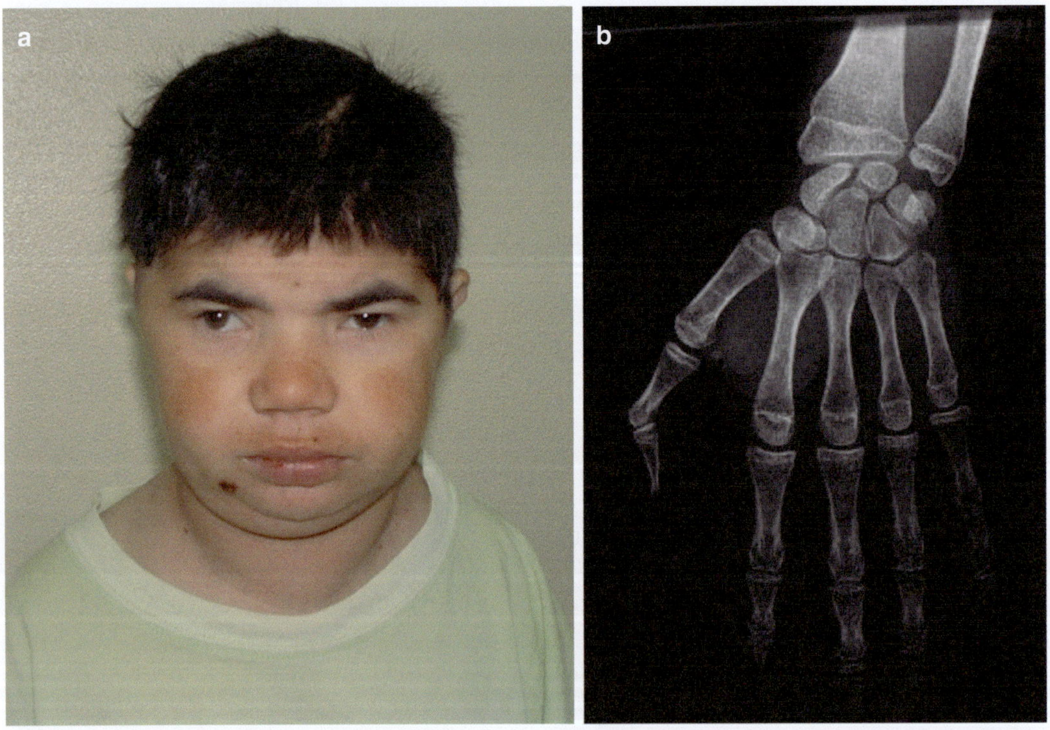

Fig. 7.4 A 26-year-old female with thyroid dyshormonogenesis due to a mutation in the thyroid peroxidase gene. (**a**) Typical clinical findings of congenital hypothyroidism were found, including dwarfism (height 118 cm), mental retardation, presence of a goiter, facial edema, evidence of a broad and flat nose, widely set eyes and strabismus. (**b**) X-ray of the left hand and wrist showing a bone age of 14 years (Courtesy of Dr. André Couto Carvalho and Dr. Cláudia Freitas)

TSH, T4 or both [185, 186]. TSH testing better detects subclinical hypothyroidism but will not identify infants with central hypothyroidism. The latter can only be recognized by measuring T4. The European Society of Paediatric Endocrinology guidelines consider that the main goal is to detect all forms of primary hypothyroidism and therefore recommend TSH screening [184]. In case of a high TSH concentration, confirmatory serum testing measuring TSH and FT4 should be performed. Thyroid ultrasound with color flow Doppler sonography and/or thyroid scan can be ordered to identify dysgenesis [187]. Some infants need genetic counseling and to perform genetic testing for the mutations associated with thyroid dyshormonogenesis [184].

Acquired Hypothyroidism

Measurement of thyroid function tests in asymptomatic patients is controversial but most experts do not favor screening the general population.

Screening individuals at risk for hypothyroidism (case finding) is recommended, including but not limited to those with autoimmune diseases, such as type 1 diabetes and pernicious anemia; patients with first-degree relatives diagnosed with an autoimmune thyroid disease; those with a history of radioiodine therapy, neck irradiation or thyroid surgery; patients with psychiatric disorders; those with an abnormal thyroid examination; patients taking drugs such as amiodarone or lithium; and those with hypercholesterolemia [16, 188]. We also suggest testing patients with Down syndrome given their risk of developing hypothyroidism (Fig. 7.5).

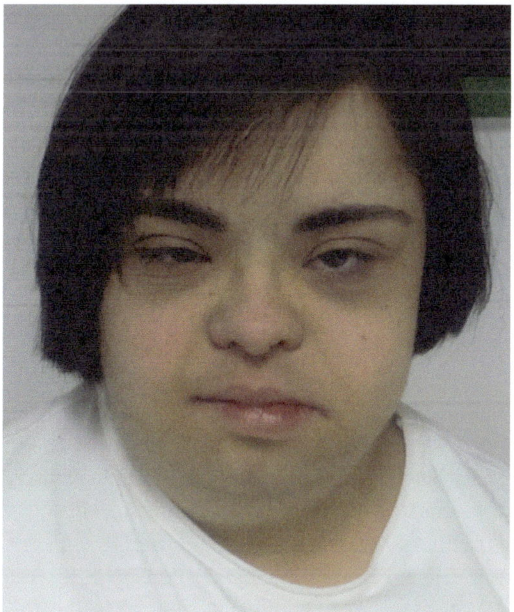

Fig. 7.5 Features of hypothyroidism in a patient with Down syndrome (Courtesy of Dr. Helder Simões)

Most organizations also recommend testing all individuals over a certain age. The American College of Physicians suggests screening in women older than 50 years of age [189]. The American Thyroid Association (ATA) recommends screening in all adults beginning at age 35 years and every 5 years thereafter [190]. Recent guidelines for hypothyroidism in adults cosponsored by the American Association of Clinical Endocrinologists (AACE) and the ATA consider screening of the population over the age of 60 [16].

TSH is the most sensitive and specific assay for detecting primary hypothyroidism and should be used for screening. However, it may not be useful if central hypothyroidism is suspected, in hospitalized patients and in those receiving drugs that affect TSH secretion [191]. If serum TSH is normal, no further testing is usually performed. In patients with a high serum TSH level, subsequent evaluation is needed including the measurement of FT4.

Diagnosis

Despite the insidious progression, hypothyroidism is usually detected at early stages, whereas severe disease is rarely seen today. This is possibly related to the availability of sensitive and specific laboratory testing and the awareness of physicians. Thus, there should be a low threshold to test patients for suspected hypothyroidism [192]. Clinical scores can help in predicting the presence of hypothyroidism [193, 194], but they are not recommended for its diagnosis given the lack of specificity of the clinical manifestations. The diagnosis relies upon thyroid function tests. Tissue markers of thyroid hormone action such as sex hormone binding globulin, osteocalcin, total and LDL cholesterol, lipoprotein(a), CK and ferritin should also not be used for the diagnosis of hypothyroidism [16].

In patients with suggestive symptoms or signs, the serum TSH should be the initial test. If an elevated level is found, the TSH measurement should be repeated along with a serum FT4. If the initial TSH level is normal but the patient has clear symptoms of hypothyroidism, a second measurement of TSH and FT4 can be performed to assess for central hypothyroidism. Furthermore, if a pituitary or hypothalamic disorder is suspected, TSH and FT4 can be initially measured. Measurements of serum total T3 and free T3 (FT3) are not indicated for the diagnosis of hypothyroidism [16].

An elevated serum TSH is usually defined as a concentration above the upper limit of the reference range for a given laboratory which typically lies between 4 and 5 mIU/L. Some authors found that more than 95 % of individuals without a thyroid disease have a TSH level less than 2.5 mIU/L, suggesting the use of a lower upper limit for the normal population [195]. TSH levels increase with age which may warrant the consideration of a higher reference range in older patients [196, 197].

Table 7.2 summarizes the thyroid function test results of the main types of hypothyroidism. In primary hypothyroidism, the first biochemical finding is a slightly elevated serum TSH value, caused by a minor decrease in T4 secretion not sufficient to produce a subnormal serum FT4 concentration (subclinical hypothyroidism). An additional decrease in T4 production results in low serum FT4 values along with higher levels of TSH (overt hypothyroidism) [198]. If performed, T3 levels are usually normal due to the preferential synthesis and secretion of T3 by the residual functioning thyroid tissue and due to the increased conversion of T4 to T3 by type 2 deiodinase (D2) in hypothyroid patients [199]. As the disease progresses serum T3 concentrations may become subnormal.

Table 7.2 Patterns of thyroid function tests in the main types of hypothyroidism

Type	Serum TSH	Serum FT4
Primary hypothyroidism		
Subclinical	High	Normal
Overt	High	Low
Central hypothyroidism	Low, normal or slightly high	Low or low-normal

FT4 free thyroxine, *TSH* thyroid-stimulating hormone

Patients with central hypothyroidism have a low-normal to low FT4 concentration and a serum TSH that is not appropriately elevated. TSH levels can be low, normal or even slightly elevated due to the secretion of biologically inactive TSH [177, 200]. A diurnal rhythm in TSH secretion with a surge late at night occurs in the normal population, whereas the nocturnal increase was found to be absent in patients with central hypothyroidism [201, 202]. Serum total T3 and FT3 levels may be normal or low [177].

After confirmation of hypothyroidism, it is mandatory to identify the etiology. Clinical history and physical examination can provide important clues, such as a previous history of thyroid surgery, cervical irradiation or radioiodine treatment, information about current and past medications and evidence of a goiter. In patients with primary hypothyroidism TPO antibodies should be measured [16]. The presence of antibodies usually indicates HT, whereas its absence suggests less common causes of hypothyroidism, such as painless or subacute thyroiditis. In addition, the finding of a low thyroid echogenicity on ultrasound usually indicates HT [203]. Measurement of radioactive iodine uptake (RAIU) is rarely required. In patients with central hypothyroidism, a pituitary magnetic resonance imaging should be performed (Fig. 7.2), along with the biochemical evaluation of other pituitary hormones to detect hormonal hypersecretion and/or combined deficiencies. Pituitary-adrenal function is usually assessed by a synacthen test. In patients with adrenal insufficiency, glucocorticoid therapy should precede treatment with L-T4 because the latter, if given alone, can precipitate an acute adrenal crisis.

Although most patients can be managed by physicians from different specialties, a subset of hypothyroid cases should be referred to endocrinologists. The guidelines cosponsored by the AACE and the ATA indicate referral in the following scenarios: children and infants, pregnancy and women planning conception, patients in whom it is difficult to achieve euthyroidism, concomitant cardiac disease, presence of goiter, nodules or other structural thyroid changes, evidence of other endocrine diseases such as adrenal and pituitary disorders, unusual combination of thyroid function tests and uncommon causes of hypothyroidism [16].

Differential Diagnosis

Primary Hypothyroidism

The differential diagnosis of primary hypothyroidism includes several conditions that present with an elevated serum TSH level.

RTH is characterized by nonsuppressed TSH levels which can be either normal or elevated. However, it can be distinguished from primary hypothyroidism due to the typical high levels of serum FT3 and FT4 and because most patients are euthyroid [93–96].

TSH-secreting pituitary adenomas are a rare cause of hyperthyroidism. The differential diagnosis with primary hypothyroidism relies on the measurement of free thyroid hormones, since these patients also present with high concentrations of FT3 and FT4 along with a measurable TSH [204, 205].

Patients with nonthyroidal illness may have transient elevations in the serum TSH concentration during recovery, sometimes presenting with TSH values above 20 mIU/L [206, 207]. Therefore, in patients with a recent illness and altered thyroid test results, measurements of serum TSH and FT4 should be repeated 4–6 weeks after recovery. In that situation normalization of the thyroid function usually occurs.

Patients with central hypothyroidism and biologically inactive TSH can present with slightly high TSH levels [177, 200]. High serum TPO antibodies suggest primary hypothyroidism, whereas abnormalities in other pituitary hormones favor the diagnosis of central hypothyroidism.

Patients with adrenal insufficiency can have a high level of serum TSH as a direct result of glucocorticoid deficiency. Thyroid function usually returns to normal after corticosteroid replacement [208].

Some individuals were found to have antibodies to the mouse immunoglobulins used in the TSH assay, causing falsely elevated TSH levels [209]. Other cases were reported to have a macromolecule formed by the binding between anti-TSH immunoglobulin and TSH, which is referred as macro-TSH. It can interfere with the laboratory measurement of TSH, leading to high results [210].

Central Hypothyroidism

Central hypothyroidism presents with low-normal to low FT4 concentrations and its differential diagnosis depends on the TSH levels [211].

As previously noted, in patients with a slightly high TSH concentration, primary hypothyroidism should be considered.

If TSH levels are normal, physicians should consider conditions related to thyroxine-binding globulin (TBG) deficiency, such as inherited mutations in the TBG gene [212], androgen ther apy [213], glucocorticoid excess [214], nephrotic syndrome [215], and therapy with L-asparaginase [216], danazol [217] or niacin [218]. Individuals with TBG deficiency usually present with low total thyroid hormone levels and normal serum TSH. However, it can be distinguished from central hypothyroidism because patients often manifest with normal serum FT4 and FT3 concentrations and have no symptoms or signs of thyroid dysfunction. Antiepileptic drugs such as phenytoin and carbamazepine may cause thyroid dysfunction by increasing thyroid hormone metabolism and competing for binding to TBG, resulting in a normal serum TSH and low total and free thyroid hormones levels [219, 220]. In patients treated with these drugs, assessment of other pituitary hormones and pituitary imaging may help to exclude central hypothyroidism. In addition, patients with drug-induced thyroid dysfunction have a normal TSH response to TRH administration, whereas those with pituitary or hypothalamic disorders have an absent or delayed response.

In patients with a low TSH concentration, subclinical hyperthyroidism may be included in the differential diagnosis [221]. A high-normal serum T3 level, a high-normal to high RAIU and the presence of focal areas of increased uptake on thyroid scan favor this diagnosis, whereas the presence of coexisting pituitary hormone abnormalities suggests central hypothyroidism. Treatment with T3 may also be considered in the setting of a low serum TSH and low or low-normal T4 values. T3 containing preparations can promote a suppression of TSH production which results in a decrease in T4 secretion by the thyroid gland.

Treatment

Primary Overt Hypothyroidism

Our therapeutic approach is in agreement with the ATA guidelines for the treatment of hypothyroidism [222] and the European Thyroid Association (ETA) guidelines [223]. The treatment of choice for hypothyroid patients is L-T4 monotherapy due to its efficacy, long-term experience, favorable side effect profile, ease of administration, good intestinal absorption, long serum half-life, and low cost. Other treatment modalities are currently not recommended [222, 223].

L-T4 Monotherapy

It has been considered the mainstay of thyroid hormone replacement for many years. Due to the peripheral conversion of the exogenous T4 into the active thyroid hormone T3, normal T3 levels are usually achieved in hypothyroid patients receiving adequate L-T4 therapy [13, 224].

Absorption of L-T4 takes place along the entire small intestine [225]. An acidic gastric pH occurring during fasting is important for a proper intestinal absorption, whereas co-administration with food reduces L-T4 absorption. Thus, L-T4 should be taken on an empty stomach [226]. The best timing of administration appears to be 60 min before breakfast or at bedtime at least 3 h after the evening meal [222, 227–229]. Another important issue to consider is patient's schedule and preferences. For example, if neither or the two previous options is feasible, taking the drug consistently 30 min before breakfast may also be reasonable and may promote treatment adherence. Approximately 80 % of the orally administered tablet is absorbed [230]. Once-daily treatment is indicated due to the long plasma half-life of L-T4 of about 7 days [231]. In addition, omission of a single pill has no significant effect. Missed doses should be administered when the omission is recognized, even on the same or subsequent day [232].

We can control thyroid function in virtually all cases. The availability in many countries of a multiplicity of tablet strengths ranging from 25 to 300 μg allows precise titration of the daily L-T4 dosage. The most common cause of treatment failure is nonadherence [233], and poorly compliant patients may be given their total weekly dose of L-T4 once per week [234]. Several formulations of T4 are available with variable absorption rates, which can explain the differences in bioequivalence between them. Either a generic or a brand-name L-T4 is acceptable. The use of brand-name products has the advantage of avoiding the switch between different formulations but will increase costs. If possible maintenance of the same generic preparation is advisable. In the case of a switch to another manufacturer, it is recommended to closely monitor the serum TSH level given the concern regarding bioequivalence [16, 222]. In addition to solid tablets that contain excipients and dyes, one brand preparation is available as an oral gel capsule that contains only L-T4, glycerin, gelatin, and water [235]. Some studies suggested that this preparation is less affected by changes in gastric pH, and may be better absorbed than standard L-T4 in selected circumstances such as the concomitant use of proton pump inhibitors or coffee consumption [236, 237]. Thus, the soft gel capsule may be an option for patients with suspected poor absorption, although long-term studies are lacking [222]. However, a less costly option is to increase the dose of the generic L-T4 tablet with periodic monitoring of serum TSH.

L-T4 requirement is dependent on lean body mass and therefore ideal body weight is usually used for dose calculations [238]. The average replacement dosage in adults is approximately 1.6–1.8 μg/kg of ideal body weight per day, which usually results in the prescription of 75–150 μg/day for women and 125–200 μg/day for men. The dose per kg is higher in infants and children. Hormone requirement may also vary according to the cause of hypothyroidism, likely reflecting the amount of residual functional thyroid tissue. Patients with HT or those submitted to radioiodine therapy may need less L-T4 than those who underwent thyroidectomy due to a thyroid cancer [239, 240]. Pretreatment serum TSH may also determine the required dose of L-T4 [241].

It is recommended to start with the fully calculated L-T4 dose in healthy young and middle-aged patients [222]. This approach leads to a more rapid normalization of serum TSH but a similar time to symptom resolution [242]. Thyroid hormone increases myocardial oxygen demand and is associated with a risk of inducing cardiac arrhythmias, angina and myocardial infarction, especially in the elderly and in patients with CHD. Thus, a low starting dose should be given to individuals older than 50–60 years (e.g. 50 μg daily) and to those with CHD (e.g. 12.5–25 μg daily). A gradual dose increase is suggested until normalization of serum TSH concentration is achieved or cardiac symptoms appear, in which case less than full replacement dose may be reasonable. Another option to allow the administration of appropriate doses of L-T4 in these patients is to consider additional cardiac medical or surgical treatments such as coronary artery revascularization [16, 222].

The goals of therapy are resolution of symptoms and signs, and normalization of the TSH secretion [222]. TSH is the most reliable marker of adequacy of replacement treatment and it should be kept within the normal reference range, which usually results in normal serum FT3 and FT4 concentrations. However, FT3 levels may be low and FT4 values are sometimes elevated [224, 243, 244]. As previously noted, the definition of a normal serum TSH is controversial and the use of age-specific cutoffs may be appropriate [195–197]. Symptoms alone lack sensitivity and specificity and are not recommended for judging adequacy of treatment [222].

Symptoms may start to improve in few weeks after the introduction of L-T4. Serum thyroid hormone concentrations increase first and produce a negative feedback action on the pituitary and hypothalamus, which results in a decrease of TSH secretion. A steady-state TSH concentration is achieved after approximately 6 weeks of therapy. Thus, TSH and FT4 levels should be measured 4–6 weeks after initiation of thyroid hormone replacement [222]. If the TSH value remains above the normal reference range, the daily dose of L-T4 can be increased by 12.5–25 μg. Thyroid function should be monitored every 4–6 weeks with additional changes in the dose of L-T4 until normal TSH levels are achieved. After identification of the proper maintenance dose, serum TSH can be measured in 4–6 months and then once yearly [222]. An increased FT4 level can be identified if the blood is drawn after L-T4 administration, and therefore it is usually suggested that collection be performed before taking the pill [245].

TSH levels may vary in the same individual by 40 % [246]. Thus, the dose of L-T4 may not be altered in clinically euthyroid patients with slightly high or low TSH levels found in a follow-up evaluation. These mild changes can be confirmed with repeat measurements of thyroid function before adjusting the therapy. There are several conditions than can interfere with the L-T4 treatment and when present may warrant a change in the dose of thyroid hormone replacement. The dose is usually increased during pregnancy or if the patient gains weight. Individuals in whom thyroid hormone absorption is diminished may also need a higher dose, including those with impaired acid secretion [247] or other gastrointestinal disorders such as celiac disease [248], and those taking calcium carbonate [249], bile acid sequestrants [250], phosphate binders [251], ferrous sulfate [252], aluminum-containing antacids [253], sucralfate [254] and proton pump inhibitors [255]. Coffee was also found to reduce L-T4 absorption [256]. In addition, some drugs increase the metabolic clearance of L-T4 and are also related to a need of higher doses, including rifampicin [257], carbamazepine [258], phenytoin [259] and sertraline [260]. Estrogen therapy in postmenopausal women is associated with a rise in serum TBG concentrations, which can result in the necessity of increasing the dose of L-T4 [261]. Thyroid function should be performed 4–8 weeks after these drugs are introduced or withdrawn [16]. However, when feasible, the best option is not to take L-T4 with interfering medications and a 4-h interval is suggested [222]. Based on our experience, hypothyroid patients who develop proteinuria due to nephrotic syndrome may also need higher dose requirements. A reduction in L-T4 dose may be needed with increasing age [262], if the patient loses weight or during androgen therapy [213]. Hormone replacement is usually performed lifelong but some etiologies of primary hypothyroidism are related to transient thyroid dysfunction, namely painless, postpartum and subacute thyroiditis.

Successful treatment with L-T4 usually reverses all the symptoms and signs of hypothyroidism. However, approximately 5–10 % of patients have persistent symptoms despite a normal TSH level [223]. Most clinical features related to thyroid dysfunction are nonspecific, and when they persist physicians should evaluate for alternative causes [222]. Suggested explanations for unresolved complaints include awareness of a chronic disorder, presence of associated autoimmune diseases, thyroid autoimmunity and inadequacy of L-T4 treatment in restoring physiological T4 and T3 concentrations in serum and tissues [223].

Adverse effects of T4 replacement are uncommonly found. Rare patients have an allergy to the dye or excipients in the tablets. For dye sensitivities, using multiples of the colorant-free 50 μg tablets is an option [263]. For allergies to excipients, the soft gel capsule can be tried [222]. Some studies suggested that about 40 % of older patients treated with L-T4 have a low TSH level [264]. Subclinical and overt hyperthyroidism due to overreplacement can be associated with atrial fibrillation and osteoporosis in the elderly and in postmenopausal women [265, 266].

General anesthesia and surgery in patients with untreated hypothyroidism are associated with minor perioperative complications [267, 268]. Thus, urgent surgery should not be postponed in hypothyroid patients, whereas it is prudent to defer elective surgical procedures until euthyroidism is achieved.

Patients treated with other therapeutic modalities should be switched to L-T4. For patients taking T4-T3 combination preparations, the equivalent dose of L-T4 can be calculated by the previous dose of T4 plus about three times the dose of T3 [269]. In general, 1 grain of desiccated thyroid extract (60 mg) is equivalent to about 88–100 μg of L-T4 [270]. In patients taking L-T4 for unclear reasons who have TSH levels in the normal range, the need for hormone replacement can be assessed by reducing the daily dose by 50 % and reevaluating the TSH and FT4 levels after 4–6 weeks. If no significant increase in TSH concentration is found and FT4 remains normal, residual thyroid function is most likely present. L-T4 can then be withdrawn and blood tests repeated in 4–6 weeks. Thyroid hormone replacement is not indicated in biochemically euthyroid individuals with symptoms of hypothyroidism, depression or obesity [222]. A systematic review showed inconclusive results regarding the effectiveness of L-T4 in weight loss [271].

A recent survey concluded that almost all physicians (mostly endocrinologists) are using L-T4 alone as the initial therapy for hypothyroid patients, and half of them prefer to use brand-name preparations. The rate of replacement was variable among the respondents with some choosing to start with a full replacement dose while others would perform a more gradual increase. Physicians preferred to use age-specific TSH targets for replacement therapy [272].

Combination T4 and T3 Therapy

Combination therapy is not recommended for the majority of patients with hypothyroidism. Whether it is beneficial in a subset of hypothyroid individuals is uncertain [16, 222, 223].

Patients who remain symptomatic during L-T4 therapy despite a normal TSH level were thought to benefit from combination therapy. However, systematic reviews and meta-analyses showed that combined T4-T3 therapy is not significantly superior to L-T4 monotherapy for the management of hypothyroid symptoms [273–276]. The ETA guidelines considered that combination therapy may be started in compliant patients treated with L-T4 who have persistent complaints despite normal serum TSH values, provided they have previously received support to deal with the chronic nature of their disorder, and associated autoimmune diseases have been excluded [223]. The authors suggested using a L-T4/liothyronine (L-T3) dose ratio between 13:1 and 20:1. Currently available combined preparations have a lower ratio and are not indicated. They therefore recommended the administration of separate L-T4 and L-T3 tablets (L-T4 once daily and L-T3 twice daily). The ATA guidelines suggested that combination therapy should not be used outside a formal clinical trial [222].

Patients with specific polymorphisms of the D2 gene, which converts T4 into T3 may be associated with better therapeutic responses to combination therapy when compared to L-T4 alone [277]. However, additional studies are needed. Genetic testing is currently not recommended as a guide to select therapy.

Furthermore, most clinical trials of combination therapy failed to mimic the physiological serum FT4-FT3 ratios. A combination of T4 and sustained-release T3 preparation may better replicate the normal ratio of T4 to T3 secretion by the thyroid gland [278, 279].

L-T3 Monotherapy

L-T3 is associated with wide fluctuations in serum T3 levels which may contribute to the development of thyrotoxic symptoms [280]. The drug half-life is approximately 1 day which requires two or three daily administrations [281].

L-T3 alone can be associated with more weight loss and improvement in the lipid profile when compared to L-T4, which could favor the use of the former in patients with obesity and dyslipidemia [282]. In addition, the use of a sustained-release T3 preparation can avoid the occurrence of serum T3 peaks [279]. However, longer-term controlled clinical trials are needed before considering this modality for clinical use. At the present time it is not recommended for the treatment of hypothyroidism [16, 222].

Desiccated Thyroid

Desiccated thyroid refers to preparations that are derived from the thyroid gland of animals. They contain both T4 and T3 in a ratio of approximately 4:1, which is significantly lower than the ratio of secretion by the human thyroid gland [283]. The relative excess of T3 results in supraphysiologic levels of serum T3 [284]. In addition, fluctuations in serum T3 levels occur throughout the day, with peaks occurring shortly after dosing [285]. A randomized clinical trial showed that desiccated thyroid was associated with more weight loss when compared to L-T4 and that some patients preferred to be treated with thyroid extracts. However, a significant improvement in quality of life was not demonstrated [270]. Since high-quality data is lacking, this modality should not be used in hypothyroid patients [16, 222].

Compounded Thyroid Hormones

Modification of the components or excipients of the thyroid hormone preparations can be performed by specialized pharmacies. This has the advantage of individualizing the medication for each patient. However, there are some concerns about safety. Errors in thyroid hormone compounding by the pharmacist have been reported which resulted in thyroid storm [286]. In addition, it was suggested that these preparations lose their potency in few weeks [287]. Therefore, they are not recommended and should only be considered in some cases of allergy to an excipient [222].

Dietary Supplements, Nutraceuticals and Other Over-the-Counter Products

Dietary supplements are substances added to the diet such as vitamins, minerals, herbs and amino acids. Nutraceuticals are dietary supplements that contain a concentrated form of a presumed bioactive substance originally derived from a food, but present in a nonfood matrix, and used to enhance health in dosages exceeding those obtainable from normal foods [288, 289].

Patients often use such products as part of the treatment of thyroid disorders [290]. Several compounds are available in the market due to the supposed capacity of enhancing thyroid function, including iodine-containing substances (e.g. kelp), tyrosine and thyroid hormone extracts or analogs such as 3,5,3′-triiodothyroacetic acid (TRIAC) [289]. These preparations are also not recommended for the treatment of hypothyroidism [16, 222].

Central Hypothyroidism

Patients with central hypothyroidism should also be treated with L-T4, using a dose of about 1.6 μg/kg [291]. Some authors suggested that they may need a higher dose when compared to patients with primary hypothyroidism caused by HT or radioiodine therapy [239]. The dose should be adjusted according to symptoms and to the serum FT4 values, aiming to maintain this biochemical parameter in the upper half of the normal range [291]. Serum TSH cannot be used to monitor therapy because it is almost always suppressed during thyroid hormone replacement [292]. A randomized controlled study comparing combination T4-T3 therapy with L-T4 alone in patients with central hypothyroidism showed that the former was associated with an improvement of ankle reflex time and a decrease in CK levels, but resulted in supraphysiological levels of FT3 [291]. There is insufficient evidence to recommend for combination therapy in this population [222]. In patients with pituitary tumors, hypothyroidism may be reversible since surgery occasionally leads to an improvement of anterior pituitary function.

Congenital Hypothyroidism

Hormone replacement is mandatory in infants after serum confirmation of overt congenital hypothyroidism and in some subclinical cases (e.g. serum TSH above 20 mIU/L). In addition, some authors consider that infants with higher screening TSH levels (e.g above 40 mIU/L) should start treatment as soon as a venous sample is obtained, without waiting for the confirmatory results [184]. As in other forms of hypothyroidism, oral L-T4 alone is the treatment of choice. Most authors recommend a starting dose of 10–15 μg/kg/day [184, 185]. The L-T4 tablet should be crushed and administered with milk or water. Although the absorption is reduced when the drug is given with food, asking the parents to administer L-T4 on an empty stomach may reduce compliance. Some authors choose to instruct the family to give the medication consistently at the same time of the day [293].

The goals of treatment are to restore adequate levels of thyroid hormones and assure normal clinical outcomes. The serum TSH level should be maintained within the age-specific reference range and the total T4 or FT4 concentrations should be kept in the upper half of the age-specific normal range. The first follow-up evaluation with measurement of serum FT4 or total T4 values and TSH levels is generally performed 1–2 weeks after the initiation of hormone replacement, and should be repeated every 2 weeks until serum TSH level is normalized [184]. The serum T4 concentration should become normal within 2 weeks and the serum TSH level is usually within the reference range after 1 month of treatment [185]. Then thyroid function may be evaluated every 1–3 months until the age of 12 months, every 2–4 months between 1 and 3 years of age and every 3–12 months thereafter until growth is complete. If the L-T4 dose is changed, thyroid function should be monitored after 4–6 weeks [184]. Regular clinical evaluation for growth, puberty, psychomotor and neurological development is also mandatory.

Lifelong treatment is usually necessary because the disorder is permanent in most cases. However, patients thought to have transient hypothyroidism may be re-evaluated, including infants with normal imaging exams of the thyroid gland, no confirmation of thyroid dyshormonogenesis, those with positive thyroid antibodies, and children who did not require an increase in L-T4 dose since infancy. In these cases L-T4 therapy is discontinued or reduced for 4–6 weeks after the age of 3 years, and thyroid function is monitored. If normal results are found, the presence of transient hypothyroidism can be assumed and no further treatment is needed. However, these patients should be monitored thereafter on a regular basis.

Some authors showed that normal development is usually achieved in children with congenital hypothyroidism treated soon after birth. However, more severely affected infants with lower serum thyroid hormone levels may develop intellectual impairment despite early treatment [294–296]. In contrast, inadequate or delayed treatment for several months may result in permanent brain damage, even if an adequate hormone replacement is started later.

Conclusion

Hypothyroidism is a common disorder that manifests with an insidious progression of nonspecific clinical features. Currently, it is usually diagnosed at early stages which allow a timely treatment. L-T4 is still the modality of choice and other therapeutic options are not recommended. The administration of an appropriate dose of L-T4 leads to a normalization of thyroid function in virtually all cases. However, patients with severe long-standing hypothyroidism can develop life-threatening complications. Therefore, physicians must be aware of the typical clinical findings in order to promptly evaluate patients with suspected hypothyroidism. Special consideration should be given to the treatment of older patients and those with CHD in whom a "start low and go slow" strategy is mandatory. Case finding is recommended for the population at risk. In addition, newborn screening of congenital hypothyroidism is crucial for the early detection and treatment of affected infants, and contributes for the prevention of severe neurodevelopmental deficits associated with late diagnosis.

Acknowledgement We thank Joan Kennedy for the assistance in preparing the chapter.

References

1. Curling TB. Two cases of absence of the thyroid body, and symmetrical swellings of fat tissue at the sides of the neck, connected with defective cerebral development. Med Chir Trans. 1850;33:303–6.
2. Gull WW. On a cretinoid state supervening in adult life in women. Trans Clin Soc Lond. 1873/1874;7:180–5.
3. Ord WM. On myxœdema, a term proposed to be applied to an essential condition in the "cretinoid" affection occasionally observed in middle-aged women. Med Chir Trans. 1878;61:57–78.5.
4. Kocher T. Ueber kropfexstirpation und ihre folgen. Arch Klin Chir. 1883;29:254–337.
5. Ord WM. Report of a committee of the Clinical Society of London nominated December 14, 1883, to investigate the subject of myxoedema. Trans Clin Soc Lond. 1888;21:1–215.
6. Murray GR. Note on the treatment of myxoedema by hypodermic injections of an extract of the thyroid gland of a sheep. Br Med J. 1891;2:796–7.
7. Hashimoto H. Zur kenntnis der lymphömatosen Veränderung der schilddrüse (Struma lymphomatosa). Archiv für Klinische Chirurgie. 1912;97:219–48.
8. Kendall E. The isolation in crystalline form of the compound containing iodin, which occurs in the thyroid. JAMA. 1915;64:2042–3.
9. Harington CR, Barger G. Chemistry of thyroxine: constitution and synthesis of thyroxine. Biochem J. 1927;21:169–83.
10. Gross J, Pitt-Rivers R. The identification of 3:5:3'-L-triiodothyronine in human plasma. Lancet. 1952;1:439–41.
11. Roitt IM, Doniach D, Campbell PN, et al. Autoantibodies in Hashimoto's disease (lymphadenoid goitre). Lancet. 1956;271:820–1.
12. Condliffe PG. Purification of human thyrotrophin. Endocrinology. 1963;72:893–6.
13. Braverman LE, Ingbar SH, Sterling K. Conversion of thyroxine (T4) to triiodothyronine (T3) in athyreotic human subjects. J Clin Invest. 1970;49:855–64.
14. Brent GA, Davies TF. Hypothyroidism and thyroiditis. In: Melmed S, editor. Williams textbook of endocrinology. 12th ed. Philadelphia: Elsevier Health Sciences; 2011. p. 406–39.
15. Roberts CG, Ladenson PW. Hypothyroidism. Lancet. 2004;363:793–803.
16. Garber JR, Cobin RH, Gharib H, et al. Clinical practice guidelines for hypothyroidism in adults: cosponsored by the American Association of Clinical Endocrinologists and the American Thyroid Association. Thyroid. 2012;22:1200–35.
17. Wiersinga WM. Adult hypothyroidism. In: Endotext. 2014. http://www.thyroidmanager.org. Accessed 21 Apr 2015.
18. Hollowell JG, Staehling NW, Flanders WD, et al. Serum TSH, T(4), and thyroid antibodies in the United States population (1988 to 1994): National

Health and Nutrition Examination Survey (NHANES III). J Clin Endocrinol Metab. 2002;87:489–99.
19. Canaris GJ, Manowitz NR, Mayor G, et al. The Colorado thyroid disease prevalence study. Arch Intern Med. 2000;160:526–34.
20. Tunbridge WM, Evered DC, Hall R, et al. The spectrum of thyroid disease in a community: the Whickham survey. Clin Endocrinol (Oxf). 1977; 7:481–93.
21. Vanderpump MP, Tunbridge WM, French JM, et al. The incidence of thyroid disorders in the community: a twenty-year follow-up of the Whickham Survey. Clin Endocrinol (Oxf). 1995;43:55–68.
22. Aoki Y, Belin RM, Clickner R, et al. Serum TSH and total T4 in the United States population and their association with participant characteristics: National Health and Nutrition Examination Survey (NHANES 1999–2002). Thyroid. 2007;17:1211–23.
23. Walsh JP, Bremner AP, Feddema P, et al. Thyrotropin and thyroid antibodies as predictors of hypothyroidism: a 13-year, longitudinal study of a community-based cohort using current immunoassay techniques. J Clin Endocrinol Metab. 2010;95:1095–104.
24. Persani L. Clinical review: Central hypothyroidism: pathogenic, diagnostic, and therapeutic challenges. J Clin Endocrinol Metab. 2012;97:3068–78.
25. Skordis N, Toumba M, Savva SC, et al. High prevalence of congenital hypothyroidism in the Greek Cypriot population: results of the neonatal screening program 1990–2000. J Pediatr Endocrinol Metab. 2005;18:453–61.
26. Harris KB, Pass KA. Increase in congenital hypothyroidism in New York State and in the United States. Mol Genet Metab. 2007;91:268–77.
27. Vanderpump MP. The epidemiology of thyroid disease. Br Med Bull. 2011;99:39–51.
28. Zimmermann MB. Iodine deficiency. Endocr Rev. 2009;30:376–408.
29. Andersson M, Karumbunathan V, Zimmermann MB. Global iodine status in 2011 and trends over the past decade. J Nutr. 2012;142:744–50.
30. Pearce EN, Andersson M, Zimmermann MB. Global iodine nutrition: where do we stand in 2013? Thyroid. 2013;23:523–8.
31. Böttcher Y, Eszlinger M, Tönjes A, et al. The genetics of euthyroid familial goiter. Trends Endocrinol Metab. 2005;16:314–9.
32. Bourdoux P, Delange F, Gerard M, et al. Evidence that cassava ingestion increases thiocyanate formation: a possible etiologic factor in endemic goiter. J Clin Endocrinol Metab. 1978;46:613–21.
33. Eastman CJ, Zimmermann M. The iodine deficiency disorders. In: Endotext. 2014. http://www.thyroidmanager.org. Accessed 21 Apr 2015.
34. Boyages SC. Clinical review 49: iodine deficiency disorders. J Clin Endocrinol Metab. 1993;77: 587–91.
35. Boyages SC, Halpern JP, Maberly GF, et al. A comparative study of neurological and myxedematous endemic cretinism in western China. J Clin Endocrinol Metab. 1988;67:1262–71.
36. Burgi H. Iodine excess. Best Pract Res Clin Endocrinol Metab. 2010;24:107–15.
37. McHenry CR, Slusarczyk SJ. Hypothyroidisim following hemithyroidectomy: incidence, risk factors, and management. Surgery. 2000;128:994–8.
38. Verloop H, Louwerens M, Schoones JW, et al. Risk of hypothyroidism following hemithyroidectomy: systematic review and meta-analysis of prognostic studies. J Clin Endocrinol Metab. 2012;97: 2243–55.
39. Kandil E, Krishnan B, Noureldine SI, et al. Hemithyroidectomy: a meta-analysis of postoperative need for hormone replacement and complications. ORL J Otorhinolaryngol Relat Spec. 2013;75:6–17.
40. Bahn RS, Burch HB, Cooper DS, et al. Hyperthyroidism and other causes of thyrotoxicosis: management guidelines of the American Thyroid Association and American Association of Clinical Endocrinologists. Thyroid. 2011;21:593–646.
41. Von Hofe SE, Dorfman SG, Carretta RF, et al. The increasing incidence of hypothyroidism within one year after radioiodine therapy for toxic diffuse goiter. J Nucl Med. 1978;19:180–4.
42. Nofal MM, Beierwaltes WH, Patno ME. Treatment of hyperthyroidism with sodium iodide I-131. JAMA. 1966;197:605–10.
43. Metso S, Jaatinen P, Huhtala H, et al. Long-term follow-up study of radioiodine treatment of hyperthyroidism. Clin Endocrinol (Oxf). 2004;61:641–8.
44. Nygaard B, Hegedüs L, Nielsen KG, et al. Long-term effect of radioactive iodine on thyroid function and size in patients with solitary autonomously functioning toxic thyroid nodules. Clin Endocrinol (Oxf). 1999;50:197–202.
45. Hancock SL, Cox RS, McDougall IR. Thyroid diseases after treatment of Hodgkin's disease. N Engl J Med. 1991;325:599–605.
46. Smolarz K, Malke G, Voth E, et al. Hypothyroidism after therapy for larynx and pharynx carcinoma. Thyroid. 2000;10:425–9.
47. Sklar C, Whitton J, Mertens A, et al. Abnormalities of the thyroid in survivors of Hodgkin's disease: data from the Childhood Cancer Survivor Study. J Clin Endocrinol Metab. 2000;85:3227–32.
48. Bogazzi F, Bartalena L, Martino E. Approach to the patient with amiodarone-induced thyrotoxicosis. J Clin Endocrinol Metab. 2010;95:2529–35.
49. Basaria S, Cooper DS. Amiodarone and the thyroid. Am J Med. 2005;118:706–14.
50. Martino E, Bartalena L, Bogazzi F, et al. The effects of amiodarone on the thyroid. Endocr Rev. 2001;22:240–54.
51. Batcher EL, Tang XC, Singh BN, et al. Thyroid function abnormalities during amiodarone therapy

for persistent atrial fibrillation. Am J Med. 2007;120:880–5.
52. Martino E, Safran M, Aghini-Lombardi F, et al. Environmental iodine intake and thyroid dysfunction during chronic amiodarone therapy. Ann Intern Med. 1984;101:28–34.
53. Martino E, Aghini-Lombardi F, Mariotti S, et al. Amiodarone iodine-induced hypothyroidism: risk factors and follow-up in 28 cases. Clin Endocrinol (Oxf). 1987;26:227–37.
54. Yagishita A, Hachiya H, Kawabata M, et al. Amiodarone-induced thyrotoxicosis late after amiodarone withdrawal. Circ J. 2013;77:2898–903.
55. Barbesino G. Drugs affecting thyroid function. Thyroid. 2010;20:763–70.
56. Lazarus JH. Lithium and thyroid. Best Pract Res Clin Endocrinol Metab. 2009;23:723–33.
57. van Melick EJ, Wilting I, Meinders AE, et al. Prevalence and determinants of thyroid disorders in elderly patients with affective disorders: lithium and nonlithium patients. Am J Geriatr Psychiatry. 2010;18:395–403.
58. Kirov G, Tredget J, John R, et al. A cross-sectional and a prospective study of thyroid disorders in lithium-treated patients. J Affect Disord. 2005;87:313–7.
59. Bocchetta A, Bernardi F, Burrai C, et al. The course of thyroid abnormalities during lithium treatment: a two-year follow-up study. Acta Psychiatr Scand. 1992;86:38–41.
60. Spaulding SW, Burrow GN, Bermudez F, et al. The inhibitory effect of lithium on thyroid hormone release in both euthyroid and thyrotoxic patients. J Clin Endocrinol Metab. 1972;35:905–11.
61. Tomer Y, Blackard JT, Akeno N. Interferon alpha treatment and thyroid dysfunction. Endocrinol Metab Clin North Am. 2007;36:1051–66.
62. Tran HA, Jones TL, Ianna EA, et al. Thyroid disease in chronic hepatitis C infection treated with combination interferon-a and ribavirin: management strategies and future perspective. Endocr Pract. 2013;19:292–300.
63. Nadeem A, Hussain MM, Aslam M, et al. Interferon-alpha induced and ribavirin induced thyroid dysfunction in patients with chronic hepatitis C. Hepat Mon. 2010;10:132–40.
64. Tomer Y. Hepatitis C, and interferon induced thyroiditis. J Autoimmun. 2010;34:J322–6.
65. Bini EJ, Mehandru S. Incidence of thyroid dysfunction during interferon alfa-2b and ribavirin therapy in men with chronic hepatitis C: a prospective cohort study. Arch Intern Med. 2004;164:2371–6.
66. Weijl NI, Van der Harst D, Brand A, et al. Hypothyroidism during immunotherapy with interleukin-2 is associated with antithyroid antibodies and response to treatment. J Clin Oncol. 1993;11:1376–83.
67. Atkins MB, Mier JW, Parkinson DR, et al. Hypothyroidism after treatment with interleukin-2 and lymphokine-activated killer cells. N Engl J Med. 1988;318:1557–63.
68. Mattijssen VJ, De Mulder PH, Van Liessum PA, et al. Hypothyroidism and goiter in a patient during treatment with interleukin-2. Cancer. 1990;65:2686–8.
69. Vialettes B, Guillerand MA, Viens P, et al. Incidence rate and risk factors for thyroid dysfunction during recombinant interleukin-2 therapy in advanced malignancies. Acta Endocrinol (Copenh). 1993;129:31–8.
70. Ahmadieh H, Salti I. Tyrosine kinase inhibitors induced thyroid dusfunction: a review of its incidence, pathophysiology, clinical relevance, and treatment. Biomed Res Int. 2013;2013:725410.
71. Wong E, Rosen LS, Mulay M, et al. Sunitinib induces hypothyroidism in advanced cancer patients and may inhibit thyroid peroxidase activity. Thyroid. 2007;17:351–5.
72. Rini BI, Tamaskar I, Shaheen P, et al. Hypothyroidism in patients with metastatic renal cell carcinoma treated with sunitinib. J Natl Cancer Inst. 2007; 99:81–3.
73. Papi G, LiVolsi VA. Current concepts on Riedel thyroiditis. Am J Clin Pathol. 2004;121:S50–63.
74. Hennessey JV. Clinical review: Riedel's thyroiditis: a clinical review. J Clin Endocrinol Metab. 2011; 96:3031–41.
75. Villa F, Dionigi G, Tanda ML, et al. Amyloid goiter. Int J Surg. 2008;6:S16–8.
76. Antonelli A, Fazzi P, Fallahi P, et al. Prevalence of hypothyroidism and Graves disease in sarcoidosis. Chest. 2006;130:526–32.
77. Oerter KE, Kamp GA, Munson PJ, et al. Multiple hormone deficiencies in children with hemochromatosis. J Clin Endocrinol Metab. 1993;76:357–61.
78. Gordon MB, Klein I, Dekker A, et al. Thyroid disease in progressive systemic sclerosis: increased frequency of glandular fibrosis and hypothyroidism. Ann Intern Med. 1981;95:431–5.
79. Chan AM, Lynch MJ, Bailey JD, et al. Hypothyroidism in cystinosis. A clinical, endocrinologic and histologic study involving sixteen patients with cystinosis. Am J Med. 1970;48:678–92.
80. Luiz HV, Pereira BD, Silva TN, et al. Thyroid tuberculosis with abnormal thyroid function – case report and review of the literature. Endocr Pract. 2013;19:e44–9.
81. Fisher DA. Second International Conference on Neonatal Thyroid Screening: progress report. J Pediatr. 1983;102:653–4.
82. Narumi S, Muroya K, Asakura Y, et al. Transcription factor mutations and congenital hypothyroidism: systematic genetic screening of a population-based cohort of Japanese patients. J Clin Endocrinol Metab. 2010;95:1981–5.
83. Grasberger H, Refetoff S. Genetic causes of congenital hypothyroidism due to dyshormonogenesis. Curr Opin Pediatr. 2011;23:421–8.
84. Sunthornthepvarakui T, Gottschalk ME, Hayashi Y, et al. Brief report: resistance to thyrotropin caused

by mutations in the thyrotropin-receptor gene. N Engl J Med. 1995;332:155–60.
85. Delange F, Dalhem A, Bourdoux P, et al. Increased risk of primary hypothyroidism in preterm infants. J Pediatr. 1984;105:462–9.
86. Bartalena L, Bogazzi F, Braverman LE, et al. Effects of amiodarone administration during pregnancy on neonatal thyroid function and subsequent neurodevelopment. J Endocrinol Invest. 2001;24: 116–30.
87. Zakarija M, McKenzie JM, Eidson MS. Transient neonatal hypothyroidism: characterization of maternal antibodies to the thyrotropin receptor. J Clin Endocrinol Metab. 1990;70:1239–46.
88. Luiz HV, Silva TN, Pereira BD, et al. Intrasellar plasmacytoma: an entity to be considered in the differential diagnosis of a pituitary mass lesion. In: Abstracts of the 97th annual meeting & expo of The Endocrine Society, San Diego, 5–8 March 2015. 2015.
89. Yamada M, Mori M. Mechanisms related to the pathophysiology and management of central hypothyroidism. Nat Clin Pract Endocrinol Metab. 2008;4:683–94.
90. Collu R, Tang J, Castagne J, et al. A novel mechanism for isolated central hypothyroidism: inactivating mutations in the thyrotropin-releasing hormone receptor gene. J Clin Endocrinol Metab. 1997; 82:1561–5.
91. Bonomi M, Proverbio MC, Weber G, et al. Hyperplastic pituitary gland, high serum glycoprotein hormone alpha-subunit, and variable circulating thyrotropin (TSH) levels as hallmark of central hypothyroidism due to mutations of the TSH beta gene. J Clin Endocrinol Metab. 2001;86:1600–4.
92. Haugen BR. Drugs that suppress TSH or cause central hypothyroidism. Best Pract Res Clin Endocrinol Metab. 2009;23:793–800.
93. Olateju TO, Vanderpump MP. Thyroid hormone resistance. Ann Clin Biochem. 2006;43:431–40.
94. Agrawal NK, Goyal R, Rastogi A, et al. Thyroid hormone resistance. Postgrad Med J. 2008;84:473–7.
95. Dumitrescu AM, Refetoff S. The syndromes of reduced sensitivity to thyroid hormone. Biochim Biophys Acta. 1830;2013:3987–4003.
96. Luiz HV, Silva TN, Pereira BD, et al. Management of differentiated thyroid carcinoma in a patient with thyroid hormone resistance: difficulties and challenges. In: Abstracts of the 16th international congress of endocrinology and 96th annual meeting & expo of The Endocrine Society, Chicago, 21–24 June 2014. 2014.
97. Huang SA, Tu HM, Harney JW, et al. Severe hypothyroidism caused by type 3 iodothyronine deiodinase in infantile hemangiomas. N Engl J Med. 2000;343:185–9.
98. Ruppe MD, Huang SA, Jan de Beur SM. Consumptive hypothyroidism caused by paraneoplastic production of type 3 iodothyronine deiodinase. Thyroid. 2005;15:1369–72.
99. Smith TJ, Bahn RS, Gorman CA. Connective tissue, glycosaminoglycans, and diseases of the thyroid. Endocr Rev. 1989;10:366–91.
100. Hall R, Scanlon MF. Hypothyroidism: clinical features and complications. Clin Endocrinol Metab. 1979;8:29–38.
101. Klein I, Ojamaa K. Thyroid hormone and the cardiovascular system. N Engl J Med. 2001;344:501–9.
102. Klein I, Danzi S. Thyroid disease and the heart. Circulation. 2007;116:1725–35.
103. Becker C. Hypothyroidism and atherosclerotic heart disease: pathogenesis, medical management, and the role of coronary artery bypass surgery. Endocr Rev. 1985;6:432–40.
104. Hussein WI, Green R, Jacobsen DW, et al. Normalization of hyperhomocysteinemia with L-thyroxine in hypothyroidism. Ann Intern Med. 1999;131:348–51.
105. Catargi B, Parrot-Roulaud F, Cochet C, et al. Homocysteine, hypothyroidism, and effect of thyroid hormone replacement. Thyroid. 1999;9: 1163–6.
106. Klein I, Mantell P, Parker M, et al. Resolution of abnormal muscle enzyme studies in hypothyroidism. Am J Med Sci. 1980;279:159–62.
107. O'Brien T, Dinneen SF, O'Brien PC, et al. Hyperlipidemia in patients with primary and secondary hypothyroidism. Mayo Clin Proc. 1993; 68:860–6.
108. Fredlund BO, Olsson SB. Long QT interval and ventricular tachycardia of "torsade de pointe" type in hypothyroidism. Acta Med Scand. 1983;213: 231–5.
109. Hardisty CA, Naik DR, Munro DS. Pericardial effudion in hypothyroidism. Clin Endocrinol (Oxf). 1980;13:349–54.
110. Santos AD, Miller RP, Mathew PK, et al. Echocardiographic characterization of the reversible cardiomyopathy of hypothyroidism. Am J Med. 1980;68:675–82.
111. Biondi B. Mechanisms in endocrinology: heart failure and thyroid dysfunction. Eur J Endocrinol. 2012;167:609–18.
112. Nordqvist P, Dhuner KG, Stenberg K, et al. Myxoedema coma and carbon dioxide-retention. Acta Med Scand. 1960;166:189–94.
113. Weg JG, Calverly JR, Johnson C. Hypothyroidism and alveolar hypoventilation. Arch Intern Med. 1965;115:302–6.
114. Rosenow F, McCarthy V, Caruso AC. Sleep apnoea in endocrine diseases. J Sleep Res. 1998;7:3–11.
115. Pelttari L, Rauhala E, Polo O, et al. Upper airway obstruction in hypothyroidism. J Intern Med. 1994;236:177–81.
116. Karmisholt J, Andersen S, Laurberg P. Weight loss after therapy of hypothyroidism is mainly caused by excretion of excess body water associated with myxoedema. J Clin Endocrinol Metab. 2011;96:E99–103.
117. Ebert EC. The thyroid and the gut. J Clin Gastroenterol. 2010;44:402–6.

118. Shafer RB, Prentiss RA, Bond JH. Gastrointestinal transit in thyroid disease. Gastroenterology. 1984;86:852–5.
119. Hohl RD, Nixon RK. Myxedema ileus. Arch Intern Med. 1965;115:145–50.
120. Rahman Q, Haboubi NY, Hudson PR, et al. The effect of thyroxine on small intestinal motility in the elderly. Clin Endocrinol (Oxf). 1991;35:443–6.
121. Kocen RS, Atkinson M. Ascites in hypothyroidism. Lancet. 1963;1:527–30.
122. Bellini MA, Cervino JM, De Buno RB, et al. Hypotonia of the gall bladder, of myxedematous origin. J Clin Endocrinol Metab. 1957;17:133–42.
123. Saha B, Maity C. Alteration of serum enzymes in primary hypothyroidism. Clin Chem Lab Med. 2002;40:609–11.
124. Amino N, Kuro R, Yabu Y, et al. Elevated levels of circulating carcinoembryonic antigens in hypothyroidism. J Clin Endocrinol Metab. 1981;52:457–62.
125. Elfström P, Montgomery SM, Kämpe O, et al. Risk of thyroid disease in individuals with celiac disease. J Clin Endocrinol Metab. 2008;93:3915–21.
126. Bernal J, Guadano-Ferraz A, Morte B. Perspectives in the study of thyroid hormone action on brain development and function. Thyroid. 2003;13:1005–12.
127. Williams GR. Neurodevelopmental and neurophysiological actions of thyroid hormone. J Neuroendocrinol. 2008;20:784–94.
128. Halpern JP, Boyages SC, Maberly GF, et al. The neurology of endemic cretinism. A study of two endemias. Brain. 1991;114:825–41.
129. Moreau T, Manceau E, Giroud-Baleydier F, et al. Headache in hypothyroidism. Prevalence and outcome under thyroid hormone therapy. Cephalalgia. 1998;18:687–9.
130. Duyff RF, Van den Bosch J, Laman DM, et al. Neuromuscular findings in thyroid dysfunction: a prospective clinical and electrodiagnostic study. J Neurol Neurosurg Psychiatry. 2000;68:750–5.
131. Kececi H, Degirmenci Y. Hormone replacement therapy in hypothyroidism and nerve conduction study. Neurophysiol Clin. 2006;36:79–83.
132. Jellinek EH, Kelly RE. Cerebellar syndrome in myxoedema. Lancet. 1960;2:225–7.
133. Beghi E, Delodovici ML, Bogliun G, et al. Hypothyroidism and polyneuropathy. J Neurol Neurosurg Psychiatry. 1989;52:1420–3.
134. Anand VT, Mann SB, Dash RJ, et al. Auditory investigations in hypothyroidism. Acta Otolaryngol. 1989;108:83–7.
135. Heinrich TW, Grahm G. Hypothyroidism presenting as psychosis: myxedema madness revisited. Prim Care Companion J Clin Psychiatry. 2003;5:260–6.
136. Tan ZS, Vasan RS. Thyroid function and Alzheimer's disease. J Alzheimers Dis. 2009;16:503–7.
137. van der Cammen TJ, Mattace-Raso F, van Harskamp F, et al. Lack of association between thyroid disorders and Alzheimer's disease in older persons: a cross-sectional observational study in a geriatric outpatient population. J Am Geriatr Soc. 2003;51:884.
138. Constant EL, de Volder AG, Ivanoiu A, et al. Cerebral blood flow and glucose metabolism in hypothyroidism: a positron emission tomography study. J Clin Endocrinol Metab. 2001;86:3864–70.
139. Ferracci F, Carnevale A. The neurological disorder associated with thyroid autoimmunity. J Neurol. 2006;253:975–84.
140. Kothbauer-Margreiter I, Sturzenegger M, Komor J, et al. Encephalopathy associated with Hashimoto thyroiditis: diagnosis and treatment. J Neurol. 1996;243:585–93.
141. Chong JY, Rowland LP, Utiger RD. Hashimoto encephalopathy: syndrome or myth? Arch Neurol. 2003;60:164–71.
142. Murphy E, Williams GR. The thyroid and the skeleton. Clin Endocrinol (Oxf). 2004;61:285–98.
143. Rivkees SA, Bode HH, Crawford JD. Long-term growth in juvenile acquired hypothyroidism: the failure to achieve normal adult stature. N Engl J Med. 1988;318:599–602.
144. Bland JH, Frymoyer JW. Rheumatic syndromes of myxedema. N Engl J Med. 1970;282:1171–4.
145. Shaw C, Shaw P. Kocher-Debre-Semelaigne syndrome: hypothyroid muscular pseudohypertrophy – a rare report of two cases. Case Rep Endocrinol. 2012;2012:153143.
146. Najjar SS, Nachman HS. The Kocher-Debre-Semelaigne syndrome; hypothyroidism with muscular "hypertrophy". J Pediatr. 1965;66:901–8.
147. Klein I, Parker M, Shebert R, et al. Hypothyroidism presenting as muscle stiffness and pseudohypertrophy: Hoffmann's syndrome. Am J Med. 1981;70:891–4.
148. Sekine N, Yamamoto M, Michikawa M, et al. Rhabdomyolysis and acute renal failure in a patient with hypothyroidism. Intern Med. 1993;32:269–71.
149. Lowe CE, Bird ED, Thomas Jr JC. Hypercalcemia in myxedema. J Clin Endocrinol Metab. 1962;22:261–7.
150. Discala VA, Kinney MJ. Effects of myxedema on the renal diluting and concentrating mechanism. Am J Med. 1971;50:325–35.
151. Iglesias P, Diez JJ. Thyroid dysfunction and kidney disease. Eur J Endocrinol. 2009;160:503–15.
152. Watanakunakorn C, Hodges RE, Evans TC. Myxedema; a study of 400 cases. Q J Med. 1960;29:513–37.
153. Tudhope GR, Wilson GM. Anaemia in hypothyroidism. Incidence, pathogenesis, and response to treatment. Q J Med. 1960;29:513–37.
154. Squizzato A, Romualdi E, Buller HR, et al. Clinical review: thyroid dysfunction and effects on coagulation and fibrinolysis: a systematic review. J Clin Endocrinol Metab. 2007;92:2415–20.
155. Manfredi E, van Zaane B, Gerdes VE, et al. Hypothyroidism and acquired von Willebrand's syndrome: a systematic review. Haemophilia. 2008;14:423–33.

156. Yamada T, Tsukui T, Ikejiri K, et al. Volume of sella turcica in normal subjects and in patients with primary hypothyroidism and hyperthyroidism. J Clin Endocrinol Metab. 1976;42:817–22.
157. Vagenakis AG, Dole K, Braverman LE. Pituitary enlargement, pituitary failure, and primary hypothyroidism. Ann Intern Med. 1976;85:195–8.
158. Yamamoto K, Saito K, Takai T, et al. Visual field defects and pituitary enlargement in primary hypothyroidism. J Clin Endocrinol Metab. 1983;57: 283–7.
159. Honbo KS, van Herle AJ, Kellett KA. Serum prolactin levels in untreated primary hypothyroidism. Am J Med. 1978;64:782–7.
160. Onishi T, Miyai K, Aono T, et al. Primary hypothyroidism and galactorrhea. Am J Med. 1977;63:373–8.
161. Valcavi R, Valente F, Dieguez C, et al. Evidence against depletion of the growth hormone (GH)-releasable pool in human primary hypothyroidism: studies with GH-releasing hormone, pyridostigmine, and arginine. J Clin Endocrinol Metab. 1993;77:616–20.
162. Gordon GG, Southren AL. Thyroid – hormone effects on steroid – hormone metabolism. Bull N Y Acad Med. 1977;53:241–59.
163. Christensen NJ. Increased levels of plasma noradrenaline in hypothyroidism. J Clin Endocrinol Metab. 1972;35:359–63.
164. Polikar R, Kennedy B, Maisel A, et al. Decreased adrenergic sensitivity in patients with hypothyroidism. J Am Coll Cardiol. 1990;15:94–8.
165. Costin G, Kershnar AK, Kogut MD, et al. Prolactin activity in juvenile hypothyroidism and precocious puberty. Pediatrics. 1972;50:881–9.
166. Louvet JP, Gouarre M, Salandini AM, et al. Hypothyroidism and anovulation. Lancet. 1979;1: 1032.
167. Krassas GE, Pontikides N, Kaltsas T, et al. Disturbances of menstruation in hypothyroidism. Clin Endocrinol (Oxf). 1999;50:655–9.
168. Smallridge RC, Ladenson PW. Hypothyroidism in pregnancy: consequences to neonatal health. J Clin Endocrinol Metab. 2001;86:2349–53.
169. Montoro M, Collea JV, Frasier SD, et al. Successful outcome of pregnancy in women with hypothyroidism. Ann Intern Med. 1981;94:31–4.
170. Carani C, Isidori AM, Granata A, et al. Multicenter study on the prevalence of sexual symptoms in male hypo- and hyperthyroid patients. J Clin Endocrinol Metab. 2005;90:6472–9.
171. Krassas GE, Papadopoulou F, Tziomalos K, et al. Hypothyroidism has an adverse effect on human spermatogenesis: a prospective, controlled study. Thyroid. 2008;18:1255–9.
172. Maratou E, Hadjidakis DJ, Kollias A, et al. Studies of insulin resistance in patients with clinical and subclinical hypothyroidism. Eur J Endocrinol. 2009;160:785–90.
173. Dimitriadis G, Mitrou P, Lambadiari V, et al. Insulin action in adipose tissue and muscle in hypothyroidism. J Clin Endocrinol Metab. 2006;91:4930–7.
174. Hecht A, Gershberg H. Diabetes mellitus and primary hypothyroidism. Metabolism. 1968;17:108–13.
175. Thvilum M, Brandt F, Brix TH, et al. Hypothyroidism is a predictor of disability pension and loss of labor market income: a Danish register-based study. J Clin Endocrinol Metab. 2014;99:3129–35.
176. Lania A, Persani L, Beck-Peccoz P. Central hypothyroidism. Pituitary. 2008;11:181–6.
177. Alexopoulou O, Beguin C, De Nayer P, et al. Clinical and hormonal characteristics of central hypothyroidism at diagnosis and during follow-up in adult patients. Eur J Endocrinol. 2004;150:1–8.
178. Vulsma T, Gons MH, de Vijlder JJ. Maternal-fetal transfer of thyroxine in congenital hypothyroidism due to a total organification defect or thyroid agenesis. N Engl J Med. 1989;321:13–6.
179. LaFranchi SH, Murphey WH, Foley Jr TP, et al. Neonatal hypothyroidism detected by the Northwest Regional Screening Program. Pediatrics. 1979;63:180–91.
180. Olivieri A, Stazi MA, Mastroiacovo P, et al. A population-based study on the frequency of additional congenital malformations in infants with congenital hypothyroidism: data from the Italian Registry for Congenital Hypothyroidism (19911998). J Clin Endocrinol Metab. 2002;87:557–62.
181. Rastogi MV, LaFranchi SH. Congenital hypothyroidism. Orphanet J Rare Dis. 2010;5:17.
182. Pantsiouou S, Stanhope R, Uruena M, et al. Growth prognosis and growth after menarche in primary hypothyroidism. Arch Dis Child. 1991;66:838–40.
183. de Vries L, Bulvik S, Phillip M. Chronic autoimmune thyroiditis in children and adolescents: at presentation and during long-term follow-up. Arch Dis Child. 2009;94:33–7.
184. Léger J, Olivieri A, Donaldson M, et al. European Society for Paediatric Endocrinology consensus guidelines on screening, diagnosis, and management of congenital hypothyroidism. Horm Res Paediatr. 2014;81:80–103.
185. Rose SR, Brown RS, Foley T, et al. Update of newborn screening and therapy for congenital hypothyroidism. Pediatrics. 2006;117:2290–303.
186. LaFranchi SH. Newborn screening strategies for congenital hypothyroidism: an update. J Inherit Metab Dis. 2010;33:S225–33.
187. Muir A, Daneman D, Daneman A, et al. Thyroid scanning, ultrasound, and serum thyroglobulin in determining the origin of congenital hypothyroidism. Am J Dis Child. 1988;142:214–6.
188. Weetman AP. Hypothyroidism: screening and subclinical disease. BMJ. 1997;314:1175–8.
189. Helfand M, Redfern CC. Clinical guideline, part 2. Screening for thyroid disease: an update. American College of Physicians. Ann Intern Med. 1998;129:144–58.

190. Ladenson PW, Singer PA, Ain KB, et al. American Thyroid Association guidelines for detection of thyroid dysfunction. Arch Intern Med. 2000;160:1573–5.
191. Spencer CA. Clinical utility and cost-effectiveness of sensitive thyrotropin assays in ambulatory and hospitalized patients. Mayo Clin Proc. 1988;63:1214–22.
192. Tachman ML, Guthrie Jr GP. Hypothyroidism: diversity of presentation. Endocr Rev. 1984;5:456–65.
193. Billewicz WZ, Chapman RS, Crooks J, et al. Statistical methods applied to the diagnosis of hypothyroidism. Q J Med. 1969;38:255–66.
194. Zulewski H, Müller B, Exer P, et al. Estimation of tissue hypothyroidism by a new clinical score: evaluation of patients with various grades of hypothyroidism and controls. J Clin Endocrinol Metab. 1997;82:771–6.
195. Wartofsky L, Dickey RA. The evidence for a narrower thyrotropin reference range is compelling. J Clin Endocrinol Metab. 2005;90:5483–8.
196. Boucai L, Hollowell JG, Surks MI. An approach for development of age-, gender-, and ethnicity-specific thyrotropin reference limits. Thyroid. 2011;21:5–11.
197. Surks MI, Hollowell JG. Age-specific distribution of serum thyrotropin and antithyroid antibodies in the US population: implications for the prevalence of subclinical hypothyroidism. J Clin Endocrinol Metab. 2007;92:4575–82.
198. Evered DC, Ormston BJ, Smith PA, et al. Grades of hypothyroidism. Br Med J. 1973;1:657–62.
199. Gereben B, Zavacki AM, Ribich S, et al. Cellular and molecular basis of deiodinase-regulated thyroid hormone signaling. Endocr Rev. 2008;29:898–938.
200. Beck-Peccoz P, Amr S, Menezes-Ferreira MM, et al. Decreased receptor binding of biologically inactive thyrotropin in central hypothyroidism. Effect of treatment with thyrotropin-releasing hormone. N Engl J Med. 1985;312:1085–90.
201. Samuels MH, Lillehei K, Kleinschmidt-Demasters BK, et al. Patterns of pulsatile pituitary glycoprotein secretion in central hypothyroidism and hypogonadism. J Clin Endocrinol Metab. 1990;70:391–5.
202. Caron PJ, Nieman LK, Rose SR, et al. Deficient nocturnal surge of thyrotropin in central hypothyroidism. J Clin Endocrinol Metab. 1986;62:960–4.
203. Pedersen OM, Aardal NP, Larssen TB, et al. The value of ultrasonography in predicting autoimmune thyroid disease. Thyroid. 2000;10:251–9.
204. Beck-Peccoz P, Lania A, Beckers A, et al. 2013 European Thyroid Association guidelines for the diagnosis and treatment of thyrotropin-secreting pituitary tumors. Eur Thyroid J. 2013;2:76–82.
205. Beck-Peccoz P, Persani L, Mannavola D, et al. Pituitary tumours: TSH-secreting adenomas. Best Pract Res Clin Endocrinol Metab. 2009;23:597–606.
206. Burman KD, Wartofsky L. Thyroid function in the intensive care unit setting. Crit Care Clin. 2001;17:43–57.
207. Adler SM, Wartofsky L. The nonthyroidal illness syndrome. Endocrinol Metab Clin North Am. 2007;36:657–72.
208. Topliss DJ, White EL, Stockigt JR. Significance of thyrotropin excess in untreated primary adrenal insufficiency. J Clin Endocrinol Metab. 1980;50:52–6.
209. Kahn BB, Weintraub BD, Csako G, et al. Factitious elevation of thyrotropin in a new ultrasensitive assay: implications for the use of monoclonal antibodies in "sandwich" immunoassay. J Clin Endocrinol Metab. 1988;66:526–33.
210. Loh TP, Kao SL, Halsall DJ, et al. Macro-thyrotropin: a case report and review of literature. J Clin Endocrinol Metab. 2012;97:1823–8.
211. Ross DS, Cooper DS, Mulder JE. Central hypothyroidism. In: Post TW, editor. UpToDate. Waltham: UpToDate; 2015. Accessed on 17 May 2015.
212. Mannavola D, Vannucchi G, Fugazzola L, et al. TBG deficiency: description of two novel mutations associated with complete TBG deficiency and review of the literature. J Mol Med (Berl). 2006;84:864–71.
213. Arafah BM. Decreased levothyroxine requirement in women with hypothyroidism during androgen therapy for breast cancer. Ann Intern Med. 1994;12:247–51.
214. Bános C, Takó J, Salamon F, et al. Effect of ACTH-stimulated glucocorticoid hypersecretion on the serum concentrations of thyroxine-binding globulin, thyroxine, triiodothyronine, reverse triiodothyronine and on the TSH-response to TRH. Acta Med Acad Sci Hung. 1979;36:381–94.
215. Afrasiabi MA, Vaziri ND, Gwinup G. Thyroid function studies in the nephrotic syndrome. Ann Intern Med. 1979;90:335–8.
216. Garnick MB, Larsen PR. Acute deficiency of thyroxine-binding globulin during L-asparaginase therapy. N Engl J Med. 1979;301:252–3.
217. Graham RL, Gambrell Jr RD. Changes in thyroid function tests during danazol therapy. Obstet Gynecol. 1980;55:395–7.
218. Shakir KM, Kroll S, Aprill BS, et al. Nicotinic acid decreases serum thyroid hormone levels while maintaining a euthyroid state. Mayo Clin Proc. 1995;70:556–8.
219. Connacher AA, Borsey DQ, Browning MC, et al. The effective evaluation of thyroid status in patients on phenytoin, carbamazepine or sodium valproate attending an epilepsy clinic. Postgrad Med J. 1987;63:841–5.
220. Lai EC, Yang YH, Lin SJ, et al. Use of antiepileptic drugs and risk of hypothyroidism. Pharmacoepidemiol Drug Saf. 2013;22:1071–9.
221. Mai VQ, Burch HB. A stepwise approach to the evaluation and treatment of subclinical hyperthyroidism. Endocr Pract. 2012;18:772–80.
222. Jonklaas J, Bianco AC, Bauer AJ, et al. Guidelines for the treatment of hypothyroidism: prepared by the American Thyroid Association task force on thyroid hormone replacement. Thyroid. 2014;24:1670–751.
223. Wiersinga WM, Duntas L, Fadeyev V, et al. 2012 ETA guidelines: the use of L-T4+L-T3 in the treatment of hypothyroidism. Eur Thyroid J. 2012;1:55–71.

224. Jonklaas J, Davidson B, Bhagat S, et al. Triiodothyronine levels in athyreotic individuals during levothyroxine therapy. JAMA. 2008;299:769–77.
225. Hays MT. Localization of human thyroxine absorption. Thyroid. 1991;1:241–8.
226. Wenzel KW, Kirschsieper HE. Aspects of the absorption of oral L-thyroxine in normal man. Metabolism. 1977;26:1–8.
227. Perez CL, Araki FS, Graf H, et al. Serum thyrotropin levels following levothyroxine administration at breakfast. Thyroid. 2013;23:779–84.
228. Bach-Huynh TG, Nayak B, Loh J, et al. Timing of levothyroxine administration affects serum thyrotropin concentration. J Clin Endocrinol Metab. 2009;94:3905–12.
229. Bolk N, Visser TJ, Nijman J, et al. Effects of evening vs morning levothyroxine intake: a randomized double-blind crossover trial. Arch Intern Med. 2010;170:1996–2003.
230. Fish LH, Schwartz HL, Cavanaugh J, et al. Replacement dose, metabolism, and bioavailability of levothyroxine in the treatment of hypothyroidism. Role of triiodothyronine in pituitary feedback in humans. N Engl J Med. 1987;316:764–70.
231. Saberi M, Utiger RD. Serum thyroid hormone and thyrotropin concentrations during thyroxine and triiodothyronine therapy. J Clin Endocrinol Metab. 1974;39:923–7.
232. Daniels GH. Response to 'How do you approach the problem of TSH elevation in a patient on high-dose thyroid hormone replacement?'. Clin Endocrinol (Oxf). 2009;71:603.
233. Walker JN, Shillo P, Ibbotson V, et al. A thyroxine absorption test followed by weekly thyroxine administration: a method to assess non-adherence to treatment. Eur J Endocrinol. 2013;168:913–7.
234. Grebe SK, Cooke RR, Ford HC, et al. Treatment of hypothyroidism with once weekly thyroxine. J Clin Endocrinol Metab. 1997;82:870–5.
235. Colucci P, DAngelo P, Mautone G, et al. Pharmacokinetic equivalence of a levothyroxine sodium soft capsule manufactured using the new food and drug administration potency guidelines in healthy volunteers under fasting conditions. Ther Drug Monit. 2011;33:355–61.
236. Benvenga S. (Soft) capsules of wisdom: preventing myo-inositol malabsorption caused by coffee. Expert Opin Drug Deliv. 2012;9:1177–9.
237. Vita R, Benvenga S. Tablet levothyroxine (L-T4) malabsorption induced by proton pump inhibitor; a problem that was solved by switching to L-T4 in soft gel capsule. Endocr Pract. 2014;20:e38–41.
238. Santini F, Pinchera A, Marsili A, et al. Lean body mass is a major determinant of levothyroxine dosage in the treatment of thyroid diseases. J Clin Endocrinol Metab. 2005;90:124–7.
239. Gordon MB, Gordon MS. Variations in adequate levothyroxine replacement therapy in patients with different causes of hypothyroidism. Endocr Pract. 1999;5:233–8.
240. Burmeister LA, Goumaz MO, Mariash CN, et al. Levothyroxine dose requirements for thyrotropin suppression in the treatment of differentiated thyroid cancer. J Clin Endocrinol Metab. 1992;75:344–50.
241. Kabadi UM, Kabadi MM. Serum thyrotropin in primary hypothyroidism: a reliable and accurate predictor of optimal daily levothyroxine dose. Endocr Pract. 2001;7:16–8.
242. Roos A, Linn-Rasker SP, van Domburg RT, et al. The starting dose of levothyroxine in primary hypothyroidism treatment: a prospective, randomized, double-blind trial. Arch Intern Med. 2005;165:1714–20.
243. Liewendahl K, Helenius T, Lamberg BA, et al. Free thyroxine, free triiodothyronine, and thyrotropin concentrations in hypothyroid and thyroid carcinoma patients receiving thyroxine therapy. Acta Endocrinol (Copenh). 1987;116:418–24.
244. Woeber KA. Levothyroxine therapy and serum free thyroxine and free triiodothyronine concentrations. J Endocrinol Invest. 2002;25:106–9.
245. Ain KB, Pucino F, Shiver TM, et al. Thyroid hormone levels affected by time of blood sampling in thyroxine-treated patients. Thyroid. 1993;3:81–5.
246. Karmisholt J, Andersen S, Laurberg P. Variation in thyroid function tests in patients with stable untreated subclinical hypothyroidism. Thyroid. 2008;18:303–8.
247. Centanni M, Gargano L, Canettieri G, et al. Thyroxine in goiter, Helicobacter pylori infection, and chronic gastritis. N Engl J Med. 2006;354:1787–95.
248. Collins D, Wilcox R, Nathan M, et al. Celiac disease and hypothyroidism. Am J Med. 2012;125:278–82.
249. Singh N, Weisler SL, Hershman JM. The acute effect of calcium carbonate on the intestinal absorption of levothyroxine. Thyroid. 2001;11:967–71.
250. Weitzman SP, Ginsburg KC, Carlson HE. Colesevelam hydrochloride and lanthanum carbonate interfere with the absorption of levothyroxine. Thyroid. 2009;19:77–9.
251. Diskin CJ, Stokes TJ, Dansby LM, et al. Effect of phosphate binders upon TSH and L-thyroxine dose in patients on thyroid replacement. Int Urol Nephrol. 2007;39:599–602.
252. Shakir KM, Chute JP, Aprill BS, et al. Ferrous sulfate-induced increase in requirement for thyroxine in a patient with primary hypothyroidism. South Med J. 1997;90:637–9.
253. Sperber AD, Liel Y. Evidence for interference with the intestinal absorption of levothyroxine sodium by aluminum hydroxide. Arch Intern Med. 1992;152:183–4.
254. Sherman SI, Tielens ET, Ladenson PW. Sucralfate causes malabsorption of L-thyroxine. Am J Med. 1994;96:531–5.
255. Sachmechi I, Reich DM, Aninyei M, et al. Effect of proton pump inhibitors on serum thyroid-stimulating hormone level in euthyroid patients treated with levothyroxine for hypothyroidism. Endocr Pract. 2007;13:345–9.

256. Benvenga S, Bartolone L, Pappalardo MA, et al. Altered intestinal absorption of L-thyroxine caused by coffee. Thyroid. 2008;18:293–301.
257. Isley WL. Effect of rifampin therapy on thyroid function tests in a hypothyroid patient on replacement L-thyroxine. Ann Intern Med. 1987;107:517–8.
258. De Luca F, Arrigo T, Pandullo E, et al. Changes in thyroid function tests induced by 2 month carbamazepine treatment in L-thyroxine-substituted hypothyroid children. Eur J Pediatr. 1986;145:77–9.
259. Faber J, Lumholtz IB, Kirkegaard C, et al. The effects of phenytoin (diphenylhydantoin) on the extrathyroidal turnover of thyroxine, 3,5,3'-triiodothyronine, 3,3',5'-triiodothyronine, and 3',5'-diiodothyronine in man. J Clin Endocrinol Metab. 1985;61:1093–9.
260. McCowen KC, Garber JR, Spark R. Elevated serum thyrotropin in thyroxine- treated patients with hypothyroidism given sertraline. N Engl J Med. 1997;337:1010–1.
261. Arafah BM. Increased need for thyroxine in women with hypothyroidism during estrogen therapy. N Engl J Med. 2001;344:1743–9.
262. Cunningham JJ, Barzel US. Lean body mass is a predictor of the daily requirement for thyroid hormone in older men and women. J Am Geriatr Soc. 1984;32:204–7.
263. Magner J, Gerber P. Urticaria due to blue dye in synthroid tablets. Thyroid. 1994;4:341.
264. Somwaru LL, Arnold AM, Joshi N, et al. High frequency of and factors associated with thyroid hormone over-replacement and under-replacement in men and women aged 65 and over. J Clin Endocrinol Metab. 2009;94:1342–5.
265. Sawin CT, Geller A, Wolf PA, et al. Low serum thyrotropin concentrations as a risk factor for atrial fibrillation in older persons. N Engl J Med. 1994;331:1249–52.
266. Bauer DC, Ettinger B, Nevitt MC, et al. Risk for fracture in women with low serum levels of thyroid-stimulating hormone. Ann Intern Med. 2001;134:561–8.
267. Ladenson PW, Levin AA, Ridgway EC, et al. Complications of surgery in hypothyroid patients. Am J Med. 1984;77:261–6.
268. Weinberg AD, Brennan MD, Gorman CA, et al. Outcome of anesthesia and surgery in hypothyroid patients. Arch Intern Med. 1983;143:893–7.
269. Celi FS, Zemskova M, Linderman JD, et al. The pharmacodynamic equivalence of levothyroxine and liothyronine: a randomized, double blind, cross-over study in thyroidectomized patients. Clin Endocrinol (Oxf). 2010;72:709–15.
270. Hoang TD, Olsen CH, Mai VQ, et al. Desiccated thyroid extract compared with levothyroxine in the treatment of hypothyroidism: a randomized, double-blind, crossover study. J Clin Endocrinol Metab. 2013;98:1982–90.
271. Kaptein EM, Beale E, Chan LS. Thyroid hormone therapy for obesity and nonthyroidal illnesses: a systematic review. J Clin Endocrinol Metab. 2009;94:3663–75.
272. Burch HB, Burman KD, Cooper DS, et al. A 2013 survey of clinical practice patterns in the management of primary hypothyroidism. J Clin Endocrinol Metab. 2014;99:2077–85.
273. Grozinsky-Glasberg S, Fraser A, Nahshoni E, et al. Thyroxine-triiodothyronine combination therapy versus thyroxine monotherapy for clinical hypothyroidism: meta-analysis of randomized controlled trials. J Clin Endocrinol Metab. 2006;91:2592–9.
274. Escobar-Morreale HF, Botella-Carretero JI, Escobar del Rey F, et al. Review: Treatment of hypothyroidism with combinations of levothyroxine plus liothyronine. J Clin Endocrinol Metab. 2005;90:4946–54.
275. Joffe RT, Brimacombe M, Levitt AJ, et al. Treatment of clinical hypothyroidism with thyroxine and triiodothyronine: a literature review and metaanalysis. Psychosomatics. 2007;48:379–84.
276. Ma C, Xie J, Huang X, et al. Thyroxine alone or thyroxine plus triiodothyronine replacement therapy for hypothyroidism. Nucl Med Commun. 2009;30:586–93.
277. Panicker V, Saravanan P, Vaidya B, et al. Common variation in the DIO2 gene predicts baseline psychological well-being and response to combination thyroxine plus triiodothyronine therapy in hypothyroid patients. J Clin Endocrinol Metab. 2009;94:1623–9.
278. Wiersinga WM. Do we need still more trials on T4 and T3 combination therapy in hypothyroidism? Eur J Endocrinol. 2009;161:955–9.
279. Hennemann G, Docter R, Visser TJ, et al. Thyroxine plus low-dose, slow-release triiodothyronine replacement in hypothyroidism: proof of principle. Thyroid. 2004;14:271–5.
280. Jackson IM, Cobb WE. Why does anyone still use desiccated thyroid USP? Am J Med. 1978;64:284–8.
281. Nicoloff JT, Low JC, Dussault JH, et al. Simultaneous measurement of thyroxine and triiodothyronine peripheral turnover kinetics in man. J Clin Invest. 1972;51:473–83.
282. Celi FS, Zemskova M, Linderman JD, et al. Metabolic effects of liothyronine therapy in hypothyroidism: a randomized, double-blind, crossover trial of liothyronine versus levothyroxine. J Clin Endocrinol Metab. 2011;96:3466–74.
283. Blumberg KR, Mayer WJ, Parikh DK, et al. Liothyronine and levothyroxine in Armour thyroid. J Pharm Sci. 1987;76:346–7.
284. Penny R, Frasier SD. Elevated serum concentrations of triiodothyronine in hypothyroid patients. Values for patients receiving USP thyroid. Am J Dis Child. 1980;134:16–8.
285. Lev-Ran A. Part-of-the-day hypertriiodothyroninemia caused by desiccated thyroid. JAMA. 1983;250:2790–1.
286. Jha S, Waghdhare S, Reddi R, et al. Thyroid storm due to inappropriate administration of a compounded thyroid hormone preparation successfully treated with plasmapheresis. Thyroid. 2012;22:1283–6.

287. Boulton DW, Fawcett JP, Woods DJ. Stability of an extemporaneously compounded levothyroxine sodium oral liquid. Am J Health Syst Pharm. 1996;53:1157–61.
288. Zeisel SH. Regulation of "nutraceuticals". Science. 1999;285:1853–5.
289. Mechanick JI, Brett EM, Chausmer AB, et al. American Association of Clinical Endocrinologists medical guidelines for the clinical use of dietary supplements and nutraceuticals. Endocr Pract. 2003;9:417–70.
290. Rosen JE, Gardiner P, Saper RB. Complementary and alternative medicine use among patients with thyroid cancer. Thyroid. 2013;23:1238–46.
291. Slawik M, Klawitter B, Meiser E, et al. Thyroid hormone replacement for central hypothyroidism: a randomized controlled trial comparing two doses of thyroxine (T4) with a combination of T4 and triiodothyronine. J Clin Endocrinol Metab. 2007;92:4115–22.
292. Shimon I, Cohen O, Lubetsky A, et al. Thyrotropin suppression by thyroid hormone replacement is correlated with thyroxine level normalization in central hypothyroidism. Thyroid. 2002;12:823–7.
293. Zeitler P, Solberg P. Food and levothyroxine administration in infants and children. J Pediatr. 2010;157:13–4.
294. Tillotson SL, Fuggle PW, Smith I, et al. Relation between biochemical severity and intelligence in early treated congenital hypothyroidism: a threshold effect. BMJ. 1994;309:440–5.
295. Glorieux J, Dussault J, Van Vliet G. Intellectual development at age 12 years of children with congenital hypothyroidism diagnosed by neonatal screening. J Pediatr. 1992;121:581–4.
296. LaFranchi SH, Austin J. How should we be treating children with congenital hypothyroidism? J Pediatr Endocrinol Metab. 2007;20:559–78.

Hyperthyroidism

8

Syed Khalid Imam

Abstract

Hyperthyroidism has multiple etiologies, manifestations, and potential therapies and untreated cases may result in significant morbidity and mortality. Appropriate treatment requires an accurate diagnosis and is influenced by age, coexisting medical conditions and patient preference. The proper treatment of hyperthyroidism depends on recognition of the signs and symptoms of the disease and determination of the etiology. The most common cause of hyperthyroidism is Graves' disease. Other common causes include toxic multinodular goiter, toxic adenomas, thyroiditis and certain medications. The diagnostic workup should begin with a thyroid-stimulating hormone level test, the most sensitive screening test. There are many therapeutic modalities of hyperthyroidism and selection of these modalities depend upon the age, cause, prevailing medical condition and patient's preference. This chapter will provide an overview of hyperthyroidism in non-pregnant adults.

Introduction

Hyperthyroidism is characterized by inappropriately increased thyroid hormone synthesis and secretion. This overactive disease has many causes, myriad of clinical manifestations, and variety of therapies. The most common forms of hyperthyroidism include diffuse toxic goiter (Graves disease), toxic multinodular goiter (Plummer disease), and toxic adenoma. Together with subacute thyroiditis, these conditions account for 85–90 % of all causes of hyperthyroidism [1, 2].

The term "thyrotoxicosis" refers to a clinical state resulting from inappropriately high thyroid hormone action in tissues generally due to inappropriately high tissue thyroid hormone levels. The term "hyperthyroidism" is a form of thyrotoxicosis due to inappropriately high synthesis and secretion of thyroid hormone(s) by the thyroid. Although, many clinicians use the terms hyperthyroidism and thyrotoxicosis interchangeably, the 2 words have distinct meanings. For

S.K. Imam, FCPS, FACE
Department of Internal Medicine, Al Mouwasat Hospital, Jubail, Kingdom of Saudi Arabia
e-mail: docimam@yahoo.com

S.K. Imam, S.I. Ahmad (eds.), *Thyroid Disorders: Basic Science and Clinical Practice*,
DOI 10.1007/978-3-319-25871-3_8

example, both exogenous thyroid hormone intake and subacute thyroiditis can cause thyrotoxicosis, but neither constitutes hyperthyroidism, because the conditions are not associated with new hormone production. It should also be noted that the elevation of free thyroid hormone levels does not always result in thyrotoxicosis.

As we know that iodine plays an important role in thyroid homeostasis (see Chap. 3 for detail description) and the incidences of Graves disease and toxic multinodular goiter, change with iodine intake. Compared with regions of the world with less iodine intake, the United States has more cases of Graves disease and fewer cases of toxic multinodular goiters. Autoimmune thyroid disease occurs with the same frequency in Caucasians, Hispanics, and Asians but at lower rates in African Americans. All thyroid diseases occur more frequently in women than in men.

Appropriate treatment of thyrotoxicosis requires an accurate diagnosis. For example, thyroidectomy is an appropriate treatment for some forms of hyperthroidism and not for others. Additionally, beta blockers, if not contraindicated, may be used in almost all forms of thyrotoxicosis, whereas antithyroid drugs are useful in only some.

Review in this chapter will mainly focus on hyperthyroidism in non-pregnant adult and subclinical hyperthyroidism, thyroid storm and pregnancy related thyroid dysfunction will be discussed separately in other chapters.

Etiology

Graves Disease

Graves disease, named after an Irish surgeon, Robert J. Graves in 1830, is classified as an autoimmune thyroid disorder [3]. In some patients, Graves disease represents a part of more extensive autoimmune processes leading to dysfunction of multiple organs (e.g., polyglandular autoimmune syndromes). Graves disease is also associated with pernicious anemia, vitiligo, type 1 diabetes mellitus, autoimmune adrenal insufficiency, systemic sclerosis, myasthenia gravis, Sjögren syndrome, rheumatoid arthritis, and systemic lupus erythematosus [4].

Epidemiology

In the United States, the prevalence of hyperthyroidism is approximately 1.2 % (0.5 % overt and 0.7 % subclinical); the most common causes include Graves' disease (GD), toxic multinodular goiter (TMNG), and toxic adenoma (TA) [1, 2]. Graves disease is the most common form of hyperthyroidism in the United States, causing approximately 60–80 % of cases of thyrotoxicosis, and in other parts of the world representing 60–90 % of all cases [5]. In the Wickham Study in the United Kingdom, the incidence was reported to be 100–200 cases per 100,000 population per year [6]. The incidence in women in the UK has been reported to be 80 cases 100,000 per year [7]. As with most autoimmune diseases, susceptibility is increased in females. Hyperthyroidism due to Graves disease has a female-to-male ratio of 7–8:1.

The female-to-male ratio for pretibial myxedema is 3.5:1. Only 7 % of patients with localized myxedema have thyroid acropachy. Unlike the other manifestations of Graves disease, the female-to-male ratio for thyroid acropachy is 1:1. Typically, Graves disease is a disease of young women, but it may occur in persons of any age. The typical age range is 20–40 years. Most affected women are aged 30–60 years. The annual incidence of Graves disease was found to be 0.5 cases per 1000 population during a 20-year period, with the peak occurrence in people aged 20–40 years [8].

Pathophysiology and Genetic Interplay

In Graves disease, B and T lymphocyte-mediated autoimmunity are known to be directed at 4 well known thyroid antigens: thyroglobulin, thyroid peroxidase, sodium-iodide symporter and the thyrotropin receptor. However, the thyrotropin receptor itself is the primary autoantigen of Graves disease and is responsible for the manifestation of hyperthyroidism. In this disease, the antibody and cell-mediated thyroid antigen-specific immune responses are well defined [9].

The thyroid gland is under continuous stimulation by circulating autoantibodies against the thyrotropin receptor, and pituitary thyrotropin secretion is suppressed because of the increased production of thyroid hormones. The stimulating activity of thyrotropin receptor antibodies is found mostly in the immunoglobulin G1 subclass. These thyroid-stimulating antibodies cause release of thyroid hormone and thyroglobulin that is mediated by 3,′5′-cyclic adenosine monophosphate (cyclic AMP), and they also stimulate iodine uptake, protein synthesis, and thyroid gland growth. The anti-sodium-iodide symporter, antithyroglobulin, and antithyroid peroxidase antibodies appear to have little role in the etiology of hyperthyroidism in Graves disease. However, they are markers of autoimmune disease against the thyroid. Intrathyroidal lymphocytic infiltration is the initial histologic abnormality in persons with autoimmune thyroid disease and can be correlated with the titer of thyroid antibodies. Besides being the source of autoantigens, the thyroid cells express molecules that mediate T cell adhesion and complement regulation that participate and interact with the immune system. Several autoimmune thyroid disease susceptibility genes have been identified such as CD40, CTLA-4, thyroglobulin, TSH receptor, and PTPN22 [10].

Some of these susceptibility genes are specific to either Graves disease or Hashimoto thyroiditis, while others confer susceptibility to both conditions. The genetic predisposition to thyroid autoimmunity may interact with environmental factors or events to precipitate the onset of Graves disease. Two new susceptibility loci were found: the RNASET2-FGFR1OP-CCR6 region at 6q27 and an intergenic region at 4p14 [11].

Several genetic syndromes have been associated with hyperthyroidism, especially autoimmune thyroid disease. McCune-Albright syndrome is caused by mutations in the *GNAS* gene. This gene encodes the stimulatory G-protein alpha subunit, which is a key component of many signal transduction pathways. Patients present with the classic triad of polyostotic fibrous dysplasia, irregular café-au-lait spots, and precocious puberty. The syndrome may also include facial asymmetry, Cushing syndrome, hyperthyroidism, and acromegaly [12].

A number of disorders of thyroid function have been found to be caused by mutations in the *TSHR* gene, which encodes the TSH receptor protein. These disorders include the following:

- Familial gestational hyperthyroidism
- One type of nonimmune hyperthyroidism
- Congenital nongoiterous thyrotoxicosis
- Toxic thyroid adenoma with somatic mutation

Other Associated Autoimmune Diseases

Type II autoimmune polyendocrine syndrome is associated with hyperthyroidism and hypothyroidism, as well as type 1 diabetes mellitus and adrenal insufficiency. Patients may also have immune deficiency, as manifested by chronic mucosal candidiasis [13].

Moreover, strong associations of thyroid-stimulating hormone receptor and major histocompatibility complex class II variants with persistently thyroid stimulating hormone receptor autoantibodies (TRAb)-positive Graves disease were found.

With the availability of genome-wide association studies, more than a dozen genes and gene regions have been found to be associated with an increased risk for development of thyrotoxicosis, particularly Graves disease [11, 14–18].

Boelaert et al investigated the prevalence of and relative risks for coexisting autoimmune diseases in patients with Graves disease (2791 patients) or Hashimoto thyroiditis (495 patients). The authors found coexisting disorders in 9.7 % of patients with Graves disease and in 14.3 % of those with Hashimoto thyroiditis, with rheumatoid arthritis being the most common of these (prevalence = 3.15 % and 4.24 % in Graves disease and Hashimoto thyroiditis, respectively). Relative risks of greater than 10 were found for pernicious anemia, systemic lupus erythematosus, Addison disease, celiac disease, and vitiligo. The authors also reported a tendency for parents of patients with Graves disease or Hashimoto thyroiditis to have a history of hyperthyroidism or hypothyroidism, respectively [19].

Graves Ophthalmopathy

An infiltrative ophthalmopathy accompanies Graves' disease in about 50 % of patients [20]. The underlying pathophysiology of Graves ophthalmopathy (also called Graves orbitopathy) is not completely characterized. It most likely involves an antibody reaction against the TSH receptor that results in activation of T cells against tissues in the retro-orbital space that share antigenic epitopes with thyroid follicular cells [21, 22].

These immune processes lead to an active phase of inflammation, with lymphocyte infiltration of the orbital tissue and release of cytokines that stimulate orbital fibroblasts to multiply and produce mucopolysaccharides (glycosaminoglycans), which absorb water. Graves disease patients a have higher rate of peripheral blood mononuclear cell conversion into CD34+ fibrocytes compared with healthy controls. These cells may contribute to the pathophysiology of ophthalmopathy by accumulating in orbital tissues and producing inflammatory cytokines, including Tumor Necrosis Factor-alha(TNF-alpha) and Interleukin-6 (IL-6) [23].

In consequence, the extraocular muscles thicken and the adipose and connective tissue of the retro-orbit increase in volume. Cigarette smoking and a high TSH receptor autoantibody level are significant risk factors for ophthalmopathy. In addition, patients who smoke appear to be more likely to experience worsening of their ophthalmopathy if treated with radioactive iodine, as do patients who have high pretreatment T3 levels and posttherapy hypothyroidism.

Other Causes of Hyperthyroidism

Toxic Multinodular Goiter (Plummer Disease)

Toxic multinodular goiter causes 5 % of the cases of hyperthyroidism in the United States and can be ten times more common in iodine-deficient areas. It typically occurs in patients older than 40 years with a long-standing goiter, and has a more insidious onset than Graves' disease [24].

While the mechanisms underlying the development of nodules are of complex nature, it has become apparent that hyperfunctioning adenomas within multinodular goiters or autonomous areas within euthyroid goiters harbor somatic gain-of-function mutations in the TSH receptor [25–27]. It is noteworthy that the mutations may differ among the adenomas within the same multinodular goiter. This observation is consistent with studies demonstrating distinct clonal origins of different thyroid adenomas within the same multinodular goiter [28]. The development of multinodular goiters had been associated with a D727E germline polymorphism in the TSH receptor, but this finding could not be corroborated in other studies [29–31].

Toxic Adenoma

Toxic adenoma is the cause of 3–5 % of cases of thyrotoxicosis and characterized by autonomously functioning nodules that are found most commonly in younger patients and in iodine-deficient areas [24]. A toxic adenoma is a monoclonal, autonomously functioning thyroid nodule (AFTN) that produces supraphysiological amounts of T4 and/or T3 resulting in suppression of serum TSH. The function of the surrounding normal thyroid tissue is often, but not always, suppressed. Approximately 1 in 10–20 solitary nodules present with hyperthyroidism. The prevalence of hyperthyroidism appears to be more common in Europe than in the USA, and it is more common in women than in men [32, 33]. Chronic stimulation of the cAMP cascade results in enhanced proliferation and function of thyrocytes [33]. Hence, any molecular alteration leading to constitutive activation of the cAMP pathway in a thyroid follicular cell is expected to result in clonal autonomous growth and function, and ultimately in a toxic adenoma [34]. In line with this concept, somatic mutations were first discovered in the *GNAS1* gene encoding the stimulatory Gs alpha subunit in toxic adenomas [34–36]. Stimulatory Gs alph amutations impair the hydrolysis of guanine triphosphate (GTP) to guanine diphosphate (GDP), resulting in persistent activation of adenylyl cyclase. The reported prevalence of TSH receptor mutations in toxic adenomas varies widely, but is as high as 80 % [35, 36].

It is now well established that somatic, constitutively activating TSH receptor mutations play a predominant role in the pathogenesis of AFTNs, while Gs alpha mutations are less common [37]. It is likely that other somatic mutations are involved in the pathogenesis of the monoclonal toxic adenomas that are negative for mutations in the TSH receptor and Gs alpha [38].

Thyroiditis

Subacute: Subacute thyroiditis produces an abrupt onset of thyrotoxic symptoms as hormone leaks from an inflamed gland. It often follows a viral illness. Symptoms usually resolve within 8 months. This condition can be recurrent in some patients [39].

Lymphocytic and Postpartum: Lymphocytic Thyroiditis and postpartum (subacute lymphocytic) thyroiditis are transient inflammatory causes of hyperthyroidism that, in the acute stage, may be clinically indistinguishable from Graves' disease. Postpartum thyroiditis can occur in up to 5–10 % of women in the first 3–6 months after delivery. A transient hypothyroidism often occurs before resolution [39].

Hashimoto's Thyroiditis: Occasionally, Hashimoto's thyroiditis is accompanied by mild symptoms of thyrotoxicosis, particularly in the early phases of the disease [40]. A detailed description of thyroiditis is provided in Chap. 6.

Drug-Induced Hyperthyroidism

Iodine-Induced: Iodine-induced hyperthyroidism can occur after intake of excess iodine in the diet, exposure to radiographic contrast media, or medications. Excess iodine increases the synthesis and release of thyroid hormone in iodine-deficient patients and in older patients with preexisting multinodular goiters [41].

Amiodarone-Induced: Amiodarone induced hyperthyroidism can be found in up to 12 % of treated patients, especially those in iodine-deficient areas, and occurs by two mechanisms. Because amiodarone contains 37 % iodine, type I is an iodine induced hyperthyroidism (see above). Amiodarone is the most common source of iodine excess in the United States. Type II is a thyroiditis that occurs in patients with normal thyroid glands. Medications such as interferon and interleukin- 2 (aldesleukin) also can cause type II Thyroiditis [41].

Thyroid Hormone-Induced: Factitious hyperthyroidism is caused by the intentional or accidental ingestion of excess amounts of thyroid hormone. Some patients may take thyroid preparations to achieve weight loss.

Tumors Induced Hyperthyroidism

Rare causes of hyperthyroidism include metastatic thyroid cancer, ovarian tumors that produce thyroid hormone (struma ovarii), trophoblastic tumors that produce human chorionic gonadotrophin and activate highly sensitive TSH receptors.

TSH-Secreting Pituitary Adenoma

TSH-secreting adenomas (TSHomas) account for less than 2 % of all pituitary adenomas and are a rare cause of thyrotoxicosis [42, 43]. The molecular mechanisms leading to the formation of TSHomas remain unknown. TSHomas have been shown to be monoclonal by X-inactivation analyses suggesting that they arise from a single cell harboring one or several mutations in genes controlling proliferation and perhaps function.

Hyperthyroidism Secondary to Thyroid Hormone Resistance

The syndrome of Resistance to Thyroid Hormone (RTH) is defined by elevated circulating levels of free thyroid hormones due to reduced target tissue responsiveness and normal, or elevated levels of TSH [44, 45].

Patients with RTH typically present with goiter. Their metabolic state may appear euthyroid or include signs of hypo- and hyperthyroidism. RTH is most commonly caused by monoallelic mutations of the *TRbeta* gene. The mutation can be inherited in an autosomal dominant manner or occur as *de novo* mutation.

Hyperthyroidism due to TSH-Receptor Mutations

Autosomal dominant familial hyperthyroidism without evidence of an autoimmune etiology has been first described by Thomas et al. in 1982.

Currently 27 families with a total of 152 affected individuals with non-autoimmune familial hyperthyroidism have been reported . The hyperthyroidism is caused by monoallelic gain-of-function germline mutations in the TSH receptor [46, 47].

Affected individuals have a suppressed TSH and elevated peripheral hormones in the absence of TSH receptor-stimulating antibodies and TPO antibodies. The family history is key in order to demonstrate familial clustering suggestive for an autosomal dominant disorder. Ultimately, the diagnosis requires sequence analysis of the *TSH receptor* gene in order to evaluate it for the presence of a monalllelic mutation.

Clinical Features

Generally, a constellation of information, including the extent and duration of symptoms, past medical history, and social and family history, in addition to the information derived from physical examination, help to guide the clinician to the appropriate diagnosis.

The family history should include careful evaluation of the autoimmune disease, thyroid disease and emigration from iodine-deficient parts of the world. Health care provider should also review a complete list of medications and dietary supplements. A number of compounds—including expectorants, amiodarone, iodinated contrast agents, and health food supplements containing seaweed or thyroid gland extracts—contain large amounts of iodine that can induce hyperthyroidism in a patient with thyroid autonomy. Rarely, iodine exposure can cause hyperthyroidism in a patient with an apparently healthy thyroid. Hyperthyroidism presents with multiple symptoms that vary according to the age of the patient, duration of illness, magnitude of hormone excess, and presence of comorbid conditions. Symptoms are related to the thyroid hormone's stimulation of catabolic enzymopathic activity and catabolism, and enhancement of sensitivity to catecholamines. Older patients often present with a paucity of classic signs and symptoms, which can make the diagnosis more difficult [41, 48].

Hyperthyroidism leads to an apparent increase in sympathetic nervous system. Younger patients tend to exhibit symptoms of sympathetic activation, such as anxiety, hyperactivity, and tremor, while older patients have more cardiovascular symptoms, including dyspnea and atrial fibrillation with unexplained weight loss [37, 49].

The clinical manifestations of hyperthyroidism do not always correlate with the extent of the biochemical abnormality.

Common symptoms of hyperthyroidism include the following:

- Nervousness
- Insomnia
- Anxiety
- Increased perspiration
- Heat intolerance
- Hyperactivity
- Palpitations
- Weight loss despite increased appetite.
- Hyperdefecation
- Reduction in menstrual flow or oligomenorrhea

Common signs of hyperthyroidism include the following:

- Diffuse goiter/toxic nodule/multinodular goiter
- Exophthalmos
- Tachycardia or atrial arrhythmia
- Systolic hypertension
- Warm, moist, smooth skin
- Lid lag
- Stare
- Hand tremor
- Proximal myopathy
- Brisk deep tendon reflexes

Features pathognomonic of Graves' disease include the following:

- Orbitopathy
- Thyroid bruit
- Pretibial myxedema
- Acropachy

Features of Graves Ophthalmopathy
Approximately 50 % of patients with Graves thy-

rotoxicosis have mild thyroid ophthalmopathy. Often, this is manifested only by periorbital edema, but it also can include conjunctival edema (chemosis), injection, poor lid closure, extraocular muscle dysfunction (diplopia), and Proptosis . Evidence of thyroid eye disease and high thyroid hormone levels confirms the diagnosis of autoimmune Grave disease.

Graves Dermopathy In rare instances, Graves disease affects the skin through deposition of glycosaminoglycans in the dermis of the lower leg. This causes nonpitting edema, which is usually associated with erythema and thickening of the skin, without pain or pruritus.

Features Related to Other Causes of Hyperthyroidism

Toxic adenomas present with signs and symptoms of hyperthyroidism and/or a thyroid nodule. The signs and symptoms of thyrotoxicosis do not differ from other etiologies. Features suggestive for Graves' disease such as endocrine ophthalmopathy, (pretibial) myxedema and acropachy are missing. The onset of hyperthyroidism is often insidious and more common in older patients, who typically have larger adenomas. Mechanical symptoms such as dysphagia or hoarseness are uncommon. Autonomously functioning nodules may remain stable in size, grow, degenerate or become gradually toxic. In one series, 10 % of patients followed for 6 years became thyrotoxic [32]. Thyrotoxicosis may develop independent of age, but is much more common in nodules over 3 cm in diameter (up to 20 %).

Toxic Multinodular Goiter In addition to the signs and symptoms associated with hyperthyroidism, patients with large toxic multinodular goiters may also have dysphagia, shortness of breath, stridor, or hoarseness.

Subacute thyroiditis often present with a history of a preceding respiratory tract infection [50]. They may have fever, malaise, and soreness, and the gland is exquisitely tender on palpation and often displays a substantially increased consistency.

Hydatiform Moles and Choriocarcinoma Most women with hydatiform moles present with uterine bleeding in the first half of pregnancy. The size of the uterus is large for the duration of gestation [51].

Many women with molar pregnancies have nausea and vomiting, some have pregnancy-induced hypertension or pre-eclampsia. The signs and symptoms of thyrotoxicosis are present in some women, but they may be obscured by toxemic signs. The characteristic features belonging to Graves' disease are missing. Hyperthyroidism is usually not severe because of a relatively short duration.

Women with choriocarcinomas present within 1 year after conception. The tumor may be confined to the uterus, more frequently it is metastatic to multiple organs such as the liver and lungs. In men, choriocarcinomas of the testes is often widely metastatic at initial presentation. Gynecomastia is a common finding.

Struma Ovarii The clinical presentation may include the finding of an abdominal mass, ascites, pelvic pain, and, rarely, a pseudo-Meigs syndrome with pleural effusions. A subset of women present with subclinical or overt thyrotoxicosis. Goiter is only presented in patients with associated thyroid disease. For example, coexistence of Graves' disease and struma ovarii has been reported [52, 53].

Apathetic Hyperthyroidism

Hyperthyroidism in the elderly is a great masquerader, and even severe, life-threatening hyperthyroidism can easily be missed in patients older than 60 years [54]. Not uncommonly, it appears in an atypical manner, and the classic symptoms are often absent. Graves disease and toxic multinodular goiter account for most cases in the elderly, while as Solitary toxic adenomas are rare in elder patients [55–58]. Again, like hypothyroidism, the symptoms of hyperthyroidism are often atypical and may mimic other common diseases in this age group. They may be absent, subtle, or may be obscured by coexisting diseases. Cardiac complications are the most common manifestations of hyperthyroidism in elderly. They are usually manifested as atrial arrhythmias (commonly atrial fibrillation with slow ventricular rates, as compared with high rates in young patients); congestive heart failure (usually high output heart failure) and angina pectoris. The underlying hyperthyroidism may not be recognized, since older patients usually do not show the classic signs/symptoms of thyroid overactivity [59]. Rather than increased appetite, weight loss with anorexia may be present. Diarrhea is common in young hyperthyroid patients; elderly patients may note a correction of preexisting constipation but will rarely complain of loose stools. Elderly patients can present with only one symptom of hyperthyroidism, sometimes referred to as monosymptomatic hyperthyroidism. Agitation and confusion can also be presenting symptoms [60].

Diagnostic Modalities

Hormonal Assays

Serum TSH The measurement of serum TSH with a sensitive third-generation assay represents the best biochemical marker to establish the diagnosis of hyperthyroidism because TSH and FT4 have an inverse log-linear relationship and a small decrease or increase in FT4 is thus associated with an exponential change in TSH levels [61].

Although measurement of the TSH level is the most reliable screening method for assessing thyroid function, the degree of hyperthyroidism cannot be estimated easily in this way. Instead, hyperthyroidism must be measured using an assay of thyroid hormone levels in the plasma. Thyroid hormone circulates as triiodothyronine (T3) and thyroxine (T4), with more than 99.9 % of the hormones bound to serum proteins (especially thyroxine-binding globulin, transthyretin or thyroxin binding prealbumin, and albumin).

Free T4 (FT4) and free T3 measurement is recommended in patients with suspected hyperthyroidism when TSH is low. Many laboratories do not measure FT4 directly, instead using a calculation to estimate the FT4 level. Serum free T4 can be estimated by several different methods such as equilibrium dialysis techniques or estimated indirectly by calculation of the free-thyroxine index (FTI):

$$\text{Free-thyroxine index (FTI)} = \text{Total } T_4 \times T_3 \text{ resin uptake } (T_3RU)\ \%.$$

The T3 resin uptake (T3RU) test indirectly estimates unsaturated binding sites on thyroid binding globulin (TBG). The patient's serum is incubated with radiolabelled T3 tracer. The unbound tracer is trapped with resin, and the value is reported as percent tracer uptake by resin. The greater the number of free TBG-binding sites, the lower the uptake of tracer by the resin. The normal range for T3RU is between 25 % and 35 %.

Since Free thyroxine (FT4) and free triiodothyronine (FT3) assays now available in most of the laboratories, therefore, FTI and T3 resin uptake measurement are rarely required.

Because nonthyroidal illness will produce temporary suppression of TSH, thyroid function tests should be repeated before therapy is instituted for subclinical disease. Hormonal changes in pregnancy can complicate the interpretation of thyroid function tests. Physiologic maximum elevation of beta human chorionic gonadotropin (β-hCG) at the end of the first trimester of pregnancy is associated with a mirror-image temporary reduction in TSH. Despite the reduction in TSH, FT4 levels usually remain normal or only slightly above the reference range. As the pregnancy progresses and β-hCG plateaus at a lower level, TSH levels return to normal.

Antibodies

Anti Thyroid Peroxidase(TPO) Antibody The most specific autoantibody test for autoimmune thyroiditis is an ELISA test for anti-Thyroid Peroxidase(TPO) antibody. The titers usually are significantly elevated in the most common type of hyperthyroidism, Graves thyrotoxicosis, and usually are low or absent in toxic multinodular goiter and toxic adenoma.

Although, antithyroid antibodies are elevated in Graves' disease and lymphocytic thyroiditis but usually are not necessary to make the diagnosis [62].

A significant number of healthy people without active thyroid disease have mildly positive anti-TPO antibody titers; thus, the test should not be performed for screening purposes.

The Thyroid-Stimulating Immunoglobulin (TSI) Level Thyroid stimulating immunoglobulins, also known as TSIs, are autoantibodies that are produced by the immune system in the setting of Graves' disease. Antibodies are molecules produced by white blood cells called B cells. B cells are stimulated to produce antibodies through a series of interactions with other white blood cells called helper T cells. These interactions transform B cells into plasma cells that secrete large amounts of antibodies. TSIs are somewhat unique in that they do not directly promote the destruc tion of any normal cells or structures in the thyroid gland. Instead they mimic the action of TSH itself, driving the TSH receptors to generate signals that stimulate the production and secretion of thyroid hormone. This process is not governed by the normal feedback mechanism that regulates the secretion of TSH from the pituitary gland. As such, TSIs that bind to TSH receptors may stimulate the production and secretion of excess amounts of thyroid hormone.

Elevated TSIs help to establish the diagnosis of Graves's disease. Thyroid-stimulating antibody levels can be used to monitor the effects of treatment with antithyroid drugs in patients with Graves' disease [63]. Circulating antithyroglobulin (anti-TG) antibodies are also present in Graves disease; however, testing for these antibodies should not be helpful, because anti-TG antibodies may be present in persons without evidence of thyroid dysfunction [64]. A high titer of serum antibodies to collagen XIII is associated with active Graves ophthalmopathy [65].

Other Relevant Investigations

Nonspecific laboratory findings can occur in hyperthyroidism, including anemia, granulocytosis, lymphocytosis, hypercalcemia, transaminase elevations, and alkaline phosphatase elevation [41].

Liver function test results should be obtained to monitor for liver toxicity caused by thioamides (antithyroid medications). A complete blood count (CBC) with differential should be obtained at baseline and with the development of fever or symptoms of infection. Graves disease may be associated with normocytic anemia, low-normal to slightly depressed total WBC count with relative lymphocytosis and monocytosis, low-normal to slightly depressed platelet count. Thionamides may rarely cause severe hematologic side effects, but routine screening for these rare events is not cost-effective.

Investigation of gynecomastia associated with Graves disease may reveal increased sex hormone–binding globulin levels and decreased free testosterone levels.

Hyperthyroidism may worsen diabetes control and may be reflected by an increase in hemoglobin A1C in diabetic patients.

A fasting lipid profile may show decreased total cholesterol levels and decreased triglyceride levels.

Measurement of serum hCG concentrations is needed for the diagnosis of moles and choriocarcinomas, and hCG serves as a sensitive and specific tumor marker during therapy and surveillance. In women, hCG concentrations are significantly higher than those found during normal pregnancies. CA125 may be found to be elevated in ovarian cancer.

Ultrasound

Ultrasounds with color-doppler evaluation have been found to be cost-effective in hyperthyroid patients and can differentiate between solitary adenoma and multinodular goiter [66, 67].

A prospective trial showed that thyroid ultrasound findings are predictive of radioiodine treatment outcome, and, in patients with

Graves disease, normoechogenic and large glands are associated with increased radioresistance [67].

In Graves disease ultrasound often shows a diffusely enlarged thyroid gland and is often hyperechoic and of heterogeneous echotexture. There is relative absence of nodularity in uncomplicated cases. Gland may become hypervascular and demonstrate a "thyroid inferno" pattern on color doppler [68]. Ultrasound will confirm the presence of a solitary nodule, adenoma and multinodular goiter. There is no indication to perform fine needle aspiration in patients with toxic adenomas because the risk of a thyroid carcinoma is extremely low and cytological evaluation will not permit distinguishing between a follicular adenoma and a follicular carcinoma [69].

Radioisotope Thyroid Scan

If the etiology of hyperthyroidism is not clear after physical examination and other laboratory tests, it can be confirmed by means of scintigraphy. A thyroid scan can be performed with 123iodine, 131iodine, or 99technetium-labeled pertechnetate . Normally, the isotope distributes homogeneously throughout both lobes of the thyroid gland. In patients with hyperthyroidism, the pattern of uptake (e.g., diffuse vs nodular) varies with the underlying disorder. The overall level of radioactive iodine uptake (RAIU) also varies with different conditions. Normal RAIU is approximately 5–20 % but is modified by the iodine content of the patient's diet.

Scintigraphically, an adenoma may be warm (uptake similar to surrounding tissue), hot (uptake increased without suppression of surrounding tissue), or toxic (uptake increased and suppression of the surrounding tissue).

Radioisotope Findings

Radionuclide uptake and scan easily distinguishes the high uptake of Graves' disease from the low uptake of thyroiditis and provides other useful anatomic information.

Following characterizes the radioisotope findings of common causes of hyperthyroidism : (see Table 8.1)

- Graves disease – Diffuse enlargement of both thyroid lobes, with uniform uptake of isotope and elevated radioactive iodine uptake.
- Toxic multinodular goiter – Irregular areas of relatively diminished and occasionally increased uptake; overall radioactive iodine uptake is mildly to moderately increased.
- Toxic adenoma- Increased tracer uptake.
- Subacute thyroiditis –Very low radioactive iodine uptake.

MRI/CT Scan

Computed tomography scanning or magnetic resonance imaging (of the orbits) may be necessary in the evaluation of proptosis. If routinely performed, most patients have evidence of orbitopathy, such as an increased volume of extraocular muscles and/or retrobulbar connective tissue. These tech-

Table 8.1 Radiotracer uptake in hyperthyroidism

Causes	24 h radioactive iodine uptake
Graves disease	Increased (moderate to high: 40–100 %)
Toxic adenoma	Increased (mild to moderate: 25–60 %)
Toxic multinodular goiter	Increased (mild to moderate: 25–60 %)
Subacute thyroiditis	Decreased (very low: <2 %)
Iodide-induced hyperthyroidism	Variable but usually low (<25 %)
Thyrotoxicosis factitia	Decreased (very low: <2 %)
Pituitary tumors producing TSH	Increased (mild to moderate: 25–60 %)
Excess human chorionic gonadotropin (molar pregnancy/choriocarcinoma)	Increased (variable: 25–100 %)
Pituitary resistance to thyroid hormone	Increased (mild to moderate: 25–60 %)
Struma ovarii with hyperthyroidism	Decreased

niques are useful to monitor changes over time or to ascertain the effects of treatment. Careful monitoring is required after using iodinated contrast agents as they may affect ongoing treatment plans. The diagnostic approach is in general similar to patients with a solitary AFTN, but cross-sectional imaging with computer tomography and pulmonary function tests need to be considered in a subset of patients in whom compression by the goiter is evident or suspected MRI pituitary may be required in ascertaining pituitary TSHoma. Cross-sectional imaging with computed tomography or magnetic resonance imaging will demonstrate uni- or bilateral ovarian masses in struma ovarii.

Treatment

If left untreated hyperthyroidism can cause thyrotoxic storm and long-standing severe thyrotoxicosis leads to severe weight loss with catabolism of bone and muscle [70].

The treatment of hyperthyroidism depends on the cause and severity of the disease, as well as on the patient's age, goiter size, comorbid conditions, and patient's preference.

The goal of therapy is to correct the hypermetabolic state with the fewest side effects and the lowest incidence of hypothyroidism. Beta blockers and iodides are used as treatment adjuncts. Antithyroid drugs, radioactive iodine, and surgery are the main treatment options for persistent hyperthyroidism [5, 20, 41, 62]. See Table 8.2.

Each therapy can produce satisfactory outcomes if properly used [71].

Following is the detailed description of therapy.

Symptomatic Relief

Beta Blockers Many of the neurologic and cardiovascular symptoms of hyperthyroidism are relieved by beta-blocker s. Before such therapy is initiated, the patient should be examined for signs and symptoms of dehydration that often occur with hyperthyroidism. After oral rehydration, beta-blocker therapy can be started. Beta-blocker therapy should not be administered to patients with a significant history of asthma or heart failure.

Beta blockers offer prompt relief of the adrenergic symptoms of hyperthyroidism such as tremor, palpitations, heat intolerance, and nervousness. Propranolol (Inderal) has been used most widely, but other beta blockers can be used. Nonselective beta blockers such as propranolol, are preferred because they have a more direct effect on hypermetabolism [72]. Therapy with propranolol should be initiated at 10–20 mg every 6 h. The dose should be increased progressively until symptoms are controlled. In most cases, a dosage of 80 320 mg per day is sufficient [41].

Calcium Channel Blockers (e.g., verapamil and diltiazem) can be used for the same purposes when beta-blockers are contraindicated or poorly tolerated. These therapies should be tapered and stopped once thyroid functions are within the normal range.

Calcium channel blockers such as diltiazem can be used to reduce heart rate in patients who cannot tolerate beta blockers [73].

Table 8.2 Treatment modalities: Pros and cons

Treatment modalities	Pros	Cons
Thioamide drug therapy	Avoiding surgery and radioactive ablation therapy	Adverse drug effects
	Less chances of life long thyroxine replacement	
131I Ablation therapy	Definitive therapy	Worsening of Graves ophthalmopathy
	Avoiding surgical risk	Life long thyroxine replacement
		Radiation exposure
		Contraindicated in pregnancy
Surgical intervention	Rapid resolution	Risk related to surgery
		Life long thyroxine replacement

Diet and Activity

No special diet must be followed by patients with thyroid disease. However, some expectorants, radiographic contrast dyes, seaweed tablets, and health food supplements contain excess amounts of iodide and should be avoided because the iodide interferes with or complicates the management of antithyroid and radioactive iodine therapies.

Exercise tolerance often is not significantly affected in otherwise healthy patients with mild to moderate hyperthyroidism. For these patients, no reduction in physical activity is necessary. For patients who are elderly or have cardiopulmonary comorbidities or severe hyperthyroidism, a decrease in activity is prudent until hyperthyroidism is medically controlled.

Antithyroid Medications

Thioamides (Cabimazole, methimazole and propylthiouracil) act principally by interfering with the organification of iodine, thereby suppressing thyroid hormone levels. Remission rates vary with the length of treatment, but rates of 60 % have been reported when therapy is continued for 2 years [63].

Relapse can occur in up to 50 % of patients who respond initially, regardless of the regimen used. A recent randomized trial indicated that relapse was more likely in patients who smoked, had large goiters, or had elevated thyroid-stimulating antibody levels at the end of therapy [74].

Methimazole and carbimazole are the antithyroid drugs most frequently used both for the preoperative and long-term medical management of hyperthyroidism because of their consistent and potent effect on lowering thyroid hormone concentrations. Both drugs are actively concentrated by the thyroid gland where they exert their effect by inhibiting thyroid hormone production. Carbimazole is actually converted to methimazole such that only methimazole accumulates in the thyroid gland. This conversion results in a 5 mg dose of carbimazole being approximately equivalent to 3 mg of methimazole (reflecting the molar ratio of the two drugs). Methimazole is available as both human and veterinary formulations (2.5 and 5 mg). Carbimazole is only available as a preparation for human use. Carbimazole/Methimazole and propylthiouracil have been used for hyperthyroidism since their introduction in the 1940s. These medications are employed for long-term control of hyperthyroidism in children, adolescents, and pregnant women. In adult men and nonpregnant women, they are used to control hyperthyroidism before definitive therapy with radioactive iodine. Antithyroid medications inhibit the formation and coupling of iodotyrosines in thyroglobulin. Because these processes are necessary for thyroid hormone synthesis, this inhibition induces a gradual reduction in thyroid hormone levels over 2–8 weeks or longer. A second action of propylthiouracil (but not methimazole) is inhibition of conversion of thyroxine (T4) to triiodothyronine (T3). T3 is more biologically active than T4; thus, a quick reduction in T3 levels is associated with a clinically significant improvement in thyrotoxic symptoms.

The antithyroid drug dose should be titrated every 4 weeks until thyroid functions normalize. Some patients with Graves disease go into a remission after treatment for 12–18 months, and the drug can be discontinued. Notably, half of the patients who go into remission experience a recurrence of hyperthyroidism within the following year. Nodular forms of hyperthyroidism (i.e., toxic multinodular goiter and toxic adenoma) are permanent conditions and will not go into remission [75].

Cabimazole/Methimazole Generally is the drug of choice in nonpregnant patients because of its lower cost, longer half-life, and lower incidence of hematologic side effects. The starting dosage is 15–30 mg per day (60 mg is the maximum dose) and it can be given in conjunction with a beta blocker [76].

Methimazole is more potent than propylthiouracil and has a longer duration of action. In addition, methimazole is taken once daily, patient compliance is often better with methimazole than with propylthiouracil. Methimazole is not recommended for use in the first trimester of pregnancy, because it has been associated, albeit rarely, with cloacal and scalp (cutis aplasia) abnormalities when given during early gestation [77, 78].

The beta blockade can be tapered after 4–8 weeks and the methimazole adjusted, according to clinical status and monthly free T4 or free T3 levels, toward an eventual maintenance dosage of 5–10 mg per day [20, 73].

TSH levels may remain undetectable for months after the patient becomes euthyroid and should not be used to monitor the effects of therapy. At 1 year, if the patient is clinically and biochemically Euthyroid and a thyroid-stimulating antibody level is not detectable, therapy can be discontinued. If the thyroid-stimulating antibody level is elevated, continuation of therapy for another year should be considered. Once antithyroid drug therapy is discontinued, the patient should be monitored every 3 months for the first year, because relapse is more likely to occur during this time, and then annually, because relapse can occur years later. If relapse occurs, radioactive iodine or surgery generally is recommended, although antithyroid drug therapy can be restarted [20].

Propylthiouracil PTU is preferred for pregnant women because methimazole has been associated with rare congenital abnormalities. The starting dosage of PTU is 100 mg three times per day (maximum dose is 600 mg/day) with a maintenance dosage of 100–200 mg daily in two to three divided doses [76].

If a nonpregnant woman who is receiving methimazole desires pregnancy, she should be switched to propylthiouracil before conception. After 12 weeks of gestation, she can be switched back to carbimazole or methimazole. Propylthiouracil remains the drug of choice in uncommon situations of life-threatening severe thyrotoxicosis (i.e., thyroid storm) because of the additional benefit of inhibition of T4 -to-T3 conversion. In this setting, propylthiouracil should be administered every 6–8 h. The reduction in T3, which is 20–100 times more potent than T4, theoretically helps reduce the thyrotoxic symptoms more quickly than methimazole would. Once thyroid levels have decreased to nearly normal values, the patient can be switched to methimazole therapy.

Adverse Effects of Thioamide Antithyroid Medications

The most common adverse effects of thioamide antithyroid drugs are allergic reactions manifesting as fever, rash, urticaria, and arthralgia, which occur in 1–5 % of patients, usually within the first few weeks of treatment. Agranulocytosis is the most serious adverse reaction of antithyroid drug therapy and is estimated to occur in 0.1–0.5 % of patients treated with these drugs [76].

The risk is higher in the first several months of therapy and may be higher with PTU than methimazole [20, 41, 63]. The onset of agranulocytosis is sometimes abrupt, so patients should be warned to stop taking the drug immediately if they develop a sudden fever or sore throat. After the drug is stopped, granulocyte counts usually start to rise within several days but may not normalize for 10–14 days. Granulocyte colony-stimulating factor (G-CSF) appears to accelerate recovery in patients with a bone marrow aspiration showing a granulocyte-to-erythrocyte ratio of 1:2 or greater than 0.5. In most cases, agranulocytosis is reversible with supportive treatment [63, 72].

Routine monitoring of white cell counts remains controversial, but results of one study showed that close monitoring of white cell counts allowed for earlier detection of agranulocytosis. In this study, patients had white cell counts every 2 weeks for the first 2 months, then monthly [79].

Minor side effects (e.g., rash, fever, gastrointestinal symptoms) sometimes can be treated symptomatically without discontinuation of the antithyroid drug; however, if symptoms of arthralgia occur, antithyroid drugs should be discontinued because arthralgia can be a precursor of a more serious polyarthritis syndrome. Other serious adverse effects include aplastic anemia, hepatitis, polyarthritis, and a lupus like vasculitis.

The FDA recommends the following measures for patients receiving propylthiouracil [80]:

- Closely monitor patients for signs and symptoms of liver injury, especially during the first 6 months after initiation of therapy.
- For suspected liver injury, promptly discontinue propylthiouracil, evaluate the patient for evidence of liver injury, and provide supportive care.
- Counsel patients to contact their health care provider promptly for the following signs or symptoms: fatigue, weakness, vague abdominal pain, loss of appetite, itching, easy bruising, or yellowing of the eyes or skin.

Radioactive Iodine 131 Ablation (RAI^{131})

Radioactive iodine therapy is the most common treatment for Graves disease and toxic multinodular goiter in adults in the United States [81].

In Europe and Japan, there has been a greater physician preference for ATDs and/or surgery [82]. Although its effect is less rapid than that of antithyroid medication or thyroidectomy, it is effective and safe and does not require hospitalization.

Radioactive iodine is administered orally as a single dose in capsule or liquid form. The iodine is quickly absorbed and taken up by the thyroid. No other tissue or organ in the body is capable of retaining the radioactive iodine; consequently, very few adverse effects are associated with this therapy. The treatment results in a thyroid-specific inflammatory response, causing fibrosis and destruction of the thyroid over weeks to many months.

Radioactive iodine therapy for TMNG results in resolution of hyperthyroidism in approximately 55 % of patients at 3 months and 80 % of patients at 6 months, with an average failure rate of 15 % [83–85]. Goiter volume is decreased by 3 months, with further reduction observed over 24 months, for a total size reduction of 40 %. Generally, the dose of ^{131} I administered is 75–200 μCi/g of estimated thyroid tissue divided by the percent of 123 I uptake in 24 h. This dose is intended to render the patient hypothyroid.

Administration of lithium in the weeks following radioactive iodine therapy may extend the retention of radioactive iodine and increase its efficacy. This may be considered in Graves disease patients with especially large Graves glands (>60 g) or in patients with extremely high thyroidal iodine uptake (>95 % in 4 h), which is associated with high iodine turnover in the gland. However, studies have yielded inconsistent results, and the benefits of using lithium with radioactive iodine must be weighed against the toxicities associated with lithium. Hypothyroidism is considered by many experts to be the expected goal of radioactive iodine therapy.

In several large epidemiologic studies of radioactive iodine therapy in patients with Graves disease, no evidence indicated that radioactive iodine therapy caused the development of thyroid carcinoma [86].

There is also no evidence that radioactive iodine therapy for hyperthyroidism results in increased mortality for any other form of cancer, including leukemia [87].

Long-term follow-up data of children and adolescents treated with radioactive iodine are lacking [62, 63].

American Thyroid Association (ATA) guidelines recommend avoiding^{131} I therapy in children younger than 5 years of age. In children 5–10 years old, ^{131} I therapy is acceptable if the calculated activity of administered^{131} I is less than 10 mCi. In children older than 10 years of age, radioactive iodine therapy is acceptable if the activity is greater than 150 μCi/g of thyroid tissue [88].

Radioactive iodine should never be administered to pregnant women, because it can cross the placenta and ablate the fetus's thyroid, resulting in hypothyroidism. Similarly, breastfeeding is a contraindication, in that the radioisotope is secreted in breast milk. Women will continue to receive increased radiation to the breast from radioactive iodine for a few months after ceasing lactation; accordingly, initiation of this therapy should be delayed. It is standard practice to check for pregnancy before starting radioactive iodine therapy and to recommend that the patient not become pregnant for at least 3–6 months after the treatment or until thyroid functions normalize. No excess fetal malformations or increased miscarriage rates have been found in women previously treated with radioactive iodine for hyperthyroidism.

Radioactive iodine usually is not administered to patients with severe ophthalmopathy, because clinical evidence suggests that worsening of thyroid eye disease occurs after radioactive iodine therapy [89]. This worsening is usually mild but occasionally severe. The risk of ophthalmopathy is greater in patients who smoke cigarettes, but it can be reduced by providing glucocorticoid therapy (prednisone 0.4 mg/kg for 1 month with subsequent taper) after radioactive iodine therapy. See algorithm for steroid treatment in Graves ophthalmopathy.

Using antithyroid drugs to achieve a euthyroid state before treatment with radioactive iodine is not recommended for most patients, but it may improve safety for patients with severe or complicated hyperthyroidism. It is unclear whether antithyroid drugs increase radioactive iodine failure rates [5, 90–92].

If used, they should be withdrawn at least 3 days before radioactive iodine and can be restarted 2–3 days later. The antithyroid drug is continued for 3 months after radioactive iodine, and then tapered.

Most of the radioactive iodine is eliminated from the body in urine, saliva, and feces within 48 h; however, double flushing of the toilet and frequent hand washing are recommended for several weeks. Close contact with others, especially children and pregnant women, should be avoided for 24–72 h [93].

Concerns about radiation exposure after therapy have led to the issuance of new recommendations by the ATA. These recommendations are compliant with Nuclear Regulatory Commission regulations and are a practical guide for patient activity after radioactive iodine therapy, with the aim of ensuring maximum radiation safety for the family and the public [94].

Other Less Commonly Used Antithyroid Medications

Iodides Iodides block the peripheral conversion of thyroxine (T4) to triiodothyronine (T3) and inhibit hormone release. Iodides also are used as adjunctive therapy before emergency nonthyroid surgery, if beta blockers are unable to control the hyperthyroidism, and to reduce gland vascularity before surgery for Graves' disease [20].

Iodides are not used in the routine treatment of hyperthyroidism because of paradoxical increases in hormone release that can occur with prolonged use. Organic iodide radiographic contrast agents (e.g., iopanoic acid or ipodate sodium) are used more commonly than the inorganic iodides (e.g., potassium iodide). The dosage of either agent is 1 g per day for up to 12 weeks [95].

A saturated solution of potassium iodide (SSKI) can be administered at a dosage of 10 drops twice daily, with a consequent rapid reduction in T3 levels.

These drugs must not be administered to patients with toxic multinodular goiter or toxic adenomas. The autonomous nature of these conditions can lead to worsening of the thyrotoxicosis in the presence of pharmacologic levels of iodide, a substrate in thyroid hormone synthesis. This phenomenon typically presents in patients living in iodine deficient areas who relocate to an iodine sufficient geographical area or upon ingestion of iodine (Jod-Basedow syndrome).

Bile Salt Sequestrant Another drug that might be considered in management of severe thyrotoxicosis would be cholestyramine, a bile salt sequestrant. It decreases thyroid hormone levels by depleting the pool by enhancing clearance from enterohepatic circulation. Doses up to 12 g in 3 divided daily doses have been used for 4 weeks.

Thyroidectomy

Subtotal thyroidectomy is the oldest form of treatment for hyperthyroidism. Total thyroidectomy and combinations of hemithyroidectomies and contralateral subtotal thyroidectomies also have been used [81, 96].

Indications for Thyroidectomy

Because of the excellent efficacy of antithyroid medications and radioactive iodine therapy in regulating thyroid function, thyroidectomy is generally reserved for special circumstances, including the following:

- Large goiter with compressive symptoms
- Pregnant women who are noncompliant with or intolerant of antithyroid drugs
- Patients who refuse radioactive iodine therapy and antithyroid treatment
- Failure to medical treatment
- Goiter with malignant potential

Preparation for Thyroidectomy

Preparation for thyroidectomy includes antithyroid medication, iodine treatment and beta-blocker therapy [96].

In severe hyperthyroidism, antithyroid drug therapy should be administered until thyroid functions normalize (4–8 weeks). Propranolol is titrated until the resting pulse rate is lower than 80 beats/min. Finally, iodide is administered as SSKI (1–2 drops twice daily for 10–14 days) before the procedure. Stable iodide therapy both reduces thyroid hormone excretion and decreases thyroid blood flow, which may help reduce intraoperative blood loss. A Swiss study found that administration of a single dose of steroid (dexamethasone 8 mg) before thyroidectomy can reduce the nausea, pain, and vomiting associated with the procedure, as well as improve voice function [97].

Adverse Effects of Thyroidectomy

During the 1800s, the mortality rate from thyroid surgery was approximately 40 %. Most deaths were caused by infection and hemorrhage [98].

Sterile surgical arenas, general anesthesia, and improved surgical techniques have made death from thyroid surgery extremely rare today. With current operative techniques, bilateral subtotal thyroidectomy should have a mortality approaching zero in patients who are properly prepared. Adverse effects of thyroidectomy include:

Postoperative Bleeding

The incidence of bleeding after thyroid surgery is low (0.3–1 %), but an unrecognized or rapidly expanding hematoma can cause airway compromise and asphyxiation [99].

Infection

Currently, postoperative infection occurs in less than 1–2 % of all thyroid surgery cases. Sterile surgical technique is the key to prevention [100];

Injury to the Recurrent Laryngeal Nerve

Recurrent laryngeal nerve (RLN) injury results in true vocal-fold paresis or paralysis. Deliberate intraoperative identification and preservation of the RLN minimizes the risk of injury [101].

Injury to the Superior Laryngeal Nerve

The external branch of the superior laryngeal nerve (SLN) is probably the nerve most commonly injured in thyroid surgery, with an injury rate estimated at 0–25 %. Trauma to the nerve results in an inability to lengthen a vocal fold and, thus, inability to create a high-pitched sound; this may be career-threatening for singers or others who rely on their voice for their profession [102].

Hypoparathyroidism

Hypoparathyroidism can result from direct trauma to the parathyroid glands, devascularization of the glands, or removal of the glands during surgery. Postoperative hypoparathyroidism, and the resulting hypocalcemia, may be permanent or transient. Hypocalcemia after thyroidectomy is initially asymptomatic in most cases [103].

Hypothyroidism

Hypothyroidism is an expected consequence of total thyroidectomy and measurement of TSH levels is the most useful laboratory test for detecting or monitoring of hypothyroidism in these patients [104].

Thyrotoxic Storm

Thyrotoxic storm is an unusual complication that may result from manipulation of the thyroid gland during surgery in patients with hyperthyroidism. It can develop intraoperatively, or postoperatively [104]. A detailed account of this entity is given in Chap. 12

Follow up After Thyroid Surgery

Patients whose thyroid functions normalize after surgery require routine follow-up because hypothyroidism, recurrent hyperthyroidism, or thyroid eye disease may develop at some time in the future. Most patients remain euthyroid after a lobectomy or lobectomy plus isthmusectomy to treat a toxic adenoma or toxic multinodular goiter with a dominant nodule. To ensure normal thyroid function, thyroid function tests should be obtained 3–4 weeks after a lobectomy. After subtotal thyroidectomy for hyperthyroidism and cessation of antithyroid therapy, most patients become hypothyroid, depending on how much functional tissue is left by the surgeon. Partial replacement (Throxine 50–75 μg/day) is recommended in these patients, beginning shortly after the procedure. Thyroid function tests should be monitored 4–8 weeks postoperatively, and the thyroxine dosage should be adjusted to maintain a normal TSH level.

Cause-Specific Treatment

Transsphenoidal surgeries, in combination with radiotherapy and somatostatin analogues in some patients with pituitary adenoma (TSHoma) are the treatment options. Hydatiform moles are treated by suction. Choriocarcinomas can be treated successfully in most patients with chemotherapy. Most patients with struma ovarii are clinically and biochemically euthyroid. Unilateral or bilateral open or laparoscopic oophorectomy is the primary therapy [105].

Thyrotoxic women with struma ovarii should be treated with antithyroid drugs and, if needed, with beta-blockers prior to surgery. In the case of malignant lesions, the patient should undergo thyroidectomy followed by treatment with 131iodine [106].

Future Directions

A promising new drug for the treatment of Graves ophthalmopathy is rituximab, an anti-CD20 monoclonal antibody causing depletion of CD20-positive B cells and thereby initially used for CD20-positive non-Hodgkin's lymphomas. Rituximab has then also been employed for several autoimmune disorders, both T cell and B cell driven. Data are too preliminary to draw any definite conclusion [107]. Other newer treatment options include endoscopic subtotal thyroidectomy [108], embolization of the thyroid arteries [109], plasmapheresis [110], and percutaneous ethanol injection of toxic thyroid nodules [111]. Autotransplantation of cryopreserved thyroid tissue may become a treatment option for postoperative hypothyroidism [112]. Nutritional supplementation with L-carnitine [113] has been shown to have a beneficial effect on the symptoms of hyperthyroidism, and L-carnitine may help prevent bone demineralization caused by the disease.

Conclusion

Hyperthyroidism has a broad spectrum of etiologies, clinical manifestations and carries significant morbidity and mortality, if left untreated. While it is most commonly caused by Graves' disease, it is of importance to recognize other etiologies in order to choose the most appropriate therapeutic option and long-term surveillance. Toxic adenomas are characterized by a single hyperactive nodule in the thyroid leading to clinical and biochemical hyperthyroidism. Older patients with a hot nodule are more likely to become toxic as compared to younger patients. The likelihood of malignancy in a toxic nodule is very low. In multinodular goiters, several nodules display an autonomous function. Administration of moderate or high doses of iodine may induce hyperthyroidism in patients with or without apparent pre-existing thyroid disease. An antiarrhythmic drug amiodarone, which may induce hyperthyroidism because of its high iodine content and/or a drug-induced thyroiditis. Any form of thyroiditis can be associated with a thyrotoxic phase because the disruption of thyroid follicles can result in an increased release of stored iodothyronines. The thyrotoxic phase may be followed by transient or permanent hypothyroidism. Hyperthyroidism in elderly may easily be missed because of atypical presentation and a high index of suspicion is required to timely diagnose and treat this life threatening condition in elderly. Graves' disease, toxic multinodular goiter, and toxic adenoma can be treated with radioactive iodine, antithyroid drugs, or surgery. Thyroidectomy is an option when other treatments fail or are contraindicated, or when a goiter is causing compressive symptoms. Special treatment consideration must be given to patients who are pregnant or breastfeeding, as well as those with Graves' ophthalmopathy. Patients' desires must be considered when deciding on appropriate therapy, and close monitoring and follow up for disease status and drug side effects are essential components of management.

Algorithm for cortico steroid (CS) treatment in Graves' ophthalmopathy

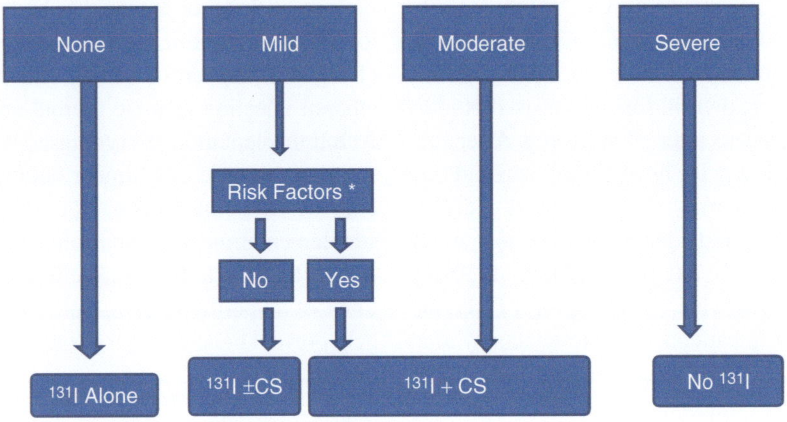

* Smoking, High T3 levels, high TRAb titers

References

1. Singer PA, Cooper DS, Levy EG, et al. (American Thyroid Association Standards of Care Committee). Treatment guidelines for patients with hyperthyroidism and hypothyroidism. JAMA. 1995;273:808–12.
2. Baskin HJ, Cobin RH, Duick DS, et al. (American Association of Clinical Endocrinologists). American Association of Clinical Endocrinologists medical guidelines for clinical practice for the evaluation and treatment of hyperthyroidism and hypothyroidism. Endocr Pract. 2002;8:457–69.
3. Ellis H. Robert Graves: 1796–1852. Br J Hosp Med (Lond). 2006;67:313.
4. Cruz AA, Akaishi PM, Vargas MA, et al. Association between thyroid autoimmune dysfunction and non-thyroid autoimmune diseases. Ophthal Plast Reconstr Surg. 2007;23:104–8.
5. Weetman AP. Graves' disease. N Engl J Med. 2000;343:1236–48.
6. Tunbridge WM, Evered DC, Hall R, et al. The spectrum of thyroid disease in a community: the Whickham survey. Clin Endocrinol (Oxf). 1977;7:481–93.
7. Vanderpump MP, Tunbridge WM, French JM, et al. The incidence of thyroid disorders in the community: a twenty-year follow-up of the Whickham survey. Clin Endocrinol (Oxf). 1995;43:55–68.
8. Davies TF, Larsen PR. Thyrotoxicosis. In: Larsen PR et al., editors. Williams textbook of endocrinology. 10th ed. Philadelphia: Saunders; 2003. p. 374–421.
9. Jacobson EM, Tomer Y. The CD40, CTLA-4, thyroglobulin, TSH receptor, and PTPN22 gene quintet and its contribution to thyroid autoimmunity: back to the future. J Autoimmun. 2007;28:85–98.
10. Iwama S, Ikezaki A, Kikuoka N, et al. Association of HLA-DR, –DQ genotype and CTLA-4 gene polymorphism with Graves' disease in Japanese children. Horm Res. 2005;63:55–60.
11. Chu X, Pan CM, Zhao SX, et al. A genome-wide association study identifies two new risk loci for Graves' disease. Nat Genet. 2011;43:897–901.

12. Lumbroso S, Paris F, Sultan C. Activating Gsalpha mutations: analysis of 113 patients with signs of McCune-Albright syndrome--an European Collaborative Study. J Clin Endocrinol Metab. 2004;89:2107–13.
13. Betterle C, Dal Pra C, Mantero F, et al. Autoimmune adrenal insufficiency and autoimmune polyendocrine syndromes: autoantibodies, autoantigens, and their applicability in diagnosis and disease prediction. Endocr Rev. 2002;23:327–64.
14. Plagnol V, Howson JM, Smyth DJ, et al. Genome-wide association analysis of autoantibody positivity in type 1 diabetes cases. PLoS Genet. 2011;7: e1002216.
15. Simmonds MJ, Brand OJ, Barrett JC, Newby PR, Franklyn JA, Gough SC. Association of Fc receptor-like 5 (FCRL5) with Graves' disease is secondary to the effect of FCRL3. Clin Endocrinol (Oxf). 2010;73:654–60.
16. Newby PR, Pickles OJ, Mazumdar S, Brand OJ, Carr-Smith JD, Pearce SH, et al. Follow-up of potential novel Graves' disease susceptibility loci, identified in the UK WTCCC genomewide nonsynonymous SNP study. Eur J Hum Genet. 2010;18: 1021–6.
17. Nakabayashi K, Shirasawa S. Recent advances in the association studies of autoimmune thyroid disease and the functional characterization of AITD-related transcription factor ZFAT. Nihon Rinsho Meneki Gakkai Kaishi. 2010;33:66–72.
18. Chu X, Dong Y, Shen M, et al. Polymorphisms in the ADRB2 gene and Graves disease: a case–control study and a meta-analysis of available evidence. BMC Med Genet. 2009;10:26.
19. Boelaert K, Newby PR, Simmonds MJ, et al. Prevalence and relative risk of other autoimmune diseases in subjects with autoimmune thyroid disease. Am J Med. 2010;123:183.e1–9.
20. Woeber KA. Update on the management of hyperthyroidism and hypothyroidism. Arch Intern Med. 2000;160:1067–71.
21. Bahn RS. Mechanisms of disease—Graves' ophthalmopathy. N Engl J Med. 2010;362:726–38.
22. Smith TJ. Pathogenesis of Graves' orbitopathy: a 2010 update. J Endocrinol Invest. 2010;33:414–21.
23. Douglas RS, Afifiyan NF, Hwang CJ, et al. Increased generation of fibrocytes in thyroid associated ophthalmopathy. J Clin Endocrinol Metab. 2010; 95:430–8.
24. Corvilain B, Dumont JF, Vassart G. Toxic adenoma and toxic multinodular goiter. In: Werner SC, Ingbar SH, Braverman LE, Utiger RD, editors. Werner & Ingbar's the thyroid: a fundamental and clinical text. 8th ed. Philadelphia: Lippincott Williams & Wilkins; 2000. p. 564–72.
25. Duprez L, Hermans J, Van Sande J, et al. Two autonomous nodules of a patient with multinodular goiter harbor different activating mutations of the thyrotropin receptor gene. J Clin Endocrinol Metab. 1997;82:306–8.
26. Holzapfel HP, Fuhrer D, Wonerow P, et al. Identification of constitutively activating somatic thyrotropin receptor mutations in a subset of toxic multinodular goiters. J Clin Endocrinol Metab. 1997;82:4229–33.
27. Tonacchera M, Chiovato L, Pinchera A, et al. Hyperfunctioning thyroid nodules in toxic multinodular goiter share activating thyrotropin receptor mutations with solitary toxic adenoma. J Clin Endocrinol Metab. 1998;83:492–8.
28. Kopp P, Kimura ET, Aeschimann S, et al. Polyclonal and monoclonal thyroid nodules coexist within human multinodular goiters. J Clin Endocrinol Metab. 1994;79:134–9.
29. Gabriel EM, Bergert ER, Grant CS, et al. Germline polymorphism of codon 727 of human thyroid-stimulating hormone receptor is associated with toxic multinodular goiter. Clin Endocrinol Metab. 1999;84:3328–35.
30. Nogueira CR, Kopp P, Arseven OK, et al. Thyrotropin receptor mutations in hyperfunctioning thyroid adenomas from Brazil. Thyroid. 1999;9:1063–8.
31. Muhlberg T, Herrmann K, Joba W, et al. Lack of association of nonautoimmune hyperfunctioning thyroid disorders and a germline polymorphism of codon 727 of the human thyrotropin receptor in a European Caucasian population. J Clin Endocrinol Metab. 2000;85:2640–3.
32. Hamburger JI. Evolution of toxicity in solitary nontoxic autonomously functioning thyroid nodules. J Clin Endocrinol Metab. 1980;50:1089–93.
33. Bransom CJ, Talbot CH, Henry L, et al. Solitary toxic adenoma of the thyroid gland. Br J Surg. 1979;66:592–5.
34. Dumont JE, Lamy F, Roger P, et al. Physiological and pathological regulation of thyroid cell proliferation and differentiation by thyrotropin and other factors. Physiol Rev. 1992;72:667–97.
35. Parma J, Van Sande J, Swillens S, et al. Somatic mutations causing constitutive activity of the thyrotropin receptor are the major cause of hyperfunctioning thyroid adenomas: identification of additional mutations activating both the cyclic adenosine 3′,5′-monophosphate and inositol phosphate-Ca2+ cascades. Mol Endocrinol. 1995;9:725–33.
36. Takeshita A, Nagayama Y, Yokoyama N, et al. Rarity of oncogenic mutations in the thyrotropin receptor of autonomously functioning thyroid nodules in Japan. J Clin Endocrinol Metab. 1995;80:2607–11.
37. Frost L, Vestergaard P, Mosekilde L. Hyperthyroidism and risk of atrial fibrillation or flutter: a population-based study. Arch Intern Med. 2004;164:1675–8.
38. Trulzsch B, Krohn K, Wonerow P, et al. Detection of thyroid-stimulating hormone receptor and Gs alpha mutations: in 75 toxic thyroid nodules by denaturing gradient gel electrophoresis. J Mol Med. 2001;78:684–91.
39. Slatosky J, Shipton B, Wahba H. Thyroiditis: differential diagnosis and management. Am Fam Physician. 2000;61:1047–52.

40. Roberts CG, Ladenson PW. Hypothyroidism. Lancet. 2004;363:793–803.
41. Fitzgerald PA. Endocrinology. In: Tierny LM, McPhee SJ, Papadakis MA, editors. Current medical diagnosis and treatment. 44th ed. New York: McGraw-Hill; 2005. p. 1102–10.
42. Beck-Peccoz P, Persani L, Mannavola D, et al. Pituitary tumours: TSH-secreting adenomas. Best Pract Res Clin Endocrinol Metab. 2009;23:597–606.
43. Beck-Peccoz P, Brucker-Davis F, Persani L, et al. Thyrotropin-secreting pituitary tumors. Endocr Rev. 1996;17:610–38.
44. Refetoff S, Weiss RE, Usala SJ. The syndromes of resistance to thyroid hormone. Endocr Rev. 1993;14:348–99.
45. Refetoff S, Dumitrescu AM. Syndromes of reduced sensitivity to thyroid hormone: genetic defects in hormone receptors, cell transporters and deiodination. Best Pract Res Clin Endocrinol Metab. 2007;21:277–305.
46. Thomas JS, Leclere J, Hartemann P, et al. Familial hyperthyroidism without evidence of autoimmunity. Acta Endocrinol (Copenh). 1982;100:512–8.
47. Gozu HI, Lublinghoff J, Bircan R, et al. Genetics and phenomics of inherited and sporadic non-autoimmune hyperthyroidism. Mol Cell Endocrinol. 2010;322:125–34.
48. Knudson PB. Hyperthyroidism in adults: variable clinical presentations and approaches to diagnosis. J Am Board Fam Pract. 1995;8:109–13.
49. Heeringa J, Hoogendoorn EH, van der Deure WM, et al. High-normal thyroid function and risk of atrial fibrillation: the Rotterdam study. Arch Intern Med. 2008;168:2219–24.
50. Ross DS. Syndromes of thyrotoxicosis with low radioactive iodine uptake. Endocrinol Metab Clin North Am. 1998;27:169–85.
51. Seckl MJ, Sebire NJ, Berkowitz RS. Gestational trophoblastic disease. Lancet. 2010;376:717–29.
52. Paladini D, Vassallo M, Sglavo G, et al. Struma ovarii associated with hyperthyroidism, elevated CA 125 and pseudo-Meigs syndrome may mimic advanced ovarian cancer. Ultrasound Obstet Gynecol. 2008;32:237–8.
53. Wong LY, Diamond TH. Severe ophthalmopathy developing after treatment of coexisting malignant struma ovarii and Graves' disease. Thyroid. 2009;19:1125–7.
54. Griffin MA, Solomon DH. Hyperthyroidism in the elderly. J Am Geriatr Soc. 1986;34:887–92.
55. Singer PA, Cooper DS, Levy EG, et al. Treatment guidelines for patients with hyperthyroidism and hypothyroidism. JAMA. 1995;273:808–12.
56. Mokshagundum SP, Barzel US. Thyroid disease in the elderly. J Am Geriatr Soc. 1993;41:1361–9.
57. Isley WL. Thyroid dysfunction in the severely ill and elderly: forget the classic signs and symptoms. Postgrad Med. 1993;94:111–8. 127–8, 139–140.
58. Henschke PJ. When to suspect thyroid disease in the elderly. Geriatrics. 1982;37:125–9.
59. Somerville W, Levine SA. Angina pectoris and thyrotoxicosis. Br Heart J. 1950;12:245.
60. Federman DD. Hyperthyroidism in geriatric population. Hosp Pract. 1991;26:61–76.
61. Baloch Z, Carayon P, Conte-Devolx B, et al. Laboratory medicine practice guidelines. Laboratory support for the diagnosis and monitoring of thyroid disease. Thyroid. 2003;13:3–126.
62. Baskin HJ, Cobin RH, Duick DS, Gharib H, Guttler RB, Kaplan MM, Segal RL, American Association of Clinical Endocrinologists. American Association of Clinical Endocrinologists medical guidelines for clinical practice for the evaluation and treatment of hyperthyroidism and hypothyroidism. Endocr Pract. 2002;8:457–69.
63. Harper MB, Mayeaux Jr EJ. Thyroid disease. In: Taylor RB, editor. Family medicine: principles and practice. 6th ed. New York: Springer; 2003. p. 1042–52.
64. Hollowell JG, Staehling NW, Flanders WD, et al. Serum TSH, T(4), and thyroid antibodies in the United States population (1988 to 1994): National Health and Nutrition Examination Survey (NHANES III). J Clin Endocrinol Metab. 2002;87:489–99.
65. Chung JO, Cho DH, Chung DJ, et al. Ultrasonographic features of papillary thyroid carcinoma in patients with Graves' disease. Korean J Intern Med. 2010;25:71–6.
66. Cappelli C, Pirola I, De Martino E, et al. The role of imaging in Graves' disease: a cost-effectiveness analysis. Eur J Radiol. 2008;65:99–103.
67. Markovic V, Eterovic D. Thyroid echogenicity predicts outcome of radioiodine therapy in patients with graves' disease. J Clin Endocrinol Metab. 2007;92:3547–52.
68. Ralls PW, Mayekawa DS, Lee KP, et al. Color-flow Doppler sonography in Graves disease: "thyroid inferno". AJR Am J Roentgenol. 1988;150:781–4.
69. Cibas ES, Ali SZ. The Bethesda system for reporting thyroid cytopathology. Am J Clin Pathol. 2009;132:658–65.
70. Riis AL, Jørgensen JO, Gjedde S, et al. Whole body and forearm substrate metabolism in hyperthyroidism: evidence of increased basal muscle protein breakdown. Am J Physiol Endocrinol Metab. 2005;288:E1067–73.
71. Torring O, Tallstedt L, Wallin G, et al. Graves' hyperthyroidism: treatment with antithyroid drugs, surgery, or radioiodine—a prospective, randomized study. J Clin Endocrinol Metab. 1996;81:2986–93.
72. Jansson S, Lie-Karlsen K, Stenqvist O, et al. Oxygen consumption in patients with hyperthyroidism before and after treatment with beta-blockade versus thyrostatic treatment: a prospective randomized study. Ann Surg. 2001;233:60–4.
73. Ginsberg J. Diagnosis and management of Graves' disease. CMAJ. 2003;168:575–85.
74. Nedrebo BG, Holm PA, Uhlving S, Sorheim JI, Skeie S, Eide GE, et al. Predictors of outcome and comparison of different drug regimens for the prevention of relapse in patients with Graves' disease. Eur J Endocrinol. 2002;147:583–9.

75. Porterfield Jr JR, Thompson GB, Farley DR, Grant CS, Richards ML. Evidence-based management of toxic multinodular goiter (Plummer's disease). World J Surg. 2008;32:1278–84.
76. Cooper DS. Antithyroid drugs. N Engl J Med. 2005;352:905–17.
77. Bahn Chair RS, Burch HB, Cooper DS, et al. Hyperthyroidism and other causes of thyrotoxicosis: management guidelines of the American Thyroid Association and American Association of Clinical Endocrinologists. Thyroid. 2011;21:593–646.
78. De Groot L, Abalovich M, Alexander EK, Amino N, Barbour L, Cobin RH, et al. Management of thyroid dysfunction during pregnancy and postpartum: an Endocrine Society clinical practice guideline. J Clin Endocrinol Metab. 2012;97:2543–65.
79. Tajiri J, Noguchi S, Murakami T, Murakami N. Antithyroid drug-induced agranulocytosis. The usefulness of routine white blood cell count monitoring. Arch Intern Med. 1990;150:621–4.
80. The Food and Drug Administration and American Thyroid Association. Propylthiouracil-related liver toxicity: public workshop. April 19, 2009; Washington, D.C.
81. Stalberg P, Svensson A, Hessman O, et al. Surgical treatment of Graves' disease: evidence-based approach. World J Surg. 2008;32:1269–77.
82. Wartofsky L, Glinoer D, Solomon B, et al. Differences and similarities in the diagnosis and treatment of Graves' disease in Europe, Japan, and the United States. Thyroid. 1991;1:129–35.
83. Erickson D, Gharib H, Li H, van Heerden JA. Treatment of patients with toxic multinodular goiter. Thyroid. 1998;8:277–82.
84. Kang AS, Grant CS, Thompson GB, et al. Current treatment of nodular goiter with hyperthyroidism (Plummer's disease): surgery versus radioiodine. Surgery. 2002;132:916–23.
85. Nygaard B, Hegedüs L, Ulriksen P, et al. Radioiodine therapy for multinodular toxic goiter. Arch Intern Med. 1999;159:1364–8.
86. Read Jr CH, Tansey MJ, Menda Y. A 36 year retrospective analysis of the efficacy and safety of radioactive iodine in treating young Graves' patients. J Clin Endocrinol Metab. 2004;89:4229–33.
87. Shore RE. Issues and epidemiological evidence regarding radiation-induced thyroid cancer. Radiat Res. 1992;131:98–111.
88. Rivkees SA. The use of radioactive iodine in the management of hyperthyroidism in children. In: Current drug targets. Immune, endocrine and metabolic disorders, vol. 1. Boca Raton: Bentham Science Publishers; 2001. p. 255–64.
89. Bartalena L, Marcocci C, Bogazzi F, Manetti L, Tanda ML, Dell'Unto E, et al. Relation between therapy for hyperthyroidism and the course of Graves' ophthalmopathy. N Engl J Med. 1998;338:73–8.
90. Braga M, Walpert N, Burch HB, Solomon BL, Cooper DS. The effect of methimazole on cure rates after radioiodine treatment for Graves' hyperthyroidism: a randomized clinical trial. Thyroid. 2002;12:135–9.
91. Andrade VA, Gross JL, Maia AL. The effect of methimazole pretreatment on the efficacy of radioactive iodine therapy in Graves' hyperthyroidism: one-year follow-up of a prospective, randomized study. J Clin Endocrinol Metab. 2001;86:3488–93.
92. Burch HB, Solomon BL, Cooper DS, Ferguson P, Walpert N, Howard R. The effect of antithyroid drug pretreatment on acute changes in thyroid hormone levels after (131) I ablation for Graves' disease. J Clin Endocrinol Metab. 2001;86:3016–21.
93. Meier DA, Brill DR, Becker DV, Clarke SE, Silberstein EB, Royal HD, et al. Society of Nuclear Medicine procedure guideline for therapy of thyroid disease with iodine-131 (sodium iodide). Accessed online 21 July 2005, at: http://interactive.snm.org/docs/pg_ch26_0403.pdf.
94. Sisson JC, Freitas J, McDougall IR, Dauer LT, Hurley JR, Brierley JD, et al. Radiation safety in the treatment of patients with thyroid diseases by radioiodine ^{131}i: practice recommendations of the American Thyroid Association. Thyroid. 2011;21(4):335–46.
95. Fontanilla JC, Schneider AB, Sarne DH. The use of oral radiographic contrast agents in the management of hyperthyroidism. Thyroid. 2001;11:561–7.
96. Shindo M. Surgery for hyperthyroidism. ORL J Otorhinolaryngol Relat Spec. 2008;70:298–304.
97. Worni M, Schudel HH, Seifert E, et al. Randomized controlled trial on single dose steroid before thyroidectomy for benign disease to improve postoperative nausea, pain, and vocal function. Ann Surg. 2008;248:1060–6.
98. Farrar WB. Complications of thyroidectomy. Surg Clin North Am. 1983;63:1353–61.
99. Schoretsanitis G, Melissas J, Sanidas E. Does draining the neck affect morbidity following thyroid surgery? Am Surg. 1998;64:778–80.
100. Johnson JT, Wagner RL. Infection following uncontaminated head and neck surgery. Arch Otolaryngol Head Neck Surg. 1987;113:368–9.
101. Gavilan J, Gavilan C. Recurrent laryngeal nerve. Identification during thyroid and parathyroid surgery. Arch Otolaryngol Head Neck Surg. 1986;112:1286–8.
102. Chandrasekhar S, Randolph G, Seidman M, et al. Clinical practice guideline: improving voice outcomes after thyroid surgery. Otolaryngol Head Neck Surg. 2013;148(6 Suppl):S1–37.
103. Wong C, Price S, Scott-Coombes D. Hypocalcaemia and parathyroid hormone assay following total thyroidectomy: predicting the future. World J Surg. 2006;30:825–32.
104. Netterville JL, Aly A, Ossoff RH. Evaluation and treatment of complications of thyroid and parathyroid surgery. Otolaryngol Clin North Am. 1990;23:529–52.
105. Ezon I, Zilbert N, Pinkney L, et al. A large struma ovarii tumor removed via laparoscopy in a 16-year-old adolescent. J Pediatr Surg. 2007;42: E19–22.

106. Wolff EF, Hughes M, Merino MJ, et al. Expression of benign and malignant thyroid tissue in ovarian teratomas and the importance of multimodal management as illustrated by a BRAF-positive follicular variant of papillary thyroid cancer. Thyroid. 2010;20:981–7.
107. Nielsen CH, El Fassi D, Hasselbalch HC, et al. B-cell depletion with rituximab in the treatment of autoimmune diseases. Graves' ophthalmopathy: the latest addition to an expanding family. Expert Opin Biol Ther. 2007;7:1061–78.
108. Yamamoto M, Sasaki A, Asahi H, Shimada Y, Sato N, Nakajima J, et al. Endoscopic subtotal thyroidectomy for patients with Graves' disease. Surg Today. 2001;31:1–4.
109. Xiao H, Zhuang W, Wang S, Yu B, Chen G, Zhou M, et al. Arterial embolization: a novel approach to thyroid ablative therapy for Graves' disease. J Clin Endocrinol Metab. 2002;87:3583–9.
110. Ozdemir S, Buyukbese M, Kadioglu P, Soyasal T, Senturk H, Akin P. Plasmapheresis: an effective therapy for refractory hyperthyroidism in the elderly. Indian J Med Sci. 2002;56:65–8.
111. Tarantino L, Giorgio A, Mariniello N, de Stefano G, Perrotta A, Aloisio V, et al. Percutaneous ethanol injection of large autonomous hyperfunctioning thyroid nodules. Radiology. 2000;214:143–8.
112. Shimizu K, Kumita S, Kitamura Y, Nagahama M, Kitagawa W, Akasu H, et al. Trial of autotransplantation of cryopreserved thyroid tissue for postoperative hypothyroidism in patients with Graves' disease. J Am Coll Surg. 2002;194:14–22.
113. Benvenga S, Ruggeri RM, Russo A, et al. Usefulness of L-carnitine, a naturally occurring peripheral antagonist of thyroid hormone action, in iatrogenic hyperthyroidism: a randomized, double-blind, placebo-controlled clinical trial. J Clin Endocrinol Metab. 2001;86:3579–94.

Autoimmune Thyroid Disease (Flajani-Parry-Graves-von Basedow Disease): An Overview of Treatment

9

Hernando Vargas-Uricoechea, Anilza Bonelo-Perdomo, Carlos Hernán Sierra-Torres, and Ivonne Meza-Cabrera

Abstract

The ideal treatment for Graves-Basedow disease should restore normal thyroid function, avoid recurrence of hyperthyroidism, prevent development of hypothyroidism and prevent the occurrence or progression of ophthalmopathy. There are basically three approaches for the treatment of GD: anti-thyroid medical treatment, I-131 therapy and surgery. Antithyroid drugs act principally by interfering with the organification of iodine, thereby suppressing thyroid hormone levels. I-131 is transported into thyroid follicular cells resulting in cell necrosis over weeks to months. Sometimes Antithyroid drugs are used before the administration of radioactive iodine to promptly achieve euthyroidism and to attenuate exacerbation of thyrotoxicosis. Surgery (thyroidectomy) results in rapid control of thyrotoxicosis and has minimal risk of recurrence when a total thyroidectomy is performed. Antithyroid drugs should be initiated before surgery to reduce the risk of thyroid storm. With experienced surgeons, the risk of permanent complications is very low. Surgery is clearly indicated in certain patients: Patients who have not responded to prolonged antithyroid drug therapy, or who develop toxic reactions to the drug and for whatever reason are unsuitable for 131-I therapy; patients with huge glands, which frequently do not regress adequately after 131-I therapy; patients who prefer surgery, and patients with thyroid nodules that raise a suspicion of carcinoma.

H. Vargas-Uricoechea, MD, MSc, Ph.Dc (✉)
Division of Endocrinology and Metabolism, Internal Medicine Department, University of Cauca, Popayán-Cauca, Colombia
e-mail: hernandovargasu10@yahoo.com

A. Bonelo-Perdomo, BSc, MSc, Ph.D
Division of Basic Immunology and Biomedical Sciences, University of Valle, Cali-Valle, Colombia

C.H. Sierra-Torres, Ph.D
Division of Genetic and Molecular Epidemiology, University of Cauca, Popayán-Cauca, Colombia

I. Meza-Cabrera, MD
Laboratory of Pathology, Hospital Universitario San José, Popayán-Cauca, Colombia

S.K. Imam, S.I. Ahmad (eds.), *Thyroid Disorders: Basic Science and Clinical Practice*,
DOI 10.1007/978-3-319-25871-3_9

Introduction

There are basically three approaches for the treatment of GD: anti-thyroid medical treatment, I-131 therapy and surgery (total or subtotal thyroidectomy). The factors that govern treatment selection are age, patient's preference, the severity of the disease; the size of the gland, traditional practice and local resources available.

Anti-thyroid Medications

Anti-thyroid medications are simple molecules called Tionamides (Metimazol, Carbimazol and Propylthiouracil). Metimazol (MTZ) is the active Carbimazol (CBZ) metabolite, and given that the conversion from CBZ into MTZ in the body is virtually complete, their effects and dose equivalence are comparable. These molecules contain a Sulfhydryl group and a thiourea trace inside a heterocyclic ring. Both Propylthiouracil –PTU- (6 propyl 2 thiouracil) and MTZ (1 Methyl 2 mercaptoimidazole) are thiourea derivatives and both are trapped inside the thyroid gland against a concentration gradient, representing the drug concentration at the site of action. MTZ is a poor protein binder, whilst PTU binds mostly to albumin up to 75 %. However, MTZ's half-life is 4–6 h, and PTU's half-life is 60 min. Since the half-life of MTZ is longer than PTU, the former is administered once or twice a day, while the latter is administered twice to thrice a day. Generally speaking, no dose adjustments are required under renal or liver failure conditions, though MTZ's clearance is decreased in patients with liver disease [1, 2].

Tionamides inhibit the thyroid hormone synthesis but not the release of the prefabricated thyroid hormones. Tionamides inhibit iodine organification and Tg tyrosine radicals binding. Tionamides also prevent Monoiodotyrosine (MIT) and Diiodotyrosine (DIT) binding to form Triiodothyronine (T3) and Tetraiodothyronine (T4), in addition to interact directly with the Tg molecule and are able to inhibit the TPO activity in vitro but not in vivo. Moreover, the PTU inhibits the T4 and T3 peripheral conversion which leads to a somewhat uncertain action, though its effect are evidenced by an acute drop in T3 and increased reverse T3. This extra-thyroid effect is dose-dependent and is increasingly marked when high doses are used (over 600 mg per day) [2, 3].

Doses and Follow-up Regimes

The usual MTZ dose is 15–30 mg, although does of up to 60 mg/day have historically been used. The PTU dose is 300 mg/day, divided into three doses. The 10:1 MTZ/PTU strength is controversial and even underestimated, since low MTZ doses may perfectly control a significant number of GD patients. Once treatment is initiated, the thyroid function should be evaluated throughout every 4–6 weeks, at least until the euthyroid status is reached or until the patient is stable. The patient may be subsequently controlled with lower doses, i.e., 5–10 mg/day of MTZ and 100–200 mg/day of PTU. After 3–6 months, the control frequency may be every 2–3 months and then every 4–6 months. The TSH levels may be continue to be suppressed, even after the T4 and T3 levels have been normalized; hence, TSH measurements is of little value at the onset of treatment. In patients with increased free T3 levels but with normal or reduced free T4 values, the approach should be to increase the tionamide dose and stop the tendency to reduce the dose administered [3–7]. Tionamides have been evaluated when administered under the "block-replacement regimen" where a high dose of tionamide is administered to block the production of thyroid hormone, in addition to a tyrosine replacement dose; the other regime evaluated is the "titration block regimen" where the tionamide dose is adjusted in accordance with the serum thyroxine concentration. The length of therapy has also been evaluated for both regimens (6 months vs. 12 months) and high (equivalent to 40 mg or more of CBZ) vs. low doses (equivalent to 30 mg of CBZ or less) in the "block-replacement regimen". The results have shown that there is some evidence –though no statistically significant- in favor of the 12–18 months therapy as compared to the 6-months therapy. The use of the "titration block regimen" yields better results than the "block-replacement regimen" and it has not been proven that extended with block-replacement, with a stronger trend to present agranulocytosis and rash. The relapse rate of hyperthyroidism following tionamide management is 50–60 % in general with a stronger occurrence 3–6 months after treatment interruption. The use of high-dose tionamides is associated with a higher incidence of agranulocytosis (12 %). It may then be concluded that based on less adverse events, the first choice for tionamide therapy in GD should be the "titration block regimen" and it should be extended for 12–18 months at a dose of <30 mg/day of CBZ, since this the dose associated with the lowest rate of adverse events and is able to effectively control thyrotoxicity. The idea of using thyroxine following the completion of tionamide therapy to prevent relapses do not seem to be real for the population in general and is not reproducible; hence its use shall not be generalized [5–8].

Adverse Reactions

The most frequently described tionamide adverse reactions are rash and pruritus, which occur in 5 % of the patients; other side effects triggered by this type of drugs are: arthralgia, fever, cervical lymphadenopathy, jaundice with cholestasis pattern, lupus-like syndrome, and hypergammaglobulinemia. The presence of arthralgia should lead to the immediate discontinuation of tionamide therapy since it could be the onset of a condition called "anti-thyroid-induced arthralgia syndrome". Fatal reactions are fortunately rare and include neutropenia and leukopenia, aplastic anemia, hepatitis, vasculitis, inter alia. Tionamide-associated liver disease and vasculitis are more often associated with the use of PTU, and be expressed with Antineutrophil Cytoplasmic Antibodies (ANCA) Positive [8–11]. The incidence of MTZ and PTU agranulocytosis is 0.36 % in average (though it may be higher in elderly patients) and the mortality secondary to agranulocytosis may be close to 22 %. The presence of fever and odynophagia should lead to the suspicion of agranulocytosis and thus be considered a red flag. Agranulocytosis induced by these agents may be mediated either by direct toxicity or by immune reaction due to IgE-mediated hypersensitivity. The theory of an allergic background has been previously described, so in patients with a history of tionamide reactions, the potential for severe reactions with further exposures has not been fully confirmed. Agranulocytosis may present at the onset of treatment or after months of tionamide exposure (even after years of using the medication) but to this date there is no real way to predict it, even with serial measurements of neutrophil count and in short periods of time. While it is thought that adverse events are MTZ-dose related, such relationship has not been established for PTU. The recommendation of frequently measuring leukocyte count while undergoing tionamide treatment is still controversial. However, in the presence of alarm signals such as fever and odynophagia, such recommendation is practically uncontested. The granulocyte count in patients that developed tionamide-induced agranulocytosis usually recovers in a few days, though sometimes may need several weeks. Anemia and thrombocytopenia may also be present. The factors leading to a poorer prognosis are: age >65 years, sepsis, and neutrophil count <100/mL. The treatment of these patients with GM-CSF (Granulocyte and Macrophage Colony Stimulating Factor) in asymptomatic agranulocytosis improves the rate of infectious complications and mortality, with a faster recovery of the neutrophil count. However, this response has not been reproduced in agranulocytosis and symptomatic patients. However, most experts recommend the use of G-CSF in tionamide-induced agranulocytosis. The use of antibiotics against germs such as *Pseudomonas aeruginosa* is usually required, in addition to the adoption of universal measures for managing febrile neutropenia [11–14].

Radioactive Iodine Treatment

Radioactive iodine therapy is a relatively safe and effective procedure but may be associated with some degree of exacerbation of ophthalmopathy and autoimmunity in GD patients. This treatment method may be used as the first choice for GD management or as second choice following failed tionamide therapy, or when hyperthyroidism persists following thyroidectomy (when tionamide has been chosen for management). Radioactive iodine is available as sodium iodide labeled as I-131 ($Na^{131}I$) in capsules and oral solution. Radioactive iodine is the result of uranium decay. The efficacy of this treatment modality for hyperthyroidism is due to radiation-induced cell damage, resulting from the high-energy beta emission. The amount of beta emission is directly proportional to the radiation dose received by the thyroid with the key effect of radiation being the disruption of the follicular cells reproductive capacity [15–17]. A lot has been written about the best mode of I-131 administration; the regimes widely accepted in the literature basically describe two ways of administration: the first takes into account the estimated gland weight (in grams) and the radioactive iodine uptake in 24 h (estimated dose regimen). The doses described in this regimen ranges from 100 to 200 μCi per gram. The other regimen establishes fixed I-131 doses based on the gland size determined by palpation (5, 10, or 15 mCi; equivalent to 185, 370 or 555 MBq, respectively). There is no general agreement about the dose that should be administered to treat GD hyperthyroidism, since the various trials have not shown any superiority of one regimen over another. According to some experts, the calculated dose regimen may also be used to help in establishing the cause of thyroiditis-related hyperthyroidism based on radioactive iodine uptake (i.e., when thyroiditis related hyperthyroidism is also suspected). In contrast, those who prefer the fixed-dose regimen argue that this method is simpler and less expensive than the estimated-dose regimen [16–18]. In general, the doses used in the fixed-dose regimen range from 350 to 600 MBq. [MBq: MegaBecquerels is the International System (IS) unit to express radioactivity; mCi: is the other measurement unit for radioactivity, where 1 mCi = 37 MBq].

Several formulae have been described to estimate the I-131 dose to be administered; for instance, one of them excludes the thyroid gland size from the calculation:

$$\left(296\text{ MBq }[8\text{ mCi}]\times 100\right) / \left(\text{Percentage of uptake in 24 h}\right)$$

Another more widely used formula to estimate the dose to be administered is based on the size of the thyroid and uptake:

$$\left(Z\times\text{thyroid size }[\text{in grams}]\times 100\right) / \left(\text{Uptake percentage at 24 h}\right)$$

In this formula, Z is the desired number of Becquerels administered per gram. The Z range varies from 3.7 to 7.4 MBq (100–200 mCi). Both formulae have a high success rate (defined as euthyroidism or hypothyroidism) after 1 year of treatment. It is difficult to determine accurately the minimum dose required to achieve a permanent euthyroidism condition. Trying to approach the regimes aimed at normalizing the patient's thyroid function may be bothersome and discouraging. Thus, the purpose of I-131 treatment is to generate a chronic hypothyroidism status using relatively high doses of I-131 (550–600 MBq: 15–16 mCi) for small to medium size glands and doses of 800–900 MBq (20–25 mCi) for large glands. Those in favor of this management regime consider that a large enough fixed dose to achieve hypothyroidism reduces the risk of hyperthyroidism relapse and hence the patient is not exposed to further I-131 doses. Moreover, hypothyroidism achieved with this modality is no different from hypothyroidism resulting from a different etiology. In patients that fail tionamide treatment, the burden of radiation from I-131 drops by about 30–50 %. In any case, you should always abide to the principle of "As Low As Reasonably Achievable" (ALARA). Notwithstanding this fact, any dose administered under a particular regime may result in a number of patients receiving I-131 mounts exceeding the minimal dose required to achieve permanent euthyroidism [16–19]. The effective half-life of radioactive iodine is defined as the period of time during which the activity of the isotope administered to the patient is cut to one half and it is considered to be around 6 to maximum 8 days. Approximately 10–15 % of patients experience a very short effective half-life, indicating fast iodine turnover in the thyroid. One way to extend the effective half-life in addition to the presence of iodine inside the gland is by increasing the biological half-life (since the physical half-life is constant). This can be achieved using hormone-release inhibitors from the thyroid that may suppress the colloid formation and Tg proteolysis using lithium Carbonate that in the long run blocks the T3 and T4 synthesis [18–20]. The ability of lithium carbonate to suppress iodine release is used in patients with a short effective radioactive iodine half-life, thus delaying its release from the thyroid, and potentiating its therapeutic effect. The use of lithium Carbonate in GD patients must be preceded by the administration of radioactive iodine 3–4 days before, at an average dose of 500–700 mg/day (10 mg/kg), leading to a blood concentration of 0.4–0.8 nmol/L. The therapy shall be maintained for 7 days following radioactive iodine treatment. This management protocol administered for the recommended number of days is unlikely to trigger any lithium-related adverse events. The use of beta blockers prior to the administration of radioactive iodine may reduce and relief the adrenergic symptoms. The use of tionamides prior to I-131 may result in a milder hyperthyroidism in the patient, and even achieve euthyroidism by the time the radioactive iodine procedure is performed. Nonetheless, when the patient is managed with tionamides the dose of I-131 should be increased to reduce the risk of treatment failure (it seems that the risk of failing increases with the use of PTU versus MTZ). Pretreatment with Tionamides prior to the administration of I-131 is reserved for elderly patients with underlying cardiovascular conditions or tachyarrhythmia and for patients with severe hyperthyroidism [20, 21]. In general, the use of tionamides prior to the administration of I-131 should be stopped 2–3 days prior to therapy and it can be reintroduced 3 days after the completion of treatment (and maintained for 4–6 weeks thereafter).

I-131 Adverse Effects and Risk of Malignancy

The use of radioactive iodine may result in radiation-related thyroiditis in up to 1 % of the patients and may lead to worsening of the symptoms of hyperthyroidism. Such symptoms may be mild and not require specific management of pain symptoms and other adrenergic-associated symptoms but often occur in cases that require using Non-Steroid Anti-Inflammatory Agents (AINEs), beta blockers, and glucocorticoids to relief the symptoms. Occasionally patients present with dysgeusia and xerostomia that may accompany the presence of pain and swelling of the submaxillary, sublingual, and parotid glands. The discomfort usually improves with adequate hydration and standard sialagogues (citric substances, chewing gum). Several trials have assessed the likelihood of developing cancer in patients that received radioactive iodine therapy for hyperthyroidism; some have not found an increased overall risk of cancer mortality, while others have described a reduced global cancer mortality rate, and still others report a small increase in the risk of thyroid cancer, particularly in patients with toxic nodular goiter. Further trials report a drop in the global risk of cancer, but with a mild increase in the risk of thyroid and colon cancer. Other groups report an increased risk of kidney, breast, and stomach cancer. The reported risk of death from cardiovascular disease following the use of radioactive iodine seems to be the result of the thyrotoxic status per se, rather than of the treatment itself [19–22]. Finally, the absolute contraindications to the use of radioactive iodine are pregnancy and breastfeeding; the relative contraindications are the presence of thyroid nodes with some risk of malignancy or malignant, and patients under 15 years of age.

Surgical Treatment for GD

Although the surgical management for GD results in fast symptom control, with low morbidity (in expert hands), it is an indication seldom indicated as initial treatment. In fact, the most frequent indications in clinical practice are those where other therapeutic options are contraindicated and in patients with giant goiter. Various surgical procedures have been document for the control of GD but two techniques have prevailed: Total Thyroidectomy (TT) and Subtotal Thyroidectomy (ST). While it has been considered that TT is the treatment of choice for patients with associated thyroid cancer, the optimal surgical approach for GD individuals without associated thyroid cancer is still subject to debate. The use of TST results –at least theoretically- in a lower risk of the recurrent laryngeal nerve injury and hypoparathyroidism in addition to an implicit higher probability of further preserving a euthyroid state as compared to TT. However, it also gives rise to a risk of persistence of the disease since the thyroid remnant may be enough to maintain the hyperthyroid status after surgery. Based on these considerations and depending on the series studied, TST is still recommended over TT. It has been thought that TT results in a predictable risk of hypothyroidism practically in every patient but it is easily managed and controlled with thyroid hormone supplementation; the risk is however variable according to the analysis of the results obtained with TST (TT has a risk of relapse or persistence of hyperthyroidism of 0 % and TST of 8 % at 5 years). Generally speaking, the surgical intervention is considered a safe and effective therapeutic option in GD patients, with low morbidity and mortality rates (particularly in the hands of experienced surgeons who perform at least 100 GD surgeries per year) and with a predictable risk of hypothyroidism virtually in every patient (particularly with TT) with a very low rate of relapses. However, the evidence is based on studies with a small number of patients, using non-standardized or inconsistent measurement techniques. Apparently the best option to surgically approach GD is through an interdisciplinary approach that identifies the risk and benefits of a particular indication and when surgery is considered the best choice, TT should be favored against TST [23, 24]. Some factors that may contraindicate surgery one-way or other for GD are: end-stage cancer, advanced cardiovascular disease, and severe lung disease. Some of the factors that influence the decision of surgery as the first line treatment in GD are: Contraindication for the use of radioactive iodine and/or tionamides, rapid symptom control, and in some pregnant women (in particular at the end of the second trimester). He most frequent complications arising for surgery in GD –in highly experienced, high-flow centers- are hypocalcemia (<2 %), recurrent laryngeal nerve injury (<1 %); both complications may be temporary or permanent; post-surgical bleeding requiring intervention (<1 %), procedure-related mortality (1 in 10.000 to 5 in 1.000.000) and all the complications inherent to general anesthesia [24, 25]. The recommendation is to take the GD patient to surgery as close to the euthyroid status as possible; hence the use of tionamides, in particular of MTZ and the additional use of potassium iodine (Lugol's solution has 8 mg of iodide per drop and the recommendation is to use 1–2 drops/0.05–0.1 mL three times per day, mixed in water for 10 days prior to the thyroidectomy procedure). Saturated Potassium Iodide solution (containing 50 mg of iodide per drop and beta blockers are key for the patient's preoperative control. In case of an emergency or a history of adverse reactions to anti-thyroid agents, the use of potassium iodide and beta-blockers are the cornerstone of treatment. The use of potassium iodide and of the saturated potassium iodide solution reduces the risk of bleeding during surgery; occasionally the use of steroids may assist in the emergency preoperative prep in patients with Graves' disease. Metimazol should be interrupted at the time of surgery and the use of beta-blockers may be downscaled in the next days, based on the adrenergic status of the patient [23–26]. Calcium and intact PTH (PTHi) measurements should be performed 6–12 h after surgery with a PTHi level <10–15 pg/mL in the immediate postop predictive of the risk of symptomatic hypocalcemia and the need for calcium and vitamin D supplementation. A calcium level >7.8 mg/dL (1.95 mmol/L) in asymptomatic patients for hypocalcemia should be considered as the lower limit to decide patient discharge fol-

Table 9.1 Surgical indications for GD patents

Indication
Giant goiter (>80 g) or compressive symptoms
Suspected or documented thyroid malignancy
Low uptake of nodules on scan imaging
Co-existing hyperparathyroidism
Short term pregnancy planning (i.e., less than 6 months)
Moderate-severe Ophthalmopathy
Rapid symptom and hyperthyroid status control
Thionamide adverse effects or relapse following thionamide use
Radioactive iodine contraindication
Express desire stated b the patient

lowing thyroidectomy. Postoperative intravenous calcium and magnesium should be managed according to the standard management protocols [27–29]. In euthyroid patients at the time of surgery, the use of levothyroxine may be started 24–48 h after surgery. Patients undergoing emergency thyroidectomy shall wait a few days to start replacement therapy, with a dose of 1.7 μg/kg/day as the reference value to begin levothyroxine treatment. TSH should be measured 6–8 weeks after surgery to adjust treatment. Table 9.1 shows some of the indications for thyroidectomy in patients with GD.

Special Conditions

Pregnancy

Hyperthyroidism results in 0.1–0.4 % pregnancy complications and 85 % of the cases are the cause of these complications is GD. The treatment of GD during pregnancy is complex due to pregnancy effect on the course of the autoimmune disease. As a general rule, subclinical hyperthyroidism is not associated with major complications, whilst florid hyperthyroidism is associated with preeclampsia, premature labor, congestive heart failure and increased rate of abortions. Uncontrolled hyperthyroidism is also associated with low birth weight and congenital malformations. The clinical diagnosis of hyperthyroidism may be difficult to pursue during pregnancy since the pregnant patient exhibits common signs and symptoms for hypothyroidism such as tachycardia, widened pulse pressure, dry skin, heat and heat intolerance. At the initial stages of pregnancy, physiological changes develop that may mimic biochemical hyperthyroidism that does not require specific management. The diagnosis of hyperthyroidism in pregnancy is done with a suppressed TSH value, with a total T4 and T3 value within a 1.5 fold adjusted reference range as compared to the non-pregnant women; or based on T3L and T4L values above the specific range of reference for each trimester. Thyroid function test ranges are different throughout pregnancy and for certain types of lab tests there may be hormonal titration variations so the recommendation is to measure the anti-TSHR titers at the time pregnancy is documented. When the titers are elevated, the tests should be repeated at week 22–26 of gestation in order to guide the fetal monitoring decisions. Human Chorionic Gonadotropin (hCG)-associated hyperthyroidism, either resulting from a molar pregnancy or because of a choriocarcinoma, may manifest as a hyperadrenergic condition with thyroid hyperactivity very similar to GD but with no ophthalmopathy or dermopathy present and with negative anti-TSHR values (whilst in GD these are usually elevated). Furthermore, serum hCG levels exceed the usual ranges present during gestation. Nevertheless, normal pregnancy may also give rise to transient hCG elevations, with TSH suppression. Overall, the two main causes of biochemical hyperthyroidism are considered to be gestational hyperthyroidism and GD. The former is hCG-mediated and indicates mild biochemical hyperthyroidism in an asymptomatic woman, usually expressed during the first trimester of pregnancy. Elevated hCG levels during the first trimester causes those changes and usually does not result in lethality. Such changes are the result of the thyrotropic hCG action through the alpha subunit late in the first trimester or early in the second trimester. A few pregnant patients with gestational hyperthyroidism develop hyperemesis with marked thyroid function changes and clinical hyperthyroidism with variable degrees of severity [29, 30]. In view of the diagnostic safety of GD during pregnancy, the need for pharmacological treatment must be established. Anti-thyroid medications are the treatment of choice, and usually PTU is preferred over MTZ (due to the higher risk of congenital malformations described with MTZ –in particular aplasia cutis congenital, choanal, and esophageal atresia- and presumably PTU crosses the placenta less readily, though this assumption has been proven wrong because both PTU and MTZ cross the placenta). Historically, the use of MTZ has been recommended after the second trimester of pregnancy and PTU could be administered throughout pregnancy, but this recommendation is questionable on the basis of the potential liver involvement (toxicity). This has led to a reevaluation of such indication so that currently the recommendation is to prescribe PTU in patients during the first trimester of pregnancy or patients who are intolerant or allergic to MTZ. Pregnant women with pre-gestational GD that have been treated with anti-thyroid medications and are euthyroid before pregnancy, exhibit a low risk of activating the hyperthyroidism during pregnancy, though the risk of relapses and post-partum thyroiditis is high. MTZ and PTU are also excreted in breast milk but in small amounts that apparently do not impact the newborn thyroid function or intellectual development. However, MTZ is preferred over PTU during breastfeeding because of the PTU-associated liver toxicity. Therefore, women receiving MTZ shall be switched over to PTU as soon as pregnancy is documented –during the first trimester- and then switchback to MTZ early in the second trimester. Likewise, if the patient received PTU prior to becoming pregnant, the recommendation is to continue the medication until the beginning of the second trimester and then switchover to MTZ. When changing from one tionamide to another, the doses should be adjusted based on the differential strength between MTZ versus PTU (refer to the information above). When PTU is maintained throughout pregnancy, liver enzymes should be monitored on a monthly basis. The goal of anti-thyroid treatment is to maintain total T3 and T4 levels barely above the upper normal range of the non-pregnant patient and free T3 and T4 levels within or slightly above the upper normal level of a non-pregnant woman. TSH values should be suppressed and thyroid function tests (TSH, free and total T3 & T4) should be measured on a monthly basis throughout pregnancy in order to meet the target with the lowest possible dose of the anti-thyroid agent of choice [31, 32]. Patients with uncontrolled hyperthyroidism, despite the use of anti-thyroid medication, or in the presence of allergies or severe reactions, should be considered for surgical management. When thyroidectomy is required, it should be performed during the second trimester of pregnancy because of the teratogenicity of anesthetics during the first trimester of pregnancy and because of the risk of premature delivery in the third trimester. Pre-surgical preparation for thyroidectomy includes a short course of potassium iodide (10 days), together with anti-thyroid agents and beta-blockers.

The administration of radioactive iodine for diagnostic or therapeutic purposes is contraindicated in pregnancy. Following week 12 of gestation, once the fetal thyroid gland develops the ability to concentrate iodine, congenital hypothyroidism may develop and has been document when inadvertently pregnant women have been exposed in the first trimester, with a 1.1 % rate of spontaneous abortion; 1.1 % of intrauterine death; 3.3 % of neonatal hypothyroidism and 2.2 % of mental retardation. This shows that hypothyroidism due to radioactive iodine exposure after week 12 of pregnancy is considerably higher than the standard incidence of congenital hypothyroidism. Towards weeks 10–12 of gestation, the increase in the Sodium/Iodine Symporter gene (NIS) the fetal thyroid is able to concentrate iodine, accumulate colloid, and produce thyroglobulin; around week 20 of gestation the TSHR responds to the TSH stimulus (as well as to the thyroid stimulating antibodies). The placenta per se is not permeable to TSH, but it is to iodine; active iodine transport through the placenta is the result of the NIS gene expression in trophoblasts. During the second trimester of pregnancy, when the fetal thyroid produces T4, the maternal intake of iodine is critical as a background for thyroid hormone synthesis. While the placental crossing of maternal antibodies to

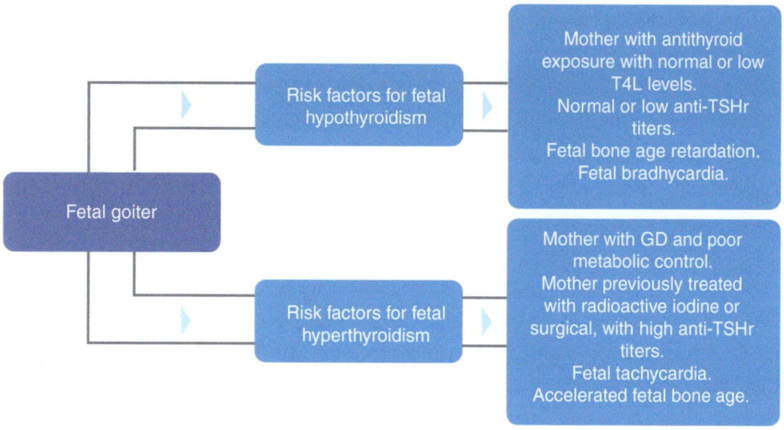

Fig. 9.1 Difference between fetal hypothyroidism and hyperthyroidism in the presence of fetal goiter

the fetus occurs very early in gestation, the fetal concentration of those antibodies is in fact low until late in the second trimester. However, placental permeability to antibodies increases substantially during the third trimester and thus the fetal levels are practically identical to the maternal levels. Such changes in maternal permeability and the ability of the fetal thyroid gland to respond to both TSH and anti-TSHR are the reason why fetal hyperthyroidism is expressed after the second half of pregnancy [33, 34]. Serial obstetric ultrasound imaging to measure the size of the thyroid is recommended, in addition to identifying the gestational age, the fetal viability, the amniotic fluid volume, the fetal anatomy, and the identification of any malformations. Fetal tachycardia (over 170 beats/min persistent for more than 10 min), growth retardation, fetal goiter (which is an early sign of fetal dysfunction, but on its own does not differentiate hyper from hypothyroidism – See Fig. 9.1), accelerated bone maturation, signs of heart failure and hydrops fetalis, are all additional considerations. The diagnosis and management of fetal hyperthyroidism should be done with a multidisciplinary approach including pediatrician, gynecologist, neonatologist, anesthesiologist, and endocrinologist. The medical record, lab tests (with anti-TSHR levels), ultrasound imaging and the clinical condition of the mother shall guide the management of fetal hyperthyroidism [34, 35]. See Chap. on 17 for further details.

Graves' Eye Disease

Many of the clinical signs and symptoms previously described in the eye manifestations of GD may be explained from a "mechanical" perspective, due to the increased volume en el of intra-orbital tissues typical of GD. Though much patients with Graves' disease exhibit an abnormal growth of the extra ocular muscles and of the orbital adipose tissue, with a potential predominant growth of one over the other, the orbital fat tissue is more prevalent among youth, while there is a stronger predisposition to extra orbital muscle growth among the elderly, with no significant changes in the orbital adipose tissue. The expansion of both the muscle and adipose tissue around the orbit leads to increased intraocular pressure, with compression of the orbital tissue contents. Intraocular pressure is relieved with the eyeball protrusion and hence proptosis and exophthalmos should be considered a natural decompression phenomenon of the orbit. The level of decompression is limited by the eyeball mobility per se. The eyeball is "fixed" in place by the rectus muscle and other eyelid structures [36]. The lymphocytic infiltration present in the orbital tissues in GD indicates the prevalence of T CD4+ and CD8+ lymphocytes, with few B cells. The retro bulbar T cells in GD patients recognize the autologous fibroblasts but fail to recognize the extracts of ocular muscles in a way restricted to HLA class I. The HLA-DR expression and the adhesion molecules in the orbital endothelial cells y fibroblasts are enhanced by cytokines such as Interleukins (IL), in particular the IL-1α, Tumor Necrosis Factor (TNF) such as TNF-α and Interferon-γ. This has led to the conclusion that the orbital fibroblast is the target of autoimmune aggression. Since the TSHr is expressed in the messenger RNA (mRNA) and in high titers in connective and adipose tissue proteins of the orbit in GD patients versus healthy individuals, TSHr is considered to be functional, as evidenced by the elevation in AMPc in response to TSH. In fact, the eye pre-adipocytes and fibroblasts differentiation in adipocytes is associated with a marked enhancement of the functional TSHr expression. This concept arises from a subpopulation of eye fibroblasts that may be the target cells in GD –called pre-adipocytes- and when these are stimulated to promote mature adipocyte differentiation, high levels of TSHr are expressed [37, 38]. Generally speaking, GD is considered to be an autoimmune disorder, triggered by autoreactive T lymphocytes that react with one or more antigens shared between the orbit and the thyroid gland. Consequently, these autoreactive lymphocytes reach the orbit, recognize the antigen (or common antigens) presented by the antigen-presenting cells (dendritic cells, macrophages, and B lymphocytes). Upon recognition of the antigen, a cascade of events leads to the secretion of cytokines that stimulate the proliferation of fibroblasts, the differentiation of pre-adipocytes to adipocytes, and the Glucosaminoglycans (GAG) secretion from fibroblasts, resulting in water retention and periocular edema. An increased orbital content mechanically explains most of the clinical manifestations in Graves' Orbitopathy –GO- [39, 40]. During the course of GO, the disease goes through several stages starting with a worsening of the signs and symptoms during the inflammatory phase. The gradual progression of the inflammatory process may lead to permanent abnormalities in function and appearance. The concept of "active" disease indicates the presence of inflammatory characteristics suggesting a potential response to anti-inflammatory therapy. "Inactive" disease defines the phase free of inflammation, though residual fibrosis may be present. Such "inactive" phase may only be changed with surgical treatment. The "activity" of eye disease refers to the presence of inflammation, while the "severity" refers to the extent of functional and cosmetic deficit at every level. It is important to determine the GO phase in order to establish proper treatment, since immune-modulator treatment may be effective in the presence of active inflammation [38–41]. There are several classifications and scores aimed at accurately defining the "activity" and the "severity" of Graves' eye disease and most of them evaluate several aspects. The acronym used is VISA:

V̲ision (the key objective is to rule out the presence of optic neuropathy).
I̲nflammation(including pain, redness, swelling, and visual function involvement).
S̲trabismus: (presence of diplopia).
A̲ppearance/exposure: (the appearance evaluates the presence of eyelid retraction, proptosis, redundant skin, and fat prolapse; the exposure evaluates the presence of opacification and corneal ulcer).

The ocular signs of GD have been described using the NONSPECS classification that described the extension of the eye disease based on the specific presentation of eye signs and symptoms, but it is of little use to monitor the disease process since a particular class does not necessarily progress to the next; in other words, the clinical characteristics considered are not always present (Table 9.2). The natural history of Graves' Orbital pathology is rapid impairment, followed by gradual improvement as time progresses. The active phase is properly described in terms of the Clinical Activity Score (CAS) that

Table 9.2 Classification of eye changes in GD (NONSPECS)

Class	Definition
0	Absence of signs or symptoms
1	Signs only, no symptoms (limited to upper lid retraction, fixed gaze)
2	With signs and symptoms (soft tissue involvement)
3	Proptosis
4	Extraocular muscle disruption
5	Corneal involvement
6	Loss of vision (optic nerve involvement)

adds one point per each clinical characteristic present (described under Table 9.3). The score ranges from 0 to 10 and predicts the response to anti-inflammatory treatment. A seven-point scale bypasses the last three items of the initial score and it is used when previous evaluations are not available. Consequently, GO is considered active with a score of ≥3. Hence, hyperthyroid patients that only present with eyelid retraction or with mild conjunctival erythema and lid edema, are not considered active GO [39–43]. The severity of the disease is better evaluated using objective and quantifiable parameters that are helpful in guiding therapy. The factors to consider when assessing severity are summarized in the European Group on Graves' Orbitopathy (EUGOGO) (See Table 9.4).

Table 9.3 GO evaluation: clinical activity score (CAS) items

Items	Each visit	Comparison against prior visits	Score
Oppressive pain over or behind the eyeball in the last 4 weeks	X		
Pain with eye movements during the last 4 weeks	X		
Eyelid redness	X		
Conjunctival redness	X		
Eyelid inflammation	X		
Chemosis (conjuntival edema)	X		
Caruncle inflammation	X		
Increased proptosis ≥2 mm		X	
Reduced eye movement ≥5° in every direction		X	
Decreased visual acuity ≥1 line on the snellen chart		X	

CAS items, a scale with the first 7 items (excluding the last 3) is used when no previous evaluations are available. The Go is considered active with a CAS ≥3

The diagnostic images for GO are basically ultrasound, Computed Tomography (CT) scan and Magnetic Resonance Imaging (MRI). Ultrasound is a non-invasive method to rule out orbital tumors and to assess the internal echogenicity of extra-ocular muscles and orbital fat. The use of mode-A 2-D ultrasound is advised. A thickening of the ventral aspect of the muscle can be detected, while the scleral attachment is barely modified. It has been hypothesized that internal reflectivity of the waves should be low in patients with active disease because of the muscle edema and high and irregular in inactive eye disease resulting from the presence of muscle fibrosis. The key advantage of mode-A ultrasound is its non-invasiveness and affordability; however, it is not as effective as CT scan. However, CT is more

Table 9.4 Evaluation of GO severity

Grade	Eyelid retraction	Soft Tissues	Proptosis	Diplopia	Corneal exposure	Optic Nerve (status)
Mild	<2 mm	Mild involvement	<3 mm	Absent or transient	Absent	Normal
Moderate	≥2 mm	Moderate involvement	≥3 mm	Inconstant	Mild	Normal
Server	≥2 mm	Severe involvement	≥3 mm	Constant	Mild	Normal
Visual threat	–	–	–	–	Severe	Compression
Upper normal limit						
Afro-Americans		M/H = 23/24 mm				
Whites		M/H = 19/21 mm				
Asians		M/H = 16/17 mm or 18.6 mm in Chinese				

Mild grades lead to lower daily life impact; the use of immunosuppressors or surgical management is usually not justified. Moderate to severe grades include vision-threatening GO-free patients, in whom the eye disease has a significant impact on daily life to justify the use of immunosuppressors (if the disease is active) or surgery (if inactive). Patients with GO a visual challenge (EX., optic neuropathy) require immediate intervention effective in the evaluation of the posterior third of the orbit due to the loss of echogenic response through the tissues (attenuation) and difficult access to evaluate the inferior rectus muscle (the structure most frequently affected) in addition to poor reproducibility. Ultrasound images of GO with muscle component will show marked thickening of the inferior, medial and lateral rectus muscles [41, 44]. CT and ultrasound are complementary techniques. When considering CT, take into account that orbital fat has a negative density, while the muscles and the optic nerve have a positive density. Consequently, there is no need to regularly use contrast agents to explore the GO, since the contrast will only be able to show muscular hyper-vascularization. The CT scan shall be performed with 3–5 mm sequence axial sections and 5 mm coronal sections from the eyelid to the sphenoid sinus, using the Salvolini-Cabanis plane (neuro-ocular view). The characteristic CE findings for GO are: exophthalmos, thickening of the muscle body, optic nerve compression at the level of the orbital apex due to thickened muscles causing neuropathy, bone bulging of the ethmoid walls, pseudo-tumoral images on the posterior orbital third produced by the thickened inferior rectus muscle. The axial views may show an increased fat volume and atrophic images within the muscle. The indications for CT-scan in GO are based on clinical judgment, the activity and the severity of the disease, as well as on the decision-making process for pharmacological and/or surgical management. MRI images do not offer any considerable advantages for the diagnosis of GO, although they allow for the differentiation between edema and fibrosis because of the high tissue water content. Likewise, MRI offers a higher sensitivity for the diagnosis of the inactive phases of the disease. Some of the advantages are the absence of ionizing radiation and the ability to differentiate orbital structures. The major disadvantages are its high cost, lower availability, and poor quality of images for studying the ethmoid bone wall since MRI does not accurately differentiate the shape of the bone [43–45]. The current therapeutic approaches for GO include local measures, glucocorticoids, orbit radiation, and surgery. Regardless of the management options, the major effort should be addressed to prevention and to avoid any progressive deterioration of the disease. The major key factors for GO are: prior use of radioactive iodine (such as hyperthyroidism treatment), smoking, elevated anti-TSHr titers, elevated T3 titers prior to treatment and uncontrolled hypothyroidism following radioactive iodine management. The euthyroid status shall always be maintained in every patient with GD and GO, or with any risk factors for the development of GO. GD patients with no clinically apparent GO, the management of their underlying hyperthyroidism can be approached with any of the universal modalities for GD management previously described. Cigarette smoking is the most modifiable risk factor for the development of GO, hence the exposure to cigarette smoking is forbidden from the time of diagnosis. The use of glucocorticoids should be considered for patients with mild activity GO and no additional risk factors, for which radioactive iodine will be the baseline therapy for hyperthyroidism. Likewise, in patients with mild GO and smoking or any other associated risk factors should be candidates for concomitant glucocorticoid use if they are going to be treated with radioactive iodine. Patients with GD and moderate to severe GO may be managed with MTZ or surgery for hyperthyroidism. However, patients with GD and inactive ophthalmopathy may be managed with tionamides, radioactive iodine, or surgery, with no need to add glucocorticoids [46–48]. Treatment of hyperthyroidism with tionamides has a neutral effect on the progression of GO, though it has an indirect positive effect on the de-escalation of anti-TSHr. Radioactive iodine is further associated with worsening and progression of GO, whilst surgery has a neutral effect or mild improvement on the progression of Graves' Orbitopathy. For patients with mild active GO, the recommendation is "watchful waiting" and the systematic use of corticosteroids is not accepted, except for those patients that will undergo radioactive iodine management. In inactive-mild GO, rehabilitation surgery for cosmetic purposes or functional reasons (orbital decompression due to exophthalmos, eye lid

	GO	Mild		Moderate to severe		Vision threatening
		Active	Inactive	Active	Inactive	
Treatment	Hyperthyroidism	AT*, I-131*, Qx*	AT, I-131, Qx	AT, I-131 Qx	AT, I-131, Qx	AT
	Orbitopathy	Watch and wait	Watch and wait	High dose Glucocorticoids	Rehabilitation Qx	Glucocorticoids and decompression QX

*AT: Anti-Thyroid agents *I-131: Radioactive iodine *Qx: Surgery

Fig. 9.2 Hyperthyroidism and GO management in various scenarios

retraction) may be required. The use of glucocorticoids is not indicated on account of their ineffectiveness; in fact, prophylactic glucocorticoid treatment is not indicated in the absence of any additional risk factors for the development of radioactive iodine-induced GO. In moderate to severe GO, the treatment choice may be controversial; these patients should receive immediate GO therapy and glucocorticoids are the treatment of choice, preferably Intravenous (IV), with or without orbit-targeted radiation therapy. All patients in this category should be euthyroid as this is a requirement for a favorable evolution in the management of GO. Patients with inactive moderate to severe GO, the baseline therapy for their hyperthyroidism is established in accordance with the individual patient criteria. If radioactive iodine management is decided, glucocorticoid therapy should only be introduced if risk factors for GO are present, particularly when there is a history of smoking. Patients with vision-threatening GO should be considered an endocrine emergency and high-dose intravenous glucocorticoids should be initiated urgently, with subsequent orbital decompression when the response to glucocorticoids is poor [44–47] Several regimes with variable IV glucocorticoid doses have been used; the response rate may range between 63 and 77 % and the use of IV glucocorticoid (methylprednisolone) is more effective than the oral prescription. The accumulated dose of intravenous glucocorticoid should not exceed 6–8 grams within 6–16 weeks. The use of cyclosporine, anti-TNF-α (Etanercept), and intravenous immunoglobulin, as well as the use of anti CD-20 monoclonal antibodies such as Rituximab, may positively impact the pathogenic mechanisms of GO by modulating the immune burden of the disease. However, no final recommendations are yet available for GO applications [47–49]. Retrobulbar radiation therapy may be an option for the treatment of moderate-severe GO, with significant benefit over eye mobility and diplopia. Usually low doses are used (1 Gy per week versus 1 or 2 Gy day) with similar efficacy in patients with moderate-severe GO. Patients with diabetes mellitus and high blood pressure have a relative contraindication for the procedure because of the high risk of post-radiation therapy retinopathy [48, 49]. Figure 9.2 illustrates an approach for the management of hyperthyroidism and GO under various clinical settings.

Pretibial Myxedema

Localized myxedema or Thyroid Dermopathy (TD) is a rare manifestation in GD. The major clinical characteristic is localized skin thickening, particularly on the pretibial area and hence the name pretibial myxedema. The key histological characteristic is the accumulation of GAG on the reticular dermis, with an exaggerated concentration of hyaluronic acid as a result of fibroblast stimulation, though the reason for the stimulation and the autoimmune origin is not totally clear, particularly because it affects mostly the pretibial area, probably because of the venous stasis. The higher probability for lower limb micro trauma leads to larger mucinous deposits or may be the fibroblasts in the body have diverse regulatory mechanisms. Another option is local edema that may enhance the secretion of cytokines that further impair the GAG concentration [50, 51]. Several therapeutic modalities have been used, ranging from compression bandages and topical steroids to steroid systemic therapy and intradermal applications. TD typically has four distinctive presentations:

(a) The edematous, indurated form without pitting accompanied by skin discolorations.
(b) In "Plaques".
(c) Nodular.
(d) Elephantiasis.

Treatment of TD is symptomatic. As a rule, the edematous and plaque presentations may be mild and not annoying for the patient; most of the time it does not require treatment but if specific management is adopted, topical steroids are enough [51–53]. The nodular and elephantiasis forms respond to management with nocturnal compressive bandaging (at the sites affected on the ankle or knee; sports bandages with a 20–40 mmHg compression may be helpful. In other areas of presentation, the use of medium compression bandages assist with management and topical steroids (i.e., 0.05–0.1 % triamcinolone acetate in cream) [52–54]. Fluocinolone acetonide and clobetasol propionate have also been used in some protocols, applied three times per day, accompanied by a soft plastic wrap over the affected area for 4–8 weeks with good response and significant improvement of the skin findings in TD. In selected cases the above protocol may be continued for an additional number of weeks or even months, keeping in mind that extended therapy may pose the risk of developing telangiectasias, ecchymosis and skin atrophy. The use of intra-lesion steroids may result in nodular skin degeneration from adipose tissue atrophy when standard needles are used, though probably the use of smaller gauge needles (mesotherapy-like) avoids the poor results described with normal needles. Overall, the use of intra-lesion and systemic steroids is increasingly being neglected because of the poor results and of their local and systemic effects. The use of immunomodulation therapies such as octreotide, azathioprine, and cyclosporine, inter alia, is not yet supported by strong evidence. TD surgery is rarely performed and in fact surgical trauma predisposes to the relapse of the disease and hence is only indicated in cases of "cosmetically" inacceptable presentations, together with topical steroid therapy [55–59].

Conclusions

Treatment of Graves-Basedow disease cannot yet be aimed at the cause because it is still unknown. There are three available forms of treatment, but there is a difference of opinion as to which of these modalities is best. Antithyroid drugs are widely used for treatment on a long- term basis. Thyroidectomy is a satisfactory form of therapy, if an excellent surgeon is available. Currently, management with I-131 is considered the best treatment in adults. There is no definitive therapy in Graves-Basedow disease; rather, the treating physician is encouraged to discuss with the patient each of the treatment options, including the logistics, benefits, expected speed of recovery, drawbacks, potential side effects and cost so that the course of action incorporates both the relevant medical considerations and the personal values and preferences of the patient.

Bibliography

1. Kumarasinghe MP, De Silva S. Pitfalls in cytological diagnosis of autoimmune thyroiditis. Pathology. 1999;31:1–8.
2. Baloch Z, LiVolsi VA. Pathology of the thyroid gland. Philadelphia: Churchill Livingstone; 2002. p. 61–88.
3. Cooper DS. Antithyroid drugs. N Engl J Med. 2005;352:905–17.

4. Nygaard B. Hyperthyroidism (primary). Clin Evid (Online). 2010;2010. pii: 0611.
5. Abraham P, Acharya S. Current and emerging treatment options for Graves' Hyperthyroidism. Ther Clin Risk Manag. 2010;6:29–40.
6. Piantanida E, Lai A, Sassi L, Gallo D, Spreafico E, Tanda ML, Bartalena L. Outcome prediction of treatment of Graves' hyperthyroidism with antithyroid drugs. Horm Metab Res. 2015;47(10):767–72.
7. Abraham P, Avenell A, McGeoch SC, Clark LF, Bevan JS. Antithyroid drug regimen for treating Graves' hyperthyroidism. Cochrane Database Syst Rev. 2010;(1):CD003420. doi:10.1002/14651858.CD003420.pub4.
8. Iagaru A, McDougall IR. Treatment of thyrotoxicosis. J Nucl Med. 2007;48:379–89.
9. Andrès E, Maloisel F, Zimmer J. The role of haematopoietic growth factors granulocyte colony-stimulating factor and granulocyte-macrophage colony-stimulating factor in the management of drug-induced agranulocytosis. Br J Haematol. 2010;150:3–8.
10. Watanabe N, Narimatsu H, Noh JY, Yamaguchi T, Kobayashi K, Kami M, Kunii Y, Mukasa K, Ito K, Ito K. Antithyroid drug-induced hematopoietic damage: a retrospective cohort study of agranulocytosis and pancytopenia involving 50,385 patients with Graves' disease. J Clin Endocrinol Metab. 2012;97:E49–53.
11. Sun MT, Tsai CH, Shih KC. Antithyroid drug-induced agranulocytosis. J Chin Med Assoc. 2009;72:438–41.
12. Nwatsock JF, Taieb D, Tessonnier L, Mancini J, Dong-A-Zok F, Mundler O. Radioiodine thyroid ablation in Grave's hyperthyroidism: merits and pitfalls. World J Nucl Med. 2012;11:7–11.
13. Ross DS. Radioiodine therapy for hyperthyroidism. N Engl J Med. 2011;364:542–50.
14. Vaidya B, Pearce SH. Diagnosis and management of thyrotoxicosis. BMJ. 2014;349:g5128. doi:10.1136/bmj.g5128.
15. Van Isselt JW, de Klerk JMH, Lips CJM. Radioiodine treatment of hyperthyroidism: fixed or calculated doses; intelligent design or science? Eur J Nucl Med Mol Imaging. 2007;34:1883–4.
16. Howarth D, Epstein M, Lan L, Tan P, Booker J. Determination of the optimal minimum radioiodine dose in patients with Graves' disease: a clinical outcome study. Eur J Nucl Med. 2001;28:1489–95.
17. Grosso M, Traino A, Boni G, Banti E, Della Porta M, Manca G, et al. Comparison of different thyroid committed doses in radioiodine therapy for Graves' hyperthyroidism. Cancer Biother Radiopharm. 2005;20:218–23.
18. Oszukowska L, Knapska-Kucharska M, Lewiński A. Effects of drugs on the efficacy of radioiodine (131I) therapy in hyperthyroid patients. Arch Med Sci. 2010;6(1):4–10.
19. de Rooij A, Vandenbroucke JP, Smit JWA, Stokkel MPM, Dekkers OM. Clinical outcomes after estimated versus calculated activity of radioiodine for the treatment of hyperthyroidism: systematic review and meta-analysis. Eur J Endocrinol. 2009;161:771–7.
20. Bonnema SJ, Hegedüs L. Radioiodine therapy in benign thyroid diseases: effects, side effects, and factors affecting therapeutic outcome. Endocr Rev. 2012;33(6):920–80.
21. Metso S, Auvinen A, Huhtala H, Salmi J, Oksala H, Jaatinen P. Increased cancer incidence after radioiodine treatment for hyperthyroidism. Cancer. 2007;109(10):1972–9.
22. Angusti T, Codegone A, Pellerito R, Favero A. Thyroid cancer prevalence after radioiodine treatment of hyperthyroidism. J Nucl Med. 2000;41:1006–9.
23. Limonard EJ, Bisschop PH, Fliers E, Nieveen van Dijkum EJ. Thyroid function after subtotal thyroidectomy in patients with Graves' hyperthyroidism. ScientificWorldJournal. 2012;2012:548796. doi:10.1100/2012/548796.
24. Palit TK, Miller 3rd CC, Miltenburg DM. The efficacy of thyroidectomy for Graves' disease: a meta-analysis. J Surg Res. 2000;90:161–5.
25. Kaplan EL, Angelos P. Surgery of the thyroid gland. Thyroid Dis Manager. Available at: www.thyroidmanager.org/Chapter21/21-frame.htm.
26. Stalberg P, Svensson A, Hessman O, Akerstrom GA, Hellman P. Surgical treatment of Graves' disease: evidence based approach. World J Surg. 2008;32(7):1269–77.
27. Sugino K, Ito K, Nagahama M, Kitagawa W, Shibuya H, Ito K. Surgical management of Graves' disease—10-year prospective trial at a single institution. Endocr J. 2008;55(1):161–7.
28. Barbuscia M, Querci A, Tonante A, Paparo D, Taranto F, Ilacqua A, Gagliano E, Milone A. Total thyroidectomy in Basedow-Graves' disease treatment: our experience. G Chir. 2015;36(3):117–21.
29. Bahn RS, Burch HB, Cooper DS, Garber JR, Greenlee MC, Klein I, et al. Hyperthyroidism and other causes of thyrotoxicosis: management guidelines of the American Thyroid Association and American Association of Clinical Endocrinologists. Thyroid. 2011;21(6):593–646.
30. Genovese BM, Noureldine SI, Gleeson EM, Tufano RP, Kandil E. What is the best definitive treatment for Graves' Disease? A systematic review of the existing literature. Ann Surg Oncol. 2012. doi:10.1245/s10434-012-2606-x.
31. Marx H, Amin P, Lazarus JH. Pregnancy plus. Hyperthyroidism and pregnancy. BMJ. 2008;336:663–7.
32. Okosieme OE, Lazarus JH. Important considerations in the management of Graves' disease in pregnant women. Expert Rev Clin Immunol. 2015;11(8):947–57.
33. Abalovich M, Amino N, Barbour LA, Cobin RH, De Groot LJ, Glinoer D, et al. Management of thyroid dysfunction during pregnancy and postpartum: an Endocrine Society clinical practice guideline. J Clin Endocrinol Metab. 2007;92(8 Suppl):S1–47.

34. Chan GW, Mandel SJ. Therapy insight: management of Graves' disease during pregnancy. Nat Clin Pract Endocrinol Metab. 2007;3:470–8.
35. Laurberg P, Andersen SL. Graves'-Basedow disease in pregnancy. New trends in the management and guidance to reduce the risk of birth defects caused by antithyroid drugs. Nuklearmedizin. 2015;54(3): 106–11.
36. Bahn RS. Graves' ophthalmopathy. New Engl J Med. 2010;362:726–38.
37. Soeters MR, van Zeijl CJJ, Boelen A, Kloos R, Saeed P, Vriesendorp TM, Mourits P. Optimal management of Graves orbitopathy: a multidisciplinary approach. Netherlands The Journal of Medicine. 2011; 69(7/8):302–8.
38. Regensburg NI, Wiersinga WM, Berendschot TT, Potgieser P, Mourits MP. Do subtypes of graves' orbitopathy exist? Ophthalmology. 2011;118(1):191–6.
39. Khalilzadeh O, Noshad S, Rashidi A, Amirzargar A. Graves' ophthalmopathy: a review of immunogenetics. Curr Genomics. 2011;12(8):564–75.
40. Maheshwari R, Weis E. Thyroid associated orbitopathy. Indian J Ophthalmol. 2012;60(2):87–93.
41. Bartalena L, Pinchera A, Marcocci C. Management of Graves' ophthalmopathy: reality and perspectives. Endocr Rev. 2000;21:168–99.
42. Bartalena L. Prevention of Graves' ophthalmopathy. Best Pract Res Clin Endocrinol Metab. 2012;26(3): 371–9.
43. Hegedüs L, Bonnema SJ, Smith TJ, Brix TH. Treating the thyroid in the presence of Graves' ophthalmopathy. Best Pract Res Clin Endocrinol Metab. 2012;26(3):313–24.
44. Marcocci C, Marinò M. Treatment of mild, moderate-to-severe and very severe Graves' orbitopathy. Best Pract Res Clin Endocrinol Metab. 2012;26(3):325–37.
45. Müller-Forell W, Kahaly GJ. Neuroimaging of Graves' orbitopathy. Best Pract Res Clin Endocrinol Metab. 2012;26(3):259–71.
46. Kirsch E, Hammer B, von Arx G. Graves' orbitopathy: current imaging procedures. Swiss Med Wkly. 2009;139(43/44):618–23.
47. Neumann S, Place RF, Krieger CC, Gershengorn MC. Future Prospects for the Treatment of Graves' Hyperthyroidism and Eye Disease. Horm Metab Res. 2015;47(10):789–96.
48. Dolman PJ. Evaluating Graves' orbitopathy. Best Pract Res Clin Endocrinol Metab. 2012;26(3): 229–48.
49. Rajendram R, Bunce C, Lee RW, Morley AM. Orbital radiotherapy for adult thyroid eye disease. Cochrane Database Syst Rev. 2012;7, CD007114. doi:10.1002/14651858.CD007114.pub2.
50. Sabih DE, Inayatullah M. Managing thyroid dysfunction in selected special situations. Thyoid research. 2013;6:2. doi:10.1186/1756-6614-6-2.
51. Li H, Want T. The autoimmunity in Graves' disease. Front Biosci. 2013;1(18):782–7.
52. Fatourechi V, Pajouhi M, Fransway AF. Dermopathy of Graves disease (pretibial myxedema). Review of 150 cases. Medicine (Baltimore). 1994;73:1–7.
53. Fatourechi V. Thyroid dermopathy and acropachy. Best Pract Res Clin Endocrinol Metab. 2012;26(4): 553–65.
54. Fatourechi V. Pretibial myxedema: pathophysiology and treatment options. Am J Clin Dermatol. 2005;6(5):295–309.
55. Reddy SV, Gupta SK, Jain M. Dermopathy of Graves' disease: Clinico-pathological correlation. Indian J Endocrinol Metab. 2012;16(3):460–2.
56. Vannucchi G, Campi I, Covelli D, Forzenigo L, Beck-Peccoz P, Salvi M. Treatment of pretibial myxedema with dexametazone injected subcutaneously by mesotherapy needles. Thyroid. 2013;23(5):626–32.
57. Schwartz KM, Fatourechi V, Ahmed DD, Pond GR. Dermopathy of Graves' disease (Pretibial myxedema): Long-term outcome. J Clin Endocrinol Metab. 2002;87:438–46.
58. Vargas-Uricoechea H, Sierra-Torres CH, Meza-Cabrera IA. Tratamiento de la Enfermedad de Graves-Basedow. Medicina (Bogotá). 2013;35(2(101)): 130–49.
59. Holahan HM, Farah RS, Swick BL. Pretibial myxedema. Cutis. 2014;94(2):60, 73–4.

Subclinical Hyperthyroidism 10

Asim Hassan

Abstract

Because of screening tests with sensitive TSH assays, subclinical hyperthyroidism is being recognized more commonly. Subclinical hyperthyroidism is defined as undectectable thyrotrophin (TSH) concentration in patients with normal levels of T4 and T3. Subtle symptoms and signs of thyrotoxicosis may be present.

It be classified as endogenous in patients with thyroid hormone production associated with nodular thyroid disease or underlying Graves' disease; and as exogenous in those with undectectable serum thyrotropin concentrations as a result of treatment with levothyroxine. Subclinical hyperthyroidism is often found in older subjects with autonomous function of a multinodular goiter or nodule.

Osteoporosis and atrial fibrillation are complications of subclinical hyperthyroidism that may be an indication for treatment. Studies suggest a possible increase in all-cause mortality in patients with subclinical hyperthyroidism with an increase beyond the age of 60, especially in aging men.

In many patients with endogeneous subclinical hyperthyroidism who do not have nodular thyroid disease or complications of excess thyroid hormone, treatment is unnecessary, but thyroid-function tests should be performed every 6 months. In older patients with atrial fibrillation or osteoporosis that could have been caused or exacerbated by the mild excess of thyroid hormone, ablative therapy with ^{131}I is the best initial option.

In patients with exogeneous subclinical hyperthyroidism, the dose of levothyroxine should be reduced, excluding those with prior thyroid cancer in whom thyrotropin suppression may be required. The dose of levothyroxine used for treating hypothyroidism may be reduced if the patient develops new atrial fibrillation, angina, cardiac failure or accelerated bone loss.

A. Hassan, FRCP, SCE/MRCP (Diab, Endo)
University Diabetes Center, King Saud University,
Riyadh, Saudi Arabia
e-mail: drahassan2@hotmail.com

S.K. Imam, S.I. Ahmad (eds.), *Thyroid Disorders: Basic Science and Clinical Practice*,
DOI 10.1007/978-3-319-25871-3_10

Introduction

The accessibility of sensitive tests for thyroid-stimulating hormone (TSH) has resulted in the diagnosis of patients who have low serum TSH concentrations (<0.5 mU/L) with normal serum free thyroxine (T4) and triiodothyronine (T3) levels; a range of biochemical findings which are described as subclinical hyperthyroidism.

> Subclinical hyperthyroidism is biochemically diagnosed by a low serum thyroid-stimulating hormone levels (TSH) but normal serum free thyroxine (T4) and triiodothyronine (T3) values. Patients with subclinical hyperthyroidism frequently have few or no symptoms of hyperthyroidism

Subclinical hyperthyroidism is biochemically described as low or undetectable serum thyroid-stimulating hormone (TSH), with normal free thyroxine (T4) and total or free triiodothyronine (T3) concentrations [1]. Presently used techniques can detect TSH as low as 0.01–0.02 mIU per L. Subclinical hyperthyroidism can be divided into two types; low but detectable TSH levels (0.1–0.4 mIU per L), and suppressed TSH levels (less than 0.1 mIU per L) [1]. It can occur due to increased endogenous secretion of thyroid hormone, prescription of thyroid hormone for treatment of thyroid carcinomas, or inadvertent excessive thyroid hormone administration. Progression to obvious hyperthyroidism is higher in persons who have suppressed thyroid-stimulating hormone concentration as opposed to those who have low but detectable levels. Subclinical hyperthyroidism is linked with an increased risk of atrial fibrillation in older patients, and with decreased bone mineral density in postmenopausal females.

> Subclinical hyperthyroidism is linked with an increased risk of atrial fibrillation and, mainly in postmenopausal women, reduced bone mineral density

Although there is convincing proof that treatment of suppressed TSH is cost-effective, especially in elderly patients, the significance of judicious detection and treatment of low but measurable TSH levels is contentious.

> The most frequent causes of subclinical hyperthyroidism are therapy with exogenous thyroxine and autonomously functioning thyroid adenomas and multinodular goiters

Causes

Subclinical hyperthyroidism may be due to endogenous excess production of thyroid hormone; or it may be exogenous as a result of deliberate administration of thyroid hormone to suppress thyroid cancer, or inadvertent excessive hormone administration in patients with hypothyroidism. Frequent causes of endogenous subclinical hyperthyroidism are Graves disease, hyper functioning thyroid adenoma, and toxic multinodular goiter. Temporary TSH suppression may occur during subacute, painless, or postpartum thyroiditis. The correlation between population iodine intake and the prevalence of autonomous thyroid dysfunction is inversely related with a higher occurrence with iodine-deficiency [2].

The differential diagnoses of subclinical hyperthyroidism are the same as that of frank hyperthyroidism and, like hyperthyroidism, subclinical hyperthyroidism can be persistent or transitory.

Exogenous Subclinical Hyperthyroidism

In the United States as many as 10 million people, and possibly 200 million persons globally, are prescribed thyroid hormone. Most of them are at risk of subclinical hyperthyroidism, either deliberate or inadvertent. Patients who are taking thyroxine (T4), about 25 % have low serum thyroid-stimulating hormone (TSH) concentration and in one study, 5.8 % had TSH under 0.1 mU/L [3–5].

Several of these patients have hypothyroidism, and subclinical hyperthyroidism in them is not the target of thyroid hormone replacement. However, subclinical hyperthyroidism is the aim of thyroxine administration in patients with thyroid cancer and in some patients with thyroid nodules, multinodular or diffuse goiters, or a history of head and neck irradiation. In these patients, the advantages of TSH suppression offset the risks of subclinical hyperthyroidism.

In the United States as many as 10 million people, and possibly 200 million persons globally, are prescribed thyroid hormone

Endogenous Subclinical Hyperthyroidism

Independently thyroid hormone producing adenomas and multinodular goiters are the most frequent causes of endogenous or internal subclinical hyperthyroidism. In persons over 55 years old, subclinical hyperthyroidism due to multinodular goiters was diagnosed in 57 % of patients, while due to Graves' disease in 6 % only [6]. One study showed that, 22 % of patients with multinodular goiter had subclinical hyperthyroidism, and 28 % had autonomous hyperfunctioning area(s) on imaging of the thyroid gland [7].

Thyroiditis can also cause subclinical hyperthyroidism, and has been shown to occur in 63 % of euthyroid cases with Graves' ophthalmopathy and 4 % of Graves' patients in remission [8–10]. It may also be seen in patients with early Graves' disease before the commencement of frank hyperthyroidism. Moreover, pregnant females, mostly in the first trimester and those with hyperemesis gravidarum or trophoblastic disease, with high serum chorionic gonadotropin concentrations, may be diagnosed to have subclinical hyperthyroidism.

Epidemiology and Natural History

Numerous large studies have looked into the prevalence of subclinical hyperthyroidism [11–17]. The data from these studies, mainly in persons over the age of 55–60 years, is presented as follows:

The reported occurrence of subclinical hyperthyroidism varies among different studies because of the variability in defining the TSH level for subclinical hyperthyroidism, age of the patient population studied, and administration of thyroid hormone. The occurrence of subclinical hyperthyroidism in the population varies from 0.7 to 12.4 %. In the U.S, the National Health and Nutrition Examination Survey (NHANES III), which did not include individuals with known thyroid disease, 0.7 % of 16,533 persons were reported to have subclinical hyperthyroidism (TSH <0.1 mU/L) [18]. Subclinical hyperthyroidism is more widespread in areas with mild to moderate iodine scarcity.

However the prevalence of subclinical hyperthyroidism has been shown to be as high as 15 % in patients older than 70 years in iodine-lacking areas [19]. It is most frequent in individuals on thyroid hormone treatment, where the prevalence may be as high as 20 % [3, 4]. Moreover, subclinical thyroid dysfunction is more frequent in females, smokers, and older persons [18, 20].

The condition is most frequent in individuals on thyroid hormone treatment, where the prevalence may be as high as 20 %. Moreover, subclinical thyroid dysfunction is more frequent in females, smokers, and older persons

Mostly subclinical hyperthyroidism will not progress to frank hyperthyroidism. The associations and the risk factors that seem to influence the natural course include the level of TSH inhibition and the primary cause. One prospective study evaluated 102 females more than 60 years old with subclinical hyperthyroidism with TSH concentrations between 0.1 and 0.4 mIU/L [21]. Amongst these women, 2.9 % developed overt hyperthyroidism; in 3.9 % TSH levels reduced to less than 0.1 mIU/L, with normal T3 and T4 values; in 23.5 % the TSH normalized; and in 69.5 % TSH levels remained within 0.1–0.4 mIU/L over an average follow-up of 41 months. This is equivalent to a 1 % development to obvious hyperthyroidism per year. The only reliable association of progression was a preliminary TSH value of less than 0.2 mIU/L. Females more than 65 years with subclinical hyperthyroidism and TSH concentrations less than 0.1 mIU/L had a 27 % chance of developing obvious hyperthyroidism over the next 2 years [22], showing that the chances of progression are higher in patients with TSH levels less than 0.1 mIU/L.

The chances of progression are higher in patients with TSH levels less than 0.1 mIU/L

A retrospective investigation of the natural course of subclinical hyperthyroidism showed that the history of disease is more unpredictable in patients with Graves disease than in toxic multinodular goiter [23]. In Graves disease, patients can go into remission, progress, or may not change in up to a 3 years of follow-up, while the majority of patients with multinodular goiter were seen to have steady thyroid function during the same period of follow-up. Multinodular goiter is more frequent in iodine-depleted areas, and administration of iodine including iodine-containing medications, such as amiodarone can precipitate subclinical hyperthyroidism [24].

When investigated prospectively, 40–60 % of subjects with subclinical hyperthyroidism have normal results [12, 13]. This is most liable to arise in persons with only slightly below normal serum TSH results (e.g., between 0.1 and 0.5 mU/L) when initially investigated. In a study of a primary care system that included 422,242 subjects without known thyroid dysfunction, 52 % who had a serum TSH level <0.35 mU/L at baseline had a normal TSH afterward without any treatment [25].

There are inconsistent data regarding the incidence of progression from subclinical to frank hyperthyroidism [11, 14, 21, 22, 26, 27]. Progression to frank hyperthyroidism appears to be associated with the level of subclinical hyperthyroidism and the underlying diagnosis.

In a community based report from Scotland, 2024 persons with at least two subnormal (<0.4 mU/L) TSH levels examined 4 months apart with normal free or total thyroxine (T4) and total triiodothyronine (T3) [27]. During the initial year of the study, the overall development from subclinical to overt hyperthyroidism was 6.1 %. In subjects with steady state subclinical hyperthyroidism who did not progress in the subsequent year, further progression rates at 2, 5, and 7 years were 0.6, 0.7, and 0.5 %, respectively. It was noted that the number of patients who progressed to clear hyperthyroidism was small, progression was around twice as common in patients with serum TSH <0.1 mU/L as compared to TSH between 0.1 and 0.4 mU/L.

In a study from New Zealand of 96 patients with endogenous subclinical thyrotoxicosis (TSH <0.25 mU/L), development of hyperthyroidism occurred in 8 % at 1 year, and amplified to 26 % at 5 years. At 5 years, overt hyperthyroidism in subclinical hyperthyroidism due to Graves' disease, nodular goiter, and autonomous nodules was seen in 9, 21, and 61 % of patients respectively [27].

In a study from Brazil of 48 women <65 years who had twice confirmed TSH ≤0.1 mU/L, 20 % with nodular disease and 40 % with Graves' disease progressed to overt hyperthyroidism over a 2-year period [22]. In another study of females ≥60 years with minimal thyrotoxicosis (TSH 0.1–0.4 mU/L), progression to overt hyperthyroidism was infrequent (approximately 1 % per year) [21].

A UK based study showed that, 20.3 % of patients with subclinical hyperthyroidism with TSH <0.1 mU/L developed overt hyperthyroidism over an average of 32 months, as compared to 6.8 % with TSH 0.1–0.39 mU/L [28].

In >60 years old in Framingham study with a TSH <0.1 mU/L, only 4.3 % of patients progressed to overt hyperthyroidism after a follow up of 4 years [11].

Clinical Findings

The major target tissues negatively affected by subclinical hyperthyroidism, are bones and the cardiovascular system although abnormalities in other systems are effected too (see Table 10.1).

Cardiovascular Mortality Risk

Cardiovascular abnormalities of subclinical hyperthyroidism include an increased heart rate, risk of atrial arrhythmias, bigger left ventricular mass, and reduced variability in heart rate [29, 30]. Decreased heart rate variability was prominent in patients with subclinical and overt hyperthyroidism as compared with control subjects, which may indicate an increased risk of later cardiac events [30]. In a retrospective analysis of adults more than 65 years old, the frequency of atrial fibrillation in persons with subclinical hyperthyroidism whose TSH concentration was less than 0.4 mIU/L was 12.7 %, as compared to 2.3 % in those with normal TSH. The age adjusted risk of atrial fibrillation is 2.8 in patients with subclinical hyperthyroidism compared with normal controls [31]. Likewise, two large cohorts of subjects 60–65 years of age found that subclinical hyperthyroidism is linked with an increased relative risk of developing atrial fibrillation over the course of 10 years [20, 32].

Table 10.1 Clinical manifestations of subclinical hyperthyroidism

Heart disease
Increased heart rate and incidence of premature atrial beats
Increased cardiac contractility
Increased left ventricular mass and septal and posterior wall thickness
Increased atrial fibrillation
Bone disease
Decreased bone density, particularly in postmenopausal women
Elevated biochemical markers of increased bone resorption
Increased urinary pyridinoline and deoxypyridinoline excretion
Increased urinary hydroxyproline excretion
Other
Disturbed sleep
Mood disorders
Laboratory abnormalities
Increased serum concentration of sex hormone-binding globulin
Increased serum concentrations of hepatic enzymes and creatine kinase
Decrease in serum total and LDL-cholesterol concentrations

Subclinical hyperthyroidism is linked with cardiovascular and all-cause mortality, even though the data are inconsistent. A prospective systematic review of cohort studies evaluating coronary heart disease and mortality in subclinical hyperthyroidism (TSH levels less than 0.3–0.5 mIU per L) found a modest trivial increase in risk [33]. Nonetheless, a meta-analysis concerning different studies reported that subclinical hyperthyroidism is associated with a 41 % increased risk of all-cause mortality compared with normal control patients, and that this risk increases with advancing age [34]. Two population based cohort studies from Germany and Brazil had incompatible results regarding the relationship between low TSH levels and mortality [35, 36]. In an 8.5-year follow-up study from Germany, adjusted all-cause mortality was not adversely effected in middle-aged subjects with TSH levels less than 0.25 mIU/L [35]. On the contrary, in Brazilian patients about 60 years of age who had TSH levels less than 0.45 mIU/L had a significant 20.3 % enhanced all-cause mortality in 7.5 years, but not elevated cardiovascular ailment [36].

Two studies looked into the cardiovascular effects of treatment of low TSH with methimazole [37] or radioactive iodine [38]. The first study showed that methimazole treatment in patients with suppressed TSH levels considerably decreased heart rate, atrial and ventricular premature beats, and left ventricular wall thickness 6 months after normalization of TSH levels, reaching same proportions to that of the normal control group [37]. Similarly in another report, treatment with radioactive iodine in persons with subclinical hyperthyroidism (TSH levels less than 0.1 mIU/L) due to multinodular goiter caused an 11 % decrease in heart rate, 19 % drop in cardiac output, and a simultaneous 30 % raised systemic vascular resistance after a mean follow-up period of 224 days after TSH normalization; though, in this study a euthyroid control group was missing [38].

Atrial Fibrillation

The collective incidence of atrial fibrillation in persons with subclinical hyperthyroidism is reported by the findings of a prospective cohort study of around 2000 subjects older than 60 years (without atrial fibrillation) followed for 10 years [17]. For patients with TSH values <0.1 mU/L, 0.1–0.4 mU/L, or within the normal range, the overall incidence of atrial fibrillation was 28, 16, and 11 %, respectively [17].

In biochemically euthyroid persons, TSH and free T4 concentrations may also be linked with atrial fibrillation risk. In a population-based study of 1426 subjects, euthyroid individuals with a TSH in the lowest levels had a higher risk of atrial fibrillation than those in the upper quartile [39]. Comparable findings were seen in another population-based study of 5519 euthyroid (normal serum TSH and free T4) elderly subjects [40]. Higher serum free T4 concentrations (but within the normal limits) were independently linked with atrial fibrillation [40].

Coronary Heart Disease, Heart Failure, and Other Cardiac Factors

In a meta-analysis consisting of 22,437 participants, 718 with endogenous subclinical hyperthyroidism, the risk of coronary heart disease was elevated in patients with endogenous subclinical hyperthyroidism (HR 1.21, 95 % CI 0.99–1.46). Similar findings were noted in a study from Scotland [41]. Endogenous subclinical hyperthyroidism was linked with an increased risk of non-fatal cardiovascular disease (HR 1.39, 95 % CI 1.22–1.58) [41].

Subclinical hyperthyroidism is also associated with an increased risk of heart failure [42–44]. In a group of males and females aged 70–82 years with a history of cardiovascular disorder (5316 participants, 71 with subclinical hyperthyroidism, five on thyroxine replacement), the risk of heart failure over 3.2 years of follow-up was more as compared with euthyroid subjects (HR 2.93, 95 % CI 1.37–6.24), and in another combined analysis of individual data from six prospective cohort studies (25,390 participants, 648 with subclinical hyperthyroidism), patients with TSH levels <0.10 mU/L had a higher risk of heart failure than euthyroid controls (16 events in 154 participants [10.4 %] versus 1762 events in 22,674 [7.8 %], HR 1.94, 95 % CI 1.01–3.72). The risk remained (HR 1.8, 95 % CI 1.04–3.13) even when those using thyroid hormone were excluded from the analysis.

Subclinical hyperthyroidism has numerous other effects on cardiac function, same but of lower severity and lower frequency than frank hyperthyroidism. These include sinus tachycardia, atrial premature beats, increased left ventricular hypertrophy, increased cardiac contractility, abnormal endothelial function, reduced exercise capacity, reduced heart rate variability, and an increase in markers of coagulopathy [45–50]. The incidence of cardiovascular findings is inconsistent, possibly due to the level of TSH suppression, the underlying disorder, and individual sensitivity to thyroid hormone excess.

The level of TSH inhibition that indicates poor cardiovascular effects is indefinite. Nevertheless, in a small study of exogenous subclinical hyperthyroidism, cardiovascular findings that were abnormal at high doses of thyroxine became normal when the dose was lowered so that the measured TSH was around 0.1 mU/L [51].

Cardiovascular Mortality

Subclinical hyperthyroidism has been associated with many cardiovascular risk factors, it is indefinite whether there is an increased mortality. In five population-based studies meta-analysis investigating the relationship between subclinical hyperthyroidism (TSH less than 0.3–0.5 mU/L) and cardiovascular and all-cause mortality, the risk for all-cause and cardiovascular mortality was not significant (relative risks [RRs] 1.12, 95 % CI 0.89–1.42 and 1.19, 95 % CI 0.81–1.76, respectively) [33]. However, another meta-analysis showed a considerably increased risk of all-cause mortality (HR 1.41, 95 % CI 1.12–1.79) [34]. Increased mortality after finding of subclinical hyperthyroidism depended upon age, with an increase beyond the age of 60 years. However, in a subsequent population-based study, subclinical hyperthyroidism was associated with reduced survival only in individuals < age 65 years [52].

The meta-analyses included both exogenous and endogenous subclinical hyperthyroidism patients. Serum triiodothyronine (T3) levels are more in persons with endogenous than exogenous subclinical hyperthyroidism, and this may give a higher mortality risk [45]. In the meta-analysis of 10 prospective cohort studies (52,674 participants, 2188 with endogenous subclinical hyperthyroidism) studying only patients with endogenous subclinical hyperthyroidism, there was an elevated risk of both all cause (HR 1.24, 95 % CI 1.06–1.46) and cardiovascular (HR 1.29, 95 % CI 1.02–1.62) mortality in patients with endogenous subclinical hyperthyroidism [53]. The risk of cardiovascular mortality was more for TSH levels <0.1 mU/L as compared to concentrations between 0.1 and 0.44 mU/L (HRs 1.84 versus 1.24).

In a study investigating patients with exogenous subclinical hyperthyroidism only, there was a higher risk of cardiovascular or all-cause mortality only in patients with totally suppressed TSH levels [54]. In this evaluation of 17,684 persons (mean age 61.6 years) on T4 replacement treatment, TSH levels were fully suppressed (<0.03 mU/L) or low (0.04–0.4 mU/L) in 6 and 21 % of subjects, respectively. In comparison to patients with normal TSH, patients with suppressed TSH levels (<0.03 mU/L) had raised cardiovascular morbidity and mortality (adjusted HR 1.37, 95 % CI 1.17–1.60), while those who had serum TSH concentration between 0.04 and 0.4 mU/L had a lesser increase in risk that was insignificant (adjusted HR 1.10 [95 % CI 0.99–1.23]). In general, the increased risk of mortality from subclinical hyperthyroidism appears to be little but rises with the extent of TSH suppression.

Bone and Mineral Metabolism

Subclinical hyperthyroidism may decrease bone mineral density (BMD), predominantly in cortical bones, though the effect is possibly influenced by the period of the disease, other associated risk factors for loss of bone, and the level of TSH inhibition. Loss of bone density with hyperthyroidism is a consequence of increased bone turnover due to imbalance between bone resorption and formation, resulting in decrease in BMD and increased bone turnover markers [55]. Though frank hyperthyroidism is linked with increased risk of fractures, the data is inconsistent for subclinical hyperthyroidism.

The effect of subclinical hyperthyroidism on BMD is significant in postmenopausal women. In a cross-sectional analysis of females with endogenous subclinical hyperthyroidism (TSH levels of 0.01–0.1 mIU/L), postmenopausal women had considerably lower BMD at the level of the femur and lumbar regions, while premenopausal women had only a modestly lower BMD in the femur area compared with corresponding euthyroid control patients [56]. A 12 studies meta-analysis also found a relationship between markedly decreased BMD in postmenopausal women, but not in premenopausal females or males [57].

There is proof that subnormal TSH results in increased bone turnover markers, particularly in postmenopausal women with exogenous subclinical hyperthyroidism. There is an inadequate data on bone turnover marker in endogenous subclinical hyperthyroidism; nonetheless the findings are similar. The data supports bone improvement from treating postmenopausal females with subclinical hyperthyroidism. In one study, postmenopausal women with subclinical hyperthyroidism (TSH levels less than 0.2 mIU/ L) due to multinodular goiter who were treated or not treated with radioactive iodine ablation, and followed up for 2 years [58]. Patients receiving radioactive iodine treatment had normal TSH levels and had no significant change in lumbar and hip BMD, while the untreated patients with low TSH levels had persistent loss of bone mass of approximately 1–2 % per year. One more study noted a prominent increase in BMD in patients with overt or subclinical hyperthyroidism (2.8 and 1.5 %, respectively) after 6 months of euthyroid status [59].

Dementia Cognitive Function

The relationship between low TSH concentration and dementia is contentious. Though data are inconsistent, subclinical hyperthyroidism may also be associated with an increased possibility of dementia [41, 60–62].

The prospective population-based Rotterdam study analyzed a random sample of 1846 patients more than 55 years old, and noted that TSH concentrations less than 0.4 mIU/L were associated with a 3.5-fold elevated risk of dementia and Alzheimer disease in a 2–4-year follow-up [63]. This association was significantly stronger for patients with both low TSH levels and positive antithyroid peroxidase antibodies, raising the likelihood of an autoimmune mechanism. Though another study among the same population did not confirm the relationship between incident dementia or Alzheimer disease and TSH levels in a follow-up of 5-year [63]. Another population-based study from Italy discovered that persons older than 65 years with TSH below 0.46 mIU/L had poorer Mini-Mental State Examination results compared with euthyroid age-matched control patients (22.61 ± 6.88 versus 24.72 ± 4.52, respectively ($P<.03$)) [62]. Moreover in multivariate regression analysis, same patients had a more than twofold increased probability of cognitive impairment compared with age-matched control patients [62]. Further studies are required to elucidate whether there is a causal link between subclinical hyperthyroidism and cognitive deterioration, or whether the relationship between low TSH and dementia is due to a higher occurrence of nonthyroidal illness in older adults.

In a prospective cohort study of 1864 subjects (mean age of 71 years and TSH of 0.1–10 mU/L), followed for an average of 12.7 years, only females whose TSH levels was in the lowest range had a 2.39 elevated risk of developing Alzheimer disease compared with the higher levels [61].

Similar data were noted in a population-based study of 1171 participants in whom subclinical hyperthyroidism (TSH <0.46 mU/L) was linked with cognitive dysfunction (HR 2.26, 95 % CI 1.32–3.91) [62].

In a community-based analysis from Scotland (n = 2004), continuous endogenous subclinical hyperthyroidism (TSH <0.4 mU/L) was associated with an increased risk of dementia (adjusted HR 1.79, 95 % CI 1.28–2.51) [45].

In another prospective population based study from Korea, 54 out of 313 patients who showed deterioration in cognitive function had lower TSH levels within the normal reference range compared with subjects whose cognitive function remained stable or got better [64].

While in contradiction, cross-sectional analysis of primary care patients in England [65], thyroid cancer subjects from Korea [66], and females taking T4-suppressive therapy in the United States [67] failed to show an association of subclinical hyperthyroidism with cognitive function.

Quality of Life

Persons with subclinical hyperthyroidism may have increased feeling of adrenergic over activity, especially those younger than 50 years. Quality of life and over activity of excess thyroid hormone were analyzed in 23 patients about 43 years old, who had TSH levels less than 0.3 mIU/L [29]. Compared with euthroid age and sex-matched control patients, those with low TSH had a higher frequency of nervousness, tremor, heat intolerance, palpitations, and sweating, and lower functional health and well-being. However, other studies did not find a relationship between TSH concentrations and health-related quality of life scores in subjects who had been treated for hyperthyroidism [68], or in a population-based study of females that included participants with subclinical hyperthyroidism [69].

In patients with exogenous subclinical hyperthyroidism, sleep disturbances and reduced functional capacity have been reported with or without considerable effect on temperament or psychological well being [65, 67, 70–72]. In a study, hypothyroid subjects at random assigned to the standard dose of T4 versus higher dose T4, the physical aspect and general health scale were worse in the subclinical hyperthyroid group [72]. While, psychological health, temperament, and physical learning were better.

In another 6-months randomized study of T4 escalated to establish continuation of TSH suppression versus normalization of TSH in 24 patients with a history of thyroid carcinoma, there were no important changes in any quality of life components in either group [71].

In another open study in which subjects were given a thyroxine dose that was 50 mcg higher or less than the normal dose, subjects on the higher dose had improved "well-being" using a visual analog scale compared with baseline [73].

In patients with endogenous subclinical hyperthyroidism, scores for both the physical and psychological health apparently are lower than in euthyroid control patients [32]. The low performance was due to clinical symptoms related to thyroid hormone excess.

Thus, quality of life may be effected in some patients with subclinical hyperthyroidism, mainly those with endogenous subclinical hyperthyroidism [45]. The inconsistency in results is possibly related to differences in duration of subclinical hyperthyroidism, degree of TSH suppression, and patient populations.

Evaluation

Patients with subclinical hyperthyroidism should be asked about symptoms of hyperthyroidism (eg, tremor, palpitations, heat intolerance), also a past history of thyroid disease, exposure to iodine-containing radiographic contrast material or iodine containing herbal products, and therapy that may suppress thyroid-stimulating hormone (thyroxine, high-dose glucocorticoids). Women of childbearing age should be inquired about the possibility of pregnancy. Moreover, all patients should be assessed for the presence of thyroid gland enlargement and nodularity.

Diagnosis

The negative feedback association between serum thyroxine and triiodothyronine and thyroid-stimulating hormone levels is directly proportional. Thus, even small elevation in serum T4 and T3 concentrations (whether caused by exogenous or endogenous thyroid hormone excess) suppresses TSH secretion [73]. There is a general consensus that measurement of serum TSH is the most sensitive indicator of thyroid hormone activity without pituitary or hypothalamic disease. Mostly the initial screening test for thyroid disease is the serum TSH.

If the serum TSH concentration is subnormal (<0.5 mU/L in many laboratories), the TSH evaluation should be repeated along with a serum free T4 and T3 to confirm the diagnosis of subclinical hyperthyroidism. The diagnosis of subclinical hyperthyroidism depends upon the combination of a low serum TSH level and normal serum free T4 and T3 level. It may be symptomatic or asymptomatic for hyperthyroidism. Because the serum TSH concentration can be temporarily reduced, a serum TSH level, together with a free T4 and T3, should be reassessed after 1–3 months to verify the diagnosis.

Subclinical hyperthyroidism should be differentiated from other diagnoses of low TSH concentrations that are not associated with relative thyroid over activity, for example, central hypothyroidism; some patients with central hypothyroidism have low serum TSH and normal (but usually low or low-normal) free T4 and T3 concentrations; nonthyroidal illness, euthyroid patients with nonthyroidal illness, especially those receiving high-dose glucocorticoids or dopamine, may have low serum TSH and low-normal free T4 and T3 concentrations; recovery from hyperthyroidism. Serum TSH concentrations may remain low for up to several months after normalization of serum T4 and T3 concentrations in patients treated for hyperthyroidism or recovering from hyperthyroidism caused by thyroiditis and psychiatric conditions, especially emotional disorders. T4 and T3 levels are generally lower in patients with these disorders, while patients with subclinical hyperthyroidism may have T4 and T3 concentrations in the mid to high normal reference range.

When the diagnosis of subclinical hyperthyroidism is doubtful, assessment of 24-h thyroid radioactive iodine uptake and scan may be supportive. A high or relatively high 24-h uptake, relative to the low serum TSH levels or a focal area of increased radionuclide uptake would support the diagnosis of subclinical hyperthyroidism.

In patients not taking T4 who have persistent subnormal TSH values and in whom treatment is considered, a radioactive iodine uptake and scan is obtained to help establish the etiology of subclinical hyperthyroidism (Table 10.2). Women of childbearing age should have a negative pregnancy test before having radioactive iodine scanning.

If the scan shows one or more focal areas of increased uptake, this could explain for the low serum TSH. If there are focal areas of increased uptake, a thyroid ultrasound would then be useful in determining the presence of distinct nodules. In patients with low or no uptake on radioiodine scan, the cause may be thyroiditis or recent iodine exposure.

In postmenopausal women or other patients at risk for osteoporosis, a bone densitometry study may be useful in making a decision to treat subclinical hyperthyroidism or observe.

Table 10.2 Causes of subclinical hyperthyroidism

Hyperthyroidism with a normal or high radioiodine uptake
Autonomous thyroid tissue (uptake may be low if recent iodine load led to iodine-induced hyperthyroidism)
Toxic adenoma
Toxic multinodular goiter
Autoimmune thyroid disease
Graves' disease
Hashitoxicosis
Human chorionic gonadotropin-mediated hyperthyroidism
Hyperemesis gravidarum
Trophoblastic disease
TSH-mediated hyperthyroidism
TSH-producing pituitary adenoma
Non-neoplastic TSH-mediated hyperthyroidism
Hyperthyroidism with a near absent radioiodine uptake
Exogenous thyroid hormone intake
Excessive replacement therapy
Intentional suppressive therapy
Factitious hyperthyroidism
Amiodarone (also may cause iodine-induced hyperthyroidism)
Thyroiditis
Subacute granulomatous (de Quervain's) thyroiditis
Painless thyroiditis (silent thyroiditis, lymphocytic thyroiditis)
Postpartum thyroiditis
Palpation thyroiditis
Radiation thyroiditis
Ectopic hyperthyroidism
Struma ovarii
Metastatic follicular thyroid cancer

Pregnancy

The diagnosis of real subclinical or frank hyperthyroidism during pregnancy may be complicated because of the changes in thyroid function that happen during normal pregnancy. Transient subclinical hyperthyroidism in the first trimester is considered a normal physiologic finding. True subclinical hyperthyroidism may occur, but it is not classically associated with negative outcomes during pregnancy [74] and does not necessitate therapy. Moreover, in pregnant women with clear hyperthyroidism, the aim of treatment is to maintain serum free T4 concentrations in the high-normal range and serum TSH concentrations in the low-normal or suppressed range (i.e. to maintain constant but minimal mild hyperthyroidism).

Screening Guidelines

There is no agreement concerning screening for subclinical hyperthyroidism in the general population. Criterion for approving a screening test should be that diagnosis and treatment of a condition in asymptomatic subjects would result in significant improvement in health outcomes compared with people who are not screened. The U.S. Preventive Services Task Force determined in 2004 that there is enough evidence that suppressed TSH concentration is a risk factor for future development of atrial fibrillation, but there is no data showing whether any therapy would prevent this complication [75]. Likewise, a group comprising of members of the American Association of Clinical Endocrinologists, the American Thyroid Association, and The Endocrine Society published the conclusions of their consensus with a proposal against population-based screening for thyroid disease [1]. Nonetheless, it is also stressed that recommendations derived from evidence-based medicine are population-based, and that doctors should use their best clinical judgment in the situation of screening the individual patients.

Management

Patients on T4 for the Treatment of Hypothyroidism

Low bone density and atrial fibrillation can both result in considerable morbidity in older patients and, therefore, subclinical hyperthyroidism should be avoided. Patients receiving thyroid replacement therapy who have thyroid-stimulating hormone (TSH) concentrations below normal should have their dose titrated to keep up a normal serum TSH level (approximately 0.5–5.0 mU/L).

> Patients receiving thyroid replacement treatment for hypothyroidism and who have TSH values below normal should have their dose titrated to maintain a normal serum TSH level(approximately 0.5–5.0 mU/L)

Patients on Suppressive Levothyroxine Therapy

Subclinical hyperthyroidism is inevitable when thyroid hormone is given to suppress TSH release in an effort to prevent or reduce goiter size or prevent relapse of thyroid cancer, since it is the aim of therapy. Nevertheless, the undesirable effects of suppressive treatment can be avoided by treatment with the lowest possible dose of thyroxine (T4) required to meet the desired goal [51, 76].

In patients with thyroid cancer, subclinical hyperthyroidism is the goal of thyroid hormone therapy, the benefits of TSH suppression outweigh the risks of subclinical hyperthyroidism.

However postmenopausal patients given suppressive doses of thyroxine should be given calcium and vitamin D supplementation, and consideration should be given to starting antiresorptive treatment to prevent bone loss.

> For patients with thyroid malignancy and in some patients with benign nodular thyroid goiter, subclinical hyperthyroidism is the aim of thyroid hormone treatment. In these patients, the benefits of TSH inhibition are thought to outweigh the risks of subclinical hyperthyroidism

Endogenous Subclinical Hyperthyroidism

There is little data to direct clinical decisions concerning the therapy of patients with endogenous subclinical hyperthyroidism. In some patients the results are normal on rechecking weeks or months later, so that treatment should not be instituted unless constantly low TSH results are confirmed [12, 14].

Latent benefits of intervention include enhancement in certain cardiovascular parameters and in bone mineral density. There is no data on long-term benefits of correcting subclinical hyperthyroidism, mainly studies with clinically important results, such as cardiovascular disease and fracture. For Instance, in a prospective but uncontrolled study of subjects with subclinical hyperthyroidism, antithyroid drugs lowered heart rate, atrial and ventricular premature beats, left ventricular mass, inter ventricular septal thickness, and left ventricular posterior wall thickness [37]. Similar benefits in hemodynamic measurements were observed in another study with radioiodine treatment [38].

Similarly in two other non-randomized trials, postmenopausal subjects with nodular goiter and subclinical hyperthyroidism given antithyroid drugs or radioiodine for 2 years had higher bone density than matched patients who were not treated [58, 77].

Thus, in certain persons with subclinical hyperthyroidism, normalization of TSH results in improvement in surrogate outcomes. Long-term clinical studies are needed to verify if correcting subclinical hyperthyroidism improves cardiovascular or skeletal outcomes. Due to deficiency of data to guide patients with endogenous subclinical hyperthyroidism for therapy, it is suggested to decide to treat on the bases of clinical risk for complications of subclinical hyperthyroidism and the degree of TSH suppression.

Patients at High Risk for Complications

In persons at increased risk for cardiac or skeletal complications (e.g., old patients >65 years of age, persons at risk factors for cardiac arrhythmias, and postmenopausal females with or at risk for osteoporosis), the following approach is suggested:

- If the TSH level is <0.1 mU/L, treat the primary cause of subclinical hyperthyroidism.
- If the TSH is 0.1–0.5 mU/L, treat if there is associated cardiovascular problem or low bone density.

Also consider treatment if a thyroid radionuclide scan shows one or more focal areas of high uptake. Subclinical hyperthyroidism due to autonomous nodule(s) is more likely to advance to frank hyperthyroidism than subclinical hyperthyroidism due to Graves' disease. Only observation is advised if the bone density is normal and the radionuclide thyroid scan fails to show a focal area of increased uptake. Observation may also be considered if a patient is on a beta-adrenergic blocker for another reason. In observed patients, check TSH, free T4, and triiodothyronine (T3) every 6 months.

> In persons with endogenous subclinical hyperthyroidism at high risk for cardiac or skeletal complications (i.e., older adults) and who have a TSH levels less than 0.1 mU/L, treatment of the underlying cause of subclinical hyperthyroidism is recommended. For comparable patients who have TSH concentrations between 0.1 and 0.5 mU/L, treatment is recommended if the bone density is low and/or if the thyroid radionuclide scan shows one or more focal areas of high uptake. If bone density is normal and the thyroid scan fails to show a focal area of increased uptake, patients are typically observed. In these patients, TSH, free T4, and T3 is measured every 6 months

Patients at Low Risk for Complications

In persons at low risk for complications of hyperthyroidism (young subjects, premenopausal patients), following approach is advised:

- If the serum TSH concentration is <0.1 mU/L, treat the main cause of subclinical hyperthyroidism if the patient is symptomatic of hyperthyroidism and/or if a radionuclide thyroid scan discovers one or more focal areas of high uptake.
- If the TSH is between 0.1 and 0.5 mU/L, observation alone is appropriate and TSH, free T4, and T3 should be measured every 6 months.

Above guidelines are in agreement with those of a clinical panel (comprised of representatives from The Endocrine Society, the American Thyroid Association [ATA], and the American Association of Clinical Endocrinologists [AACE]) [1].

For patients with endogenous subclinical hyperthyroidism at low risk for cardiac or skeletal complications (young individuals, premenopausal women) and TSH values less than 0.1 mU/L, treatment is advised if the radionuclide scan shows one or more focal areas of high uptake. For low risk patients who have a TSH value between 0.1 and 0.5 mU/L, only observation is advised. TSH, free T4, and T3 is measured every 6 months

Treatment Options

Therapy options for patients with subclinical hyperthyroidism are similar to those for frank hyperthyroidism and depend upon the basic etiology. Beta-blockers are useful for symptomatic control of adrenergic hyperactivity (eg, palpitations, tremor).

In persons with Graves' disease or nodular thyroid disease with autonomy, treatment options include thionamides, radioiodine, or surgery.

In patients with low or no uptake on thyroid radioiodine scan, the etiology of subclinical hyperthyroidism may be thyroiditis or exogenous thyroid hormone intake (Table 10.2). Majority of patients with thyroiditis need no treatment since thyroid dysfunction is infrequently severe and is temporary. Nevertheless, thyroid functions should be repeated, at the outset every 4–8 weeks, until normalized. Symptomatic patients may benefit from beta-blockade.

The treatment options for patients with subclinical hyperthyroidism are similar as those for frank hyperthyroidism and depend upon the basic etiology

Summary and Recommendations

- Subclinical hyperthyroidism is biochemically diagnosed by a low serum thyroid-stimulating hormone levels (TSH) but normal serum free thyroxine (T4) and triiodothyronine (T3) values. Patients with subclinical hyperthyroidism frequently have few or no symptoms of hyperthyroidism.
- The most frequent causes of subclinical hyperthyroidism are therapy with exogenous thyroxine and autonomously functioning thyroid adenomas and multinodular goiters.
- Subclinical hyperthyroidism is linked with an increased risk of atrial fibrillation and, mainly in postmenopausal women, reduced bone mineral density.
- Patients receiving thyroid replacement treatment for hypothyroidism and who have TSH values below normal should have their dose titrated to maintain a normal serum TSH level (approximately 0.5–5.0 mU/L).
- For patients with thyroid malignancy and in some patients with benign nodular thyroid goiter, subclinical hyperthyroidism is the aim of thyroid hormone treatment. In these patients, the benefits of TSH inhibition are thought to outweigh the risks of subclinical hyperthyroidism.
- In persons with endogenous subclinical hyperthyroidism at high risk for cardiac or skeletal complications (ie, older adults) and who have a TSH levels less than 0.1 mU/L, treatment of the underlying cause of subclinical hyperthyroidism is recommended.
- For comparable patients who have TSH concentrations between 0.1 and 0.5 mU/L, treatment is recommended if the bone density is low and/or if the thyroid radionuclide scan shows one or more focal areas of high uptake. If bone density is normal and the thyroid scan fails to show a focal area of increased

uptake, patients are typically observed. In these patients, TSH, free T4, and T3 are measured every 6 months.

- For patients with endogenous subclinical hyperthyroidism at low risk for cardiac or skeletal complications (young individuals, premenopausal women) and TSH values less than 0.1 mU/L, treatment is advised if the radionuclide scan shows one or more focal areas of high uptake. For low risk patients who have a TSH value between 0.1 and 0.5 mU/L, only observation is advised. TSH, free T4, and T3 are measured every 6 months.
- The treatment options for patients with subclinical hyperthyroidism are similar as those for frank hyperthyroidism and depend upon the basic etiology.

Conclusion

Subclinical hyperthyroidism is defined by low or undetectable serum thyroid-stimulating hormone levels, with normal free thyroxine and total or free triiodothyronine levels. It can be caused by increased endogenous production of thyroid hormone, administration of thyroid hormone for treatment of malignant thyroid disease, or unintentional excessive thyroid hormone therapy. The rate of development of overt hyperthyroidism is elevated in subjects who have suppressed thyroid-stimulating hormone levels compared with those who have low but detectable levels. Subclinical hyperthyroidism is linked with higher risk of atrial fibrillation in older adults, and with reduced bone mineral density in postmenopausal females. Possible relationships between subclinical hyperthyroidism and quality of life factors, cognition, and increased mortality rates are controversial. Prospective randomized controlled trials are required to address the results of early treatment on potential morbidities to help determine whether screening should be advocated in the asymptomatic general population.

References

1. Surks MI, Ortiz E, Daniels GH, Sawin CT, Col NF, Cobin RH, et al. Subclinical thyroid disease: scientific review and guidelines for diagnosis and management. JAMA. 2004;291:228–38.
2. Bülow Pedersen I, Knudsen N, Jørgensen T, Perrild H, Ovesen L, Laurberg P. Large differences in incidences of overt hyper- and hypothyroidism associated with a small difference in iodine intake: a prospective comparative register-based population survey. J Clin Endocrinol Metab. 2002;87:4462–9.
3. De Whalley P. Do abnormal thyroid stimulating hormone level values result in treatment changes? A study of patients on thyroxine in one general practice. Br J Gen Pract. 1995;45:93–5.
4. Canaris GJ, Manowitz NR, Mayor G, Ridgway EC. The Colorado thyroid disease prevalence study. Arch Intern Med. 2000;160:526–34.
5. Taylor PN, Iqbal A, Minassian C, Sayers A, Draman MS, Greenwood R, et al. Falling threshold for treatment of borderline elevated thyrotropin levels-balancing benefits and risks: evidence from a large community-based study. JAMA Intern Med. 2014; 174:32–9.
6. Díez JJ. Hyperthyroidism in patients older than 55 years: an analysis of the etiology and management. Gerontology. 2003;49:316–23.
7. Rieu M, Bekka S, Sambor B, Berrod JL, Fombeur JP. Prevalence of subclinical hyperthyroidism and relationship between thyroid hormonal status and thyroid ultrasonographic parameters in patients with non-toxic nodular goitre. Clin Endocrinol (Oxf). 1993;39:67–71.
8. Charkes ND. The many causes of subclinical hyperthyroidism. Thyroid. 1996;6:391–6.
9. Kasagi K, Hatabu H, Tokuda Y, Iida Y, Endo K, Konishi J. Studies on thyrotrophin receptor antibodies in patients with euthyroid Graves' disease. Clin Endocrinol (Oxf). 1988;29:357–66.
10. Murakami M, Koizumi Y, Aizawa T, Yamada T, Takahashi Y, Watanabe T, et al. Studies of thyroid function and immune parameters in patients with hyperthyroid Graves' disease in remission. J Clin Endocrinol Metab. 1988;66:103–8.
11. Sawin CT, Geller A, Kaplan MM, Bacharach P, Wilson PW, Hershman JM. Low serum thyrotropin (thyroid-stimulating hormone) in older persons without hyperthyroidism. Arch Intern Med. 1991;151:165–8.
12. Eggertsen R, Petersen K, Lundberg PA, Nyström E, Lindstedt G. Screening for thyroid disease in a primary care unit with a thyroid stimulating hormone assay with a low detection limit. BMJ. 1988;297:1586–92.
13. Bagchi N, Brown TR, Parish RF. Thyroid dysfunction in adults over age 55 years. A study in an urban US community. Arch Intern Med. 1990;150:785–7.
14. Parle JV, Franklyn JA, Cross KW, Jones SC, Sheppard MC. Prevalence and follow-up of abnormal thyrotrophin (TSH) concentrations in the elderly in the

United Kingdom. Clin Endocrinol (Oxf). 1991;34: 77–83.
15. Franklyn JA, Black EG, Betteridge J, Sheppard MC. Comparison of second and third generation methods for measurement of serum thyrotropin in patients with overt hyperthyroidism, patients receiving thyroxine therapy, and those with nonthyroidal illness. J Clin Endocrinol Metab. 1994;78:1368–71.
16. Sundbeck G, Jagenburg R, Johansson PM, Edén S, Lindstedt G. Clinical significance of low serum thyrotropin concentration by chemiluminometric assay in 85-year-old women and men. Arch Intern Med. 1991;151:549–56.
17. Sawin CT, Geller A, Wolf PA, Belanger AJ, Baker E, Bacharach P, et al. Low serum thyrotropin concentrations as a risk factor for atrial fibrillation in older persons. N Engl J Med. 1994;331:1249–52.
18. Hollowell JG, Staehling NW, Flanders WD, Hannon WH, Gunter EW, Spencer CA, et al. Serum TSH, T(4), and thyroid antibodies in the United States population (1988 to 1994): National Health and Nutrition Examination Survey (NHANES III). J Clin Endocrinol Metab. 2002;87:489–99.
19. Aghini-Lombardi F, Antonangeli L, Martino E, Vitti P, Maccherini D, Leoli F, et al. The spectrum of thyroid disorders in an iodine-deficient community: the Pescopagano survey. J Clin Endocrinol Metab. 1999;84:561–6.
20. Belin RM, Astor BC, Powe NR, Ladenson PW. Smoke exposure is associated with a lower prevalence of serum thyroid autoantibodies and thyrotropin concentration elevation and a higher prevalence of mild thyrotropin concentration suppression in the third National Health and Nutrition Examination Survey (NHANES III). J Clin Endocrinol Metab. 2004;89:6077–86.
21. Rosario PW. Natural history of subclinical hyperthyroidism in elderly patients with TSH between 0.1 and 0.4 mIU/l: a prospective study. Clin Endocrinol (Oxf). 2010;72:685–8.
22. Rosario PW. The natural history of subclinical hyperthyroidism in patients below the age of 65 years. Clin Endocrinol (Oxf). 2008;68:491–2.
23. Woeber KA. Observations concerning the natural history of subclinical hyperthyroidism. Thyroid. 2005;15:687–91.
24. Stanbury JB, Ermans AE, Bourdoux P, Todd C, Oken E, Tonglet R, et al. Iodine-induced hyperthyroidism: occurrence and epidemiology. Thyroid. 1998;8: 83–100.
25. Meyerovitch J, Rotman-Pikielny P, Sherf M, Battat E, Levy Y, Surks MI. Serum thyrotropin measurements in the community: five-year follow-up in a large network of primary care physicians. Arch Intern Med. 2007;167:1533–8.
26. Schouten BJ, Brownlie BEW, Frampton CM, Turner JG. Subclinical thyrotoxicosis in an outpatient population - predictors of outcome. Clin Endocrinol (Oxf). 2011;74:257–61.
27. Vadiveloo T, Donnan PT, Cochrane L, Leese GP. The Thyroid Epidemiology, Audit, and Research Study (TEARS): the natural history of endogenous subclinical hyperthyroidism. J Clin Endocrinol Metab. 2011;96:E1–8.
28. Das G, Ojewuyi TA, Baglioni P, Geen J, Premawardhana LD, Okosieme OE. Serum thyrotrophin at baseline predicts the natural course of subclinical hyperthyroidism. Clin Endocrinol (Oxf). 2012;77:146–51.
29. Biondi B, Palmieri EA, Fazio S, Cosco C, Nocera M, Saccà L, et al. Endogenous subclinical hyperthyroidism affects quality of life and cardiac morphology and function in young and middle-aged patients. J Clin Endocrinol Metab. 2000;85:4701–5.
30. Petretta M, Bonaduce D, Spinelli L, Vicario ML, Nuzzo V, Marciano F, et al. Cardiovascular haemodynamics and cardiac autonomic control in patients with subclinical and overt hyperthyroidism. Eur J Endocrinol. 2001;145:691–6.
31. Auer J, Scheibner P, Mische T, Langsteger W, Eber O, Eber B. Subclinical hyperthyroidism as a risk factor for atrial fibrillation. Am Heart J. 2001;142: 838–42.
32. Cappola AR, Fried LP, Arnold AM, Danese MD, Kuller LH, Burke GL, et al. Thyroid status, cardiovascular risk, and mortality in older adults. JAMA. 2006;295:1033–41.
33. Ochs N, Auer R, Bauer DC, Nanchen D, Gussekloo J, Cornuz J, et al. Meta analysis: subclinical thyroid dysfunction and the risk for coronary heart disease and mortality. Ann Intern Med. 2008;148:832–45.
34. Haentjens P, Van Meerhaeghe A, Poppe K, Velkeniers B. Subclinical thyroid dysfunction and mortality: an estimate of relative and absolute excess all-cause mortality based on time-to-event data from cohort studies. Eur J Endocrinol. 2008;159:329–41.
35. Ittermann T, Haring R, Sauer S, Wallaschofski H, Dörr M, Nauck M, et al. Decreased serum TSH levels are not associated with mortality in the adult northeast German population. Eur J Endocrinol. 2010;162: 579–85.
36. Sgarbi JA, Matsumura LK, Kasamatsu TS, Ferreira SR, Maciel RMB. Subclinical thyroid dysfunctions are independent risk factors for mortality in a 7.5-year follow-up: the Japanese-Brazilian thyroid study. Eur J Endocrinol. 2010;162:569–77.
37. Sgarbi JA, Villaça FG, Garbeline B, Villar HE, Romaldini JH. The effects of early antithyroid therapy for endogenous subclinical hyperthyroidism in clinical and heart abnormalities. J Clin Endocrinol Metab. 2003;88:1672–7.
38. Faber J, Wiinberg N, Schifter S, Mehlsen J. Haemodynamic changes following treatment of subclinical and overt hyperthyroidism. Eur J Endocrinol. 2001;145:391–6.
39. Heeringa J, Hoogendoorn EH, van der Deure WM, Hofman A, Peeters RP, Hop WCJ, et al. High-normal thyroid function and risk of atrial fibrillation: the Rotterdam study. Arch Intern Med. 2008;168: 2219–24.
40. Gammage MD, Parle JV, Holder RL, Roberts LM, Hobbs FDR, Wilson S, et al. Association between

serum free thyroxine concentration and atrial fibrillation. Arch Intern Med. 2007;167:928–34.
41. Vadiveloo T, Donnan PT, Cochrane L, Leese GP. The Thyroid Epidemiology, Audit, and Research Study (TEARS): morbidity in patients with endogenous subclinical hyperthyroidism. J Clin Endocrinol Metab. 2011;96:1344–51.
42. Nanchen D, Gussekloo J, Westendorp RGJ, Stott DJ, Jukema JW, Trompet S, et al. Subclinical thyroid dysfunction and the risk of heart failure in older persons at high cardiovascular risk. J Clin Endocrinol Metab. 2012;97:852–61.
43. Gencer B, Collet T-H, Virgini V, Bauer DC, Gussekloo J, Cappola AR, et al. Subclinical thyroid dysfunction and the risk of heart failure events: an individual participant data analysis from 6 prospective cohorts. Circulation. 2012;126:1040–9.
44. Selmer C, Olesen JB, Hansen ML, von Kappelgaard LM, Madsen JC, Hansen PR, et al. Subclinical and overt thyroid dysfunction and risk of all-cause mortality and cardiovascular events: a large population study. J Clin Endocrinol Metab. 2014;99:2372–82.
45. Biondi B, Cooper DS. The clinical significance of subclinical thyroid dysfunction. Endocr Rev. 2008;29:76–131.
46. Cooper DS, Biondi B. Subclinical thyroid disease. Lancet. 2012;379:1142–54.
47. Yavuz DG, Yazici D, Toprak A, Deyneli O, Aydin H, Yüksel M, et al. Exogenous subclinical hyperthyroidism impairs endothelial function in nodular goiter patients. Thyroid. 2008;18:395–400.
48. Dörr M, Robinson DM, Wallaschofski H, Schwahn C, John U, Felix SB, et al. Low serum thyrotropin is associated with high plasma fibrinogen. J Clin Endocrinol Metab. 2006;91:530–4.
49. Demir T, Akinci B, Comlekci A, Karaoglu O, Ozcan MA, Yener S, et al. Levothyroxine (LT4) suppression treatment for benign thyroid nodules alters coagulation. Clin Endocrinol (Oxf). 2009;71:446–50.
50. Eustatia-Rutten CFA, Corssmit EPM, Heemstra KA, Smit JWA, Schoemaker RC, Romijn JA, et al. Autonomic nervous system function in chronic exogenous subclinical thyrotoxicosis and the effect of restoring euthyroidism. J Clin Endocrinol Metab. 2008;93:2835–41.
51. Mercuro G, Panzuto MG, Bina A, Leo M, Cabula R, Petrini L, et al. Cardiac function, physical exercise capacity, and quality of life during long-term thyrotropin-suppressive therapy with levothyroxine: effect of individual dose tailoring. J Clin Endocrinol Metab. 2000;85:159–64.
52. Van de Ven AC, Netea-Maier RT, de Vegt F, Ross HA, Sweep FCGJ, Kiemeney LA, et al. Associations between thyroid function and mortality: the influence of age. Eur J Endocrinol. 2014;171:183–91.
53. Collet T-H, Gussekloo J, Bauer DC, den Elzen WPJ, Cappola AR, Balmer P, et al. Subclinical hyperthyroidism and the risk of coronary heart disease and mortality. Arch Intern Med. 2012;172:799–809.
54. Flynn RW, Bonellie SR, Jung RT, MacDonald TM, Morris AD, Leese GP. Serum thyroid-stimulating hormone concentration and morbidity from cardiovascular disease and fractures in patients on long-term thyroxine therapy. J Clin Endocrinol Metab. 2010;95:186–93.
55. Abe E, Marians RC, Yu W, Wu XB, Ando T, Li Y, et al. TSH is a negative regulator of skeletal remodeling. Cell. 2003;115:151–62.
56. Rosario PW. Bone and heart abnormalities of subclinical hyperthyroidism in women below the age of 65 years. Arq Bras Endocrinol Metabol. 2008;52: 1448–51.
57. Uzzan B, Campos J, Cucherat M, Nony P, Boissel JP, Perret GY. Effects on bone mass of long term treatment with thyroid hormones: a meta-analysis. J Clin Endocrinol Metab. 1996;81:4278–89.
58. Faber J, Jensen IW, Petersen L, Nygaard B, Hegedüs L, Siersbaek-Nielsen K. Normalization of serum thyrotrophin by means of radioiodine treatment in subclinical hyperthyroidism: effect on bone loss in postmenopausal women. Clin Endocrinol (Oxf). 1998;48:285–90.
59. Greenlund LJS, Nair KS, Brennan MD. Changes in body composition in women following treatment of overt and subclinical hyperthyroidism. Endocr Pract. 2008;14:973–8.
60. Kalmijn S, Mehta KM, Pols HA, Hofman A, Drexhage HA, Breteler MM. Subclinical hyperthyroidism and the risk of dementia. The Rotterdam study. Clin Endocrinol (Oxf). 2000;53:733–7.
61. Tan ZS, Beiser A, Vasan RS, Au R, Auerbach S, Kiel DP, et al. Thyroid function and the risk of Alzheimer disease: the Framingham Study. Arch Intern Med. 2008;168:1514–20.
62. Ceresini G, Lauretani F, Maggio M, Ceda GP, Morganti S, Usberti E, et al. Thyroid function abnormalities and cognitive impairment in elderly people: results of the Invecchiare in Chianti study. J Am Geriatr Soc. 2009;57:89–93.
63. De Jong FJ, den Heijer T, Visser TJ, de Rijke YB, Drexhage HA, Hofman A, et al. Thyroid hormones, dementia, and atrophy of the medial temporal lobe. J Clin Endocrinol Metab. 2006;91:2569–73.
64. Moon JH, Park YJ, Kim TH, Han JW, Choi SH, Lim S, et al. Lower-but-normal serum TSH level is associated with the development or progression of cognitive impairment in elderly: Korean Longitudinal Study on Health and Aging (KLoSHA). J Clin Endocrinol Metab. 2014;99:424–32.
65. Roberts LM, Pattison H, Roalfe A, Franklyn J, Wilson S, Hobbs FDR, et al. Is subclinical thyroid dysfunction in the elderly associated with depression or cognitive dysfunction? Ann Intern Med. 2006;145:573–81.
66. Moon JH, Ahn S, Seo J, Han JW, Kim KM, Choi SH, et al. The effect of long-term thyroid-stimulating hormone suppressive therapy on the cognitive function of elderly patients with differentiated thyroid carcinoma. J Clin Endocrinol Metab. 2014;99:3782–9.

67. Samuels MH, Kolobova I, Smeraglio A, Peters D, Janowsky JS, Schuff KG. The effects of levothyroxine replacement or suppressive therapy on health status, mood, and cognition. J Clin Endocrinol Metab. 2014;99:843–51.
68. Abraham-Nordling M, Wallin G, Lundell G, Törring O. Thyroid hormone state and quality of life at long-term follow-up after randomized treatment of Graves' disease. Eur J Endocrinol. 2007;156:173–9.
69. Bell RJ, Rivera-Woll L, Davison SL, Topliss DJ, Donath S, Davis SR. Well-being, health-related quality of life and cardiovascular disease risk profile in women with subclinical thyroid disease – a community-based study. Clin Endocrinol (Oxf). 2007;66:548–56.
70. Schlote B, Schaaf L, Schmidt R, Pohl T, Vardarli I, Schiebeler H, et al. Mental and physical state in subclinical hyperthyroidism: investigations in a normal working population. Biol Psychiatry. 1992;32:48–56.
71. Eustatia-Rutten CFA, Corssmit EPM, Pereira AM, Frölich M, Bax JJ, Romijn JA, et al. Quality of life in longterm exogenous subclinical hyperthyroidism and the effects of restoration of euthyroidism, a randomized controlled trial. Clin Endocrinol (Oxf). 2006;64:284–91.
72. Samuels MH, Schuff KG, Carlson NE, Carello P, Janowsky JS. Health status, mood, and cognition in experimentally induced subclinical thyrotoxicosis. J Clin Endocrinol Metab. 2008;93:1730–6.
73. Carr D, McLeod DT, Parry G, Thornes HM. Fine adjustment of thyroxine replacement dosage: comparison of the thyrotrophin releasing hormone test using a sensitive thyrotrophin assay with measurement of free thyroid hormones and clinical assessment. Clin Endocrinol (Oxf). 1988;28:325–33.
74. Casey BM, Dashe JS, Wells CE, McIntire DD, Leveno KJ, Cunningham FG. Subclinical hyperthyroidism and pregnancy outcomes. Obstet Gynecol. 2006;107:337–41.
75. Helfand M. U.S. Preventive Services Task Force. Screening for subclinical thyroid dysfunction in non-pregnant adults: a summary of the evidence for the U.S. Preventive Services Task Force. Ann Intern Med. 2004;140:128–41.
76. Biondi B, Cooper DS. Benefits of thyrotropin suppression versus the risks of adverse effects in differentiated thyroid cancer. Thyroid. 2010;20:135–46.
77. Mudde AH, Houben AJ, Nieuwenhuijzen Kruseman AC. Bone metabolism during anti-thyroid drug treatment of endogenous subclinical hyperthyroidism. Clin Endocrinol (Oxf). 1994;41:421–4.

Subclinical Hypothyroidism 11

Asim Hassan

Abstract

Subclinical hypothyroidism, is defined as normal serum levels of FT4 and T3, but mildly elevated serum TSH levels, usually less than 10 mU/L. This represents the mildest form of hypothyroidism and is a consequence of the very sensitive feedback relationship between the thyroid and the pituitary gland. In this situation, a small decrement in thyroid hormone output by the thyroid gland, in which serum T4 levels are still within the normal range, results in a serum TSH level that is elevated, albeit usually less than 10 mU/L.

Whether subclinical hypothyroidism is a significant health problem that warrants therapy is a matter of debate. Some patients may have mild symptoms of hypothyroidism as well as increased lipid levels and other risk factors for atherosclerotic cardiovascular disease. There may be progression to overt hypothyroidism over time, especially if serum levels of antithyroid antibodies are high. On the other hand, most patients are asymptomatic, especially when TSH serum levels are less than 10 mU/L, and the link between atherosclerosis is still controversial.

Subclinical hypothyroidism is usually due to underlying Hashimoto thyroiditis. The major complication of Hashimoto thyroiditis is progressive hypothyroidism. Most patients with Hashimoto thyroiditis initially have a small goiter and subclinical hypothyroidism. This is in contrast to overt hypothyroidism, in which FT4 levels are subnormal. The clinical picture of fully developed myxedema is usually quite clear, but the symptoms and signs of mild or subclinical hypothyroidism may be very subtle or absent. This has led to the recommendation by some professional organizations that screening for hypothyroidism be undertaken, especially in

A. Hassan, FRCP, SCE/MRCP (Diab, Endo)
University Diabetes Center, King Saud University,
Riyadh, Saudi Arabia
e-mail: drahassan2@hotmail.com

S.K. Imam, S.I. Ahmad (eds.), *Thyroid Disorders: Basic Science and Clinical Practice*,
DOI 10.1007/978-3-319-25871-3_11

high-risk groups, such as older women where the prevalence is high (up to 20 % in women >age 65), and in pregnant women, where untreated hypothyroidism may cause adverse outcomes in the child.

The treatment of subclinical hypothyroidism is a matter of debate but is often instituted because of (1) mild symptoms; (2) dyslipidemia which could be ameliorated by T4 therapy; and (3) positive antithyroid antibody titers, which predicts a higher chance of progression to overt hypothyroidism over time. Sufficient T4 is given to normalize TSH and allow regression of the goiter.

Introduction

Subclinical hypothyroidism (SCH) is diagnosed when thyroid hormone levels are within normal range but serum thyroid-stimulating hormone (TSH) levels are mildly elevated. Biochemically subclinical hypothyroidism (SCH) is defined as a serum thyroid-stimulating hormone (TSH) level above the upper limit of normal with normal serum free thyroxine [1]. Serum TSH has a log-linear relationship with serum thyroid hormone levels (a twofold change in free thyroxine will produce a 100-fold change in TSH). Hence, serum TSH evaluation is the essential test for diagnosis of SCH when the serum thyroid hormone levels are within normal reference range [1]. The individual range for circulating thyroid hormones is narrower than the population reference range; hence, a slight reduction within the normal range will result in a rise of serum TSH above normal range.

> Subclinical hypothyroidism is biochemically defined as a normal serum free thyroxine (T4) level with elevated serum thyroid-stimulating hormone (TSH) levels

Epidemiology

Subclinical hypothyroidism or mild thyroid failure is a frequent problem, with a prevalence of 3–8 % in the population without known thyroid disorder [2, 3]. The prevalence rises with age and is higher in women [2]. Eighty percent of patients with SCH, have a serum TSH of less than 10 mIU/L. The most important consequence of SCH is high probability of development of overt hypothyroidism.

> A significant number of subjects with subclinical hypothyroidism finally progress to overt hypothyroidism

In NHANES III survey, which did not include patients with known thyroid disorder, 3 % of 16,533 people found to have developed subclinical hypothyroidism [2]. The prevalence is less in blacks than in whites. Though, the prevalence is determined by the upper limit of normal for serum thyroid-stimulating hormone (TSH). If the upper limit of normal increases with age, as suggested, then the prevalence may not be as high as has been previously thought.

In European population, where iodine intake is inconsistent, subclinical hypothyroidism is more common in areas of iodine adequacy. In one study, the occurrence of subclinical hypothyroidism ranged from 4.2 % in iodine scarce areas to 23.9 % in an area of abundant iodine intake, despite a similar incidence of patients with high serum levels of antithyroid peroxidase (anti-TPO) antibodies [4].

Beyond the sixth decade of life, the occurrence in males reaches that of females, with a collective prevalence of 10 % [2]. Antithyroid antibodies can be detected in 80 % of subjects with SCH.

Etiology

Majority of patients have chronic autoimmune (Hashimoto's) thyroiditis with elevated serum levels of antithyroid peroxidase (anti-TPO, previously known as antithyroid microsomal) antibodies [5]. Other major diagnoses include prior radioactive iodine ablation or antithyroid drug treatment for hypterthyroidism; previous partial thyroidectomy, external radiation therapy in subjects with Hodgkin lymphoma, leukemia, or brain tumors; insufficient thyroxine replacement for frank hypothyroidism; and drugs effecting thyroid function.

> Antithyroid antibodies can be detected in 80 % of subjects with SCH, and 80 % of persons with SCH have a serum TSH of less than 10 mIU/L.

Before confirmation of SCH, other causes of raised TSH concentration, such as healing from nonthyroidal illness, assay inconsistency, presence of heterophile antibodies interfering with the TSH evaluation, and some patients with central hypothyroidism with biologically inactive TSH and thyroid hormone resistance, should be considered. Nevertheless, the most common cause of raised TSH is autoimmune thyroid disotder [1]. Earlier radioiodine therapy, thyroid gland surgery, and external neck radiation can also cause mild thyroid dysfunction. Temporary SCH may result after granulomatous, silent, and postpartum Thyroiditis [1, 6]. The causes of subclinical hypothyroidism are the same as those of frank hypothyroidism (Table 11.1).

The clinical significance of and treatment for mild increase of serum TSH (<10 mIU/L) and the exact upper level of normal for the serum TSH level remain controversial [7–10]. When the TSH concentration is above 10 mIU/L, levothyroxine therapy is usually approved to be appropriate [11, 12]. However, management of subjects with a serum TSH level of less than 10 mIU/L is controversial [13]. Some investigators argue for routine and some for selective treatment [11, 12].

Table 11.1 Etiology of subclinical hypothyroidism

Hashimoto's thyroiditis (Associations: personal or family history of other autoimmune disorders, family history of autoimmune thyroid disorder, Turner's syndrome, Down syndrome)
Thyroid damage: partial thyroidectomy or other neck surgery, radioactive iodine treatment, head and neck external radiotherapy
Constant TSH rise in postpartum thyroiditis, subacute thyroiditis, painless thyroiditis
Medications causing thyroid dysfunction: iodine, iodine-containing drugs (radiological contrast media, amiodarone), lithium carbonate, interferon α, sulfonamides, sulfonylureas, aminoglutethimide, and ethionamide
Insufficient replacement for obvious hypothyroidism (not enough dosage, noncompliance, drug interactions [calcium carbonate, iron, cholestyramine, dietary fiber, soy, etc.], raised T_4 metabolism [phenobarbital, phenytoin, carbamazepine, etc.], poor absorption)
Secondary hypothyroidism with reduced TSH bioactivity
Infiltration of thyroid (amyloidosis, hemochromatosis, sarcoidosis, cystinosis, Riedel's thyroiditis, AIDS, primary thyroid lymphoma)
TSH receptor gene alterations; Gα gene mutations
Lethal substances: environmental and industrial agents

A meta-analysis of 14 randomized clinical trials including a total of 350 patients concluded that levothyroxine replacement for SCH does not result in enhanced survival or reduced cardiovascular morbidity. Results on health-related quality of life and symptoms did not show marked differences among intervention groups. Some data suggests that levothyroxine therapy improves some aspects of lipid profiles and left ventricular function [14].

Screening for Subclinical Hypothyroidism

"Screening" refers to the evaluation of thyroid function tests in asymptomatic subjects at risk of having thyroid disease who are currently not known to have thyroid disease. The primary advantage of screening is the recognition of hypothyroidism before the occurrence of symptoms.

Consistent national guidelines for screening for thyroid disease with serum TSH levels have not been developed. However, due to the high occurrence of SCH and related metabolic risk issues such as hyperlipidemia, the American Thyroid Association advocates screening by checking serum TSH starting at the age of 35 years and every 5 years afterwards [15]. The proof in favor of screening is specially convincing in females, but it can also be justified for males as a moderately cost-effective measure in the context of the regular health evaluation. Patients with symptoms and signs potentially related to thyroid dysfunction and those with risk factors for its occurrence may need more frequent serum TSH testing [15]. The American College of Physicians recognizes that treatment for subclinical thyroid dysfunction is contentious but recommends that screening to detect thyroid dysfunction may be indicated in females more than 50 years old [16]. Because of potential consequences of SCH for unfavorable outcome of pregnancy and neurological and psychiatric development of the fetus, intensive case finding in pregnant women or in females planning pregnancy has been advised [11, 17, 18]. However, depending only on intensive case finding results in missing a third of women with frank hypothyroidism or SCH [19].

Before recommending routine screening of the general population, large-scale randomized trials are needed to prove that treatment will improve quality of life in otherwise healthy patients who have mildly elevated TSH level (5–10 mIU/L) typical of most SCH cases. For the time being, physicians should keep a low threshold for requesting a serum TSH level in females who have vague suggestive symptoms, who are pregnant or anticipating pregnancy, or who have a strong family history of autoimmune thyroid disorder. Many endocrinologist advise routine screening before and during pregnancy [19].

> Physicians should keep a low threshold for requesting a serum TSH level in females who have vague suggestive symptoms, who are pregnant or anticipating pregnancy, or who have a strong family history of autoimmune thyroid disorder.

SCH is frequent in the adult population [20]. However, there is no clear proof that early diagnosis and therapy with thyroxine (T4) improves outcomes in patients with hypothyroidism diagnosed by screening. Although thyroxine replacement treatment has few side effects when properly given, over-replacement with thyroxine is common and may be linked with adverse skeletal and cardiovascular outcomes, particularly in older persons.

There are two methods for screening asymptomatic persons: testing all persons over a specific age (when risk of hypothyroidism rises) or evaluating only those persons with clinical risk factors for hypothyroidism. In the absence of evidence favoring any screening strategy, it is advised testing patients at increased risk for hypothyroidism, including persons with goiter, history of autoimmune disorder, past history of radioactive iodine therapy, head and neck irradiation, family history of thyroid disorder, and use of drugs that may adversely affect thyroid function.

It is recommended to measure serum thyroid-stimulating hormone (TSH) as a screening test for hypothyroidism.

> It is advised testing patients at increased risk for hypothyroidism, including persons with goiter, history of autoimmune disorder, past history of radioactive iodine therapy, head and neck irradiation, family history of thyroid disorder, and use of drugs that may adversely affect thyroid function.

Diagnosis

The detection of SCH depends upon biochemical evaluation alone. Subclinical hypothyroidism is defined as a normal serum free thyroxine (T4) and raised thyroid-stimulating hormone (TSH) [21–23]. It may be symptomatic or asymptomatic for mild symptoms of hypothyroidism. Majority of patients have serum TSH levels <10 mU/L and have no symptoms.

> It is recommended to measure serum thyroid-stimulating hormone (TSH) as a screening test for hypothyroidism.

In the majority of patients, the first screening test for thyroid disorder is the serum TSH. If the serum TSH level is raised, the TSH measurement should be repeated along with a serum free T4 to confirm the diagnosis of SCH. Because the serum TSH can be temporarily elevated, a serum TSH measurement should be repeated after 1–3 months to confirm the diagnosis. However, in situation where there is a strong indication for thyroxine therapy, such as pregnancy or infertility, thyroxine replacement should be started if the serum TSH is raised when repeated along with the serum free T4.

For pregnant females, elevated TSH should be defined using trimester-specific TSH reference ranges However in non-pregnant adults, raised serum TSH is defined as a TSH concentration above the upper level of the normal TSH reference range, which is classically 4–5 mU/L in most cases. There is significant disagreement over the appropriate upper level of normal for serum TSH. Some experts have advised that the true upper limit is only 2.5 or 3 mU/L in healthy subjects without thyroid disorder, while others suggest that the serum TSH level shifts towards higher values with age, irrespective of the presence of antithyroid antibodies [7]. In such situation, the upper limit of normal could be as high as 6–8 mU/L in healthy elderly patients.

What Is the Upper Limit of Normal for the Serum TSH Level?

Reducing the upper limit of normal for the serum TSH level from 5.0 to 3.0 or even 2.5 mIU/L has been suggested [8, 10] but such suggestions have been met with a lot of criticism [7, 9]. The strongest support in favor of reducing the upper limit of normal for the serum TSH level is the higher level of antithyroid antibodies found in patients with a serum TSH level between 3.0 and 5.0 mIU/L and the higher rate of development of clinical thyroid disease [10]. After exclusion of subjects with antithyroid antibodies, goiter, and a family history of thyroid disease, the mean serum TSH is found to be 1.5 mIU/L. The serum TSH distribution curve is not a typical bell shaped; there is a tail end at the upper limits of normal. If the distribution is extrapolated to be Gaussian, then the upper limit for the 97.5th percentile will be 2.5 mIU/L [10]. The reason against lowering the upper level of normal for TSH value is that 22–28 million more Americans would be diagnosed with hypothyroidism without any clinical or therapeutic benefit from this diagnosis [9].

Furthermore other data also suggests that lowering the upper limit of the TSH reference range to 3.0 mIU/L would result in more than a fourfold increase in diagnosis of hypothyroidism among persons without history of thyroid disorder seen in a tertiary care center [24]. No obvious data supports a benefit for intervention at these concentration of TSH. Moreover, reducing the level of TSH from the upper level of normal to lower normal range by adjustment of levothyroxine dose does not improve any quality of life [25]. Scrutiny of the statistics from the National Health and Nutrition Examination Survey III study has indicated that serum TSH distribution continuously moves toward higher levels (NHANES) with age and that the occurrence of SCH may be considerably overestimated with advancing age groups unless an age-specific range for TSH is determined [7]. In an analysis of 766 persons with inconclusive findings on antithyroid antibody tests, normal results on thyroid ultrasonography, and no proof of thyroid disease, Hamilton et al. [26] decided that a serum TSH level of 4.1 mIU/L to be the upper normal level. This number is more acceptable clinically and practically.

Although patients with a TSH level within 3.0 and 5.0 mIU/L are more probable to have positive antithyroid antibodies and future thyroid disease, the lack of substantiation for a benefit from levothyroxine treatment at these concentrations makes keeping the upper limit of TSH at 4.0–5.0

more rational. For patients more than 70 years, levels up to 6.0 or even 7.0 mIU/L with negative antithyroid antibodies should not be diagnosed to be hypothyroid [7]. Whatever the preferred upper limit of normal, a credible case can be made for closer follow-up of patients with a TSH concentration of 3–5 mIU/L, especially if anti thyroid antibodies are positive.

Different pregnancy specific normal TSH values are suggested. The normal limits of serum TSH levels in the first trimester of pregnancy is 0.03–2.3 mIU/L; the upper limit of normal is 3.5 mIU/L in the second and third trimesters. Pregnancy related thyroid dysfunction will be covered in separate chapters.

Differential Diagnosis

There are many reasons of an elevated serum TSH values that do not exactly fit the description of subclinical hypothyroidism. These consist of the following situations:

- During the period of recovery from nonthyroidal illness, where a momentarily raised serum TSH level is detected after a stage of TSH repression.
- After the hyperthyroid period of subacute, painless, or postpartum thyroiditis, when mild hypothyroidism is frequently encountered.
- Inconsistency of test assays.
- The occurrence of heterophilic antibodies can hinder with TSH measurements in immunometric assays. These human anti-mouse gamma globulins can cause falsely elevated results [27]. Conversely, heterophilic antibodies obstruct binding of one of the mouse monoclonal antibodies to TSH and result in falsely low analysis for TSH.
- Rheumatoid factors may result in same hindrance in immunometric tests [27].
- Autoantibodies to TSH have also been detected which generate TSH-anti-TSH immunoglobulin G (IgG) complexes, also called macro-TSH, which lacks biologic action but may be immunoreactive, and cause falsely high TSH concentration (often >100 mU/L) in euthyroid (normal free T4 and triiodothyronine [T3] levels) persons [22, 28, 29]. Autoantibodies to TSH can be identified by elimination of the IgG-TSH complexes and then retesting [30].
- Non diagnosed and untreated adrenal deficiency.
- Pituitary TSH-producing adenomas, thyroid hormone resistance, and rare TSH receptor mutations. In patients with pituitary TSH-producing adenomas or thyroid hormone resistance, the high TSH is associated with raised serum free T4 and/or T3 levels. On the contrary, subjects with subclinical hypothyroidism have normal free T4 levels. Patients with TSH resistance due to abnormality in the TSH receptor have high serum TSH values and normal or low serum free T4 and T3 levels.
- Central hypothyroidism, where up to 25 % of subjects have a mildly raised serum TSH (approximately 10 mU/L) and a low or low-normal free T4.

Evaluation

A number of persons with subclinical hypothyroidism have few non-specific symptoms of hypothyroidism, such as fatigue and constipation. Therefore, individuals with subclinical hypothyroidism should be inquired about symptoms of hypothyroidism, in addition to previous treatment for hyperthyroidism, past history of frank hypothyroidism, and use of drugs that may disturb thyroid hormone absorption or function (Table 11.2). Moreover, they should also be examined for the presence of thyroid gland enlargement [31].

Antithyroid peroxidase (anti-TPO) antibodies are not routinely measured in patients with subclinical hypothyroidism. However, the detection of antibodies may be helpful in deciding to treat or monitor, and thus may be practical in individuals when the decision to treat or to monitor is not clear.

Table 11.2 Drugs causing hypothyroidism

Inhibition of thyroid hormone synthesis and/or release – thionamides, lithium, perchlorate, aminoglutethimide, thalidomide, and iodine and iodine-containing drugs including amiodarone, radiographic agents, expectorants (Organidin, Combid), kelp tablets, potassium iodine solutions (SSKI), Betadine douches, topical antiseptics
Decreased absorption of T4 – cholestyramine, colestipol, colesevelam, aluminum hydroxide, calcium carbonate, sucralfate, iron sulfate, raloxifene, omeprazole, lansoprazole, and possibly other medications that impair acid secretion, sevelemer, lanthanum carbonate, and chromium; malabsorption syndromes can also diminish T4 absorption
Immune dysregulation – interferon-alfa, interleukin-2, ipilimumab, alemtuzumab, pembrolizumab
Suppression of TSH – dopamine
Possible destructive thyroiditis – sunitinib
Increased type 3 deiodination – sorafenib
Increased T4 clearance and suppression of TSH – bexarotene

T4 thyroxine, *TSH* thyroid-stimulating hormone, *TBG* thyroxine-binding globulin, *T3* triiodothyronine

Consequences of Subclinical Hypothyroidism

Though studies have indicated to some undesirable effects of SCH, no agreement exists as to the clinical significance of the unfavorable effects and the benefits of levothyroxine treatment, mainly for the 80 % of individuals with SCH who have a TSH of less than 10 mIU/L, because of the different concentrations of TSH and severity of thyroid dysfunction in these studies [13, 32]. Following is a discussion of some of the anticipated adverse effects of SCH.

Systemic Symptoms of Hypothyroidism

Many randomized trials related to the effects of levothyroxine therapy in persons with SCH are available. One study related to persons with serum TSH levels from 5 to 10 mIU/L did not show any advantage [33]. Some data (range of TSH level, 3–32 mIU/L) showed better symptom scores or enhanced memory in one fourth of patients. Several studies have not shown significant improvement in anxiety, mood, and cognition in older patients [34–36]. In another review available data was considered inadequate to support a benefit for levothyroxine treatment in patients with SCH, specially for the cohort with TSH less than 10 mIU/ L, and a similar conclusion was again reached later [11].

Progression to Overt Hypothyroidism

Persons with SCH have a high incidence of development of clinically frank hypothyroidism, 2.6 % every year if thyroperoxidase (TPO) antibodies are negative and 4.3 % if they are positive [37]. Nevertheless, some patients do not progress any further and a number of individuals normalize. A TSH level more than 10 mIU/L predicts an elevated risk of progression, and a concentration of less than 6 mIU/L predicts a lower probability of any further progression. In a study in both males and females older than 55 years with a mean follow-up of 32 months, the TSH level normalized in 52 % of subjects with a serum TSH of lower than 10 mIU/L [38].

A significant percentage of patients with subclinical hypothyroidism ultimately develop frank hypothyroidism. In prospective studies with nearly 10–20 years of follow-up, the collective incidence of overt hypothyroidism ranges from 33 to 55 % [23, 37, 39]. The rate of further progression is associated with the preliminary serum thyroid-stimulating hormone (TSH) level (higher with TSH values >12 to >15 mU/L) and the detection of antithyroid peroxidase (anti-TPO) antibodies, [38–40]. In a study of more than 1700 individuals followed for 20 years, for instance, females with both elevated serum TSH and high thyroid antibody levels developed hypothyroidism at a rate of 4.3 % per year (cumulative incidence 55 %) [37]. In a different study in which 82 females were followed for 9.2 years, the overall incidence of frank hypothyroidism was zero percent for individuals with initial TSH levels of 4–6 mU/L [39].

The primary disorder also may be a determining factor for the risk of development of overt hypothyroidism [23]. Subjects who have autoimmune thyroid disease or received radioiodine therapy or high-dose external radiation are liable to progress to overt hypothyroidism. On the contrary, subclinical hypothyroidism is likely to continue in those who have had thyroid surgery for reasons other than hyperthyroidism, or in those who were given external radiation during childhood.

Natural recovery has also been seen in subjects with subclinical hypothyroidism, although the incidence of this occurrence is not clear [38, 39, 41, 42]. In a data of 422,242 subjects without known thyroid disease, serum TSH was elevated (5.5 to ≤10 mU/L) in 3 % [42]. In a 5-year follow-up period, TSH levels normalized without treatment in 62 % of patients. Reversal of serum TSH levels is more likely to occur in persons with negative antithyroid antibodies, serum TSH concentration <10 mU/I, and within the first 2 years of the diagnosis [41].

Cardiovascular Disease

The Rotterdam Study found an association of SCH with myocardial infarction and aortic calcification [43]. In contrast, the Wickham study [44] showed no higher cardiac mortality in a 20-year follow-up. Another observational study also did not show any link between undetected SCH and cardiovascular incidents or mortality [45]. However, a number of meta-analyses of observational studies showed a relationship between SCH and coronary artery disease [46–48]. The risk was lower when higher quality data were shared [47]. An analysis of 7 cohort studies concluded that the relative risk of all-cause mortality was higher compared with euthyroid controls, mainly in subjects with other comorbidities [49]. Another meta-analysis showed an increased occurrence and incidence of cardiovascular mortality only in comparatively younger patients [50]. Overall, the results of these 6 meta-analyses indicate that a cardiovascular risk exists for individuals less than 70 years with no effect on those aged 70–80 years and a perhaps a protective effect for those more than 80 years [5]. Therefore, the cardiovascular risk effect remains contentious and further robust trials are required to assess the value of levothyroxine therapy in risk reduction.

In persons with subclinical hypothyroidism, the results are inconsistent, possibly related to differences in the patient populations and study designs. A number of but not every observational study report a higher risk of coronary heart disease (CHD) in patients with subclinical hypothyroidism [43, 45, 51–56]. A meta-analysis of seven prospective cohort studies (25,977 participants, 2020 with subclinical hypothyroidism) showed a noteworthy tendency of increased rate of CHD events (nonfatal myocardial infarction, CHD death, hospitalization for angina or coronary revascularization) with elevated serum TSH levels [57]. In comparison with euthyroid individuals, subjects with TSH ≥10 mU/L had a significant rise in CHD events (38.4 versus 20.3 events/1000 person years, hazard ratio [HR] 1.89, 95 % CI 1.28–2.80). On the contrary, minimum TSH rise (4.5–6.9 mU/L) were not related with an increased risk (HR 1.00, 95 % CI 0.96–1.43). The risk rates did not differ according to age, gender, or preexisting CVD.

In a combined analysis data from six prospective cohort studies (25,390 participants, 2068 with subclinical hypothyroidism), there was also an important trend for higher risk of heart failure at higher TSH levels [58]. In comparison with euthyroid subjects, individuals with a TSH between 10 and 19.9 mU/L had a significant rise in heart failure (40 events in 224 participants [17.9 %] versus 1762 events in 22,674 controls [7.8 %], HR 1.86, 95 % CI 1.27–2.72) [59]. The elevated risk of heart failure in patients with a serum TSH between 7.0 and 9.9 mU/L was not statistically important [53], events in 422 participants [12.8 %], (HR 1.65, 95 % CI 0.84–3.23), and minimal TSH elevations (4.5–6.9 mU/L) were not connected with an increased risk (HR 1.01, 95 % CI 0.81–1.26).

A number of, but not all, studies show a link between raised TSH and total and low-density lipoprotein (LDL) cholesterol levels [5]. In one of the biggest cross-sectional data so far (25,862 participants, median age 56 years), patients with modest rise in serum TSH (between 5.1 and 10 mU/L) had considerably raised mean total cholesterol concentrations than those who had normal TSH (223 versus 216 mg/dL [5.6 versus 5.8 mmol/L]) [37]. Though, cholesterol levels were not adjusted for age. Moreover, it is not clear whether this difference is clinically significant concerning CHD risk.

Additionally, subclinical hypothyroidism has been linked with an increase in a number of other cardiovascular risk factors and surrogate cardiovascular endpoints, including markers of inflammation, vascular reactivity, endothelial function, and carotid intima media thickness [59–64]. Some individuals with subclinical hypothyroidism also have diastolic dysfunction and raised peripheral vascular resistance, as shown in patients with frank hypothyroidism [65]. On the contrary, another study showed no change in left ventricular mass or function in persons with serum TSH concentrations between 3.5 and 10 mU/L in comparison to those with normal TSH [66].

> Subclinical hypothyroidism may possibly be linked with an elevated risk of cardiovascular disease (CVD) (eg, heart failure, coronary heart disease [CHD]), mostly when the serum TSH level is above 10 mU/L.

Studies have also shown slowed left ventricular relaxation time, increased vascular tone at rest, and left ventricular systolic dysfunction with exercise and abnormal endothelial function [67]. A number of studies have shown improvement of cardiac contractibility and systolic time interval with levothyroxine treatment [67]. No proof exists to support the link between heart failure and a serum TSH level of less than 10.0 mIU/L. Yet again, most studies were not classified for degrees of TSH elevation, and data remain inadequate for a TSH concentration less than 10 mIU/L but strongly indicative for a TSH level higher than 10 mIU/L.

Cardiovascular Mortality

In a number of [52, 53] but not all [35, 45, 68, 69] studies, subjects with subclinical hypothyroidism have a higher risk of cardiovascular and/or all-cause mortality. In a data from 11 prospective cohort studies, the risk of cardiovascular mortality, but not all-cause mortality, increased with higher concentrations of TSH and was appreciably higher in individuals with TSH concentrations ≥10 mU/L (HR 1.58, 95 % CI 1.10–2.27) [57]. On the contrary, minimum rise of TSH (4.5 to 6.9 mU/L) were not related with cardiovascular or all-cause mortality.

In one prospective data, older participants (>85 years) in the Netherlands with untreated subclinical hypothyroidism (the majority with TSH between 4.8 and 10 mU/L) in fact had a lower rate of cardiovascular and all-cause mortality [35]. Similar results were found in a retrospective cohort study from Denmark; subclinical hypothyroidism with a TSH of 5–10 mIU/L was associated with a reduced all-cause mortality [70]. Though, in a prospective cohort study from the US, older persons with untreated subclinical hypothyroidism had neither higher nor lower mortality over a median follow-up period of 5 years [71].

Subsequently data using the NHANES III, subclinical hypothyroidism (median TSH 6.3 mU/L) compared with euthyroidism was linked with higher mortality in those with heart failure but not in those without heart failure [72].

Non-alcoholic Fatty Liver Disease

In an observational study, non-alcoholic fatty liver disease (NAFLD) was associated with raised serum TSH levels. One third of the subjects with subclinical hypothyroidism revealed classic ultrasonographic features of NAFLD (versus 20 % of controls) while 20 and 26 % of subjects with subclinical or overt hypothyroidism had abnormal liver enzymes [73].

Neuropsychiatric Symptoms

Data linked to provocation of depression, bipolar disorder, and effect on cognitive function have been demonstrated [74]. A study has indicated no relationship with anxiety, depression, or cognitive dysfunction [34]. However, it is still rational to have a low threshold for treatment for SCH in patients with depression, bipolar disorder, and cognitive dysfunction.

Many studies indicate that subclinical hypothyroidism is linked with neuropsychiatric diseases [75–78]. Nevertheless, additional data (together with a large study of primary care subjects in England that failed to show an association of subclinical hypothyroidism with depression, anxiety, or cognitive dysfunction) does not support these findings [22, 34–36, 79].

Neuromuscular Dysfunction

It has been proposed that neuromuscular symptoms and dysfunction are frequent in persons with SCH and can be reversed by levothyroxine therapy [80]. A conclusive decision will need more trials with TSH concentrations stratified to less than or more than 10 mIU/L.

Potential Consequences

- In a number of [81–83] but not all [84, 85] studies in middle-aged persons, increasing serum TSH levels within the normal levels or slightly above normal were linked with a modest increase in body weight. In older females (>65 years), subclinical hypothyroidism (mean TSH 6.7 mU/L) as compared with euthyroidism (TSH 2.2 mU/L) was related with a slightly higher baseline weight (0.51 kg higher baseline weight per 1 mU/L higher TSH level) but with no change over time [86]. There was no link between TSH and weight in older males.
- In one study, 21 of 33 patients (64 %) with subclinical hypothyroidism had a raised incidence of neuromuscular complaints (weakness, fatigue, paresthesias, cramps), in comparison with 6 of 44 normal persons (14 %) [87]. Conversely, in another study of more than 2000 older persons, functional mobility (walking endurance and gait speed) was better in those with mild elevations in TSH (4.5 to <7.0 mU/L) than in those with TSH concentration within the normal limits (0.4 to <4.5 mU/L) [88].
- Subclinical hypothyroidism may also be linked with shortcomings in vocal memory and managerial functioning [89, 90]. These defects correct with T4 therapy and are thought to reflect abnormal hippocampal function rather than general cognitive impairment.
- In a cross sectional study, subclinical hypothyroidism was related with an higher risk of Alzheimer disease (AD) in females but not in males [91].
- In one study, subjects with spontaneous deep venous thrombosis were more liable to have subclinical hypothyroidism [92].
- In a study, individuals with subclinical hypothyroidism were more prone to have common bile duct stones, probably secondary to sphincter of Oddi dysfunction [93].

Pregnancy

Subclinical hypothyroidism is more common than frank hypothyroidism, occurring in 2.0–2.5 % of screened females in the US [94, 95]. Undiagnosed subclinical hypothyroidism in pregnancy is a risk factor for miscarriage and low birth weight infants, and possibly poor developmental outcome in the offspring.

Undiagnosed subclinical hypothyroidism in pregnancy is a risk factor for miscarriage and low birth weight infants, and possibly poor developmental outcome in the offspring

An original study by Haddow et al. [18] showed a 7-point drop in intelligence quotient in children aged 7–9 years whose mothers had SCH during pregnancy compared with the children of mothers with normal thyroid function. Even though this was a single study, it nonetheless points to the need for screening of pregnant women and treatment for mild thyroid dysfunction in women who are pregnant or planning to become pregnant.

Effects of Thyroid Hormone Replacement

The primary clinical issue concerning individuals with subclinical hypothyroidism is whether they should be treated with thyroid hormone. On the basis of the natural history only, one might suggest that therapy should be initiated to prevent frank hypothyroidism, mainly in patients with serum thyroid-stimulating hormone (TSH) concentration ≥10 mU/L. The treatment of individuals with TSH results between 4.5 and 10 mU/L remains contentious, as studies have not demonstrated a steady benefit with therapy.

Hypothyroid Signs and Symptoms

The information concerning the association between T4 therapy and improvement in hypothyroid symptoms are contradictory, probably due to differences among the patient populations investigated, such as age, TSH values, detection of antithyroid antibodies, and history of previous thyroid disorder. In some [96–98] but not all [33, 36, 99] studies, T4 treatment resulted in better hypothyroid symptoms and/or intellectual functions. The improvement seems to be restricted to individuals with baseline serum TSH concentration ≥10 mU/L. In 12 clinical trials meta-analysis (nine trials with TSH concentrations <10 to <15 mU/L), there was no disparity in hypothyroid signs or symptoms, quality of life, or unfavorable effects between the T4 therapy and placebo groups [14].

Successive trials and a systematic review looking into the results of T4 on hypothyroid symptoms and/or cognitive function suggest minimal benefit [100]. For instance, in a double blind randomized cross-over trial of 100 subjects with serum TSH between 3.7 and 15.8 mU/L, replacement with a fixed dose of levothyroxine 0.100 mg daily resulted in an improvement in the percentage of individuals complaining of fatigue (89–79 %), but no major improvement in other quality of life parameters [101]. In this study, TSH values were below normal in some individuals (range 0.01–12.1 mU/L).

In persons with subclinical hypothyroidism and goiter, T4 therapy may reduce the size of the goiter. In a study of 13 subjects with subclinical hypothyroidism, therapy with T4 was associated with a considerable reduction (median 80 %) in thyroid volume as assessed by ultrasound [102].

Cardiovascular Disease

Even though T4 therapy has been found to improve many of cardiovascular risk aspects and surrogate cardiovascular markers in subjects with subclinical hypothyroidism, including dyslipidemia, markers of inflammation, vascular smooth muscle proliferation, vascular reactivity, ventricular function, endothelial function, and carotid intima media thickness, statistics indicating its ability to decrease cardiovascular events are lacking [59, 63, 65, 101, 103–109]. In a study of the UK General Practitioner Research Database, ischemic heart disease endpoints were less frequent in those individuals aged 40–70 years given levothyroxine (68 events in 1634 treated patients [4.2 %] versus 97 events in 1459 untreated patients [6.6 %], hazard ratio [HR] 0.61 [95 % CI 0.39–0.95]) [110]. On the other hand in subjects over age 70 years there was no benefit of therapy (104 events in 819 treated patients [12.7 %] versus 88 events in 823 untreated patients [10.7 %], HR 0.99) [110]. The risk of unfavorable cardiovascular events linked with over treatment when thyroxine is given, mainly in older adults, is unknown. Therefore, studies are required to evaluate whether thyroid hormone treatment lowers cardiovascular disease (CVD) events in subjects with subclinical hypothyroidism.

Serum Lipid and Apoprotein Concentrations

The consequences of T4 treatment on lipids is not clear. A number of studies show benefit, but the results are conflicting and the extent of the effect is of vague clinical significance [100]. In 12 clinical trials meta-analysis (nine trials with TSH concentrations <10 or 15 mU/L), seven of the studies analyzed lipid concentration after therapy of subclinical hypothyroidism [14]. There were no major effects of T4 treatment on total cholesterol, high-density lipoprotein (HDL), low-density lipoprotein (LDL), triglycerides, apolipoprotein A and B, or lipoprotein (a). Though, in many studies of patients with subclinical hypothyroidism treated with thyroxine versus placebo, serum total and LDL cholesterol [59, 98, 101, 111–113] and apoprotein B-100 concentrations [98, 101, 112] reduced appreciably, while serum HDL cholesterol, triglyceride, and lipoprotein (a) levels did not change [98, 113]. All except one of these studies included subjects with serum TSH levels >10 mU/L.

Other Benefits

There may be other benefits of thyroid hormone therapy, as demonstrated by the following data:

- In a study of 113 patients with chronic kidney disease and subclinical hypothyroidism, development of renal failure was slowed by treatment with levothyroxine [114].
- Patients with concomitant iron-deficiency anemia and subclinical hypothyroidism had a higher rise in hemoglobin when given both iron and thyroid hormone treatment as compared with those given only iron [115].

Management of Subclinical Hypothyroidism

Treatment of SCH differs based on whether the serum TSH concentration is 3–5 mIU/L, 5.1–10 mIU/L, or more than 10 mIU/L.

Serum TSH Concentration of 3–5 mIu/l

Reducing the upper level of normal for the serum TSH concentration from 5.0 to 3.0 mIU/L is still contentious. Concentration between 3 and 5 mIU/L are unlikely to point toward a clinically significant impairment, and levothyroxine treatment at these concentration may or may not provide any improvement. Though individuals with a serum TSH level of 3–5 mIU/L may be at higher risk of development of hypothyroidism, [37] no clear proof of health effect exists. Actually, in a randomized, crossover, 12-week trial of persons with symptoms indicating hypothyroidism with serum TSH in the upper normal limit, no difference in psychological and cognitive function was shown between levothyroxine-replacement and control groups [25]. Given these results, treatment cannot be proposed for this group, but follow-up by serum TSH testing in 1 year would be a sensible approach, mainly if anti-thyroid antibodies are positive.

Serum TSH Concentration of 5.1–10 mIu/l

Major randomized trials to convincingly demonstrate lowering of cholesterol with levothyroxine replacement in this subgroup are deficient. Most studies are not classified for various levels of serum TSH concentrations, and even though improvement of symptoms and lipid concentration have been demonstrated for mild thyroid dysfunction as a group, results cannot be extrapolated to most subjects with SCH who are in this subgroup [98]. Another trial of TSH concentration of 5.0–10.0 mIU/L did not demonstrate any improvement [33].

Moreover, cognitive, neuropsychiatric, cardiac, and muscle impairment found in studies including a wide range of TSH concentration in SCH should be established by better randomized trials. The likelihood that a raised serum TSH concentration is a cardiovascular risk factor is still very contentious. Therefore choice for levothyroxine treatment for this cluster should be individualized and should be based on the age of the patient (in favor of treatment for younger subjects), comorbid medical conditions, degree of TSH concentration, constant and slow rise of TSH, detection of antithyroid antibodies, existence of goiter, and hypothyroid symptoms. Given both the findings of reduced intelligence quotient in the children in females who had SCH during pregnancy and the undesirable effects of mild thyroid dysfunction on pregnancy result, levothyroxine replacement should be suggested for pregnant women and women anticipating pregnancy. Due of the benefits of thyroxine on growth and development, levothyroxine replacement for children and adolescents is also practical. Treatment may be proposed for persons with a constant serum TSH concentration of more than 8 mIU/L because these levels are linked with a 70 % development to a TSH level of 10 mIU/L in 4 years.

Serum TSH Concentration Greater Than 10 mlu/l

Majority of endocrinologist are in agreement that all persons with SCH and a TSH concentration over 10 mIU/L must be given levothyroxine [13, 32]. Support is more convincing for the unfavorable effects of mild thyroid dysfunction in this group. Trials have demonstrated that levothyroxine replacement results in an 8 mg lowering of low-density lipoprotein levels [98, 116]. Amongst the causes that predict response of lipid concentration to levothyroxine replacement are higher results of TSH, insulin resistance, higher concentration of pretreatment cholesterol, and type III hyperlipidemia. Some data suggests that mild thyroid dysfunction can worsen bipolar disorder and depression [117] and that it is related with impairment of muscle function, nerve conduction, cardiac function [118], and cognitive and psychological function, with benefit after levothyroxine treatment [96–99, 118].

Candidates for T4 Replacement

Although almost all experts advocate therapy of persons with serum thyroid-stimulating hormone (TSH) levels >10 mU/L, the regular treatment of asymptomatic persons with TSH results between 4.5 and 10 mU/L remains uncertain [1, 12, 22, 31, 32]

> For persons with subclinical hypothyroidism and TSH values ≥10 mU/L, treatment with thyroid hormone (T4) is proposed

In view of evidence linking subclinical hypothyroidism with atherosclerosis and myocardial infarction, and the elevated risk of development of overt hypothyroidism, it is proposed that treatment of individuals with subclinical hypothyroidism and TSH concentrations more than 10 mU/L. This recommendation is in agreement with that of a clinical consensus panel (comprised of representatives from the Endocrine Society, American Thyroid Association (ATA), and the American Association of Clinical Endocrinologists) [31].

There is some evidence to show benefit or risk of thyroxine (T4) therapy in persons with TSH concentration between 4.5 and 10 mU/L. The recommending panel did not advocate routine replacement for such individuals, but proposed monitoring TSH concentrations and replacement based upon individual features (e.g., symptoms of hypothyroidism, positive thyroid peroxidase [TPO] antibodies). Though, others have proposed replacement for individuals with TSH results in this range because undetectable symptoms may get better, improvement of abnormal serum lipid levels are potentially cardioprotective, and there is little risk linked with controlled T4 therapy [1, 12, 32, 119].

Thyroid hormone therapy is proposed in younger persons with serum TSH values of 4.5–10 mU/L who are symptomatic for hypothyroidism. Subjects with elevated titers of anti-TPO antibodies, who may swiftly progress to overt hypothyroidism, and persons with goiter may also improve from early intervention. Many physicians propose that the detection of risk factors for cardiovascular disease (CVD) is reasonable for commencing treatment [5]. Others warn that over treatment with T4 is frequent, happening in as many as 41 % of subjects ≥65 years of age, and that overtreatment may result in adverse outcomes, such as cardiac dysrhythmias, particularly in older persons [120]. Thus, older patients (over age 70 years) with subclinical hypothyroidism and TSH between 4.5 and 8 mU/L are not candidates for replacement therapy.

> For older persons (over age 70 years) with subclinical hypothyroidism and TSH between 4.5 and 8 mU/L, no treatment is suggested, considering the doubtful benefits and the possibility of both cardiovascular and skeletal risks related with unintentional excess treatment

It is suggested to start T4 therapy in pregnant ladies with subclinical hypothyroidism (TSH concentrations above trimester-specific normal reference limit with normal free T4) and in patients with subclinical hypothyroidism who are contemplating to become pregnant or have ovulatory abnormalities and infertility. Because of the alteration in thyroid physiology during gestation, trimester-specific reference levels for TSH should be followed.

> T4 treatment in women with subclinical hypothyroidism (TSH values >2.5 mU/L) who are pregnant, who wish to become pregnant, or have ovulatory dysfunction and infertility is recommended.

Anecdotal evidence suggest that T4 replacement may be useful in persons with symptoms of hypothyroidism but normal thyroid function results. Though, in a crossover trial of 22 such patients, T4 was no more beneficial than placebo in improving cognitive function and psychological health [25]. Therefore, therapies should not be initiated for persons with hypothyroid symptoms but normal thyroid function tests.

Thyroid Peroxidase Antibodies

A high rate of fetal loss, perinatal mortality, and large-for-gestational-age babies has been shown in euthyroid subjects with raised serum antithyroid peroxidase antibody (TPO antibodies) levels [121–123]. In various studies, the detection of thyroid autoantibodies in euthyroid females is linked with an elevated risk of spontaneous abortions which is two to three times more than in subjects without antibodies [124, 125]. In addition, the risk of premature delivery is approximately two times higher [124, 126].

In a number of patients, therapy with thyroxine (T4) may improve abortion rates. In a prospective data of 115 TPO antibody positive individuals, half were randomly assigned to thyroxine (median dose 50 mcg daily) and half were not given any treatment, and compared with 869 TPO antibody negative subjects. Spontaneous abortion rates were 3.5 % in TPO antibody positive treated patients, 2.4 % in the TPO antibody negative patients, and 13.8 % in TPO antibody positive untreated patients. Premature delivery rates were 7 %, 8.2 %, and 22.4 %, respectively [127].

In the same study, a number of euthyroid patients with TPO antibodies progressed to subclinical hypothyroidism. In early gestation, the TPO positive patients had considerably raised serum thyrotropin (TSH) concentrations than TPO negative patients, even though the concentration was within the normal range. Around 20 % of TPO positive women later developed subclinical hypothyroidism by term if not treated.

Euthyroid females with TPO positive antibodies getting in vitro fertilization (IVF) also have increased miscarriage rates. In four observational studies meta-analysis (1098 women undergoing

IVF), the risk rate of miscarriage was two times higher in euthyroid women with than without positive TPO antibodies (relative risk [RR] 1.99, 95 % CI 1.42–2.78) [128]. However, in an intervention study of thyroxine versus placebo in 72 euthyroid subfertile patients with positive TPO antibodies having assisted reproductive treatment (ART), thyroid hormone treatment did not lower the risk of early fetal loss [129]. Though, these outcomes are confounded by accompanying additional infertility risks in women getting ART.

It is uncertain if the detection of TPO antibodies in euthyroid pregnant patients affects the behavioral or cognitive development of their offspring. In a community -based cohort data from the Netherlands, 4770 pregnant patients had blood extracted at 13.5 weeks of pregnancy and cord blood was taken directly after birth in 2121 of the neonates [130]. All samples were tested immediately after delivery for TSH, free T4, and thyroid peroxidase antibodies. TPO antibodies were raised in 4.7 %. TSH levels were more elevated in TPO positive than negative women (3.8 versus 1.5 mU/L), but TSH concentration in the cord blood did not vary between positive and negative women. Raised levels of TPO antibodies during gestation did not predict the vocal and non vocal cognitive function of the offspring when tested at 2.5 years. Nevertheless, offspring of euthyroid mothers with positive TPO antibodies were at elevated risk of attention deficit/hyperactivity disorder (odds ratio [OR] 1.77, 95 % CI 1.15–2.72). When the results were adjusted for maternal TSH level, the association was reduced but remained significant (OR 1.56).

The choice to treat euthyroid patients with raised TPO antibodies with levothyroxine (T4) or to watch for the progression of hypothyroidism during pregnancy is unclear. The majority of pregnant patients are not likely to know their antithyroid antibody results because routine screening is not generally done. The ATA decided there was inadequate data to propose for or against thyroxine treatment in Euthyroid antibody positive pregnant patients; though, monitoring for the progression for hypothyroidism was proposed [131].

Since closely observed thyroid hormone therapy is safe, a number of experts, propose levothyroxine treatment (T4, 50 mcg daily) in TPO positive euthyroid patients who have had repeated miscarriage, until additional evidence emerges. On the other hand, many experts do not regularly treat euthyroid TPO positive patients with T4 because of inadequate proof of benefit.

In antibody positive euthyroid pregnant female who are not given thyroid hormone, TSH should be tested every month during the first half of pregnancy and at least once during the last trimester to detect for the progression of hypothyroidism. Thyroid hormone should be started if TSH is raised above the trimester-specific reference level (2.5 mU/L for first, and 3.0 mU/L for second and third trimesters).

Arguments for Treatment

Therapy will avert development of overt hypothyroidism, particularly in those with serum TSH concentrations higher than 10 to 15 mU/L and elevated serum anti-TPO antibody levels. Replacement in persons with minor elevations in serum TSH levels may probably improve uncer tain symptoms of hypothyroidism, such as constipation, depression, or fatigue, and may reduce the size of goiter. Treatment may also benefit cardiac contractility and serum lipid levels in some individuals and additionally lower the risk of atherosclerosis.

Arguments Against Treatment

Point of view against T4 therapy include its expenditure (for both the treatment and monitoring), the lifetime obligation to daily treatment in asymptomatic individuals, the potential risk of excessive treatment and producing symptoms from extra thyroid hormone, and the likely development or worsening of angina pectoris or cardiac rhythm disturbances in vulnerable individuals [13] particularly considering data from a population based survey demonstrating that 41 % of subjects over age 65 years on thyroxine replacement had below normal serum TSH [120]. Even though these apprehensions are not usually enough to offset the possible benefits of treatment in younger subjects, a higher TSH threshold is proposed for treating older persons, especially since the upper limit of normal for serum TSH may be higher in this age group. If the patient is not treated, regular follow-up is indicated.

Goals of Treatment

The target of treatment is to lower the patient's serum TSH levels within the normal reference values. As the average serum TSH for the general population is approximately 1.4 mU/L, with 90 % with serum TSH values <3.0 mU/L, several physicians propose a clinical TSH target of 0.5–2.5 mU/L in young and middle-aged persons. A TSH goal of 3–5 mU/L may be suitable in individuals over 70 years of age.

Every person with SCH and a serum TSH level over 10 mIU/L and for subjects with serum TSH levels of 5.1–10.0 mIU/L in whom individualized choice for treatment is made, replacement should be initiated with levothyroxine. Combination of T4 plus T3 therapy is not recommended. The typical required daily levothyroxine dose is 50–75 μg [132]. In anticipation of future development of thyroid dysfunction, some physicians recommend a full replacement dose. A daily dose of 25–75 μg, is suggested based on the age of the subject, the results of free thyroxine, and the serum TSH concentration. Serum TSH should be tested after 8 weeks, and the dose should be titrated. When a normal serum TSH concentration has been reached, TSH should be analyzed again after 6 months and then every year.

Dose Modification Strategy

The advantages of modification of levothyroxine replacement to achieve lower concentration of TSH should be assessed with the prospect of undesirable effects of aggressive levothyroxine treatment resulting in suppressed TSH. There are two ways of starting T4 treatment. One approach is to initiate with the lowest dose required to control the serum TSH level, usually 25–50 mcg daily. This strategy will prevent excess treatment and is most suitable in older subjects or in patients with accompanying CVD.

For younger persons with Hashimoto's thyroiditis who do not have autonomy (e.g., a prior history of toxic adenoma or Graves' disease treated with radioiodine) and who have usual negative feedback response, another strategy is to start replacement at somewhat lower than full therapeutic doses (1.6 mcg/kg/day). This strategy prevents the need for repeated dose adjustment, in case there is further autoimmune damage of the thyroid gland. On the other hand, younger persons can be initiated on low dose replacement, as is proposed for older subjects. Dose titration and further follow up adjustment are similar to the management of overt hypothyroidism.

Conclusion

Subclinical hypothyroidism arises in the clinical scenario of a serum TSH concentration over the upper level of normal in spite of a normal serum free thyroxine level. Starting levothyroxine treatment is advocated for all persons with a TSH higher than 10 mIU/L, even if the free thyroxine level is within normal limits. Though, therapy of individuals with a serum TSH concentration between 5 and 10 mIU/L remains uncertain. The strongest reasonings for levothyroxine replacement are the high rate of development of frank hypothyroidism, the potential improvement of quality of life, and the prospect that SCH is a cardiovascular risk factor. Data shows that any potential elevated cardiovascular risk would be to patients less than 70 years; those between 70 and 80 years have no added risk, and those more than 80 years may in fact have potential protective benefit. High quality trials are required to evaluate the effectiveness of levothyroxine replacement in the subset with TSH concentration of less than 10 mIU/L. In the meantime, treatment of this subgroup should be individualized based on presence of symptoms, age, patient preference, and associated medical conditions.

Summary and Recommendations

- Subclinical hypothyroidism is biochemically defined as a normal serum free thyroxine (T4) level with elevated serum thyroid-stimulating hormone (TSH) levels. Subclinical hypothyroidism may be symptomatic or asymptomatic for hypothyroidism. For non-pregnant patients, a raised serum TSH is defined as a TSH level higher than the upper level of the normal TSH reference level, which is usually 4–5 mU/L in the majority of laboratories. For pregnant females, elevated levels in TSH should be distinct using trimester-explicit TSH reference ranges.
- A significant number of subjects with subclinical hypothyroidism finally progress to overt hypothyroidism.
- Subclinical hypothyroidism may possibly be linked with an elevated risk of cardiovascular disease (CVD) (e.g., heart failure, coronary heart disease [CHD]), mostly when the serum TSH level is above 10 mU/L.
- For persons with subclinical hypothyroidism and TSH values ≥10 mU/L, treatment with thyroid hormone (T4) is proposed. For younger persons with TSH values within 4.5 and 10 mU/L who are symptomatic of hypothyroidism treatment with T4 is suggested. Therapy with thyroid hormone T4 can also be contemplated in younger persons with TSH within 4.5 and 10 mU/L who have raised levels of thyroid peroxidase (TPO) antibodies, which predict development of overt hypothyroidism, or goiter.
- For older persons (over age 70 years) with subclinical hypothyroidism and TSH between 4.5 and 8 mU/L, no treatment is suggested, considering the doubtful benefits and the possibility of both cardiovascular and skeletal risks related with unintentional excess treatment.
- T4 treatment in women with subclinical hypothyroidism (TSH values >2.5 mU/L) who are pregnant, who wish to become pregnant, or have ovulatory dysfunction and infertility is recommended.
- Synthetic T4 is the treatment of choice for replacement of hypothyroidism. For older persons and those with associated CVD, the starting dose of T4 is usually 25–50 mcg/day. This strategy will prevent overtreatment. For younger subjects without a previous history of thyroid autonomy, another approach is to start therapy at somewhat below the full replacement doses (1.6 mcg/kg/day). The target of treatment is to lower the patient's serum TSH values into the lower half of the age-adjusted normal reference range.
- Due to the high occurrence of SCH and related metabolic risk issues such as hyperlipidemia, the American Thyroid Association advocates screening by checking serum TSH starting at the age of 35 years and every 5 years afterwards.

References

1. Cooper DS. Clinical practice. Subclinical hypothyroidism. N Engl J Med. 2001;345:260–5.
2. Hollowell JG, Staehling NW, Flanders WD, Hannon WH, Gunter EW, Spencer CA, et al. Serum TSH, T(4), and thyroid antibodies in the United States population (1988 to 1994): National Health and Nutrition Examination Survey (NHANES III). J Clin Endocrinol Metab. 2002;87:489–99.
3. Karmisholt J, Andersen S, Laurberg P. Variation in thyroid function tests in patients with stable untreated subclinical hypothyroidism. Thyroid Off J Am Thyroid Assoc. 2008;18:303–8.
4. Szabolcs I, Podoba J, Feldkamp J, Dohan O, Farkas I, Sajgó M, et al. Comparative screening for thyroid disorders in old age in areas of iodine deficiency, long-term iodine prophylaxis and abundant iodine intake. Clin Endocrinol (Oxf). 1997;47:87–92.

5. Biondi B, Cooper DS. The clinical significance of subclinical thyroid dysfunction. Endocr Rev. 2008;29:76–131.
6. Fatourechi V. Subclinical hypothyroidism: When to treat, when to watch? Consultant. 2004;44:533–9.
7. Surks MI, Hollowell JG. Age-specific distribution of serum thyrotropin and antithyroid antibodies in the US population: implications for the prevalence of subclinical hypothyroidism. J Clin Endocrinol Metab. 2007;92:4575–82.
8. Spencer CA, Hollowell JG, Kazarosyan M, Braverman LE. National Health and Nutrition Examination Survey III thyroid-stimulating hormone (TSH)-thyroperoxidase antibody relationships demonstrate that TSH upper reference limits may be skewed by occult thyroid dysfunction. J Clin Endocrinol Metab. 2007;92:4236–40.
9. Surks MI, Goswami G, Daniels GH. The thyrotropin reference range should remain unchanged. J Clin Endocrinol Metab. 2005;90:5489–96.
10. Wartofsky L, Dickey RA. The evidence for a narrower thyrotropin reference range is compelling. J Clin Endocrinol Metab. 2005;90:5483–8.
11. Surks MI, Ortiz E, Daniels GH, Sawin CT, Col NF, Cobin RH, et al. Subclinical thyroid disease: scientific review and guidelines for diagnosis and management. JAMA. 2004;291:228–38.
12. Gharib H, Tuttle RM, Baskin HJ, Fish LH, Singer PA, McDermott MT, et al. Consensus Statement #1: Subclinical thyroid dysfunction: a joint statement on management from the American Association of Clinical Endocrinologists, the American Thyroid Association, and The Endocrine Society. Thyroid Off J Am Thyroid Assoc. 2005;15:24–8.
13. Chu JW, Crapo LM. The treatment of subclinical hypothyroidism is seldom necessary. J Clin Endocrinol Metab. 2001;86:4591–9.
14. Villar HCCE, Saconato H, Valente O, Atallah AN. Thyroid hormone replacement for subclinical hypothyroidism. Cochrane Database Syst Rev. 2007;(3):CD003419.
15. Ladenson PW, Singer PA, Ain KB, Bagchi N, Bigos ST, Levy EG, et al. American Thyroid Association guidelines for detection of thyroid dysfunction. Arch Intern Med. 2000;160:1573–5.
16. Helfand M, Redfern CC. Clinical guideline, part 2. Screening for thyroid disease: an update. American College of Physicians. Ann Intern Med. 1998;129:144–58.
17. Hollowell JG, LaFranchi S, Smallridge RC, Spong CY, Haddow JE, Boyle CA. 2004 where do we go from here?–summary of working group discussions on thyroid function and gestational outcomes. Thyroid Off J Am Thyroid Assoc. 2005;15:72–6.
18. Haddow JE, Palomaki GE, Allan WC, Williams JR, Knight GJ, Gagnon J, et al. Maternal thyroid deficiency during pregnancy and subsequent neuropsychological development of the child. N Engl J Med. 1999;341:549–55.
19. Vaidya B, Anthony S, Bilous M, Shields B, Drury J, Hutchison S, et al. Detection of thyroid dysfunction in early pregnancy: Universal screening or targeted high-risk case finding? J Clin Endocrinol Metab. 2007;92:203–7.
20. Canaris GJ, Manowitz NR, Mayor G, Ridgway EC. The Colorado thyroid disease prevalence study. Arch Intern Med. 2000;160:526–34.
21. Cooper DS, Biondi B. Subclinical thyroid disease. Lancet. 2012;379:1142–54.
22. Rix M, Laurberg P, Porzig C, Kristensen SR. Elevated thyroid-stimulating hormone level in a euthyroid neonate caused by macro thyrotropin-IgG complex. Acta Paediatr Oslo Nor. 2011;100:e135–7.
23. Kabadi UM. "Subclinical hypothyroidism". Natural course of the syndrome during a prolonged follow-up study. Arch Intern Med. 1993;153:957–61.
24. Fatourechi V, Klee GG, Grebe SK, Bahn RS, Brennan MD, Hay ID, et al. Effects of reducing the upper limit of normal TSH values. JAMA. 2003;290:3195–6.
25. Pollock MA, Sturrock A, Marshall K, Davidson KM, Kelly CJ, McMahon AD, et al. Thyroxine treatment in patients with symptoms of hypothyroidism but thyroid function tests within the reference range: randomised double blind placebo controlled cross-over trial. BMJ. 2001;323:891–5.
26. Hamilton TE, Davis S, Onstad L, Kopecky KJ. Thyrotropin levels in a population with no clinical, autoantibody, or ultrasonographic evidence of thyroid disease: implications for the diagnosis of subclinical hypothyroidism. J Clin Endocrinol Metab. 2008;93:1224–30.
27. Després N, Grant AM. Antibody interference in thyroid assays: a potential for clinical misinformation. Clin Chem. 1998;44:440–54.
28. Loh TP, Kao SL, Halsall DJ, Toh S-AES, Chan E, Ho SC, et al. Macro-thyrotropin: a case report and review of literature. J Clin Endocrinol Metab. 2012;97:1823–8.
29. Sakai H, Fukuda G, Suzuki N, Watanabe C, Odawara M. Falsely elevated thyroid-stimulating hormone (TSH) level due to macro-TSH. Endocr J. 2009;56:435–40.
30. Gurnell M, Halsall DJ, Chatterjee VK. What should be done when thyroid function tests do not make sense? Clin Endocrinol (Oxf). 2011;74:673–8.
31. Garber JR, Cobin RH, Gharib H, Hennessey JV, Klein I, Mechanick JI, et al. Clinical practice guidelines for hypothyroidism in adults: cosponsored by the American Association of Clinical Endocrinologists and the American Thyroid Association. Thyroid Off J Am Thyroid Assoc. 2012;22:1200–35.
32. McDermott MT, Ridgway EC. Subclinical hypothyroidism is mild thyroid failure and should be treated. J Clin Endocrinol Metab. 2001;86:4585–90.
33. Kong WM, Sheikh MH, Lumb PJ, Naoumova RP, Freedman DB, Crook M, et al. A 6-month randomized trial of thyroxine treatment in women

with mild subclinical hypothyroidism. Am J Med. 2002;112:348–54.
34. Roberts LM, Pattison H, Roalfe A, Franklyn J, Wilson S, Hobbs FDR, et al. Is subclinical thyroid dysfunction in the elderly associated with depression or cognitive dysfunction? Ann Intern Med. 2006;145:573–81.
35. Gussekloo J, van Exel E, de Craen AJM, Meinders AE, Frölich M, Westendorp RGJ. Thyroid status, disability and cognitive function, and survival in old age. JAMA. 2004;292:2591–9.
36. Jorde R, Waterloo K, Storhaug H, Nyrnes A, Sundsfjord J, Jenssen TG. Neuropsychological function and symptoms in subjects with subclinical hypothyroidism and the effect of thyroxine treatment. J Clin Endocrinol Metab. 2006;91:145–53.
37. Vanderpump MP, Tunbridge WM, French JM, Appleton D, Bates D, Clark F, et al. The incidence of thyroid disorders in the community: a twenty-year follow-up of the Whickham Survey. Clin Endocrinol (Oxf). 1995;43:55–68.
38. Díez JJ, Iglesias P. Spontaneous subclinical hypothyroidism in patients older than 55 years: an analysis of natural course and risk factors for the development of overt thyroid failure. J Clin Endocrinol Metab. 2004;89:4890–7.
39. Huber G, Staub J-J, Meier C, Mitrache C, Guglielmetti M, Huber P, et al. Prospective study of the spontaneous course of subclinical hypothyroidism: prognostic value of thyrotropin, thyroid reserve, and thyroid antibodies. J Clin Endocrinol Metab. 2002;87:3221–6.
40. Rosenthal MJ, Hunt WC, Garry PJ, Goodwin JS. Thyroid failure in the elderly. Microsomal antibodies as discriminant for therapy. JAMA. 1987;258:209–13.
41. Díez JJ, Iglesias P, Burman KD. Spontaneous normalization of thyrotropin concentrations in patients with subclinical hypothyroidism. J Clin Endocrinol Metab. 2005;90:4124–7.
42. Meyerovitch J, Rotman-Pikielny P, Sherf M, Battat E, Levy Y, Surks MI. Serum thyrotropin measurements in the community: five-year follow-up in a large network of primary care physicians. Arch Intern Med. 2007;167:1533–8.
43. Hak AE, Pols HA, Visser TJ, Drexhage HA, Hofman A, Witteman JC. Subclinical hypothyroidism is an independent risk factor for atherosclerosis and myocardial infarction in elderly women: the Rotterdam Study. Ann Intern Med. 2000;132:270–8.
44. Vanderpump MP, Tunbridge WM, French JM, Appleton D, Bates D, Clark F, et al. The development of ischemic heart disease in relation to autoimmune thyroid disease in a 20-year follow-up study of an English community. Thyroid Off J Am Thyroid Assoc. 1996;6:155–60.
45. Cappola AR, Fried LP, Arnold AM, Danese MD, Kuller LH, Burke GL, et al. Thyroid status, cardiovascular risk, and mortality in older adults. JAMA. 2006;295:1033–41.
46. Rodondi N, Aujesky D, Vittinghoff E, Cornuz J, Bauer DC. Subclinical hypothyroidism and the risk of coronary heart disease: a meta-analysis. Am J Med. 2006;119:541–51.
47. Ochs N, Auer R, Bauer DC, Nanchen D, Gussekloo J, Cornuz J, et al. Meta-analysis: subclinical thyroid dysfunction and the risk for coronary heart disease and mortality. Ann Intern Med. 2008;148:832–45.
48. Singh S, Duggal J, Molnar J, Maldonado F, Barsano CP, Arora R. Impact of subclinical thyroid disorders on coronary heart disease, cardiovascular and all-cause mortality: a meta-analysis. Int J Cardiol. 2008;125:41–8.
49. Haentjens P, Van Meerhaeghe A, Poppe K, Velkeniers B. Subclinical thyroid dysfunction and mortality: an estimate of relative and absolute excess all-cause mortality based on time-to-event data from cohort studies. Eur J Endocrinol Eur Fed Endocr Soc. 2008;159:329–41.
50. Razvi S, Shakoor A, Vanderpump M, Weaver JU, Pearce SHS. The influence of age on the relationship between subclinical hypothyroidism and ischemic heart disease: a metaanalysis. J Clin Endocrinol Metab. 2008;93:2998–3007.
51. Lindeman RD, Romero LJ, Schade DS, Wayne S, Baumgartner RN, Garry PJ. Impact of subclinical hypothyroidism on serum total homocysteine concentrations, the prevalence of coronary heart disease (CHD), and CHD risk factors in the New Mexico Elder Health Survey. Thyroid Off J Am Thyroid Assoc. 2003;13:595–600.
52. Imaizumi M, Akahoshi M, Ichimaru S, Nakashima E, Hida A, Soda M, et al. Risk for ischemic heart disease and all-cause mortality in subclinical hypothyroidism. J Clin Endocrinol Metab. 2004;89:3365–70.
53. Walsh JP, Bremner AP, Bulsara MK, O'Leary P, Leedman PJ, Feddema P, et al. Subclinical thyroid dysfunction as a risk factor for cardiovascular disease. Arch Intern Med. 2005;165:2467–72.
54. Razvi S, Weaver JU, Vanderpump MP, Pearce SHS. The incidence of ischemic heart disease and mortality in people with subclinical hypothyroidism: reanalysis of the Whickham Survey cohort. J Clin Endocrinol Metab. 2010;95:1734–40.
55. Rodondi N, Newman AB, Vittinghoff E, de Rekeneire N, Satterfield S, Harris TB, et al. Subclinical hypothyroidism and the risk of heart failure, other cardiovascular events, and death. Arch Intern Med. 2005;165:2460–6.
56. Hyland KA, Arnold AM, Lee JS, Cappola AR. Persistent subclinical hypothyroidism and cardiovascular risk in the elderly: the cardiovascular health study. J Clin Endocrinol Metab. 2013;98:533–40.
57. Rodondi N, den Elzen WPJ, Bauer DC, Cappola AR, Razvi S, Walsh JP, et al. Subclinical hypothyroidism and the risk of coronary heart disease and mortality. JAMA. 2010;304:1365–74.

58. Gencer B, Collet T-H, Virgini V, Bauer DC, Gussekloo J, Cappola AR, et al. Subclinical thyroid dysfunction and the risk of heart failure events: an individual participant data analysis from 6 prospective cohorts. Circulation. 2012;126:1040–9.
59. Monzani F, Caraccio N, Kozàkowà M, Dardano A, Vittone F, Virdis A, et al. Effect of levothyroxine replacement on lipid profile and intima-media thickness in subclinical hypothyroidism: a double-blind, placebo- controlled study. J Clin Endocrinol Metab. 2004;89:2099–106.
60. Nagasaki T, Inaba M, Kumeda Y, Hiura Y, Shirakawa K, Yamada S, et al. Increased pulse wave velocity in subclinical hypothyroidism. J Clin Endocrinol Metab. 2006;91:154–8.
61. Kvetny J, Heldgaard PE, Bladbjerg EM, Gram J. Subclinical hypothyroidism is associated with a low-grade inflammation, increased triglyceride levels and predicts cardiovascular disease in males below 50 years. Clin Endocrinol (Oxf). 2004;61:232–8.
62. Cikim AS, Oflaz H, Ozbey N, Cikim K, Umman S, Meric M, et al. Evaluation of endothelial function in subclinical hypothyroidism and subclinical hyperthyroidism. Thyroid Off J Am Thyroid Assoc. 2004;14:605–9.
63. Owen PJD, Rajiv C, Vinereanu D, Mathew T, Fraser AG, Lazarus JH. Subclinical hypothyroidism, arterial stiffness, and myocardial reserve. J Clin Endocrinol Metab. 2006;91:2126–32.
64. Choi SH, Lee YJ, Park YJ, Kim KW, Lee EJ, Lim S, et al. Retinol binding protein-4 elevation is associated with serum thyroid-stimulating hormone level independently of obesity in elderly subjects with normal glucose tolerance. J Clin Endocrinol Metab. 2008;93:2313–8.
65. Biondi B, Fazio S, Palmieri EA, Carella C, Panza N, Cittadini A, et al. Left ventricular diastolic dysfunction in patients with subclinical hypothyroidism. J Clin Endocrinol Metab. 1999;84:2064–7.
66. Iqbal A, Schirmer H, Lunde P, Figenschau Y, Rasmussen K, Jorde R. Thyroid stimulating hormone and left ventricular function. J Clin Endocrinol Metab. 2007;92:3504–10.
67. Biondi B. Cardiovascular effects of mild hypothyroidism. Thyroid Off J Am Thyroid Assoc. 2007;17:625–30.
68. Atzmon G, Barzilai N, Surks MI, Gabriely I. Genetic predisposition to elevated serum thyrotropin is associated with exceptional longevity. J Clin Endocrinol Metab. 2009;94:4768–75.
69. Waring AC, Harrison S, Samuels MH, Ensrud KE, LeBLanc ES, Hoffman AR, et al. Thyroid function and mortality in older men: a prospective study. J Clin Endocrinol Metab. 2012;97:862–70.
70. Selmer C, Olesen JB, Hansen ML, von Kappelgaard LM, Madsen JC, Hansen PR, et al. Subclinical and overt thyroid dysfunction and risk of all-cause mortality and cardiovascular events: a large population study. J Clin Endocrinol Metab. 2014;99:2372–82.
71. Waring AC, Arnold AM, Newman AB, Bùzková P, Hirsch C, Cappola AR. Longitudinal changes in thyroid function in the oldest old and survival: the cardiovascular health study all-stars study. J Clin Endocrinol Metab. 2012;97:3944–50.
72. Rhee CM, Curhan GC, Alexander EK, Bhan I, Brunelli SM. Subclinical hypothyroidism and survival: the effects of heart failure and race. J Clin Endocrinol Metab. 2013;98:2326–36.
73. Chung GE, Kim D, Kim W, Yim JY, Park MJ, Kim YJ, et al. Non-alcoholic fatty liver disease across the spectrum of hypothyroidism. J Hepatol. 2012;57:150–6.
74. Haggerty JJ, Garbutt JC, Evans DL, Golden RN, Pedersen C, Simon JS, et al. Subclinical hypothyroidism: a review of neuropsychiatric aspects. Int J Psychiatry Med. 1990;20:193–208.
75. Baldini IM, Vita A, Mauri MC, Amodei V, Carrisi M, Bravin S, et al. Psychopathological and cognitive features in subclinical hypothyroidism. Prog Neuropsychopharmacol Biol Psychiatry. 1997;21:925–35.
76. Monzani F, Del Guerra P, Caraccio N, Pruneti CA, Pucci E, Luisi M, et al. Subclinical hypothyroidism: neurobehavioral features and beneficial effect of L-thyroxine treatment. Clin Investig. 1993;71:367–71.
77. Haggerty JJ, Stern RA, Mason GA, Beckwith J, Morey CE, Prange AJ. Subclinical hypothyroidism: a modifiable risk factor for depression? Am J Psychiatry. 1993;150:508–10.
78. Tappy L, Randin JP, Schwed P, Wertheimer J, Lemarchand-Béraud T. Prevalence of thyroid disorders in psychogeriatric inpatients. A possible relationship of hypothyroidism with neurotic depression but not with dementia. J Am Geriatr Soc. 1987;35:526–31.
79. Engum A, Bjøro T, Mykletun A, Dahl AA. An association between depression, anxiety and thyroid function – a clinical fact or an artefact? Acta Psychiatr Scand. 2002;106:27–34.
80. Christ-Crain M, Meier C, Huber PR, Staub J-J, Müller B. Effect of l-thyroxine replacement therapy on surrogate markers of skeletal and cardiac function in subclinical hypothyroidism. Endocrinologist. 2004;14:161–6.
81. Knudsen N, Laurberg P, Rasmussen LB, Bülow I, Perrild H, Ovesen L, et al. Small differences in thyroid function may be important for body mass index and the occurrence of obesity in the population. J Clin Endocrinol Metab. 2005;90:4019–24.
82. Fox CS, Pencina MJ, D'Agostino RB, Murabito JM, Seely EW, Pearce EN, et al. Relations of thyroid function to body weight: cross-sectional and longitudinal observations in a community-based sample. Arch Intern Med. 2008;168:587–92.
83. Asvold BO, Bjøro T, Vatten LJ. Association of serum TSH with high body mass differs between smokers and never-smokers. J Clin Endocrinol Metab. 2009;94:5023–7.

84. Makepeace AE, Bremner AP, O'Leary P, Leedman PJ, Feddema P, Michelangeli V, et al. Significant inverse relationship between serum free T4 concentration and body mass index in euthyroid subjects: differences between smokers and nonsmokers. Clin Endocrinol (Oxf). 2008;69:648–52.
85. Manji N, Boelaert K, Sheppard MC, Holder RL, Gough SC, Franklyn JA. Lack of association between serum TSH or free T4 and body mass index in euthyroid subjects. Clin Endocrinol (Oxf). 2006;64:125–8.
86. Garin MC, Arnold AM, Lee JS, Tracy RP, Cappola AR. Subclinical hypothyroidism, weight change, and body composition in the elderly: the Cardiovascular Health Study. J Clin Endocrinol Metab. 2014;99:1220–6.
87. Monzani F, Caraccio N, Del Guerra P, Casolaro A, Ferrannini E. Neuromuscular symptoms and dysfunction in subclinical hypothyroid patients: beneficial effect of L-T4 replacement therapy. Clin Endocrinol (Oxf). 1999;51:237–42.
88. Simonsick EM, Newman AB, Ferrucci L, Satterfield S, Harris TB, Rodondi N, et al. Subclinical hypothyroidism and functional mobility in older adults. Arch Intern Med. 2009;169:2011–7.
89. Samuels MH, Schuff KG, Carlson NE, Carello P, Janowsky JS. Health status, mood, and cognition in experimentally induced subclinical hypothyroidism. J Clin Endocrinol Metab. 2007;92:2545–51.
90. Correia N, Mullally S, Cooke G, Tun TK, Phelan N, Feeney J, et al. Evidence for a specific defect in hippocampal memory in overt and subclinical hypothyroidism. J Clin Endocrinol Metab. 2009;94:3789–97.
91. Tan ZS, Beiser A, Vasan RS, Au R, Auerbach S, Kiel DP, et al. Thyroid function and the risk of Alzheimer disease: the Framingham Study. Arch Intern Med. 2008;168:1514–20.
92. Squizzato A, Romualdi E, Piantanida E, Gerdes VEA, Büller HR, Tanda M, et al. Subclinical hypothyroidism and deep venous thrombosis. A pilot cross-sectional study. Thromb Haemost. 2007;97:803–6.
93. Laukkarinen J, Kiudelis G, Lempinen M, Räty S, Pelli H, Sand J, et al. Increased prevalence of subclinical hypothyroidism in common bile duct stone patients. J Clin Endocrinol Metab. 2007;92:4260–4.
94. Allan WC, Haddow JE, Palomaki GE, Williams JR, Mitchell ML, Hermos RJ, et al. Maternal thyroid deficiency and pregnancy complications: implications for population screening. J Med Screen. 2000;7:127–30.
95. Klein RZ, Haddow JE, Faix JD, Brown RS, Hermos RJ, Pulkkinen A, et al. Prevalence of thyroid deficiency in pregnant women. Clin Endocrinol (Oxf). 1991;35:41–6.
96. Cooper DS, Halpern R, Wood LC, Levin AA, Ridgway EC. L-Thyroxine therapy in subclinical hypothyroidism. A double-blind, placebo-controlled trial. Ann Intern Med. 1984;101:18–24.
97. Jaeschke R, Guyatt G, Gerstein H, Patterson C, Molloy W, Cook D, et al. Does treatment with L-thyroxine influence health status in middle-aged and older adults with subclinical hypothyroidism? J Gen Intern Med. 1996;11:744–9.
98. Meier C, Staub JJ, Roth CB, Guglielmetti M, Kunz M, Miserez AR, et al. TSH-controlled L-thyroxine therapy reduces cholesterol levels and clinical symptoms in subclinical hypothyroidism: a double blind, placebo-controlled trial (Basel Thyroid Study). J Clin Endocrinol Metab. 2001;86:4860–6.
99. Nyström E, Caidahl K, Fager G, Wikkelsö C, Lundberg PA, Lindstedt G. A double-blind crossover 12-month study of L-thyroxine treatment of women with "subclinical" hypothyroidism. Clin Endocrinol (Oxf). 1988;29:63–75.
100. Rugge JB, Bougatsos C, Chou R. Screening and treatment of thyroid dysfunction: an evidence review for the U.S. Preventive Services Task Force. Ann Intern Med. 2015;162:35–45.
101. Razvi S, Ingoe L, Keeka G, Oates C, McMillan C, Weaver JU. The beneficial effect of L-thyroxine on cardiovascular risk factors, endothelial function, and quality of life in subclinical hypothyroidism: randomized, crossover trial. J Clin Endocrinol Metab. 2007;92:1715–23.
102. Romaldini JH, Biancalana MM, Figueiredo DI, Farah CS, Mathias PC. Effect of L-thyroxine administration on antithyroid antibody levels, lipid profile, and thyroid volume in patients with Hashimoto's thyroiditis. Thyroid Off J Am Thyroid Assoc. 1996;6:183–8.
103. Adrees M, Gibney J, El-Saeity N, Boran G. Effects of 18 months of L-T4 replacement in women with subclinical hypothyroidism. Clin Endocrinol (Oxf). 2009;71:298–303.
104. Taddei S, Caraccio N, Virdis A, Dardano A, Versari D, Ghiadoni L, et al. Impaired endothelium-dependent vasodilatation in subclinical hypothyroidism: beneficial effect of levothyroxine therapy. J Clin Endocrinol Metab. 2003;88:3731–7.
105. Ozcan O, Cakir E, Yaman H, Akgul EO, Erturk K, Beyhan Z, et al. The effects of thyroxine replacement on the levels of serum asymmetric dimethylarginine (ADMA) and other biochemical cardiovascular risk markers in patients with subclinical hypothyroidism. Clin Endocrinol (Oxf). 2005;63:203–6.
106. Milionis HJ, Tambaki AP, Kanioglou CN, Elisaf MS, Tselepis AD, Tsatsoulis A. Thyroid substitution therapy induces high-density lipoprotein-associated platelet-activating factor-acetylhydrolase in patients with subclinical hypothyroidism: a potential antiatherogenic effect. Thyroid Off J Am Thyroid Assoc. 2005;15:455–60.
107. Turhan S, Tulunay C, Ozduman Cin M, Gursoy A, Kilickap M, Dincer I, et al. Effects of thyroxine therapy on right ventricular systolic and diastolic function in patients with subclinical hypothyroidism: a study by pulsed wave tissue Doppler imaging. J Clin Endocrinol Metab. 2006;91:3490–3.
108. Faber J, Petersen L, Wiinberg N, Schifter S, Mehlsen J. Hemodynamic changes after levothyroxine treat-

ment in subclinical hypothyroidism. Thyroid Off J Am Thyroid Assoc. 2002;12:319–24.
109. Shakoor SKA, Aldibbiat A, Ingoe LE, Campbell SC, Sibal L, Shaw J, et al. Endothelial progenitor cells in subclinical hypothyroidism: the effect of thyroid hormone replacement therapy. J Clin Endocrinol Metab. 2010;95:319–22.
110. Razvi S, Weaver JU, Butler TJ, Pearce SHS. Levothyroxine treatment of subclinical hypothyroidism, fatal and nonfatal cardiovascular events, and mortality. Arch Intern Med. 2012;172:811–7.
111. Caraccio N, Ferrannini E, Monzani F. Lipoprotein profile in subclinical hypothyroidism: response to levothyroxine replacement, a randomized placebo-controlled study. J Clin Endocrinol Metab. 2002;87:1533–8.
112. Iqbal A, Jorde R, Figenschau Y. Serum lipid levels in relation to serum thyroid-stimulating hormone and the effect of thyroxine treatment on serum lipid levels in subjects with subclinical hypothyroidism: the Tromsø Study. J Intern Med. 2006;260:53–61.
113. Mikhail GS, Alshammari SM, Alenezi MY, Mansour M, Khalil NA. Increased atherogenic low-density lipoprotein cholesterol in untreated subclinical hypothyroidism. Endocr Pract Off J Am Coll Endocrinol Am Assoc Clin Endocrinol. 2008;14:570–5.
114. Shin DH, Lee MJ, Lee HS, Oh HJ, Ko KI, Kim CH, et al. Thyroid hormone replacement therapy attenuates the decline of renal function in chronic kidney disease patients with subclinical hypothyroidism. Thyroid Off J Am Thyroid Assoc. 2013;23:654–61.
115. Cinemre H, Bilir C, Gokosmanoglu F, Bahcebasi T. Hematologic effects of levothyroxine in iron-deficient subclinical hypothyroid patients: a randomized, double-blind, controlled study. J Clin Endocrinol Metab. 2009;94:151–6.
116. Danese MD, Ladenson PW, Meinert CL, Powe NR. Clinical review 115: effect of thyroxine therapy on serum lipoproteins in patients with mild thyroid failure: a quantitative review of the literature. J Clin Endocrinol Metab. 2000;85:2993–3001.
117. Haggerty JJ, Prange AJ. Borderline hypothyroidism and depression. Annu Rev Med. 1995;46:37–46.
118. Biondi B, Palmieri EA, Lombardi G, Fazio S. Effects of subclinical thyroid dysfunction on the heart. Ann Intern Med. 2002;137:904–14.
119. McDermott MT. In the clinic. Hypothyroidism. Ann Intern Med. 2009;151:ITC61.
120. Somwaru LL, Arnold AM, Joshi N, Fried LP, Cappola AR. High frequency of and factors associated with thyroid hormone over-replacement and under-replacement in men and women aged 65 and over. J Clin Endocrinol Metab. 2009;94:1342–5.
121. Bussen S, Steck T. Thyroid autoantibodies in euthyroid non-pregnant women with recurrent spontaneous abortions. Hum Reprod Oxf Engl. 1995;10:2938–40.
122. Prummel MF, Wiersinga WM. Thyroid autoimmunity and miscarriage. Eur J Endocrinol Eur Fed Endocr Soc. 2004;150:751–5.
123. Männistö T, Vääräsmäki M, Pouta A, Hartikainen A-L, Ruokonen A, Surcel H-M, et al. Perinatal outcome of children born to mothers with thyroid dysfunction or antibodies: a prospective population-based cohort study. J Clin Endocrinol Metab. 2009;94:772–9.
124. Thangaratinam S, Tan A, Knox E, Kilby MD, Franklyn J, Coomarasamy A. Association between thyroid autoantibodies and miscarriage and preterm birth: meta-analysis of evidence. BMJ. 2011;342:d2616.
125. Chen L, Hu R. Thyroid autoimmunity and miscarriage: a meta-analysis. Clin Endocrinol (Oxf). 2011;74:513–9.
126. Korevaar TIM, Schalekamp-Timmermans S, de Rijke YB, Visser WE, Visser W, de Muinck K-SSMPF, et al. Hypothyroxinemia and TPO-antibody positivity are risk factors for premature delivery: the generation R study. J Clin Endocrinol Metab. 2013;98:4382–90.
127. Negro R, Formoso G, Mangieri T, Pezzarossa A, Dazzi D, Hassan H. Levothyroxine treatment in euthyroid pregnant women with autoimmune thyroid disease: effects on obstetrical complications. J Clin Endocrinol Metab. 2006;91:2587–91.
128. Toulis KA, Goulis DG, Venetis CA, Kolibianakis EM, Negro R, Tarlatzis BC, et al. Risk of spontaneous miscarriage in euthyroid women with thyroid autoimmunity undergoing IVF: a meta-analysis. Eur J Endocrinol Eur Fed Endocr Soc. 2010;162:643–52.
129. Negro R, Mangieri T, Coppola L, Presicce G, Casavola EC, Gismondi R, et al. Levothyroxine treatment in thyroid peroxidase antibody-positive women undergoing assisted reproduction technologies: a prospective study. Hum Reprod Oxf Engl. 2005;20:1529–33.
130. Ghassabian A, Bongers-Schokking JJ, de Rijke YB, van Mil N, Jaddoe VWV, de Muinck K-SSMPF, et al. Maternal thyroid autoimmunity during pregnancy and the risk of attention deficit/hyperactivity problems in children: the Generation R Study. Thyroid Off J Am Thyroid Assoc. 2012;22:178–86.
131. Stagnaro-Green A, Abalovich M, Alexander E, Azizi F, Mestman J, Negro R, et al. Guidelines of the American Thyroid Association for the diagnosis and management of thyroid disease during pregnancy and postpartum. Thyroid Off J Am Thyroid Assoc. 2011;21:1081–125.
132. Fatourechi V, Lankarani M, Schryver PG, Vanness DJ, Long KH, Klee GG. Factors influencing clinical decisions to initiate thyroxine therapy for patients with mildly increased serum thyrotropin (5.1-10.0 mIU/L). Mayo Clin Proc. 2003;78:554–60.

Thyroid Emergencies

12

Syed Abbas Raza

Abstract

Thyroid gland plays a pivotal role in keeping biochemical harmony and maintaining appropriate functioning of vital organs. Therefore any abnormality in thyroid hormone regulation, can lead to wide ranging detrimental effects. This chapter is assigned for identifying and managing thyroid conditions, which require emergent or urgent interventions. It's not only the biochemical status of the patient which determines this, but also the clinical presentation can make it urgent vs emergent. This is discussed in condition such as Thyroid storm and myxedema coma. Also, thyroid hormone abnormalities during pregnancy, ICU setting, involving vital organ (CNS, cardiovascular) or related to medicine use (lithium/amiodarone) may pose certain acute management challenges and hence discussed in this chapter.

True Thyroid Emergencies

Thyroid Storm

Pathophysiology

Pathophysiology behind this acute release/responsiveness of thyroid hormone along with catecholamine surge/responsiveness is not clearly understood [1]. Levels of suppression of TSH, Elevation of thyroxine level and thyroid scan uptake are usually not helpful in differentiating uncomplicated thyrotoxicosis and thyroid storm, but it's the clinical presentation.

Signs/Symptoms

Incidence of thyroid disorders varies in regional observational studies. Thyroid storm usually happens at the back ground of thyroid conditions such as Graves' disease, toxic multinodular goiter, solitary toxic adenoma.

Thyroid storm is a clinical diagnosis supported by biochemical evidence.

- Physical finding Include Goiter with opthalmopathy (Exophthalmos, lid lag and photosensitivity).

S.A. Raza, MD, FACE
Department of Internal Medicine, Shaukat Khanum Hospital and Research Center, Lahore, Pakistan
e-mail: sabbasraza@hotmail.com

S.K. Imam, S.I. Ahmad (eds.), *Thyroid Disorders: Basic Science and Clinical Practice*,
DOI 10.1007/978-3-319-25871-3_12

- Cardiovascular Symptoms: Tachycardia (Usually >1.5 times the resting heart rate). This may further deteriorate into hypotension, cardiac arrhythmia and cardiovascular collapse [2].
- Neurological Symptoms: confusion, anxiety, stupor progressing to coma.
- Central/constitutional: Hyperpyrexia (104–106 °F), moist skin and tremors.
- Others: GI symptoms (Vomiting, diarrhea, hepatic dysfunction and abdominal pain), Hyperglycemia, Hemeconcentration, Hypercalcemia [3].

Establishing Diagnosis

Although not universally accepted but most used scoring system in evaluation of Thyroid storm was postulated by Burch and Wartofsky [3, 4]. This scoring system helps in confirming (score of >45) vs unlikely (Score of <25). (See table below)

Scoring System

A score of 45 or greater is highly suggestive of thyroid storm; a score of 25–44 is suggestive of impending storm, and a score below 25 is unlikely to represent thyroid storm.

Treatment

Management of Thyroid storm is in same lines of thyrotoxicosis but dosages of medication are higher due to higher mortality and urgency of treatment [5].

- Antithyroid Medication: No one drug (Thionamide) is better in management in any of the clinical trials. Thionamide block thyroid hormone synthesis (Onset of action <2 h) but don't effect on the release of preformed hormone. Initially, there may be required in higher doses to control of thyroid hormone. Dosage required is in range of 200 mg every 4 h for Propylthiouracil (PTU) and 20 mg every 6 h for Methimazole/Carbimazole.
- PTU has additional benefit of preventing conversion of T4 to T3, hence sometimes preferred in acute setting/storm [6] but less hepato toxicity and better therapeutic control of Methimazole/Carbimazole makes them preferred choice in other situation/chronic use. Preparation in the form of suppository for rectal administration and intravenous preparation (Methimazole) can be requested in specialized pharmacy.
- Beta blockers: May require higher doses due to increased metabolism. They are used to control increased adrenergic response and potentially inhibit T4 to T3 conversion (Propranolol). Usually dosage of propranolol

Burch and Wartofsky scoring system for thyroid storm

Diagnostic parameters	Scoring points
Thermoregulatory dysfunction	
Temperature °F (°C)	
99–99.9 (37.2–37.7)	5
100–100.9 (37.8–38.2)	10
101–101.9 (38.3–38.8)	15
102–102.9 (38.9–39.2)	20
103–103.9 (39.3–39.9)	25
≥104.0 (≥40.0)	30
Central nervous system effects	
Absent	0
Mild (agitation)	10
Moderate (delirium, psychosis, extreme lethargy)	20
Severe (seizures, coma)	30
Gastrointestinal-hepatic dysfunction	
Absent	0
Moderate (diarrhea, nausea/vomiting, abdominal pain)	10
Severe (unexplained jaundice)	20
Cardiovascular dysfunction	
Tachycardia (beats/minute)	
90–109	5
110–119	10
120–129	15
130–139	20
≥140	25
Congestive heart failure	
Absent	0
Mild (pedal edema)	5
Moderate (bibasilar rales)	10
Severe (pulmonary edema)	15
Atrial fibrillation	
Absent	0
Present	10
Precipitating event	
Absent	0
Present	10

is in range of 60–80 mg every 6 h (Provided patient tolerates). Intravenous administration is an option but only if hemodynamic status is continuously being monitored (Propranolol 0.5–1 mg over 10 min) [7]. Esmolol is another short acting beta blocker which can be used and the usual dosage is 250–500 mcg/kg, followed by an infusion at 50–100 mcg/kg per minute. In reactive Airway disease patient option of cardio selective beta-blockers such as Metoprolol or Atenolol could be considered.

- Iodine: Iodine solutions are sometime used to block release of thyroid hormone (Only after initiation of Thionamide). Dosage could be administered as SSKI, five drops orally every 6 h, or Lugol's solution, 10 drops every 8 h [2]. Higher doses of Iodine (>960 mg iodine/day) have been linked with Esophageal/duodenal ulceration/hemorrhage [8]. Iopanoic acid and other iodinated radiocontrast agents were used for treatment in acute cases but now rarely used.
- Steroids: Steroid are used for their ability to promote vasomotor stability (especially in condition of relative adrenal Insufficiency) [9] and reduce T4 to T3 conversion. Usual dosage is Hydrocortisone 100 mg intravenously every 8 h.
- Fluid Management: Depends on fluid overload (Congestive heart failure) vs fluid resuscitation (Dehydration).
- Treatment on underlying/Precipitating Cause:
  - Fever/Pain: Acetaminophen is preferred choice. Aspirin can potentially interfere in protein binding of T4/T3 leading to increased circulating levels.
  - Antibiotics: Use antibiotic as indicated to treat possible infection as triggering factor. Infectious should be evaluated carefully in back ground of thyroid storm.
  - Others:
  - For heart rate control Diltiazem could be considered as alternative to Beta blocker such as asthmatic patient [10].
- Lithium use is limited by its neurological and renal side effects. The mechanism of action include blocking the release of thyroid hormone.
- Plasmapheresis has been tried when traditional therapy has not been successful [11].

Do and Don'ts/Things Not to Be Missed

- Don't under estimate the mortality associated with Thyroid storm. Thyroid storm is one of few life threatening endocrine emergencies [1]. Mortality associated with hyroid storm is ranges between 10 and 30 % [12].
- Don't miss the precipitating factor. Thyroid storm can be in a setting of precipitating event such infection, iodine exposure, acute stress or myocardial infarction.
- Don't use Iodine without blocking with Thionamide.
- Don't use beta blocker in setting of Severe Airway disease or contraindication.
- Do monitor the patient under cardiac surveillance.
- Use of Acetaminophen is preferred over Aspirin in acute thyroid emergency
- Do use steroid, intravenous fluids, antibiotics and calcium channel blocker when indicated in proper setting.

Follow Up of Patients

- Discontinuation of Iodine and steroids after improvement of clinical parameters.
- Reduction in dosage of beta blocker and thionamide with stability in thyroid function test.
- Switching Propylthiouracil to Methimazole/Carbimazole due to PTU safety concerns.
- Planning for RAI therapy on achieving good control over thyroid symptoms/biochemical status.
- Surgery is an option for patients but not usually recommended due to cost and association with more complication/longer recovery time. Surgery is considered in patient with a very large or obstructive goiter or severe orbitopathy.

Myxedema Coma

Pathophysiology

Diagnosis is made based on the severity of hypothyroidism symptoms. Level of elevation of TSH levels and suppression of thyroxine level are not help in differentiating uncomplicated hypothyroidism from Myxedema. Although its pathophysiology is unclear, but it is a rare entity due to wide spread availability of TSH testing and universal screening for thyroid disorders.

Establishing Diagnosis

Myxedema is defined as hypothyroidism presenting with severe signs/symptoms including mental status changes, hypothermia and multiorgan involvement. These symptoms are usually reported as progressively getting worse. Myxedema coma is a clinical diagnosis substantiated by biochemical evidence (Elevated TSH and Low Free T4). There is a need to evaluate for possible precipitating factors behind this presentation including cardiac decompensation, infection, cold exposure or use of medications such as sedative especially opioids, lithium and amiodarone [13, 14]. Delay in diagnosis and treatment may result in even higher mortality, which ranges from 30 to 40 % [15–17]

Signs/Symptoms

General/Metabolic: Myxedema is manifested in slowing down/down regulation of metabolic function of virtually all organs/systems. Hypothermia (this may limit fever response of precipitating infection), hypoglycemia (Relative Adrenal insufficiency and hypothyroidism) and generalized swelling (swollen lips and enlarged tongue) accompanied by non-pitting edema (Mucin deposit in skin) are other significant presentations. Biochemically, reversible hyponatremia may be seen in more than 50 % of patient (Inappropriate excess vasopressin secretion or/and impaired renal function leading to free water excretion defect). Severity of hypothermia is sometime reflective of higher mortality.

Cardiac: Hypothyroid is manifested by cardiac abnormalities which are reversible on treatment. Mild disease presents with diastolic hypertension with a narrowed pulse pressure. These are superadded by bradycardia, decreased myocardial contractility, a low cardiac output in severe hypothyroidism [18]. Pericardial effusion may be present resulting in low voltage on electrocardiogram, poor cardiac sounds and a large cardiac silhouette on chest x-ray.

Neurological: Slowing down/sub optimal mental functioning progressing rarely into coma. Seizures leading to status epilepticus have been reported in myxedema, which are also precipitated by hyponatremia [19, 20]. CSF finding in this condition may reveal elevated protein.

Pulmonary: Central Hypoventilation, poor respiratory efforts (decreased response to hypoxia and hypercapnia) leading to respiratory distress and respiratory acidosis.

Treatment

Time is a major factor in treatment of Myxedema due to its high mortality.

- Identifying precipitating factors such as Infection, cardiac etc. is important as they might be masked due to nature of hypothyroidism.
- Supportive Care: Treatment on hypothermia (passive rewarming blanket) fluid resuscitation, hypotension (consider vasopressor drugs for resistant severe hypotension), ventilator support in respiratory compromised and correction of electrolyte abnormality (Dilute fluids should be avoided in hyponatremia) and infection should be aggressively treated by antibiotic.
- Thyroxine Replacement: Due to sparse clinical data on this rare disorder, there is no consensus on right dosage of loading and replacing thyroxine in this myxedema. Also, danger of exacerbating the underlying comorbid condition (Cardiac/adrenal insufficiency) sometime limit aggressive replacement/bolus dosage. Similarly use of T3, T4 or combination is not universally agreed upon. It is usually recommended neither to over dose T4 (exceed >500 mcg, T3 ($\geq$75 mcg) nor under dose in this situation [21–24]. Loading dosage of thyroxine (500 mcg) followed by maintenance dosage has some

benefit over starting and continuing same dosage (100 mcg) [25]. Using T3 as initial dosage has some added benefit of having rapid onset of action and possibly bypassing delay in T4 to T3 conversion (delayed due to decreased de-iodinase activity seen in severe hypothyroidism although this has not been proven by studies). There is also a theoretic risk of higher mortality with high T3 level [15]. Also lower dosage may be considered for patient with cardiac arrhythmias and failure.

- Steroid: Usual dosage is hydrocortisone intravenously, 100 mg every 8 h. Due to autoimmunity nature of hypothyroidism, adrenal insufficiency should always be considered.

Do and Don't/What Not to Miss

- Do timely investigation and diagnostic test for potentially fatal condition.
- Do provide Respiratory support by mechanical ventilation in respiratory compromised patient (myxedematous infiltration of the pharynx, mechanical difficulties in tongue enlargement or hypo ventilation)
- Do send for biochemical evaluation (TSH, free T4 and cortisol) before initiation of treatment.
- Do consider other autoimmune disorders such adrenal insufficiency when faced with patient with hypothyroidism. Treat empirically with steroid before the laboratory results are obtained.
- Do initiate aggressive supportive care initially as it can make better outcome and lesser mortality.
- Do use aggressively Thyroxine T4 (With or without bolus) although bolus has some additional beneficial effect. Use of T3 is limited to initial management.
- Don't use regular doses in patient with cardiac arrhythmias and failure.

Follow Up of Patients

- Discontinuation of steroids and intravenous thyroxine after improvement of clinical parameters.
- Planning for follow up laboratory and adjusting dosage accordingly.
- Patient education and outpatient follow up.

Thyroid Dysfunction Requiring Urgent Measures

Thyroid Dysfunction During Pregnancy

Urgency in diagnosis and treatment: There are some unique aspects of thyroid disease during pregnancy vs. non pregnant females. This distinctive situation calls for urgency in diagnosis and treatment.

Hyperthyroidism

- Hyperthyroidism during pregnancy is mostly attributed to Graves' disease and hCG-mediated hyperthyroidism. Urgency of diagnosis and treatment during pregnancy is due to effects in fetal outcome (management of these are discussed in respective chapter).
- Do use Propylthiouracil – PTU as preferred drug during first trimester due to concerns of aplasia cutis, tracheoesophageal fistulas, patent vitellointestinal duct, and choanal atresia with use of methimazole/Carbimazole [26–31]. PTU can be switched to Carbimazole/Methimazole during second and third trimester.
- Don't use beta blockers for more than 6 weeks for symptomatic relief/tachycardia due to concerns of fetal growth retardation and hypoglycemia [32–34].
- Don't opt for radioactive iodine, as it is absolute contraindication and thyroidectomy during pregnancy is rarely necessary.
- In situation where other options cannot be utilized, Plasmapheresis has also been used to rapidly control hyperthyroidism [35, 36].

Hypothyroidism

- Hypothyroidism results in deleterious effect of pregnancy out come and mental/physical growth of fetus.
- Don't plan pregnancy till person (mother to be) is biochemically Euthyroid
- Do increase dosage of thyroxine by 30 % at the time of conception

- Do monitor thyroid function every 4–6 weeks during pregnancy and adjust dosage accordingly.
- Post-partum the Thyroxine dosage will need to be adjusted and reduced again.

Neurological Presentation of Thyroid Disease

Any thyroid condition becomes an urgent one when systemic symptoms including palpitations, heat intolerance, and weight loss are accompanied by central and peripheral nervous system manifestations.

Cognitive Disorders and Seizures

- Cognitive impairment is common in hyperthyroidism, especially in elderly population and may present as one or more different syndromes. Study by Martin et al revealed incidence of dementia (33 %) and confusion (18 %) [37]. These rates were higher than noted in studies looking into younger population [38, 39].
- It becomes a medical emergency/urgency, when thyrotoxic patient experience seizures along with encephalopathy. Seizure could vary from focal to generalize in clinical presentation [40–43]. Seizures are more prominent in this setting and may include status epilepticus [40, 41, 43–45].
- Confirming Diagnosis: Investigation including magnetic resonance imaging (MRI) or computed tomography (CT) neuroimaging studies and electroencephalography (EEG) may help differentiate/diagnose thyroid condition with others [43, 46, 47]. Other investigation such as single photon emission CT (SPECT) demonstrated diffusely reduced cerebral uptake with an accentuation in the temporoparietal regions bilaterally, which improved following resolution of the hyperthyroid state [47].
- Treatment: Treating hyperthyroidism usually lead to resolution of cognitive and behavioral impairments. Some symptoms resolve earlier (Agitation, inattention, and frontal lobe impairment) than others (cognitive functions) [37]. Although Seizures associated with Thyrotoxicosis should with improvement in thyroid function but anti-seizure medication are sometime required.

Movement Disorders

- Presentation: Tremor of Thyrotoxicosis should be differentiated from movement disorders. Benign tremors are typically noticed with high frequency and low amplitude [48].
- Myoclonus/Ballism have been reported although rarely in hyperthyroidism [49, 50]. Chorea occurs in less than 2 % of patient effected by hyperthyroidism [51]. Chorea usually present as gradual onset. It is presented as unilateral, bilateral, or multifocal and involves the extremities predominantly and less often the trunk or facial muscles [52–54]. Chorea's pathophysiology include reduction in the production and turnover of the level of homovanillic acid (metabolite of dopaminein the cerebrospinal fluid in hyperthyroid patients) which results in increased sensitivity of dopamine receptors and a resulting decrease in dopamine turnover [55]. Management of chorea includes correction of hyperthyroid state and use of dopamine antagonist (Haloperidol), beta-blockers and reserpine.

Cerebrovascular Disease

Ischemic cerebrovascular disease is a rare but recognizable complication of hyperthyroidism. In a prospective cohort study by Sheu et al revealed cumulative incidence of ischemic stroke was 1.0 % compared to 0.6 % in a control group over 5 years (HR = 1.44) [56]. Atrial fibrillation remains a recognizable risk factor for cerebral infarction related to hyperthyroidism [57]. In clinical scenario of atrial fibrillation (AF), anticoagulation remains mainstay of treatment to prevent cerebrovascular accidents (CVA).

Another rare condition seen in thyrotoxic patient with a very high mortality and morbidity is cerebral venous sinus thrombosis. This usually occurs in backdrop of dehydration, central nervous system infection, or hypercoagulable states [58–61].

Some of the other rare thyroid urgencies include fatal stroke and bilateral carotid artery dissection [62], intracranial stenosis [63], some autoimmune disorders (Antiphospholipid syndrome, giant cell arteritis, and Takayasu arteritis) are more common in patient with thyroid autoimmunity (although not proven) [64–67].

Neuromuscular Emergencies

Thyrotoxic patient may present with a muscular condition with unknown etiology which has acute onset of muscle weakness, muscle atrophy and myalgias. The prevalence of these conditions could be as high as 80 % in untreated patients [68, 69]. Possible explanation of these manifestations is increased cellular metabolism and energy utilization, increased catabolism and protein degradation, reduced carnitine and inefficient energy utilization [70–74].

Others condition presenting in emergency room with muscular weakness include Rhabdomyolysis [75–77]. Hypokalemic periodic paralysis present in its acquired form as Thyrotoxic periodic paralysis. This condition is usually preceded by generalized weakness, often following a strenuous exercise or a high-carbohydrate diet. Asian race and male gender are risk factor for this condition.

Peripheral neuropathy may be presenting complaint in hyperthyroidism; these could vary from carpel tunnel syndrome to sensory polyneuropathy. Common presentation is symmetric distal sensory disturbance and reduced Achilles reflexes. Carpel tunnel could be seen more commonly in hypothyroidism than hyperthyroidism [78]. Axonal damage of thyrotoxic patient is seen in diagnostic testing with nerve conduction studies and EMG [79–81]. Some of the other rare presentations seen in acute thyrotoxic/thyroid storm include Basedow's paraplegia (acute and severe leg weakness and areflexia) and recovery is with improvement in hyperthyroid state [82]. Other condition manifesting due to autoimmunity nature of thyrotoxicosis is Guillain-Barré syndrome and chronic inflammatory demyelinating polyneuropathy. They are autoimmune disorders rarely presenting along with hyperthyroidism [83].

One of the other emergencies in hyperthyroidism is involvement of peripheral nerves in myasthenia gravis. Prevalence of this condition varies from 2 to 17 % when prevalence in general population is 1 in 10,000 [84–86]. Common genetic susceptibility (HLA antigen type, HLA-DQ3) may explain higher prevalence [87]. The treatment of Myasthenia gravis remains same regarding of coexistence with thyroid state, which includes acetylcholinesterase inhibitors, thymectomy and immunosuppressive therapy [88].

Although Graves' opthalmopathy has a slow progressive presentation but sometime can have acute phase exacerbation. This relatively common in Graves' disease, occurring in 20–25 % of cases. Another uncommon urgent scenario may result from thyroid gland enlargement causing compression of recurrent laryngeal nerve compression (respiratory stridor, vocal cord paralysis, and dysphonia) and sympathetic chain (Horner's syndrome) [89, 90],

Cardiovascular Emergencies

Thyroid condition presenting with cardiovascular manifestation becomes an emergency due to high risk and mortality. These effects are carried by the triiodothyronine (T3) on heart. T3 binds with nuclear receptors and transported into the cardiac myocyte, leading to increases in heart rate, cardiac contractility, systolic and mean pulmonary artery pressure, cardiac output, diastolic relaxation, and increased myocardial oxygen consumption. These result in reductions in systemic vascular resistance and diastolic pressure [91, 92]. Some other effects on heart are produced by direct beta-adrenergic stimulation of T3 [93]. These positive chronotropic and ionotropic effects lead to cardiac output increases by as much as 250 % and pulse pressure widens.

Patient may present with resting tachycardia which is exacerbated by exercise and systolic hypertension with widened pulse pressure [94]. Women, more than men may present with angina-like chest pain, with EKG changes suggesting myocardial ischemia. This scenario is attributed to coronary vasospasm and responds to treatment with orally administered calcium channel blockers.

Another acute presentation of thyrotoxicosis is atrial fibrillation, premature supraventricular depolarization, atrial premature contractions (APCs), more non-sustained supraventricular tachycardia, increased heart rate and reduced heart rate variability [95]. A detailed account of arrhythmias is given in another chapter.

Thyrotoxic patient may present with heart failure, especially with co-existing with atrial fibrillation or prolonged tachycardia [96]. Usually the clinical picture improves after sinus rhythm is restored and restoration of Euthyroid status. Other condition which may result in heart failure include cardiomyopathy (rate related), which too disappears after restoration of euthyroidism. Treatment is primarily on rate control by beta-adrenergic blockade.

Medication Exposure and Thyroid Emergencies

Acute Iodine Exposure: Jod-Basedow Phenomenon/Wolff-Chaikoff Effect

Excessive iodine exposure in patient with nodular goiter and having underlying iodine deficiency (Living in areas with iodine deficiency) may result in acute onset of thyrotoxicosis. This effect is due to underlying areas of autonomy within the thyroid gland. Jod-Basedow phenomenon, autonomous areas producing thyroid hormone independent of normal regulatory mechanisms, results in thyrotoxic state. These individuals may be thyrotoxic even before iodine repletion [97, 98]. This Iodine-induced thyrotoxicosis rarely occurs in patients without underlying thyroid disease (e.g., iodine-induced thyroiditis). Common presentation of this thyrotoxic state is seen after iodine exposure in medication (Amiodarone), iodine based contrast (radiological procedure and cardiac catherizaton) [99–103].

Contrast to above presentation, iodine exposure may result in development of rapid iodine-induced hypothyroidism. Pathophysiology behind this phenomenon is unusually sensitive to the inhibitory effects of iodide upon its own organification, in part due to a sustained activity of the sodium/iodide symporter. This sustained activity of the symporter results in a prolonged inhibition of thyroid hormone synthesis and an increase in TSH. Hypothyroidism ensues in these patients because of failure to escape from the acute Wolff-Chaikoff effect. This Condition associated with patient with chronic autoimmune thyroiditis, painless/postpartum/subacute granulomatous thyroiditis and with Graves' hyperthyroidism previously treated either with radioactive iodine or subtotal thyroidectomy [104–106].

Condition such as cystic fibrosis and thalassemia major undergoing blood transfusion places individual under increased risk of developing iodine induced hypothyroidism [107, 108].

Lithium Intoxication

Lithium exposure has been reported to cause hypothyroidism as well as hyperthyroidism. Pathophysiology of this inhibition of thyroid hormone release in not clearly known, although animal and human studies have revealed that lithium increases intrathyroidal iodine content, inhibits the coupling of iodotyrosine residues to form iodothyronines (thyroxine and triiodothyronin) and inhibits release of T4 and T3 [109–111]. Lithium induced hypothyroidism may present with or without goiter, but usually occurs during first 2 years of lithium use, back ground of chronic autoimmune hyroiditis and older age [112–114]. It is this effect of lithium which makes it useful in treatment of hyperthyroidism. Lithium in dosage of 600–1000 mg/day quantitatively similar to those of iodide in rapid correction of hyperthyroidism in patient allergic to iodine or thionamide [115, 116].

Miller et all and Kristensen et all have published data regarding two to three fold increase risk of hyperthyroidism in patient using lithium than general population [116, 117].

Lithium induced goiter may lead acute complication (compression). Approximately 40–50% of individuals may experience goiter formation

[118–121]. The treatment of goiter in patients taking lithium is the same as for goiter of any etiology.

Amiodarone-Induced Thyroid Emergencies

Amiodarone is implicated with thyroid dysfunction including both hypo as well as hyperthyroidism. These conditions can present as an acute event. This effect is attributed to amiodarone' s high iodine content (6 mg of iodine associated with a 200 mg dose of amiodarone) and its direct toxic effect on the thyroid. Iodine load can result in the Wolff-Chaikoff effect or (hypothyroidism) or Jod-Basedow (excessive thyroid hormone synthesis and thyrotoxicosis). Both of these are already discussed above.

Based on the underlying thyroid status, dietary iodine intake and/or subclinical thyroid disorders, there is 2–30 % risk of amiodarone-induced thyroid dysfunction [122–124].

Amiodarone-induced thyrotoxicosis is of two types. In type 1, there is increased synthesis of thyroid hormone, seen in patient with pre-existing multinodular goiter or latent Graves' disease; whereas in type 2 there is excess release of T4 and T3 due to a destructive thyroiditis caused by a direct toxic effect of amiodarone on thyroid follicular epithelial cells [125–127].

Treatments of these disorders are based on the clinical scenario. In hypothyroid state thyroid function can be easily normalized by replacement with thyroxine. Amiodarone should be continued.

Thionamide used in Patients with type I hyperthyroidism usually respond slowly and large doses (30–40 mg daily) may be required. This is due to very high intrathyroidal iodine stores [128]. Perchlorate, which blocks further iodine uptake by the thyroid, may be of beneficial but its association with aplastic anemia limits its use [129]. Sometimes lithium has been used to expedite recovery of hyperthyroidism [130]. RAI Therapy is only used if radioactive uptake is high enough for ablation. Patient with refractory disease to antithyroid drug therapy may be considered for thyroidectomy, but realizing that these patient are usually high risk.

Steroids remain the mainstay for treatment of type II hyperthyroidism. The dosage required is prednisone 40–60 mg/day and amiodarone could be continued [131]. Although iopanoic acid can be used but it is less effective than steroids [132]. Diagnosis could be challenging and possibility of "mixed" form of thyrotoxicosis or the underlying cause (type I or type II) may be uncertain. It is better to treat for both with combination of prednisone (40 mg/day) and methimazole/ Carbimazole (40 mg/day).

Post RAI

There could be a transient exacerbation of hyperthyroidism after radioiodine exposure. This clinical emergency may be eliminated by pretreatment and controlling hyperthyroidism clinically and biochemically before referring for RAI therapy [133–135]. Patient with severe intolerance to hyperthyroid symptoms, having underlying cardiac condition and elderly would qualify for pretreatment before RAI is offered to these individuals. Coincidental use of Lithium with RAI may also be help full reducing transient increase in serum thyroid hormone concentrations following radioiodine, but may not be recommended due to inconsistent data and lithium toxicity [136].

Thyroxine Overdose

Ingestion of excessive amounts of thyroxine can lead to exogenous hyperthyroidism. It could range from intentional (i.e., suppressive doses of thyroxine to treat thyroid cancer) or inadvertent (i.e., contamination of dietary supplements) or surreptitious ingestion (thyrotoxicosis factitia). These individuals present clinically as hyperthyroid except exophthalmos and goiter (unless present since the beginning). Acute thyroxine overdose can present with all acute complication of thyrotoxicosis such as myocardial infarction, especially in elderly patients, and seizures in children [137–139]. Chronic thyroxine overdose can cause chronic overt (low serum TSH, high free T4 and/or T3) or subclinical (low serum TSH with normal free T4) hyperthyroidism. Laboratory investigation will reveal low serum TSH concentrations with elevated serum thyroxine (T4) and/or triiodothyronine (T3). Serum thyroglobulin on the other hand is suppressed unlike other thyrotoxic conditions (Graves' and thyroiditis). 24-h radioiodine uptake is low due to suppression of TSH secretion. Treatment could be challenging in different scenario. Discontinuation or reduction in the dose of thyroid hormone is usually the only treatment needed. Half of the circulating dosage is removed from circulation in 7 days' time. T4 may take longer than T3 in clearance (serum half-life of about 1 day). Symptomatic treatment is offered in form of Beta-adrenergic antagonist drugs. Cholestyramine can be given to bind T4 and T3 in the intestine, thereby interrupting the normal enterohepatic circulation of the two hormones (Usual dose of cholestyramine is 4 g four times a day). Radiographic contrast agents ipodate or iopanoic acid, induction of emesis, gastric lavage, and intragastric instillation of charcoal and plasmapheresis have been used to treat massive thyroid hormone overdose [140].

Conclusion

Thyroid hormone is responsible for controlling biochemical status of the body and this is regulated by targeting all the cells of the body. Therefore any abnormality in thyroid regulation can have wide ranging effects. Diverse metabolic effects of this hormone make it peculiar and essential in regulating metabolic activities through our body. The effects of thyroid encompass activities which help in regulating body temperature, cholesterol and carbohydrate metabolism, body growth, neurological development (alteration in mental status), cardiovascular stability (heart rate, cardiac contractility and cardiac output regulation) and also reproductive health (behavioral and fertility effects). Person may require different approach of management even when biochemical status is same but clinically manifestations are different (Hyperthyroidism vs thyroid storm, hypothyroidism vs Myxedema coma).

Management of these conditions poses medical dilemmas which can be very challenging at times. Best example could be thyroid disease caused by certain medicine (amiodarone/lithium); in these scenarios decision regarding cessation of medication vs. continuation is to be made evaluating the need for these medication. Another example is titration of doses after resolution of acute presentation in thyroid storm and myxedema coma.

References

1. Sarlis NJ, Gourgiotis L. Thyroid emergencies. Rev Endocr Metab Disord. 2003;4:129.
2. Ngo SY, Chew HC. When the storm passes unnoticed – a case series of thyroid storm. Resuscitation. 2007;73:485.
3. Nayak B, Burman K. Thyrotoxicosis and thyroid storm. Endocrinol Metab Clin North Am. 2006;35:663.
4. Burch HB, Wartofsky L. Life-threatening thyrotoxicosis. Thyroid storm. Endocrinol Metab Clin North Am. 1993;22:263.
5. Bahn Chair RS, Burch HB, Cooper DS, et al. Hyperthyroidism and other causes of thyrotoxicosis: management guidelines of the American Thyroid Association and American Association of Clinical Endocrinologists. Thyroid. 2011;21:593.
6. Cooper DS, Saxe VC, Meskell M, et al. Acute effects of propylthiouracil (PTU) on thyroidal iodide organification and peripheral iodothyronine deiodination: correlation with serum PTU levels measured by radioimmunoassay. J Clin Endocrinol Metab. 1982;54:101.
7. Das G, Krieger M. Treatment of thyrotoxic storm with intravenous administration of propranolol. Ann Intern Med. 1969;70:985.
8. Benua RS, Becker DV, Hurley JR. Thyroid storm. In: Bardin CW, editor. Current therapy in endocrinology and metabolism. St. Louis: Mosby; 1994. p. 75.
9. Roti E, Robuschi G, Gardini E, et al. Comparison of methimazole, methimazole and sodium ipodate, and methimazole and saturated solution of potassium iodide in the early treatment of hyperthyroid Graves' disease. Clin Endocrinol (Oxf). 1988;28:305.
10. Nabil N, Miner DJ, Amatruda JM. Methimazole: an alternative route of administration. J Clin Endocrinol Metab. 1982;54:180.

11. Mazzaferri EL, Skillman TG. Thyroid storm. A review of 22 episodes with special emphasis on the use of guanethidine. Arch Intern Med. 1969;124:684.
12. Sherman SI, Simonson L, Ladenson PW. Clinical and socioeconomic predispositions to complicated thyrotoxicosis: a predictable and preventable syndrome? Am J Med. 1996;101:192.
13. Mazonson PD, Williams ML, Cantley LK, et al. Myxedema coma during long-term amiodarone therapy. Am J Med. 1984;77:751.
14. Waldman SA, Park D. Myxedema coma associated with lithium therapy. Am J Med. 1989;87:355.
15. Hylander B, Rosenqvist U. Treatment of myxoedema coma – factors associated with fatal outcome. Acta Endocrinol (Copenh). 1985;108:65.
16. Dutta P, Bhansali A, Masoodi SR, et al. Predictors of outcome in myxoedema coma: a study from a tertiary care centre. Crit Care. 2008;12:R1.
17. Beynon J, Akhtar S, Kearney T. Predictors of outcome in myxoedema coma. Crit Care. 2008;12:111.
18. Klein I. Thyroid hormone and the cardiovascular system. Am J Med. 1990;88:631.
19. Westphal SA. Unusual presentations of hypothyroidism. Am J Med Sci. 1997;314:333.
20. Kwaku MP, Burman KD. Myxedema coma. J Intensive Care Med. 2007;22:224.
21. Arlot S, Debussche X, Lalau JD, et al. Myxoedema coma: response of thyroid hormones with oral and intravenous high-dose L-thyroxine treatment. Intensive Care Med. 1991;17:16.
22. MacKerrow SD, Osborn LA, Levy H, et al. Myxedema-associated cardiogenic shock treated with intravenous triiodothyronine. Ann Intern Med. 1992;117:1014.
23. Holvey DN, Goodner CJ, Nicoloff JT. Treatment of Myxedema coma with intravenous thyroxine. Arch Intern Med. 1964;113:89.
24. Yamamoto T, Fukuyama J, Fujiyoshi A. Factors associated with mortality of myxedema coma: report of eight cases and literature survey. Thyroid. 1999;9:1167.
25. Rodríguez I, Fluiters E, Pérez-Méndez LF, et al. Factors associated with mortality of patients with myxoedema coma: prospective study in 11 cases treated in a single institution. J Endocrinol. 2004;180:347.
26. Foulds N, Walpole I, Elmslie F, Mansour S. Carbimazole embryopathy: an emerging phenotype. Am J Med Genet A. 2005;132A:130.
27. Bowman P, Osborne NJ, Sturley R, Vaidya B. Carbimazole embryopathy: implications for the choice of antithyroid drugs in pregnancy. QJM. 2012;105:189.
28. Wilson LC, Kerr BA, Wilkinson R, et al. Choanal atresia and hypothelia following methimazole exposure in utero: a second report. Am J Med Genet. 1998;75:220.
29. Di Gianantonio E, Schaefer C, Mastroiacovo PP, et al. Adverse effects of prenatal methimazole exposure. Teratology. 2001;64:262.
30. Wing DA, Millar LK, Koonings PP, et al. A comparison of propylthiouracil versus methimazole in the treatment of hyperthyroidism in pregnancy. Am J Obstet Gynecol. 1994;170:90.
31. Bowman P, Vaidya B. Suspected spontaneous reports of birth defects in the UK associated with the use of carbimazole and propylthiouracil in pregnancy. J Thyroid Res. 2011;2011:235130.
32. Butters L, Kennedy S, Rubin PC. Atenolol in essential hypertension during pregnancy. BMJ. 1990;301:587.
33. Lydakis C, Lip GY, Beevers M, Beevers DG. Atenolol and fetal growth in pregnancies complicated by hypertension. Am J Hypertens. 1999;12:541.
34. Lip GY, Beevers M, Churchill D, et al. Effect of atenolol on birth weight. Am J Cardiol. 1997;79:1436.
35. Adali E, Yildizhan R, Kolusari A, et al. The use of plasmapheresis for rapid hormonal control in severe hyperthyroidism caused by a partial molar pregnancy. Arch Gynecol Obstet. 2009;279:569.
36. Azezli A, Bayraktaroglu T, Topuz S, Kalayoglu-Besisik S. Hyperthyroidism in molar pregnancy: rapid preoperative preparation by plasmapheresis and complete improvement after evacuation. Transfus Apher Sci. 2007;36:87.
37. Martin FI, Deam DR. Hyperthyroidism in elderly hospitalised patients. Clinical features and treatment outcomes. Med J Aust. 1996;164:200.
38. Yudiarto FL, Muliadi L, Moeljanto D, Hartono B. Neuropsychological findings in hyperthyroid patients. Acta Med Indones. 2006;38:6.
39. Wu T, Flowers JW, Tudiver F, et al. Subclinical thyroid disorders and cognitive performance among adolescents in the United States. BMC Pediatr. 2006;6:12.
40. Li Voon Chong JS, Lecky BR, Macfarlane IA. Recurrent encephalopathy and generalised seizures associated with relapses of thyrotoxicosis. Int J Clin Pract. 2000;54:621.
41. Safe AF, Griffiths KD, Maxwell RT. Thyrotoxic crisis presenting as status epilepticus. Postgrad Med J. 1990;66:150.
42. Jabbari B, Huott AD. Seizures in thyrotoxicosis. Epilepsia. 1980;21:91. Lee TG, Ha CK, Lim BH. Thyroid storm presenting as status epilepticus and stroke. Postgrad Med J. 1997;73:61.
43. Newcomer J, Haire W, Hartman CR. Coma and thyrotoxicosis. Ann Neurol. 1983;14:689.
44. Jabbari B, Huott AD. Seizures in thyrotoxicosis. Epilepsia. 1980;21:91.
45. Lee TG, Ha CK, Lim BH. Thyroid storm presenting as status epilepticus and stroke. Postgrad Med J. 1997;73:61.
46. Stern RA, Robinson B, Thorner AR, et al. A survey study of neuropsychiatric complaints in patients with Graves' disease. J Neuropsychiatry Clin Neurosci. 1996;8:181.
47. Fukui T, Hasegawa Y, Takenaka H. Hyperthyroid dementia: clinicoradiological findings and response to treatment. J Neurol Sci. 2001;184:81.

48. Duyff RF, Van den Bosch J, Laman DM, et al. Neuromuscular findings in thyroid dysfunction: a prospective clinical and electrodiagnostic study. J Neurol Neurosurg Psychiatry. 2000;68:750.
49. Teoh HL, Lim EC. Platysmal myoclonus in subclinical hyperthyroidism. Mov Disord. 2005;20:1064.
50. Loh LM, Hum AY, Teoh HL, Lim EC. Graves' disease associated with spasmodic truncal flexion. Parkinsonism Relat Disord. 2005;11:117.
51. Ristić AJ, Svetel M, Dragasević N, et al. Bilateral chorea-ballism associated with hyperthyroidism. Mov Disord. 2004;19:982.
52. Fischbeck KH, Layzer RB. Paroxysmal choreoathetosis associated with thyrotosicosis. Ann Neurol. 1979;6:453.
53. Yen DJ, Shan DE, Lu SR. Hyperthyroidism presenting as recurrent short paroxysmal kinesigenic dyskinesia. Mov Disord. 1998;13:361.
54. Puri V, Chaudhry N. Paroxysmal kinesigenic dyskinesia manifestation of hyperthyroidism. Neurol India. 2004;52:102.
55. Klawans Jr HL, Shenker DM. Observations on the dopaminergic nature of hyperthyroid chorea. J Neural Transm. 1972;33:73.
56. Sheu JJ, Kang JH, Lin HC, Lin HC. Hyperthyroidism and risk of ischemic stroke in young adults: a 5-year follow-up study. Stroke. 2010;41:961.
57. Squizzato A, Gerdes VE, Brandjes DP, et al. Thyroid diseases and cerebrovascular disease. Stroke. 2005;36:2302.
58. Ra CS, Lui CC, Liang CL, et al. Superior sagittal sinus thrombosis induced by thyrotoxicosis. Case report. J Neurosurg. 2001;94:130.
59. Siegert CE, Smelt AH, de Bruin TW. Superior sagittal sinus thrombosis and thyrotoxicosis. Possible association in two cases. Stroke. 1995;26:496.
60. Molloy E, Cahill M, O'Hare JA. Cerebral venous sinus thrombosis precipitated by Graves' disease and Factor V Leiden mutation. Ir Med J. 2003;96:46.
61. Verberne HJ, Fliers E, Prummel MF, et al. Thyrotoxicosis as a predisposing factor for cerebral venous thrombosis. Thyroid. 2000;10:607.
62. Campos CR, Basso M, Evaristo EF, et al. Bilateral carotid artery dissection with thyrotoxicosis. Neurology. 2004;63:2443.
63. Nakamura K, Yanaka K, Ihara S, Nose T. Multiple intracranial arterial stenoses around the circle of Willis in association with Graves' disease: report of two cases. Neurosurgery. 2003;53:1210.
64. Thomas RD, Croft DN. Thyrotoxicosis and giant-cell arteritis. Br Med J. 1974;2:408.
65. Marongiu F, Conti M, Murtas ML, et al. Anticardiolipin antibodies in Grave's disease: relationship with thrombin activity in vivo. Thromb Res. 1991;64:745.
66. Bowness P, Shotliff K, Middlemiss A, Myles AB. Prevalence of hypothyroidism in patients with polymyalgia rheumatica and giant cell arteritis. Br J Rheumatol. 1991;30:349.
67. Hofbauer LC, Spitzweg C, Heufelder AE. Graves' disease associated with the primary antiphospholipid syndrome. J Rheumatol. 1996;23:1435.
68. Ramsay ID. Electromyography in thyrotoxicosis. Q J Med. 1965;34:255.
69. Havard CW, Campbell ED, Ross HB. Electromyographic and histological findings in the muscles of patients with thyrotoxicosis. Q J Med. 1963;32:145.
70. Sinclair C, Gilchrist JM, Hennessey JV, Kandula M. Muscle carnitine in hypo- and hyperthyroidism. Muscle Nerve. 2005;32:357.
71. Kaminski HJ, Ruff RL. Endocrine myopathies (hyper- and hypofunction of adrenal, thyroid, pistuitary, and parathyroid glands and iatrogenic corticosteroid myopathy. In: Myology, 2nd ed, Enngel, AG, Franzini-Armstrong, C (Eds), McGraw-Hill, New York 1994. p.1726
72. Horak HA, Pourmand R. Endocrine myopathies. Neurol Clin. 2000;18:203.
73. Kissel JT, Mendell JR. The endocrine myopathies. In: Rowland LP, Dimauro S, editors. Handbook of clinical neurology myopathies. New York: Elsevier Science; 1992. p. 527.
74. Erkintalo M, Bendahan D, Mattéi JP, et al. Reduced metabolic efficiency of skeletal muscle energetics in hyperthyroid patients evidenced quantitatively by in vivo phosphorus-31 magnetic resonance spectroscopy. Metabolism. 1998;47:769.
75. Bennett WR, Huston DP. Rhabdomyolysis in thyroid storm. Am J Med. 1984;77:733.
76. Lichtstein DM, Arteaga RB. Rhabdomyolysis associated with hyperthyroidism. Am J Med Sci. 2006;332:103.
77. Alshanti M, Eledrisi MS, Jones E. Rhabdomyolysis associated with hyperthyroidism. Am J Emerg Med. 2001;19:317.
78. Roquer J, Cano JF. Mononeuropathies in thyrotoxicosis. J Neurol Neurosurg Psychiatry. 1992;55:332.
79. Fisher M, Mateer JE, Ullrich I, Gutrecht JA. Pyramidal tract deficits and polyneuropathy in hyperthyroidism, Combination clinically mimicking amyotrophic lateral sclerosis. Am J Med. 1985;78:1041.
80. Feibel JH, Campa JF. Thyrotoxic neuropathy (Basedow's paraplegia). (. J Neurol Neurosurg Psychiatry. 1976;39:491.
81. Sözay S, Gökçe-Kutsal Y, Celiker R, et al. Neuroelectrophysiological evaluation of untreated hyperthyroid patients. Thyroidology. 1994;6:55.
82. Pandit L, Shankar SK, Gayathri N, Pandit A. Acute thyrotoxic neuropathy–Basedow's paraplegia revisited. J Neurol Sci. 1998;155:211.
83. Bronsky D, Kaganiec GI, et al. An association between the Guillain-barr'e syndrome and hyperthyroidism. Am J Med Sci. 1964;247:196.
84. Kiessling WR, Pflughaupt KW, Ricker K, et al. Thyroid function and circulating antithyroid antibodies in myasthenia gravis. Neurology. 1981;31:771.
85. Ratanakorn D, Vejjajiva A. Long-term follow-up of myasthenia gravis patients with hyperthyroidism. Acta Neurol Scand. 2002;106:93.

86. Weissel M, Mayr N, Zeitlhofer J. Clinical significance of autoimmune thyroid disease in myasthenia gravis. Exp Clin Endocrinol Diabetes. 2000;108:63.
87. Sekiguchi Y, Hara Y, Takahashi M, Hirata Y. Reverse 'see-saw' relationship between Graves' disease and myasthenia gravis; clinical and immunological studies. J Med Dent Sci. 2005;52:43.
88. Téllez-Zenteno JF, Cardenas G, Estañol B, et al. Associated conditions in myasthenia gravis: response to thymectomy. Eur J Neurol. 2004;11:767.
89. Ríos A, Rodríguez JM, Canteras M, et al. Surgical management of multinodular goiter with compression symptoms. Arch Surg. 2005;140:49.
90. Anders HJ. Compression syndromes caused by substernal goitres. Postgrad Med J. 1998;74:327.
91. Davis PJ, Davis FB. Nongenomic actions of thyroid hormone on the heart. Thyroid. 2002;12:459.
92. Brent GA. The molecular basis of thyroid hormone action. N Engl J Med. 1994;331:847.
93. Klein I. Endocrine disorders and cardiovascular disease. In: Bonow RO, Mann DL, Zipes DP, Libby P, editors. Braunwald's heart disease: a textbook of cardiovascular medicine. 9th ed. Philadelphia: Elsevier Saunders; 2012. p. 1829.
94. Iglesias P, Acosta M, Sánchez R, et al. Ambulatory blood pressure monitoring in patients with hyperthyroidism before and after control of thyroid function. Clin Endocrinol (Oxf). 2005;63:66.
95. Wustmann K, Kucera JP, Zanchi A, et al. Activation of electrical triggers of atrial fibrillation in hyperthyroidism. J Clin Endocrinol Metab. 2008;93:2104.
96. Siu CW, Yeung CY, Lau CP, et al. Incidence, clinical characteristics and outcome of congestive heart failure as the initial presentation in patients with primary hyperthyroidism. Heart. 2007;93:483.
97. Roti E, Uberti ED. Iodine excess and hyperthyroidism. Thyroid. 2001;11:493.
98. Stanbury JB, Ermans AE, Bourdoux P, et al. Iodine-induced hyperthyroidism : occurrence and epidemiology. Thyroid. 1998;8:83.
99. Skare S, Frey HM. Iodine induced thyrotoxicosis in apparently normal thyroid glands. Acta Endocrinol (Copenh). 1980;94:332.
100. Hintze G, Blombach O, Fink H, et al. Risk of iodine-induced thyrotoxicosis after coronary angiography: an investigation in 788 unselected subjects. Eur J Endocrinol. 1999;140:264.
101. Fradkin JE, Wolff J. Iodide-induced thyrotoxicosis. Medicine (Baltimore). 1983;62:1.
102. Rhee CM, Bhan I, Alexander EK, Brunelli SM. Association between iodinated contrast media exposure and incident hyperthyroidism and hypothyroidism. Arch Intern Med. 2012;172:153.
103. Burman KD, Wartofsky L. Iodine effects on the thyroid gland: biochemical and clinical aspects. Rev Endocr Metab Disord. 2000;1:19.
104. Clark OH, Cavalieri RR, Moser C, Ingbar SH. Iodide-induced hypothyroidism in patients after thyroid resection. Eur J Clin Invest. 1990;20:573.
105. Roti E, Minelli R, Gardini E, et al. Impaired intrathyroidal iodine organification and iodine-induced hypothyroidism in euthyroid women with a previous episode of postpartum thyroiditis. J Clin Endocrinol Metab. 1991;73:958.
106. Kämpe O, Jansson R, Karlsson FA. Effects of L-thyroxine and iodide on the development of autoimmune postpartum thyroiditis. J Clin Endocrinol Metab. 1990;70:1014.
107. Costigan DC, Holland FJ, Daneman D, et al. Amiodarone therapy effects on childhood thyroid function. Pediatrics. 1986;77:703.
108. Alexandrides T, Georgopoulos N, Yarmenitis S, Vagenakis AG. Increased sensitivity to the inhibitory effect of excess iodide on thyroid function in patients with beta-thalassemia major and iron overload and the subsequent development of hypothyroidism. Eur J Endocrinol. 2000;143:319.
109. Burrow GN, Burke WR, Himmelhoch JM, et al. Effect of lithium on thyroid function. J Clin Endocrinol Metab. 1971;32:647.
110. Bagchi N, Brown TR, Mack RE. Studies on the mechanism of inhibition of thyroid function by lithium. Biochim Biophys Acta. 1978;542:163.
111. Berens SC, Bernstein RS, Robbins J, Wolff J. Antithyroid effects of lithium. J Clin Invest. 1970;49:1357.
112. Kirov G, Tredget J, John R, et al. A cross-sectional and a prospective study of thyroid disorders in lithium-treated patients. J Affect Disord. 2005;87:313.
113. Bocchetta A, Loviselli A. Lithium treatment and thyroid abnormalities. Clin Pract Epidemiol Ment Health. 2006;2:23.
114. Van Melick EJ, Wilting I, Meinders AE, Egberts TC. Prevalence and determinants of thyroid disorders in elderly patients with affective disorders: lithium and nonlithium patients. Am J Geriatr Psychiatry. 2010;18:395.
115. Ng YW, Tiu SC, Choi KL, et al. Use of lithium in the treatment of thyrotoxicosis. Hong Kong Med J. 2006;12:254.
116. Kristensen O, Andersen HH, Pallisgaard G. Lithium carbonate in the treatment of thyrotoxicosis. A controlled trial. Lancet. 1976;1:603.
117. Miller KK, Daniels GH. Association between lithium use and thyrotoxicosis caused by silent thyroiditis. Clin Endocrinol (Oxf). 2001;55:501.
118. Lazarus JH. Lithium and thyroid. Best Pract Res Clin Endocrinol Metab. 2009;23:723.
119. Perrild H, Hegedüs L, Baastrup PC, et al. Thyroid function and ultrasonically determined thyroid size in patients receiving long-term lithium treatment. Am J Psychiatry. 1990;147:1518.
120. Lee S, Chow CC, Wing YK, Shek CC. Thyroid abnormalities during chronic lithium treatment in Hong Kong Chinese: a controlled study. J Affect Disord. 1992;26:173.
121. Bocchetta A, Bernardi F, Pedditzi M, et al. Thyroid abnormalities during lithium treatment. Acta Psychiatr Scand. 1991;83:193.

122. Batcher EL, Tang XC, Singh BN, et al. Thyroid function abnormalities during amiodarone therapy for persistent atrial fibrillation. Am J Med. 2007;120:880.
123. Tsadok MA, Jackevicius CA, Rahme E, et al. Amiodarone-induced thyroid dysfunction: brand-name versus generic formulations. CMAJ. 2011;183, E817.
124. Martino E, Safran M, Aghini-Lombardi F, et al. Environmental iodine intake and thyroid dysfunction during chronic amiodarone therapy. Ann Intern Med. 1984;101:28.
125. Lambert M, Unger J, De Nayer P, et al. Amiodarone-induced thyrotoxicosis suggestive of thyroid damage. J Endocrinol Invest. 1990;13:527.
126. Bartalena L, Brogioni S, Grasso L, et al. Treatment of amiodarone-induced thyrotoxicosis, a difficult challenge: results of a prospective study. J Clin Endocrinol Metab. 1996;81:2930.
127. Martino E, Bartalena L, Bogazzi F, Braverman LE. The effects of amiodarone on the thyroid. Endocr Rev. 2001;22:240.
128. Bogazzi F, Bartalena L, Martino E. Approach to the patient with amiodarone-induced thyrotoxicosis. J Clin Endocrinol Metab. 2010;95:2529.
129. Martino E, Aghini-Lombardi F, Mariotti S, et al. Treatment of amiodarone associated thyrotoxicosis by simultaneous administration of potassium perchlorate and methimazole. J Endocrinol Invest. 1986;9:201.
130. Dickstein G, Shechner C, Adawi F, et al. Lithium treatment in amiodarone-induced thyrotoxicosis. Am J Med. 1997;102:454.
131. Bogazzi F, Tomisti L, Rossi G, et al. Glucocorticoids are preferable to thionamides as first-line treatment for amiodarone-induced thyrotoxicosis due to destructive thyroiditis: a matched retrospective cohort study. J Clin Endocrinol Metab. 2009;94:3757.
132. Bogazzi F, Bartalena L, Cosci C, et al. Treatment of type II amiodarone-induced thyrotoxicosis by either iopanoic acid or glucocorticoids: a prospective, randomized study. J Clin Endocrinol Metab. 2003;88:1999.
133. Shafer RB, Nuttall FQ. Acute changes in thyroid function in patients treated with radioactive iodine. Lancet. 1975;2:635.
134. Stensvold AD, Jorde R, Sundsfjord J. Late and transient increases in free T4 after radioiodine treatment for Graves' disease. J Endocrinol Invest. 1997;20:580.
135. Burch HB, Solomon BL, Cooper DS, et al. The effect of antithyroid drug pretreatment on acute changes in thyroid hormone levels after (131)I ablation for Graves' disease. J Clin Endocrinol Metab. 2001;86:3016.
136. Bogazzi F, Bartalena L, Campomori A, et al. Treatment with lithium prevents serum thyroid hormone increase after thionamide withdrawal and radioiodine therapy in patients with Graves' disease. J Clin Endocrinol Metab. 2002;87:4490.
137. Shammas NW, Richeson JF, Pomerantz R. Myocardial dysfunction and necrosis after ingestion of thyroid hormone. Am Heart J. 1994;127:232.
138. Gorman RL, Chamberlain JM, Rose SR, Oderda GM. Massive levothyroxine overdose: high anxiety–low toxicity. Pediatrics. 1988;82:666.
139. Locker GJ, Kotzmann H, Frey B, et al. Factitious hyperthyroidism causing acute myocardial infarction. Thyroid. 1995;5:465.
140. Cohen 3rd JH, Ingbar SH, Braverman LE. Thyrotoxicosis due to ingestion of excess thyroid hormone. Endocr Rev. 1989;10:113.

Thyroid Nodule

13

Syed Hunain Riaz, Muhammad Zaman Khan Assir, Ali Jawa, and Javed Akram

Abstract

Thyroid nodules are not an uncommon clinical problem, even in iodine sufficient areas. The incidence is 2–4 per 100,000 people per year, being more common in women and the elderly. The evaluation of thyroid nodule is aimed at differentiating benign from malignant thyroid nodules and comprises of detailed history (irradiation, family history etc), examination and biochemical, radiological and cytological investigations. Most common diagnoses are colloid cysts and nodules (80 % of cases), benign follicular neoplasms (10–15 % of cases) and thyroid cancer (5 % of cases). Measurement of serum TSH is the first step in the work-up. Subnormal TSH warrants radio-isotope scanning to exclude hyper functioning thyroid nodule. Patients with normal or high serum TSH undergo imaging studies and FNA. A number of radiological modalities are used including simple (USG) and advanced imaging studies (CT,MRI,PET). Thyroid USG is still considered the radiological modality of choice for initial work-up. FNA is the procedure of choice and all non-palpable/palpable nodules of >1 cm in size warrant FNA. The indications for FNA in sub-centimeter nodules include solid hypoechoic nodule with microcalcifications, nodules with abnormal cervical lymph nodes detected on physical examination or imaging, high risk history. Treatment of thyroid nodule depends on whether the

S.H. Riaz, MBBS, FCPS (✉)
Department of Endocrinology, Allama Iqbal Medical College, Lahore, Pakistan
e-mail: syedhunain@gmail.com

M.Z.K. Assir, MBBS, FCPS
Department of Medicine, Allama Iqbal Medical College, Lahore, Pakistan

A. Jawa, MD, MPH, DABIM, DABIM (Endo)
J. Akram, MRCP, FRCP, FACC, FACP, FASIM
Department of Endocrinology, Shaheed Zulfiqar Ali Bhutto Medical University, PIMS, Islamabad, Pakistan

S.K. Imam, S.I. Ahmad (eds.), *Thyroid Disorders: Basic Science and Clinical Practice*,
DOI 10.1007/978-3-319-25871-3_13

nodule is benign or malignant. Surgery is generally the treatment of choice for nodules that have high risk clinical or cytological features. Radio-iodine treatment is indicated for nodules with biochemical hyperthyroidism. Percutaneous ethanol injection is indicated for benign functioning/non-functioning solid nodules and also for cystic nodules.

Introduction

Epidemiology

Studies have shown thyroid nodules to be present in 5 % of women and 1 % of men in areas which are iodine sufficient [1, 2], and is not an uncommon clinical problem. In the United states, 4–7 % of people have palpable thyroid nodules [3] with an incidence of around 2–4 per 100,000 people per year and constitute about 1 % of all the cancers [4]. Approximately 23 % of solitary nodules are actually dominant nodules within a multinodular goiter [5]. Thyroid nodules are more commonly seen in women and the elderly [6]. After exposure to ionizing radiation, thyroid nodules develop at a rate of 2 % annually [5]. The prevalence of thyroid nodules is increased when those nodules are included which are detected by Ultrasonography or at autopsy [7].

Clinical Problem

The clinical spectrum ranges from small, incidental asymptomatic nodules to large ones which can cause pressure symptoms. The clinical relevance of thyroid nodules rests in the detection of or ruling out thyroid cancer depending on age, sex, radiation exposure history, family history, and other factors [8]. The most common diagnoses according to approximate distribution are colloid nodules, cysts, and thyroiditis (in 80 % of cases); benign follicular neoplasms (in 10–15 %); and thyroid carcinoma (in 5 %) [8]. Differentiated thyroid cancer (DTC), which includes papillary and follicular cancer, comprises the majority (90 %) of all thyroid cancers [9]. The incidence of thyroid cancers has increased over the years mainly due to increase in the incidence of papillary thyroid cancer (PTC) around 2.9 fold between 1988 and 2002 [10]. The increasing incidence is partly due to increasing use of ultrasonography of neck for diagnostics and also due to changing trends which lay emphasis on early diagnosis and treatment of Thyroid cancer [11]. Certain factors associated with increased risk for thyroid nodules are smoking, alcohol consumption and IGF-1 levels [12, 13]. Oral contraceptives and statins are possibly associated with a reduced risk of nodule formation [14, 15].

Clinical Evaluation

History and physical examination are integral to the further workup of a thyroid nodule as the suspicion of a malignancy is increased or decreased with a properly taken history and appropriately done physical examination. It is to be noted though that non-palpable nodules detected on ultrasonography or other imaging techniques are termed 'incidentilomas' and the risk of malignancy in these nodules is the same as for palpable nodules of same size [16].

History

Factors in history predicting malignancy in a thyroid nodule include [17, 18]:

1. Childhood history of head and neck irradiation
2. Whole body irradiation for bone marrow transplantation
3. Family history suggestive of thyroid cancer
4. History of exposure to radiation fallout in childhood or adolescence
5. Thyroid cancer syndromes (Familial polyposis, Cowden's syndrome, Multiple endocrine neoplasia type 2 [MEN-2], Werner syndrome) in a first degree relative

6. Rapidly increasing size of nodule/growth.
7. Symptoms of compression including dysphagia, dysphonia, hoarseness, cough and dyspnea.

Physical Examination

A thorough physical examination of the head and neck region is essential to gauge the risk of malignancy in the thyroid nodule. However, in a small number of patients, findings suggestive of malignancy are present in patients with benign thyroid nodules. Inter-examiner variations do exist, leading to an increasing trend towards using imaging as part of evaluation [4, 19].

Palpation of the thyroid lobes and isthmus along with careful palpation of the anterior and posterior triangles of the neck for lymphadenopathy is necessary to clinically assess the nature of the thyroid nodule. Thyroid nodules should be assessed for several parameters such as dimensions, surface, consistency, mobility, overlying skin and tenderness. They are described individually as follows:

- ***Dimensions***: Can be of varying sizes, though nodules >1 cm should undergo further workup. Nodules <1 cm are generally not palpable unless they are in the anterior lobe. Those less than <1 cm should undergo workup only if there is associated lymphadenopathy, suggestive high risk history or suspicious ultrasonography findings.
- ***Surface:*** Can range from smooth to irregular suggesting benign and malignant nature of nodule respectively
- ***Consistency:*** Can range from soft, firm to hard suggesting diagnoses such as colloid cysts, adenomas to carcinomas respectively
- ***Mobility:*** Nodules fixed to underlying tissues generally are suggestive of cancer
- ***Overlying skin:*** Can be freely mobile or fixed in case of cancer.
- ***Tenderness:*** Tenderness suggests recent hemorrhage.

Factors suggesting high and moderate risk of malignancy on physical examination as follows:

High Suspicion for Malignancy

1. Nodule that is firm or hard
2. Fixation of nodule to adjacent structures
3. Regional lymphadenopathy
4. Distant metastasis
5. Vocal cord paralysis (on indirect laryngoscopy)

Moderate Suspicion for Malignancy

1. Nodule >4 cm or partially cystic
2. Age <20 or >70 years

It should be noted though that ultrasound neck detects nodules in more than half of patients with normal clinical examination. This fact highlights the low sensitivity and specificity of neck clinical examination [20]. Although when two or more risk factors for high suspicion are present, the likelihood that the nodule is malignant approaches almost 100 % [21].

Investigations

The objective of evaluation of thyroid nodule is to differentiate benign from a malignant lesion and to assess the functional status of the nodule. The work up of a thyroid nodule includes thyroid function tests, radionuclide scanning, radiological studies including thyroid USG, Computed Tomography (CT), Magnetic Resonance Imaging (MRI), Positron-Emission Tomography, and fine needle aspiration (Fig. 13.1). ATA has published detailed guidelines on the workup of thyroid nodule and a summary of these recommendations is presented below (Table 13.1).

Indications for Evaluation [22]

1. Since non-palpable nodules have the same risk of malignancy as palpable nodules with the same size [16], thyroid nodules detected on clinical examination or incidentally on radiological examination (incidentalomas) need evaluation.
2. Generally, only nodules >1 cm should be evaluated, since they have a greater potential to be clinically significant cancers. Occasionally,

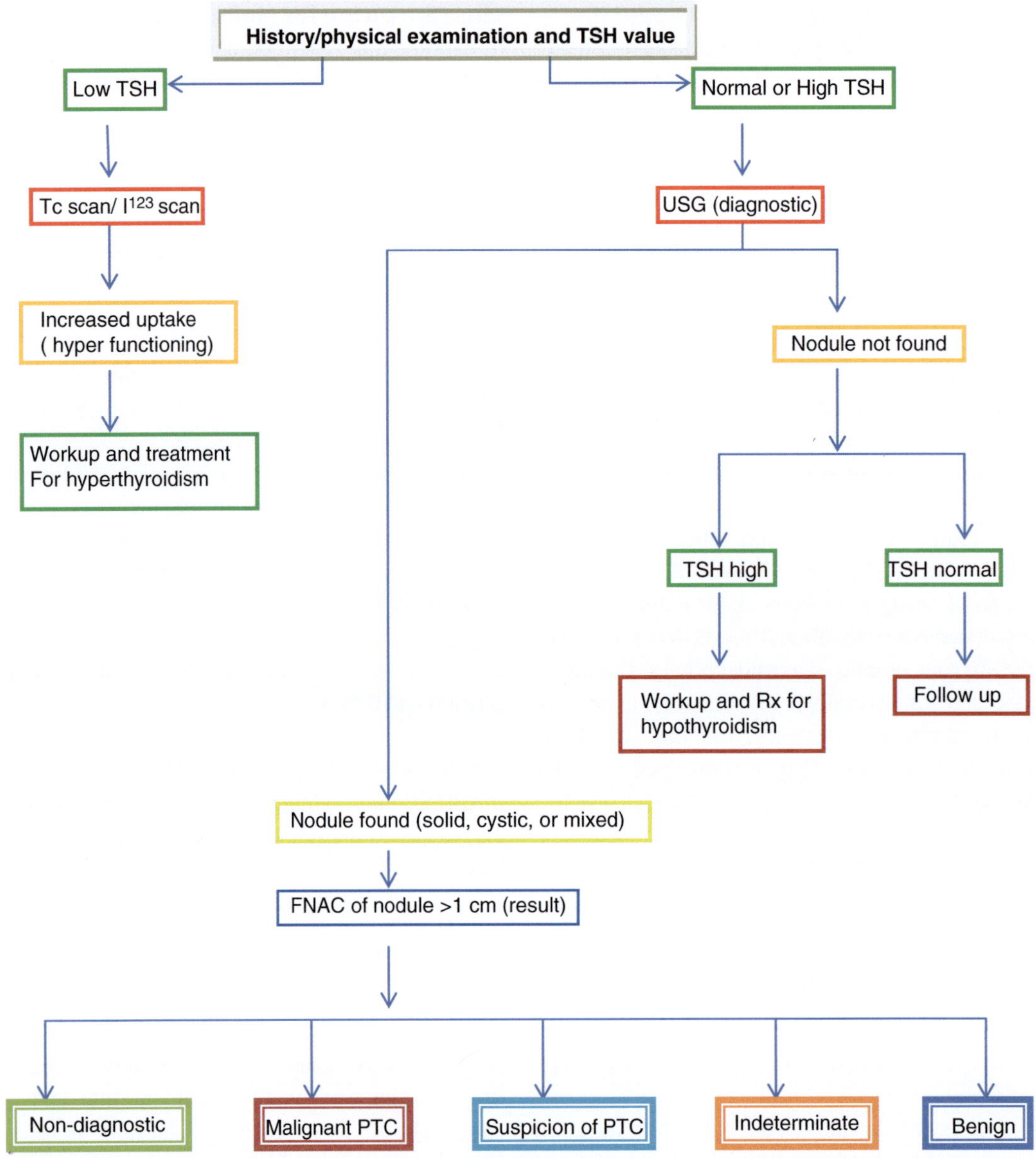

Fig. 13.1 Diagnostic algorithm for evaluation of thyroid nodule. *US* ultrasound, *PTC* papillary thyroid cancer

there may be nodules <1 cm that require evaluation because of suspicious USG findings, associated lymphadenopathy, a history of head and neck irradiation, or a history of thyroid cancer or thyroid cancer syndrome (e.g. Cowden Syndrome, familial polyposis, Carney complex, multiple endocrine neoplasia [MEN] 2, Werner syndrome) in one or more first-degree relatives.

3. Approximately 1–2 % of people undergoing 2-deoxy-2[18F] fluoro-d-glucose positron emission tomography (18FDG-PET) imaging for other reasons have thyroid nodules discovered incidentally. Since the risk of malignancy in these 18FDG-positive nodules is about 33 % and the cancers may be more aggressive [23], such lesions require prompt evaluation [24–26].

Table 13.1 Summary of revised American Thyroid Association 2009 recommendations on the evaluation of thyroid nodule

Sr #	Investigation/ condition	Recommendation	Recommendation rating
1	Serum TSH	Measure serum TSH in the initial evaluation of a patient with a thyroid nodule. If the serum TSH is subnormal, a radionuclide thyroid scan should be performed using either technetium 99mTc pertechnetate or 123I	A
2	Thyroid sonography	Thyroid sonography should be performed in all patients with known or suspected thyroid nodules	A
3	Serum thyroglobulin (Tg)	Routine measurement of serum Tg for initial evaluation of thyroid nodules is not recommended	F
4	Serum calcitonin	The panel cannot recommend either for or against the routine measurement of serum calcitonin	I
5	FNA	(a) FNA is the procedure of choice in the evaluation of thyroid nodules	A
		(b) US guidance for FNA is recommended for those nodules that are nonpalpable, predominantly cystic, or located posteriorly in the thyroid lobe	B
		(c) US guidance should be used when repeating the FNA procedure for a nodule with an initial nondiagnostic cytology result	A
6	Cytology: diagnostic of or suspicious for PTC	(a) If a cytology result is diagnostic of or suspicious for PTC, surgery is recommended	A
		(b) If the reading is "suspicious for papillary carcinoma" or "Hurthle cell neoplasm," a radionuclide scan is not needed, and either lobectomy or total thyroidectomy is recommended, depending on the lesion's size and other risk factors	A
7	Cytology: indeterminate	(a) The use of molecular markers (e.g., BRAF, RAS, RET=PTC, Pax8-PPARg, or galectin-3) may be considered for patients with indeterminate cytology on FNA to help guide management	C
		(b) The panel cannot recommend for or against routine clinical use of 18FDG-PET scan to improve diagnostic accuracy of indeterminate thyroid nodules	I
8	Cytology: follicular neoplasm	If the cytology reading reports a follicular neoplasm, a 123I thyroid scan may be considered, if not already done, especially if the serum TSH is in the low-normal range. If a concordant autonomously functioning nodule is not seen, lobectomy or total thyroidectomy should be considered	C
9	Cytology: benign	(a) If the nodule is benign on cytology, further immediate diagnostic studies or treatment are not routinely required	A
		(b) It is recommended that all benign thyroid nodules be followed with serial US examinations 6–18 months after the initial FNA. If nodule size is stable (i.e., no more than a 50 % change in volume or <20 % increase in at least two nodule dimensions in solid nodules or in the solid portion of mixed cystic–solid nodules), the interval before the next follow-up clinical examination or US may be longer, e.g., every 3–5 years	C
		(c) If there is evidence for nodule growth either by palpation or sonographically (more than a 50 % change in volume or a 20 % increase in at least two nodule dimensions with a minimal increase of 2 mm in solid nodules or in the solid portion of mixed cystic–solid nodules), the FNA should be repeated, preferably with US guidance	B

(continued)

Table 13.1 (continued)

Sr #	Investigation/ condition	Recommendation	Recommendation rating
10	Two or more thyroid nodules	(a) In the presence of two or more thyroid nodules >1 cm, those with a suspicious sonographic appearance should be aspirated preferentially	A
		(b) If none of the nodules has a suspicious sonographic appearance and multiple sonographically similar coalescent nodules with no intervening normal parenchyma are present, the likelihood of malignancy is low and it is reasonable to aspirate the largest nodules only and observe the others with serial US examinations	C
		(c) A low or low-normal serum TSH concentration may suggest the presence of autonomous nodule(s). A technetium 99mTc pertechnetate or 123I scan should be performed and directly compared to the US images to determine functionality of each nodule >1–1.5 cm. FNA should then be considered only for those isofunctioning or nonfunctioning nodules, among which those with suspicious sonographic features should be aspirated preferentially	B

Biochemical Tests

Serum TSH

First step in the evaluation of thyroid nodule is measurement of serum TSH levels. Most patients presenting with a solitary thyroid nodule are euthyroid. If serum TSH is subnormal, levels of free thyroxine or free triiodothyronine should be measured to document the presence and degree of hyperthyroidism. Thyroid scintigraphy should be performed in these patients to document whether the nodule is hyperfunctioning (i.e., tracer uptake is greater than the surrounding normal thyroid), is functioning or "warm" (i.e., tracer uptake is equal to the surrounding thyroid), or nonfunctioning (i.e., has uptake less than the surrounding thyroid tissue). Approximately 10 % of patients with a solitary nodule have a suppressed level of serum TSH, which suggests a benign hyperfunctioning nodule. Since a hyperfunctioning nodule rarely harbors malignancy, FNA is not required in these cases [22].

On the other hand if the serum TSH concentration is normal or elevated, and the nodule meets criteria for sampling, then fine needle aspiration biopsy is indicated. Serum TSH is an independent risk factor for predicting malignancy in a thyroid nodule. In a study of 1500 patients presenting to a thyroid practice, the prevalence of malignancy was 2.8, 3.7, 8.3, 12.3, and 29.7 % for patients with serum TSH concentrations <0.4 mU/L, 0.4–0.9 mU/L, 1.0–1.7 mU/L, 1.8–5.5 mU/L, and >5.5 mU/L, respectively [27]. In addition, a serum anti-thyroperoxidase (anti TPO) antibody level should be obtained in hypothyroid patients to confirm Hashimoto's thyroiditis. However, the finding of an elevated level of anti TPO antibodies does not obviate the need for a fine-needle aspiration biopsy, since lymphoma which accounts for 5 % of thyroid cancers is associated with Hashimoto's thyroiditis [8].

Serum Thyroglobulin

Serum Tg is frequently elevated in thyroid diseases, however measurement of serum Tg does not differentiate benign from malignant thyroid disease [28]. Therefore, routine measurement of serum Tg for initial evaluation of thyroid nodules is not recommended.

Serum Calcitonin

Basal serum calcitonin levels should be obtained in any patient with a family history of medullary thyroid carcinoma, multiple endocrine neoplasia types 2a or b, pheochromocytoma, or hyperparathyroidism. Since only 1 in 250 nodules represent medullary thyroid carcinoma, serum calcitonin testing is reserved for high risk patients only [29].

Serum calcitonin levels are also elevated in C-cell hyperplasia and hence calcitonin levels alone are unable to distinguish between benign and malignant disease [30]. However, if basal (unstimulated) serum calcitonin level is greater than 100 pg/mL, medullary thyroid cancer is likely present [31].

Imaging

Radionuclide Scanning

A radionuclide scan is useful in determining if a thyroid nodule is functioning and is recommended in patients with sub-normal serum TSH. Radioisotopes that have been used are technetium (99 mTc), I^{123}, and I^{131}, and though similar information is obtained with similar amounts of radiation exposure, radioiodine is preferred [32]. Iodine isotopes, which are both trapped and bound organically in the thyroid, are preferred, since 3–8 % of nodules that appear functioning on pertechnetate scanning may appear nonfunctioning on radioiodine scanning, and a few of those nodules may be thyroid cancers [33]. Hot nodules account for 5 % of thyroid nodules and carry less than 1 % risk of malignancy. Therefore, when a functioning thyroid nodule is found, FNA is not required. On the other hand about 80–85 % of thyroid nodules are cold, and about 10 % of these nodules represent a malignancy. Radionuclide scan does not provide an accurate measurement of size and is performed much more commonly in Europe than in United States. Taken together, the sensitivity for the diagnosis of thyroid cancer is 89–93 %, specificity is 5 %, and the positive predictive value of malignancy is only 10 % [34].

Thyroid Ultrasound

Ultrasonography is the imaging study of choice for thyroid nodules. Diagnostic thyroid US should be performed in all patients with a suspected thyroid nodule, nodular goiter, or radiographic abnormality; e.g., a nodule found incidentally on computed tomography (CT) or magnetic resonance imaging (MRI) or thyroidal uptake on 18FDG-PET scan [22]. Ultrasonography can accurately detect non palpable nodules, estimate the size of the nodule and the volume of the goiter, and differentiate simple cysts, which have a low risk of being malignant, from solid nodules or from mixed cystic and solid nodules, which have a 5 % risk of being malignant. Thyroid ultrasound is also useful in detecting cervical lymphadenopathy and provides accurate measurements of nodule diameter for interval monitoring.

Sonographic findings cannot reliably distinguish between benign and cancerous lesions; however it is useful in selecting the site within a nodule for fine needle aspirate biopsy (FNAB) in order to improve diagnostic yield, or to select appropriate nodules to aspirate within a multinodular thyroid. There are certain characteristics on Ultrasonography of Thyroid nodule that can predict the presence of malignancy such as micro-calcifications, irregular margins, surrounding invasion, hypoechogenicity, an absent halo, and a shape taller than the width measured in the transverse dimension, presence of lymphadenopathy and increased blood flow on Doppler flow scan. The most common sonographic appearances of papillary and follicular thyroid cancer differ. A PTC is generally solid or predominantly solid and hypoechoic, often with infiltrative irregular margins and increased nodular vascularity. Microcalcifications, if present, are highly specific for PTC, but differentiation from colloid may be difficult, while Follicular cancer is more often iso- to hyperechoic and has a thick and irregular halo, but does not have microcalcifications [8, 35]. Certain sonographic appearances may also be highly suggestive of a benign nodule. A pure cystic nodule, although rare (<2 % of all nodules), is highly unlikely to be malignant [36]. In addition, a spongiform appearance, defined as an aggregation of multiple micro-cystic components in more than 50 % of the nodule volume, is 99.7 % specific for identification of a benign thyroid nodule [37]. Other features suggestive of a benign nodule include macrocalcifications, comet-tail shadowing and hyperechoic mass with peripheral vascularity.

Diagnostic Ultrasound of the thyroid provides useful information as whether the nodule is cystic, solid or mixed (solid plus cystic). Cystic nodules were earlier on thought to be predominantly benign and conservative management was suggested [38]. However it has been seen recently that cystic thyroid nodules also carry an equal or even greater risk than solid nodules to harbor malignancy [39]. Cysts that are larger in size (>33 mm), have a blood component in them, have recurrences after repeated aspirations and previous history of neck irradiation are all considerations for surgery. To improve the accuracy of the FNAC in such nodules, it should be carried out under Ultrasound guidance because when done blindly, there is possibility of geographically missing the area with malignancy [40, 41]. Similarly the diagnostic accuracy of FNA performed by palpation is low in posteriorly located nodules and in these cases, ultrasound guided FNA of thyroid nodule is recommended. Additionally, US guidance should be used when repeating the FNA procedure for a nodule with an initial non-diagnostic cytology result. The rate of malignancy in nodules in thyroid glands involved with Hashimoto's thyroiditis is as least as high as or possibly higher than normal thyroid gland. The nodularity of thyroid gland in the setting of Hashimoto's thyroiditis may represent focal enlargement from lymphocytic infiltrates, TSH-induced hyperplasia of follicular tissue, or a thyroid tumor and thyroid ultrasound may help to distinguish among these possibilities.

Other Imaging Studies

Computed tomography (CT) and magnetic resonance imaging (MRI) are not routinely recommended for the work up of a thyroid nodule. They are useful in the evaluation of retro-sternal thyroid. It is important to note that iodinated contrast material utilized for CT scan should be avoided because its use prevents scintigraphy or administration of radioactive iodine (RAI) therapy for a period of 1–2 months. Gadolinium contrast used with MRI does not interfere with thyroid uptake of radiotracer, but it is significantly more expensive than CT or ultrasound.

18F-fluorodeoxyglucose positron emission tomography-computed tomography (18FDG-PET/CT) can be used to improve diagnostic accuracy of indeterminate thyroid nodules. ATA guidelines do not recommend for or against the use of 18FDG-PET scan.

Fine Needle Aspiration

The American Thyroid Association recommends FNA biopsy as the procedure of choice for evaluating thyroid nodules and selecting candidates for surgery. FNA is the most accurate and cost-effective method for evaluating thyroid nodules. It has advantages of cost-effectiveness, easy to learn and can be performed on outpatient basis. FNA is performed with or without local lidocaine anesthesia [42], by repetitively moving a 23–27-gauge (most commonly 25-gauge) needle through the nodule. Biopsy can be guided by palpation only or by ultrasound. Ultrasound guidance is recommended in case of posteriorly located nodule, nodule with mixed solid and cystic components and repeat FNA. Fine-needle capillary sampling (FNC, also called fine-needle non-aspiration biopsy) is a variation of FNA in which the sample is obtained by repetitively moving within the nodule a 25–27-gauge needle that is not attached to a syringe [43, 44]. After the needle is removed from the nodule, a syringe containing air is used to express the sample on a slide, which is smeared, stained, and submitted for cytologic interpretation. If FNA is scheduled antiplatelets and anticoagulants should ideally be discontinued 5–7 days before the procedure, however clinician should weigh the risk of discontinuing these drugs and current use of these medications does not preclude FNA. FNA is a simple and safe procedure. Local pain and hematomas are the most common complications, while serious adverse events are rare.

Routine FNA is not recommended for nodules <1 cm in size. The indications for FNA in subcentimeter nodules include solid hypoechoic nodule with microcalcifications, nodules with abnormal cervical lymph nodes detected on physical examination or imaging, high risk history (family history of PTC [45]; history of external beam radiation exposure as a child [46]; exposure to ionizing radiation in childhood or adolescence [47]; history of prior hemi thyroidectomy with discovery of thyroid cancer) and 18FDGPET–positive thyroid nodules (Fig. 13.2).

Criteria for cytological adequacy of FNA include the presence of at least six follicular cell groups, each containing 10–15 cells derived from at least two aspirates of a nodule [48].

FNA biopsy results are divided into six categories: Non-diagnostic, benign, follicular lesion of

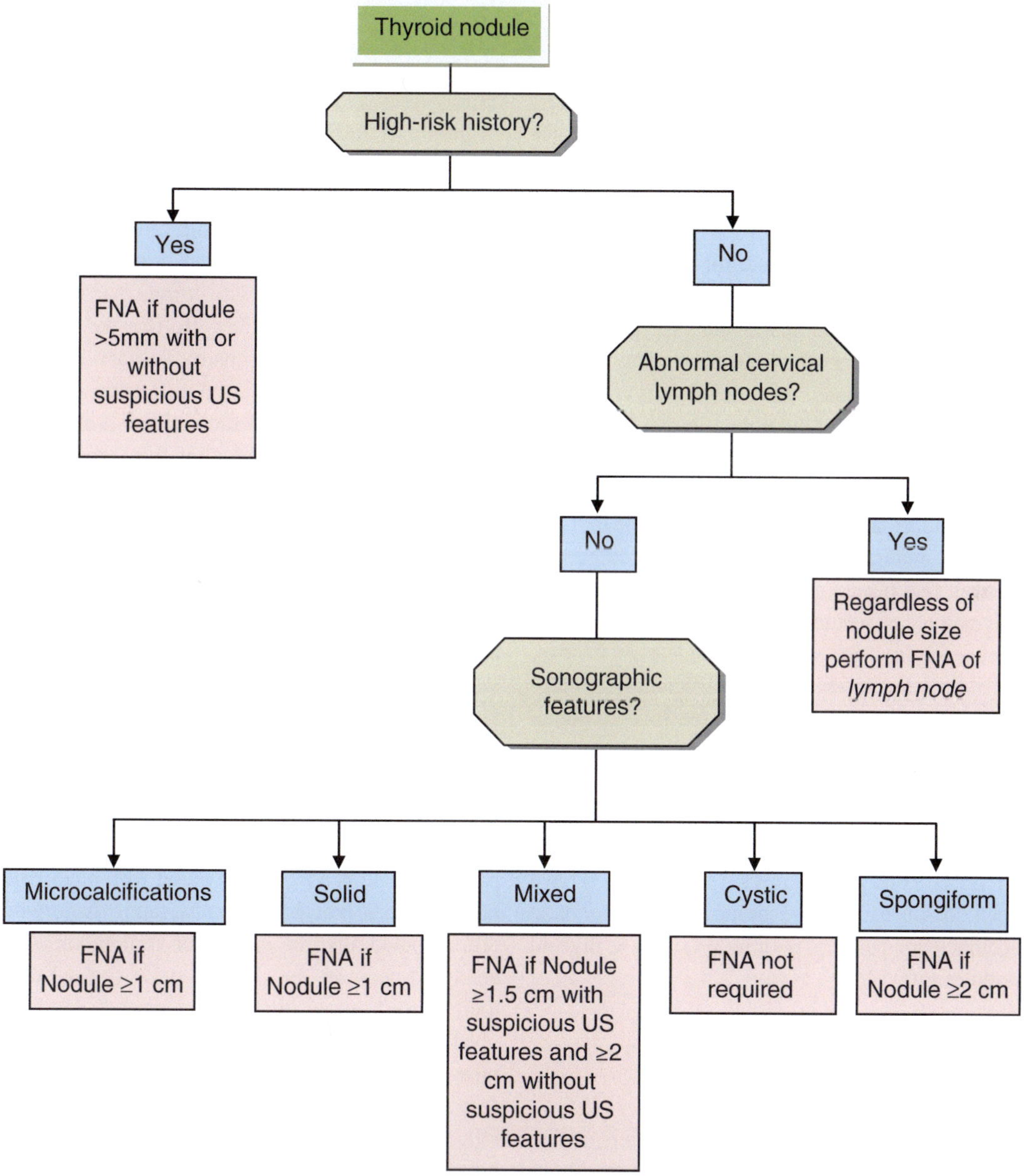

Fig. 13.2 A step wise approach to the decision of FNA in a thyroid nodule based on ATA guidelines. The decision to obtain FNA in a thyroid nodule takes into consideration both the size and high risk characteristics (high risk history, physical examination and suspicious ultrasonographic findings)

undetermined significance, follicular neoplasm, suspicious for malignancy and malignant. Non-diagnostic biopsies are those that fail to meet specified criteria for cytologic adequacy. In case of non-diagnostic FNA biopsy results, ultrasound guided repeat biopsy is indicated. It is important to note that absence of malignant cells should not be interpreted as 'negative'. Benign lesions include macrofollicular or "colloid" adenomas, chronic lymphocytic (Hashimoto's) thyroiditis, or subacute granulomatous thyroiditis. Follicular lesions of undetermined significance are those lesions that are not convincingly benign but do not have definitive features of a follicular neoplasm and are not highly suspicious of malignancy. This category includes lesions with mild atypia, mixed macro- and microfollicular lesions where the proportion of micro- and macrofollicles is similar, and specimens that are compromised because of poor fixation or obscuring blood. Follicular lesions include microfollicular or cellular adenomas. The category 'suspicious for malignancy' includes lesions with some features suggestive of but not definitive for thyroid cancer. The malignant category includes papillary cancer, medullary cancer, thyroid lymphoma, anaplastic cancer, and cancer metastatic to the thyroid. The only malignant pathology reliably diagnosed through fine needle aspiration is papillary thyroid carcinoma, as features such as 'Orphan Annie' nuclei, nuclear grooves, intra-nuclear inclusions, and psammoma bodies can be sufficient for a diagnosis. Medullary carcinoma, anaplastic carcinoma, lymphoma, poorly differentiated carcinoma, and metastatic disease have also been reported to be classified on the basis of cytology [49].

A number of genetic markers (BRAF, Ras, RET/PTC) and protein markers (galectin-3) have been shown to improve preoperative diagnostic accuracy for patients with indeterminate thyroid nodules [50–52].

Treatment

The management of a thyroid nodule depends on decisions taken on basis of thorough history taking, physical examination, TSH values, thyroid radionuclide scan, ultrasonography of thyroid and FNAC of thyroid nodule. The next step in management depends on whether the nodule is benign, malignant or has suspicious features on any of the diagnostic modalities. The following algorithm shows the approach to diagnosis of a solitary Thyroid Nodule (Fig. 13.1).

Overview of Treatment Options for Solitary Thyroid Nodules

Thyroid nodules with gross presentations like rapidly increasing size, pressure symptoms or suspicion of malignancy on FNAC warrant treatment without ambiguity, however solitary thyroid nodule which are quiescent are the ones which represent a diagnostic dilemma at times. It has been seen that majority of non-functioning benign nodules grow with time, particularly those which are solid [53]. Before we have a look at the treatment options for solitary Thyroid nodule, we will look at the differentiation of these nodules on basis of their nature (solid/cystic/mixed) and also on whether they are benign or malignant.

We will now discuss the treatment options for small thyroid nodule:

Surgery

Surgery is generally the treatment of choice for nodules which have high risk clinical or cytological features or have symptoms suggestive of cancer [54]. Near total or total thyroidectomy is preferred for patients with diagnosis of malignancy on histopathology and is >1 cm [55] along with other risk factors such as lymphadenopathy, family history of differentiated thyroid cancer or radiotherapy to head and neck region. A large study showed that total thyroidectomy improved recurrence and survival rates in nodules >1 cm [55]. Comprehensive bilateral central lymph node dissection is done (especially in PTC) which improves survival and reduces recurrences [56]. In those patients where histology is indeterminate (follicular or Hurthle cell neoplasm) or non-diagnostic, Thyroid Lobectomy is the initial approach. However when there are high risk features of size >4 cm and atypia, total thyroidectomy can be performed [22].

For those patients of cystic thyroid nodules with subsequent recurrent symptomatic cystic fluid accumulation, surgical removal, generally by hemi thyroidectomy is an option.

Pro's and Con's There is complete relief of symptoms and histological diagnosis while on the hind side there is need for hospitalization and the risks associated with surgery such as vocal cord palsy (<1 %), hypoparathyroidism and hypothyroidism (both <1 %) [16].

Radio-Iodine

It is an option for a functioning thyroid nodule with or without biochemical hyperthyroidism. There is normalization of thyroid nuclide scanning and serum thyrotropin levels in up to 75 % cases and the thyroid volume decreases up to 40 % from baseline after a single dose of iodine-131 aiming at a level of 100 Gy, independent of pretreatment thyroid function [57, 58]. There is risk of developing hypothyroidism post-treatment in 10 % of patients in 5 years, and the frequency of risk increases with time. Post treatment, the thyroid function should be monitored on a yearly basis to diagnose hypothyroidism. Post-treatment, thyroid nodules rarely grow. If they do, then a biopsy should be done to assess histology. Radio-iodine is contraindicated in pregnant or breast feeding women.

Pro's and Con's There is no need for hospitalization and the cost is less. There is significant reduction in thyroid volume. However the reduction in thyroid volume is very gradual and there is a risk of radiation induced thyroiditis or thyrotoxicosis. Fertile women will need contraception before and after treatment [8].

Percutaneous Ethanol Injection

This involves injection of Ethanol under ultrasound guidance in benign functioning/non-functioning solid nodules and also in cystic nodules [59]. The mechanism proposed for its use is local coagulative necrosis and thrombosis of small vessels. However this procedure requires skill and experience and obviously a benign cytology to begin with [7]. There is risk of local pain and other side effects.

The current data suggests that multiple injections of ethanol (a median of four) can achieve a complete cure (i.e., a normalization of results of radionuclide scanning and serum thyrotropin measures) in majority of the patients with hyperfunctioning nodules and functioning nodules without hyperthyroidism. In solid non-functioning benign nodules, a single ethanol injection can reduce the size of a thyroid nodule by up to half [53]. Evidence shows that there is no recurrence on ultrasonography following treatment [60].

Pro's and Con's There is no need for hospitalization and the cost is less. There is around half reduction in size of thyroid nodules following treatment in 6 months. It requires considerable skill and experience. There is local pain, risk of vocal cord paralysis (in up to 2 %) and thyrotoxicosis. After treatment, histology interpretation of the nodule is obscured [8].

Levothyroxine

Treatment with levothyroxine is based on the principle that suppression of thyrotropin prevents growth of benign thyroid nodule. However definitive evidence for its support is lacking. The objective of treatment is to suppress thyrotropin to <0.3 mU/l.

A meta-analysis suggested that after 6–12 months of suppressive therapy, there was no significant difference in nodule growth in patients on levothyroxine and those on no treatment [61]. The chances of nodule size reduction are greater with suppression of thyrotropin to <0.1 mU/l as compared to <0.3 mU/l [61]. In a randomized trial, levothryroxine suppression showed decrease in the frequency of appearance of new thyroid nodules when thyrotropin was suppressed to <0.1 mU [62]. Of note is the fact that nodule regrowth occurs after cessation of treatment and it does not have effect on cyst recurrence after aspiration [63]. However, suppression to such a low level of thyrotropin does not come without hazards of developing complications such as atrial fibrillation.

Pro's and Con's Does not need hospitalization and the cost is less. It 'may' reduce nodule size and prevent new nodule formation. However the gross drawback is that the nodules regrow after cessation of treatment and there is high risk of developing atrial fibrillation and osteoporosis with this degree of thyrotropin suppression. And lastly, it is of no utility in those patients who already have a suppressed or low thyrotropin [8].

Conclusion

The purpose of evaluation of thyroid nodule is to identify the malignant lesions on the basis of detailed history, physical examination, biochemical, radiological and cytological investigations. Clinical evaluation alone is insufficient in identification of malignant lesions. The risk of harboring a malignancy in nodules with subnormal serum TSH and high radio-isotope uptake is low and FNA is not required in these cases. Patients with normal or high serum TSH are evaluated with thyroid ultrasound and FNA. FNA is the investigation of choice for initial workup and is indicated in nodules >1 cm, nodules with high risk history, examination and suspicious ultrasound findings. Surgery is generally the treatment of choice for nodules which have high risk clinical or cytological features or have symptoms suggestive of cancer.

References

1. Tunbridge WM, Evered DC, Hall R, Appleton D, Brewis M, Clark F, et al. The spectrum of thyroid disease in a community: the Whickham survey. Clin Endocrinol (Oxf). 1977;7(6):481–93.
2. Vander JB, Gaston EA, Dawber TR. The significance of nontoxic thyroid nodules. Final report of a 15-year study of the incidence of thyroid malignancy. Ann Intern Med. 1968;69(3):537–40.
3. Singer PA, Cooper DS, Daniels GH, Ladenson PW, Greenspan FS, Levy EG, et al. Treatment guidelines for patients with thyroid nodules and well-differentiated thyroid cancer. American Thyroid Association. Arch Intern Med. 1996;156(19):2165–72.
4. Wong CK, Wheeler MH. Thyroid nodules: rational management. World J Surg. 2000;24(8):934–41.
5. Mazzaferri EL. Management of a solitary thyroid nodule. N Engl J Med. 1993;328(8):553–9.
6. Tan GH, Gharib H. Thyroid incidentalomas: management approaches to nonpalpable nodules discovered incidentally on thyroid imaging. Ann Intern Med. 1997;126(3):226–31.
7. Hegedus L, Bonnema SJ, Bennedbaek FN. Management of simple nodular goiter: current status and future perspectives. Endocr Rev. 2003;24(1):102–32.
8. Hegedüs L. The thyroid nodule. N Engl J Med. 2004;351(17):1764–71.
9. Sherman SI. Thyroid carcinoma. Lancet. 2003;361(9356):501–11.
10. Davies L, Welch HG. Increasing incidence of thyroid cancer in the United States, 1973–2002. JAMA. 2006;295(18):2164–7.
11. Leenhardt L, Bernier MO, Boin-Pineau MH, Conte Devolx B, Marechaud R, Niccoli-Sire P, et al. Advances in diagnostic practices affect thyroid cancer incidence in France. Eur J Endocrinol. 2004;150(2):133–9.
12. Valeix P, Faure P, Bertrais S, Vergnaud AC, Dauchet L, Hercberg S. Effects of light to moderate alcohol consumption on thyroid volume and thyroid function. Clin Endocrinol (Oxf). 2008;68(6):988–95.
13. Volzke H, Friedrich N, Schipf S, et al. Association between serum insulin-like growth factor-I levels and thyroid disorders in a population-based study. J Clin Endocrinol Metabol. 2007;92(10):4039–45.
14. Knudsen N, Bülow I, Laurberg P, et al. Low goitre prevalence among users of oral contraceptives in a population sample of 3712 women. Clinical Endocrinol (Oxf). 2002;57:71.
15. Cappelli C, Castellano M, Pirola I, De Martino E, Gandossi E, Delbarba A, et al. Reduced thyroid volume and nodularity in dyslipidaemic patients on statin treatment. Clin Endocrinol (Oxf). 2008;68(1):16–21.
16. Hagag P, Strauss S, Weiss M. Role of ultrasound-guided fine-needle aspiration biopsy in evaluation of nonpalpable thyroid nodules. Thyroid. 1998;8(11):989–95.
17. Curtis RE, Rowlings PA, Deeg HJ, Shriner DA, Socie G, Travis LB, et al. Solid cancers after bone marrow transplantation. N Engl J Med. 1997;336(13):897–904.
18. Pacini F, Vorontsova T, Demidchik EP, Molinaro E, Agate L, Romei C, et al. Post-Chernobyl thyroid carcinoma in Belarus children and adolescents: comparison with naturally occurring thyroid carcinoma in Italy and France. J Clin Endocrinol Metab. 1997;82(11):3563–9.
19. Jarlov AE, Nygard B, Hegedus L, Karstrup S, Hansen JM. Observer variation in ultrasound assessment of the thyroid gland. Br J Radiol. 1993;66(787):625–7.

20. Hegedus L. Thyroid ultrasound. Endocrinol Metab Clin North Am. 2001;30(2):339–60, viii–ix.
21. Hamming JF, Goslings BM, van Steenis GJ, van Ravenswaay Claasen HH, Hermans JJ, van de Velde CH. THe value of fine-needle aspiration biopsy in patients with nodular thyroid disease divided into groups of suspicion of malignant neoplasms on clinical grounds. Arch Intern Med. 1990;150(1):113–6.
22. American Thyroid Association Guidelines Taskforce on Thyroid N, Differentiated Thyroid C, Cooper DS, Doherty GM, Haugen BR, Kloos RT, et al. Revised American Thyroid Association management guidelines for patients with thyroid nodules and differentiated thyroid cancer. Thyroid. 2009;19(11):1167–214.
23. Are C, Hsu J, Ghossein R, Schoder H, Shah J, Shaha A. Histological aggressiveness of fluorodeoxyglucose positron-emission tomogram (FDG-PET)-detected incidental thyroid carcinomas. Ann Surg Oncol. 2007;14(11):3210–5.
24. Bogsrud TV, Karantanis D, Nathan MA, Mullan BP, Wiseman GA, Collins DA, et al. The value of quantifying 18F-FDG uptake in thyroid nodules found incidentally on whole-body PET-CT. Nucl Med Commun. 2007;28(5):373–81.
25. Kang KW, Kim S-K, Kang H-S, Lee ES, Sim JS, Lee IG, et al. Prevalence and risk of cancer of focal thyroid incidentaloma identified by 18F-fluorodeoxyglucose positron emission tomography for metastasis evaluation and cancer screening in healthy subjects. J Clin Endocrinol Metab. 2003;88(9):4100–4.
26. Choi JY, Lee KS, Kim H-J, Shim YM, Kwon OJ, Park K, et al. Focal thyroid lesions incidentally identified by integrated 18F-FDG PET/CT: clinical significance and improved characterization. J Nucl Med. 2006;47(4):609–15.
27. Boelaert K, Horacek J, Holder RL, Watkinson JC, Sheppard MC, Franklyn JA. Serum thyrotropin concentration as a novel predictor of malignancy in thyroid nodules investigated by fine-needle aspiration. J Clin Endocrinol Metab. 2006;91(11):4295–301.
28. Pacini F, Pinchera A, Giani C, Grasso L, Doveri F, Baschieri L. Serum thyroglobulin in thyroid carcinoma and other thyroid disorders. J Endocrinol Invest. 1980;3(3):283–92.
29. Elisei R, Bottici V, Luchetti F, Coscio GD, Romei C, Grasso L, et al. Impact of routine measurement of serum calcitonin on the diagnosis and outcome of medullary thyroid cancer: experience in 10,864 patients with nodular thyroid disorders. J Clin Endocrinol Metab. 2004;89(1):163–8.
30. Gleich LL, Gluckman JL, Nemunaitis J, et al. Clinical experience with hla-b7 plasmid dna/lipid complex in advanced squamous cell carcinoma of the head and neck. Arch Otolaryngol Head Neck Surg. 2001;127(7):775–9.
31. Gagel RF, Huang A, Cote GJ. Medullary thyroid carcinoma. In: Braverman LE Utiger R, editor. Werner and Ingbar's the thyroid. 9th ed. Philadelphia: Lippincott Williams & Wilkins; 2005. p. 967.
32. Shibuya TYKS, Nguyen K, Parikh P, Wadhwa A, Brockardt C, Do J. Covalent linking of proteins and cytokines to suture: enhancing the immune response of head and neck cancer patients. Laryngoscope. 2003;113(11):1870–84.
33. Shambaugh 3rd GE, Quinn JL, Oyasu R, Freinkel N. Disparate thyroid imaging: Combined studies with sodium pertechnetate tc 99m and radioactive iodine. JAMA. 1974;228(7):866–9.
34. Cases JASM, Surks M. The changing role of scintigraphy in the evaluation of thyroid nodules. Semin Nucl Med. 2000;30(2):81–7.
35. S-k J, Jung SL, Kim BS, Lee YS. Evaluating the degree of conformity of papillary carcinoma and follicular carcinoma to the reported ultrasonographic findings of malignant thyroid tumor. Korean J Radiol. 2007;8(3):192–7.
36. Frates MC, Benson CB, Doubilet PM, Kunreuther E, Contreras M, Cibas ES, et al. Prevalence and distribution of carcinoma in patients with solitary and multiple thyroid nodules on sonography. J Clin Endocrinol Metab. 2006;91(9):3411–7.
37. Moon W-J, Jung SL, Lee JH, Na DG, Baek J-H, Lee YH, et al. Benign and malignant thyroid nodules: US differentiation—multicenter retrospective study. Radiology. 2008;247(3):762–70.
38. Crile G. Treatment of thyroid cysts by aspiration. Surgery. 1966;59:210–2.
39. Nygaard B, Nygaard T, Court-Payen M, Jensen LI, Søe-Jensen P, Gerhard Nielsen K, et al. Thyroid volume measured by ultrasonography and CT. Acta Radiol. 2002;43(3):269–74.
40. McHenry CR, Walfish P, Rosen IB. Non-diagnostic fine needle aspiration biopsy: a dilemma in management of nodular thyroid disease. Am Surg. 1993;7(59):415–9.
41. Rosen IB, Azadian A, Walfish PG, Salem S, Lansdown E, Bedard YC. Ultrasound-guided fine-needle aspiration biopsy in the management of thyroid disease. Am J Surg. 1993;166(4):346–9.
42. Gursoy A, Ertugrul DT, Sahin M, Tutuncu NB, Demirer AN, Demirag NG. Needle-free delivery of lidocaine for reducing the pain associated with the fine-needle aspiration biopsy of thyroid nodules: time-saving and efficacious procedure. Thyroid. 2007;17(4):317–21.
43. Mair S, Dunbar F, Becker PJ, Du Plessis W. Fine needle cytology – is aspiration suction necessary? A study of 100 masses in various sites. Acta Cytol. 1989;6(33):809–13.
44. Kate MS, Kamal MM, Bobhate SK, Kher AV. Evaluation of fine needle capillary sampling in superficial and deep-seated lesions. An analysis of 670 cases. Acta Cytol. 1998;42(3):679–84.
45. Hemminki K, Eng C, Chen B. Familial Risks for Nonmedullary Thyroid Cancer. J Clin Endocrinol Metab. 2005;90(10):5747–53.
46. Schneider AB, Ron E, Lubin J, Stovall M, Gierlowski TC. Dose–response relationships for radiation-induced thyroid cancer and thyroid nodules: evidence

for the prolonged effects of radiation on the thyroid. J Clin Endocrinol Metab. 1993;77(2):362–9.
47. Shibata Y, Yamashita S, Masyakin VB, Panasyuk GD, Nagataki S. 15 years after Chernobyl: new evidence of thyroid cancer. Lancet. 2001;358(9297):1965–6.
48. Mandel SJ. A 64-year-old woman with a thyroid nodule. JAMA. 2004;292(21):2632–42.
49. Baloch ZW, LiVolsi VA, Asa SL, Rosai J, Merino MJ, Randolph G, et al. Diagnostic terminology and morphologic criteria for cytologic diagnosis of thyroid lesions: a synopsis of the national cancer institute thyroid fine-needle aspiration state of the science conference. Diagn Cytopathol. 2008;36(6):425–37.
50. Bartolazzi A, Orlandi F, Saggiorato E, Volante M, Arecco F, Rossetto R, et al. Galectin-3-expression analysis in the surgical selection of follicular thyroid nodules with indeterminate fine-needle aspiration cytology: a prospective multicentre study. Lancet Oncol. 2008;9(6):543–9.
51. Nikiforov YE, Steward DL, Robinson-Smith TM, Haugen BR, Klopper JP, Zhu Z, et al. Molecular testing for mutations in improving the fine-needle aspiration diagnosis of thyroid nodules. J Clin Endocrinol Metab. 2009;94(6):2092–8.
52. Franco C, Martinez V, Allamand JP, Medina F, Glasinovic A, Osorio M, et al. Molecular markers in thyroid fine-needle aspiration biopsy: a prospective study. Appl Immunohistochem Mol Morphol. 2009;17(3):211–5.
53. Bennedbæk FN, Nielsen LK, Hegedüs L. Effect of percutaneous ethanol injection therapy versus suppressive doses of l-thyroxine on benign solitary solid cold thyroid nodules: a randomized trial. J Clin Endocrinol Metab. 1998;83(3):830–5.
54. Bennedbaek FN, Perrild H, Hegedus L. Diagnosis and treatment of the solitary thyroid nodule. Results of a European survey. Clin Endocrinol (Oxf). 1999;50(3):357–63.
55. Bilimoria KY, Bentrem DJ, Ko CY, Stewart AK, Winchester DP, Talamonti MS, et al. Extent of surgery affects survival for papillary thyroid cancer. Ann Surg. 2007;246(3):375–81; discussion 81–4.
56. Tisell LE, Nilsson B, Molne J, Hansson G, Fjalling M, Jansson S, et al. Improved survival of patients with papillary thyroid cancer after surgical microdissection. World J Surg. 1996;20(7):854–9.
57. Ferrari C, Reschini E, Paracchi A. Treatment of the autonomous thyroid nodule: a review. Eur J Endocrinol. 1996;135(4):383–90.
58. Nygaard B, Hegedus L, Nielsen KG, Ulriksen P, Hansen JM. Long-term effect of radioactive iodine on thyroid function and size in patients with solitary autonomously functioning toxic thyroid nodules. Clin Endocrinol (Oxf). 1999;50(2):197–202.
59. Lippi F, Ferrari C, Manetti L, Rago T, Santini F, Monzani F, et al. Treatment of solitary autonomous thyroid nodules by percutaneous ethanol injection: results of an Italian multicenter study. The Multicenter Study Group. J Clin Endocrinol Metab. 1996;81(9):3261–4.
60. Kim DW, Rho MH, Kim HJ, Kwon JS, Sung YS, Lee SW. Percutaneous ethanol injection for benign cystic thyroid nodules: is aspiration of ethanol-mixed fluid advantageous? AJNR Am J Neuroradiol. 2005;26(8):2122–7.
61. Castro MR, Caraballo PJ, Morris JC. Effectiveness of thyroid hormone suppressive therapy in benign solitary thyroid nodules: a meta-analysis. J Clin Endocrinol Metab. 2002;87(9):4154–9.
62. Papini E, Petrucci L, Guglielmi R, Panunzi C, Rinaldi R, Bacci V, et al. Long-term changes in nodular goiter: a 5-year prospective randomized trial of levothyroxine suppressive therapy for benign cold thyroid nodules. J Clin Endocrinol Metab. 1998;83(3):780–3.
63. McCowen KD, Reed JW, Fariss BL. The role of thyroid therapy in patients with thyroid cysts. Am J Med. 1980;68(6):853–5.

Thyroid Cancer

14

Zakir Alavi

Abstract

The incidence of thyroid cancer is rising in most regions of the world. This rise is mostly made up of small, low risk papillary thyroid cancers with little effect on mortality. Overall the mortality for differentiated thyroid cancers is low, with a 10 year survival greater than 95 %. Although there is debate regarding the extent of surgery, need for lymph node dissection and the need for or dose of radioactive iodine, the traditional triad of treatment for differentiated thyroid cancer i.e. surgery, radioactive iodine ablation and TSH suppression with thyroxine, is still the standard recommendation. In the absence of strong trial evidence it is difficult to judge the benefits of these treatment modalities against the potential harm of over treatment.

Recent times have seen an explosion in our understanding of the molecular mechanism involved in thyroid cancer. Molecular analysis of FNA biopsy has lead to better preoperative diagnosis. Novel new tyrosine kinase inhibiting drugs such as sorafinib and sunitinib (for non-iodine avid progressive differentiated thyroid cancers) and vanditinib (for medullary thyroid cancers) have helped halt the progress of these cancers and improved survival rates.

Genetic screening of family members of patients with the familial type of medullary thyroid cancer (either without associated endocrine disease or as part of multiple endocrine neoplasia syndromes), and prophylactic surgery have resulted in survival comparable to differentiated thyroid cancer.

Introduction

The normal thyroid gland is composed of two types of cells. Follicular cells line the follicles and are responsible for the production of thyroid hormones. The other cell type are the C or parafollicular cells which produce the hormone

Z. Alavi
National Medical Center, Defense Housing Authority, Karachi, Pakistan
e-mail: zmalavi@gmail.com

S.K. Imam, S.I. Ahmad (eds.), *Thyroid Disorders: Basic Science and Clinical Practice*,
DOI 10.1007/978-3-319-25871-3_14

calcitonin. The follicular cells give rise to well-differentiated thyroid cancers i.e. papillary thyroid cancer (PTC), follicular thyroid cancer (FTC) as well as Hurthle cell cancer (HCC) and anaplastic thyroid cancers. The parafollicular cells are the cells of origin for medullary thyroid carcinoma.

Thyroid cancer is the most common endocrine malignancy and is one of fastest growing diagnosis. Worldwide thyroid cancer is 16th most common cancer, with around 298,000 new cases diagnosed in 2012 (2 % of total), with highest incidence reported in North America and lowest in Western Africa [1].

The incidence of thyroid cancer specifically PTC has increased rapidly over last three decades [2], the majority of these are small PTCs however increased incidences have been exhibited for all sizes and stages of PTC in both genders and all ethnic groups [3]. It has been suggested that this surge of new cases is due to development and use of imaging technologies capable of detecting a large reservoir of subclinical disease [4]. This notion is supported by cadaveric studies, where a third of patients who died from non-thyroid related conditions were found to have thyroid cancer [5].

Despite its high prevalence thyroid cancer is an uncommon cause of death. The discrepancy between high number of cases and relatively low deaths reflects the indolent nature and excellent long-term survival associated with thyroid malignancies. Overall greater than 90 % of patients are alive 10 years after diagnosis.

Calcification

(A) Differentiated thyroid cancer
  (a) Papillary adenocarcinoma (Variants: Follicular variant of papillary carcinoma, Tall cell, columnar cells, Oxyphyl, Solid sclerosing)
  (b) Follicular adenocarcinoma (variants: Hurthle cell carcinoma, Clear cell carcinoma, Insular carcinoma)

(B) Medullary Carcinoma

(C) Undifferentiated (Anaplastic Carcinoma)

(D) Miscellaneous including:
  (a) Lymphoma
  (b) Fibrosarcoma
  (c) Squamous cell carcinoma
  (d) Teratoma
  (e) Metastatic lesions

Differentiated Thyroid Cancers

Papillary Cell Carcinoma

Epidemiology

Papillary thyroid cancer (PTC) is the most common endocrine malignancy. PTC constitutes about 80 % of all thyroid cancers including 85 % of those induced by radiation. However in countries where the incidence of endemic goiter is high, a greater portion are follicular or anaplastic.

PTC largely accounts for the increase in new diagnosis of thyroid cancer. As stated earlier the reason for this increase is believed to be largely due to wide spread use of radiology tests done for other reasons that detect small none palpable thyroid cancers. Consistent with this theory is that death rate from thyroid cancer has remained stable despite the increase in cases. However a recent analysis suggests that all stages of thyroid cancer are increasing, a finding that may not be explained by surveillance alone [6]. It has been suggested that the increase in the incidence of thyroid cancer might also reflect a new risk factor not yet identified, it could be increased exposure to low dose ionizing radiation from radiographic imaging as well as hormonal or nutritional factors. However the association of these risk factors with low risk thyroid cancer is weak and inconsistent.

Pathology

Papillary carcinoma typically presents as a nodule that is firm and solid on ultrasound, sometimes with internal calcifications. It is usually the dominant nodule in a multi-nodular goiter and with suspicious ultrasound characteristics. However, especially in children it may sometimes present with enlarged cervical lymph nodes. Occasionally there is hemorrhage, necrosis and cyst formation in a malignant nodule on ultrasound. In such cases FNAC of the solid component will reveal the underlying malignancy. It may also be found incidentally when the gland is removed for another reason.

PTCs usually are nonencapsulated, sharply circumscribed tumors. A small percentage may spread directly through the thyroid capsule into the surrounding structures.

The size of the primary lesion is important for prognosis. Tumors <1.5 cm rarely metastasize and virtually never cause death [7].

Microscopically, papillary cancer usually consists of single layer of thyroid cells arranged in vascular stocks, with papillary projections extending into microscopic cyst like spaces. The nuclei of the cells are large and pale ("Orphan Annie Eye" nuclei) and frequently contain clear, glassy intranuclear inclusion bodies. Psammoma bodies are calcified concentric laminated spheres within or near the tumor and in nearby lymph nodes, these occur in about half the cases and are pathognomic of papillary carcinoma.

A tumors is designated as follicular variant of PTC if the lining cells of the neoplastic follicles have the same nuclear features as typical PTC and the follicular predominance over the papillae is complete.

Most PTCs remain confined to the thyroid gland and local lymph nodes. However these cancers can exhibit intraglandular metastasis and lymph node spread. More aggressive tumors especially in older patients can spread locally into adjacent muscles nerves and the trachea. In later stages it may metastasize to the lungs, brain, bones and other organs.

Anaplastic transformation may occur in well differentiated PTC resulting in aggressive local invasion of tumor and widespread rapidly fatal metastasis.

Follicular Thyroid Carcinoma

Epidemiology

Follicular thyroid carcinoma (FTC) is an unusual thyroid cancer comprising approximately 5–10 % of thyroid cancers in nonendemic goiter areas of the world [8]. It tended to be more common in areas of iodine deficiency and endemic goiter. However owing to changing diagnostic criteria, rising incidence of PTC and iodine supplementation, it frequency is decreasing. It occurs at a slightly older age group than PTC and is rare in children. It occurs infrequently after radiation exposure and is not commonly found at autopsy as an occult inconsequential tumor.

Pathology

FTC is characterized histologically by the presence of small follicles with poor colloid formation. 'Minimally invasive' FTC is an encapsulated tumor whose growth pattern resembles that of a trabecular or solid, microfollicular, or atypical adenoma. FTC is distinguished from benign adenoma microscopically by the presence of capsule and/or vascular invasion within the tumor capsule. Such tumors have an indolent course similar to low-grade PTC. "Widely invasive" form of FTC may be partially encapsulated, however the margins are infiltrative even on gross examination and vascular invasion is often extensive. Such cancers are aggressive and have the potential for distant metastasis to bone, brain, lung and other organs.

When more than 75 % of cells in an FTC exhibit Hurthle cell or oncocytic features (characterized by large individual cells with pink staining cytoplasm filled with mitochondria) the tumor is classified as Hurthle cell neoplasm.

Molecular Biology of Differentiated Thyroid Cancer

Two intracellular pathways have been identified that play a role in thyroid cancer – the MAPK (mitogen activated protein kinase) and PI3-AKT-MTOR (phosphatidylinositide 3-kinase-protein kinase B-mammalian target of rapamycin) pathways. Aberrant activation of MAPK pathway results in tumor promotion, whereas mutations in the PI3K-AKT-MTOR pathway decrease expression of tumor suppressor genes [9].

PTC is likely caused by mutations in genes in the MAPK signaling pathway, especially the BRAF mutation. Another common finding in PTCs, especially after radiation exposure, are gene rearrangements in which a portion of the RET gene (a receptor tyrosine kinase not normally expressed in the thyroid), is linked to a portion of one of several unrelated genes, producing a constitutively active chimeric RET receptor. Subsequently loss of P53 suppressor gene may allow progression to anaplastic carcinoma.

Activating mutations of RAS oncogene and loss of function of PTEN a tumor suppressor gene, are common in benign follicular adenomas. Progression to follicular carcinoma may occur after another genetic event involving a chromosomal translocation forming a fusion gene between the thyroid transcription factor PAX8 and PPARɣ gene (PAX8-PPARɣ). Further loss of suppressor gene P53 may allow progression to anaplastic carcinoma.

Diagnosis

Most thyroid cancers present as a lump in the thyroid region detected by the patient or detected by physician on examination or incidentally found on radiological examination of the neck done for an unrelated reason. There is a 5–10 % chance of a nodule to be malignant, most are benign. High risk factors for malignancy are, extremes of age, family history of thyroid cancer, history of rapid increase in size of nodule, dyspnea, dysphagia, hoarseness of voice. On examination large size of the nodule, hard nodule, lack of mobility, adherence to structures, and ipsilateral lymphadenopathy.

Investigations

Thyroid Function Tests when a thyroid nodule is discovered a Serum TSH should be obtained to identify thyroid dysfunction but not to differentiate between benign and malignant. If the TSH is suppressed, a radionuclide thyroid scan should be performed to document whether the nodule is hyper-functioning, or non-functioning. Since hyper-functioning nodules rarely harbor malignancy, no cytological evaluation is necessary [10]

Thyroid Ultrasound diagnostic ultrasound is one of the most useful adjunct to clinical exam for assessing thyroid nodules. It should be performed in all patients with known or suspected thyroid nodule [10]. It helps in determining if the nodule is solid, or cystic with solid component or purely cystic (unlikely to be malignant), measures the size of the nodule, and identifies features suspicious of malignancy and the presence or absence of cervical lymphadenopathy. Sonographic characteristics suspicious of malignancy include nodule ecogenecity, increased nodular vascularity, irregular infiltrating margins, the presence of microcalcifications, absent halo and a shape which is taller than width. Typically sonographic features of PTC and FTC differ. A PTC is generally solid or predominantly solid and hyperechoic, often with infiltrative irregular margins and increased vascularity. Microcalcifications if present are highly specific for PTC. Conversely FTC is more often isoechoic and has a thick irregular halo but no microcalcification. Certain sonographic characteristics may also be highly predictive of a benign nature of a nodule.

Fine Needle Aspiration (FNA) Biopsy FNA is the procedure of choice for evaluating a thyroid nodule [10]. Ultrasound directed FNA is recommended for those nodules which are non-palpable, predominantly cystic or located posteriorly in the thyroid gland. FNA biopsy is the most accurate, safe and cost effective method of evaluating a thyroid nodule. Traditionally FNA results are divided into four categories, non-diagnostic, malignant, intermediate or suspicious and benign.

Routine FNA is not recommended for subcentimeter nodules. In suspicious subcentimeter nodules sonography of lateral neck and central neck lymph nodes must be performed. Detection of abnormal lymph nodes should lead to FNA of the lymph nodes. Other groups of patient for whom consideration of FNA of subcentimeter node include, patients with high risk history; family history of PTC, history of external beam irradiation exposure as a child, exposure to ionizing radiation in childhood or adolescence, prior history of hemithyroidectomy with discovery of carcinoma, FDG-PET-positive nodules.

Molecular Markers molecular markers (eg BRAF, RET/PTC, PAX8-PPARɣ, galactin-3) may be considered for patients with intermediate cytology on FNA to help guide management.

Treatment of Differentiated Thyroid Cancer

The mainstay in the treatment of DTCs is surgery ± radioactive iodine therapy and lifelong TSH suppression. The goals of treatment, as stated in the recent American Thyroid Association management guidelines [10], are as follows;

(1) To remove the primary tumor, disease that has extended beyond the thyroid capsule, and involved cervical lymph nodes. Completeness of surgical resection is an important determinant of outcome, while residual metastatic lymph nodes represent the most common site of disease persistence/recurrence.
(2) To minimize treatment-related morbidity. The extent of surgery and the experience of the surgeon both play important roles in determining the risk of surgical complications.
(3) To permit accurate staging of the disease. Because disease staging can assist with initial prognostication, disease management, and follow-up strategies, accurate postoperative staging is a crucial element in the management of patients with DTC.
(4) To facilitate postoperative treatment with radioactive iodine, where appropriate. For patients undergoing RAI remnant ablation, or RAI treatment of residual or metastatic disease, removal of all normal thyroid tissue is an important element of initial surgery. Near total or total thyroidectomy also may reduce the risk for recurrence within the contralateral lobe.
(5) To permit accurate long-term surveillance for disease recurrence. Both RAI whole-body scanning (WBS) and measurement of serum Tg are affected by residual normal thyroid tissue. Where these approaches are utilized for long-term monitoring, near-total or total- thyroidectomy is required.
(6) To minimize the risk of disease recurrence and metastaticspread. Adequate surgery is the most important treatment variable influencing prognosis, while radioactive iodine treatment, TSH suppression, and external beam irradiation each play adjunctive roles in at least some patients.

Surgery

There is agreement that surgery is the definite form of treatment for DTC, however there is controversy regarding the extent of surgery. Increased extent of primary surgery may improve survival for high-risk and low risk patients. A study of 50,000 patients with PTC found on multivariate analysis that total thyroidectomy significantly improved recurrence and survival rates for tumors >1 cm [11]. Other studies have shown that rates of recurrence are reduced by total or near-total thyroidectomy among low risk patients [12–14]. Hence the recommendation is that the initial surgical procedure should be total or near-total thyroidectomy if the primary tumor is >1 cm, there are contralateral thyroid nodules, have regional or distant metastasis, patient has history of radiation to head and neck or the patient has a first degree relative with history of DTC. Older patients (>45 years) even with tumors 1–1.5 cm would also require total or near-total thyroidectomy. Increased extent of initial surgery improves survival for both high-risk and low risk patients. Therapeutic central compartment neck dissection for patients with clinically involved central or lateral neck lymph nodes should accompany total or near-total thyroidectomy to provide disease clearance from the central compartment. Prophylactic central compartment neck dissection (ipsilateral or bilateral) may be performed in patients with PTC with clinically involved lymph nodes, especially for advanced primary tumors. Near-total or total thyroidectomy without prophylactic central neck dissection may be appropriate for small (T1 or T2), non-invasive, clinically node-negative PTCs and most follicular cancers.

For patients with extra-thyroidal extension, *en bloc* resection of involved structures should be performed when possible.

Staging Postoperative staging is recommended to permit prognostication for an individual patient, to individualize decisions regarding treatment and to make decisions regarding intensity and frequency of follow-up. TNM classification system for differentiated thyroid cancer is the recommended staging for all patients with DTC (Table 14.1).

Table 14.1 TNM classification for differentiated thyroid carcinoma

	Definition	
T1	Tumor diameter 2 cm or smaller	
T2	Primary tumor diameter >2–4 cm	
T3	Primary tumor diameter >4 cm limited to the thyroid or minimal extrathyroidal extension	
T4a	Tumor of any size extending beyond the thyroid capsule to invade subcutaneous soft tissues, larynx, trachea, esophagus, or recurrent laryngeal nerve	
T4b	Tumor invades prevertebral fascia or encases carotid artery or mediastinal vessels	
TX	Primary tumor size unknown, but without extrathyroidal invasion	
N0	No metastatic nodes	
N1a	Metastases to level VI (pretracheal, paratracheal, and prelaryngeal/Delphian lymph nodes)	
N1b	Metastasis to unilateral, bilateral, contralateral cervical or superior mediastinal nodes	
NX	Nodes not assessed at surgery	
M0	No distant metastasis	
M1	Distant metastasis	
MX	Distance metastasis not assessed	
Stages	**Patient age <45**	**Patient age >45**
Stage I	Any T, any N, M0	T1, N0, M0
Stage II	Any T, any N, M1	T2, N0, M0
Stage III		T3, N0, M0
		T1, N1a, M0
		T2, N1a, M0
		T3, N1a, M0
Stage IVA		T4a, N0, M0
		T4a, N1a, M0
		T1, N1b, M0
		T2, N1b, M0
		T3, N1b, M0
		T4a, N1b, M0
Stage IVB		T4b, any N, M0
Stage IVC		Any T, any N, M1

The source of this material is the AJCC Cancer Staging Manual, Sixth Edition

Radioactive Iodine (RAI)

A small amount of thyroid tissue, called the thyroid remnant, is often left after total thyroidectomy. RAI can be administered postoperatively to destroy any remaining thyroid cells, normal or malignant. RAI improves the specificity of future surveillance imaging to detect recurrent disease. It also allows clinicians to monitor serum thyroglobulin, a protein made by thyroid follicular cells, as a marker of disease.

RAI ablation is recommended for all patients with known distant metastases, gross extrathyroidal extension of the tumor regardless of tumor size, or primary tumor size >4 cm even in the absence of other higher risk features. RAI ablation is also recommended for selected patients with 1–4 cm thyroid cancers confined to the thyroid, who have documented lymph node metastases, or other higher risk features when the combination of age, tumor size, lymph node status, and individual histology predicts an intermediate to high risk of recurrence or death from thyroid cancer.

RAI ablation is not recommended for patients with unifocal cancer <1 cm without other higher risk features or for patients with multifocal cancer when all foci are <1 cm in the absence other higher risk features.

Preparation for RAI Thyroid stimulating hormone (TSH) stimulation increases iodine uptake in the thyroid cell hence an elevated TSH is required to achieve maximal uptake of RAI into the remnant. This can be achieved by using injection of recombinant human TSH (rhTSH*Thyrogen*^{TM}) given to the patient in the euthyroid state. Alternatively, TSH stimulation can be achieved by withdrawing the patient from thyroxine therapy which causes transient clinical hypothyroidism (in such a case T_3 is often prescribed temporarily at a dose of 25–50 μg daily in divided doses for 2–4 weeks; the medication is then withdrawn for 2 week, and the patient quickly becomes hypothyroid prior to RAI). In general rhTSH is preferred, since hypothyroidism is avoided and whole body radiation exposure is lower as radioiodine is cleared from the body more rapidly. *Thyrogen*^{TM} injection (0.9 mg) is given as an intramuscular injection on two consecutive days followed by RAI on third day. Regardless of how the patient achieves the elevated TSH a low iodine diet is prescribed for 2 weeks to enhance uptake of RAI.

Pretherapy scan may be useful when the extent of thyroid remnant cannot be accurately ascertained or when results would alter the decision to treat or the RAI dose. Following thyroid hormone withdrawal or rhTSH stimulation, the serum thyroglobulin level is determined, and the patient is scanned 24–72 h after a low dose RAI (1–4 mCi of ^{131}I or 1–2 mCi of ^{123}I). If the decision is to give ablative RAI then ^{131}I is administered in a dose of 30–100 mCi depending on the size and invasiveness of the primary tumor.

A posttherapy scan is recommended following RAI remnant ablation. This is typically done 2–10 days after the therapeutic dose is administered, to be sure no additional areas of radioiodine uptake are revealed.

TSH Suppression Therapy

Similar to normal follicular cells, thyroid cancer cells express thyrotropin receptors and respond to TSH by increasing cell growth. Lifelong suppression of TSH using supra-physiological doses of thyroxine, is commonly used to treat patients with thyroid cancer in an effort to decrease the risk of recurrence. Initial TSH suppression to below 0.1 mU/L is recommended for high risk and intermediate risk thyroid cancer patients, while maintaining a TSH slightly below normal (0.1–0.5 mU/L) is appropriate for low risk patients.

Long Term Management

Nine to twelve months later rhTSH is administered or thyroid hormone therapy is withdrawn, and a radioiodine scan and thyroglobulin are repeated to document ablation of all functioning thyroid tissue. An undetectable thyroglobulin at a time when TSH is elevated is the most sensitive evidence that all thyroid tissue has been eradicated.

If the patients TSH stimulated thyroglobulin (usually achieved by giving rhTSH) is less than 1 ng/ml and the whole body radioiodine scan is negative, the patient is considered to be disease free. On the other hand, if the serum thyroglobulin concentration rises above 2 ng/ml and/or if the radioiodine scan is positive, the patient is likely to have either persistent thyroid tissue or residual thyroid cancer. Neck sonography, CT or MRI should be done to look for residual cancer, and if found, additional surgery may be warranted. If stimulated thyroglobulin is greater than 20 ng/ml and other imaging studies are negative, some experts recommend empiric RAI therapy because of the high suspicion of residual disease.

Follow-up at intervals of 6–12 months should include local neck exam, sometimes including ultrasound exam looking for recurrent mass or cervical lymph nodes. If abnormal lymph nodes are discovered an FNAB is indicated. The patients TSH should be checked to see if adequately suppressed. The serum thyroglobulin should be periodically checked to be certain it is undetectable. A rise in serum thyroglobulin while the TSH is suppressed suggests tumor recurrence and imaging studies such as ultrasound, CT, MRI should be done. A PET scan can be especially useful in such situations when other imaging studies are negative.

Thyroglobulin antibodies interfere with the thyroglobulin assay and result in falsely low thyroglobulin result. Hence patients who are positive for these antibodies should be followed up with ultrasound or CT.

Treatment Options for Advanced DTC

Patients with progressive DTCs that are not responsive to standard treatment require additional therapy. Neck dissection should be considered even in metastatic disease. External beam radiation (EBRT) may help provide local control. Doxorubicin is approved for treatment of thyroid cancer, however response rates are low and short lived. Doxorubicin may act as a radiation sensitizer in some cancers of thyroid origin.

Novel Therapies

In recent years, new targeted agents for the treatment of advanced thyroid cancer have emerged. The rationale for these agents is that they target and block known aberrancies in thyroid carcinoma, namely constitutive activation of the MAPK and/or PI3 pathway and vascular endothelial growth factor receptors (VEGFRs). Most of these novel agents are tyrosine kinase inhibitors and include Axitinib, Motesanib, Sorafenib, Sunitinib and Pazopanib. Thalidomide and Lenalidomide are inhibitors of angiogenesis.

Some of these agents are still in phase II and phase III trials while others have established efficacies. The role of these agents in the management of advanced radioiodine refractory cancers is emergent and needs to be clarified as to which patients may benefit most from these agents.

Medullary Thyroid Cancer

Epidemiology and Pathology

Medullary thyroid cancer (MTC) account for 3–6 % of thyroid cancer [8]. It arises from the parafollicular or C cell of the thyroid gland. MTC tumors are usually firm and non-encapsulated. On histologic examination the tumor is composed of cells that vary in their morphologic features and arrangements. Round polyhedral and spindle shaped cells form solid and trabecular glandular like structures. An amyloid like stroma is commonly present [15]. Gross or microscopic foci of carcinoma may be present in other parts of the gland, and blood vessels may be invaded. The tumors typically produces early biochemical signals and are capable of secreting calcitonin, carcinoembryonic antigen (CEA), histamine, prostaglandins, serotonin, VIP, corticotrophin and other peptides.

MTC is typically more aggressive than DTC, extending locally to cervical lymph nodes and into surrounding tissues. It may also invade lymphatics and blood vessels, and metastasize to other viscera. Serum calcitonin (which is invariably secreted by the tumor) and CEA are useful markers for diagnosis and follow up.

MTC occurs in both sporadic and familial forms. The familial form make up approximately 20 % of the total. There are three familial forms; (1) Familial medullary cancer without associated endocrine disease; (2) Multiple endocrine neoplasia 2A (MEN 2A), consisting of medullary thyroid carcinoma, pheochromocytoma and hyperparathyroidism; and (3) MEN 2B, consisting of medullary thyroid cancer, pheochromocytoma, multiple mucosal neuromas (bumpy lip syndrome), as well as intestinal ganglioneuromatosis. These familial syndromes are due to RET protooncogene mutations mostly in exon 10, 11 or 16.

Presentation and Diagnosis

The clinical symptoms at the time of presentation vary. MTC usually appears as a hard nodule or mass in the thyroid gland or as an enlargement of the regional lymph nodes. The neck mass is frequently painful and often located in the upper two thirds of each lobe of the gland, reflecting the anatomic location of the parafollicular cells. Patients with familial MTC who are identified on screening are usually identified before development of macroscopic disease. Differentiation of sporadic MTC from other types of thyroid nodules on clinical grounds may be difficult. In a patient with a family history of thyroid cancer associated with hypertension or hyperparathyroidism, the MEN 2A syndrome should be suspected. In MEN2A hyperparathyroidism occurs late. Pheochromocytomas invariably occur later than MTC and are often bilateral and may be clinically silent. In MEN 2B, MTC and pheochromocytoma are associated with multiple mucosal neuromas ('Bumpy lip syndrome'), a Marfinoid habitus and typical facies, but they do not have hyperparathyroidism.

FNAB has made it possible to diagnose MTC prior to surgery. Positive immunocytochemical staining for calcitonin allows confirmation of diagnosis. Basal plasma calcitonin levels are elevated in virtually all the patients with MTC. If MTC is diagnosed in a patient on FNAB or at surgery, it is essential that the patient be screened for one of the familial MTC syndromes by DNA analysis for mutations in the RET protooncogene. If screening is negative then the tumor is most likely sporadic and other family members need not be screened. On the other hand family members of a patient with an RET oncogene should be screened.

Treatment

Early and adequate initial thyroidectomy and regional node dissection is the best therapy for MTC. More extensive surgery may be warranted, depending on the extent and invasiveness of the tumor. Patient with MTC should be evaluated for a pheochromocytoma and hyperparathyroidism. In patients with the MEN syndrome surgery for pheochromocytoma (if found) should be performed prior to surgery for MTC.

As stated above first degree relatives of patients with MEN syndrome or familial MTC should undergo testing for RET gene. Gene carriers should undergo prophylactic total thyroidectomy at an age that depends on the mutations. Within the first year of life for those with MEN 2B and before 5 years of age for those with other mutations. Some cases may be delayed to beyond the age of 5 years depending upon the mutations type and normal calcitonin level.

Follow up; Patients with MTC should be followed post operatively with periodic measurement of serum markers, calcitonin and CEA that indicate residual disease. If a patient after total thyroidectomy and regional node dissection has persistently elevated calcitonin levels then neck ultrasound, CT, MRI and selective venous catheterization may reveal location of metastasis. Metastatic foci may also be revealed by PET scan, octreotide scan or sestamibi scan. If these fail to locate the metastatic foci the patient must be followed until lesions become evident on clinical examinations or imaging.

For metastatic disease external beam radiation therapy (EBRT) may be useful locally. Cytotoxic drugs have short lived and low response rates. In recent times tyrosine kinase inhibitors (TKI) especially inhibitors of RET and VEGFR tyrosine kinases have had good results in advanced disease. Of these, treatment with vanditanib and cabozantinib can be used as single agent first line systemic therapy. However it is not clear whether either of these improves overall survival and when treatment with TKIs should be terminated. Resistance to TKIs may also be problem and the mechanisms of resistance needs further elucidation.

Prognosis The introduction of genetic screening and prophylactic surgery has improved the survival of patients with MTC. Recent studies show 5 year survival between 80–90 % and 10 year survival between 70–80 % for combined series of familial and sporadic MTC [16].

Anaplastic Thyroid Carcinoma

Anaplastic thyroid carcinoma (ATC) is one of the most aggressive and difficult human malignancies to treat. It is also one of the most lethal malignancies and accounts for 1–2 % of all thyroid cancers. Closely related to PTC and FTC, which may be the precursors of ATC. Mutations of P 53 gene are present in many ATC but not present in residual differentiated component suggesting that this mutation may play a key role in tumor transformation from DTC to ATC. This carcinoma is highly malignant, is nonencapsulated and extends widely. Invasion of adjacent structures such as skin, muscles, nerves, blood vessels, larynx and esophagus, and metastasizes early to distant organs.

Clinically it represents as a rapid, often painful enlargement of a mass which may have been present in the thyroid gland for many years. As a result of invasion of surrounding structures patient may also complain of hoarseness, inspiratory stridor, dysphagia or hemoptysis. On examination the overlying skin is often warm and discolored. The mass is tender and fixed to adjoining structures. It is stony hard but may have soft or fluctuant areas. Regional lymph nodes are usually enlarged.

Treatment consists of surgical resection if feasible, followed by a combination of EBRT and chemotherapy. The cytotoxic drug doxorubicin is the single most effective chemotherapeutic agent for ATC and combination with platinum is more effective than doxorubicin alone. However survival is very poor, usually less than 5 months with very few patients reaching 1 year.

Melignant Thyroid Lymphoma

Primary lymphomas of the thyroid are rare and account for 2.5 % of all non-Hodgkin's lymphomas and less than 2 % of thyroid tumors. Male to female ratio is 3:1, peak incidence is in the 7th decade of life.

Thyroid lymphomas are of B-cell lineage. Most are of mucosa associated lymphoid tissue (MALT) origin and usually arise in a background of Hashimoto's thyroiditis. They present as rapidly enlarging painless swelling of the gland. Some patients also have compressive symptoms. The mass is often fixed and neck lymph nodes are frequently palpable. It is usually hypoechoic on ultrasound and depicts a characteristic ultrasonic feature. Serum antiperoxidase and anti-thyroglobulin are mostly present.

Diagnosis can be established on FNAC. Staging of disease is essential to treatment and requires a physical exam, complete blood count, LDH, liver function tests, bone marrow trephine biopsy, and CT of neck, thorax, abdomen and pelvis. Gastrointestinal involvement may be present and an endoscopy may be required.

Treatment is usually with chemotherapy although small lymphomas may be treated initially with surgery, additional radiotherapy may be required in case of indolent lymphomas. Usual chemotherapy consist of four to six cycles of CHOP (cyclophosphamide, doxorubicin, vincristine and prednisolone) combined with rituximab.

Conclusion

Recent times have seen a large rise in the incidence of thyroid cancer worldwide, however there are important geographic variations. This rise is largely made up of PTCs and is mainly due to high pick up from widespread radiological imaging detecting small PTCs which might not have been otherwise clinically important. Although generally treatment plans are effective there is disagreement regarding the extent of surgery for DTCs and the place of RAI in the treatment plan. New novel agents such as TKIs have greatly improved the outlook for patients with progressive DTCs. Our understanding of the genetic mutations associated with various types of familial MTCs have greatly improved our ability to identify patients at risk before the clinical onset of the disease. Early detection and prophylactic surgery have resulted in improved survival which is now comparable to PTC patients.

References

1. Ferlay J, Soerjomataram I, Ervik M, et al. GLOBOCAN 2012 v1.0, Cancer incidence and mortality worldwide: IARC Cancer Base No. 11 [Internet]. Lyon: International Agency for Research on Cancer; 2013. Available from: http://globocan.iarc.fr(link is external).
2. Davis L, Welch HG. Increasing incidence of thyroid cancer in the United States, 1973–2002. JAMA. 2006;295:2164–7.
3. Zhu C, Zheng T, Kilfoy BA, et al. A birth cohort analysis of the incidence of papillary thyroid cancer in the United States, 1973–2004. Thyroid. 2009;10:1061–6.
4. Brito JP, Morris JC, Montori VM. Thyroid cancer: zealus imaging has increased detection and treatment of low risk tumors. BMJ. 2013;347:f4706.
5. Harach HR, Franssila KO, Vasenius VM. Occult papillary carcinoma of the thyroid. "A normal" finding in Finland. A systematic autopsy study. Cancer. 1985;56:531–8.
6. Chen AY, Jemal A, Ward EM. Increasing incidence of differentiated thyroid cancer in the United States, 1988–2005. Cancer. 2009;115(16):3801–7.
7. Mazzaferri E, Young RL. Papillary thyroid carcinoma: a ten year follow-up report of the impact of therapy in 576 patients. Am J Med. 1981;70:511.
8. LiVolsi VA, Asa SL. The demise of follicular carcinoma of the thyroid gland. Thyroid. 1994;4(2):233–6.
9. Xing M, Haugen BR, Schlumberger M. Progress in molecular-based management of differentiated thyroid cancer. Lancet. 2013;381:1058–69.
10. Cooper DS, Doherty GM, Haugen BR, Kloos RT, Lee SL, Mandel SJ, et al. Revised American Thyroid Association management guidelines for patients with thyroid nodules and differentiated thyroid cancer. Thyroid. 2009;19:1167–214.
11. Bilimoria KY, Bentrem DJ, Ko CY, et al. Extent of surgery affects survival for papillary thyroid cancer. Ann Surg. 2007;246:375–81.
12. Hay ID, Thompson GB, Grant CS, et al. Papillary thyroid carcinoma managed at the Mayo Clinic during six decades (1940–1999): temporal trends in initial therapy and long-term outcome in 2444 consecutively treated patients. World J Surg. 2002;26:879–85.
13. Shaha AR, Shah JP, Loree TR. Differentiated thyroid cancer presenting initially with distant metastasis. Am J Surg. 1997;174:474–6.
14. Sanders LE, Cady B. Differentiated thyroid cancer: reexamination of risk groups and outcome of treatment. Arch Surg. 1998;133:419–25.
15. Hedringer C, William ED, Sobin LH. Histological typing of thyroid tumors. 2nd ed. originally published by WHO as no 11 in the international histological classification of tumors series. New York: Springer; 1988. p. 1–20.
16. Modigliani E, Cohen R, Campos JM, et al. Prognostic factors for survival and for biochemical cure in medullary thyroid carcinoma: results of 899 patients. The GETC study group. Groupede'etude des tumeurs a calcitonine. Clin Endocrinol. 1998;48:265–73.

Thyroid Dysfunction and Mental Disorders

15

Elnasser Elmaghraby

Abstract

Psychiatric manifestations are not uncommon presentation of thyroid dysfunction. Although, depression and anxiety are likely to occur in both hypo and hyperthyroidism, there are much more mental symptoms which may take place within a course of thyroid dysfunction. Those symptoms may present as a mood, psychotic, cognitive and anxiety in character. The mechanism of such mental symptoms in relation to thyroid abnormalities is still unclear. Proper management is expected to bring about good outcome.

Introduction

The relationship between and the interest in the brain and the thyroid function was established long time ago. According to Esposito et al., this connection was first recorded by Parry in 1786 [1].

Only approximately one century after that, in 1873, Gull demonstrated the association between myxedema and psychosis. He was one of the first to understand that the cause of myxoedema is atrophy of the thyroid gland. In his seminal paper related the changed appearance of one of his patients he wrote "There had been a distinct change in the mental state. The mind, which had previously been active and inquisitive, assumed a gentle, placid indifference, corresponding to the muscular languor, but the intellect was unimpaired…" [2].

The Committee of the Clinical Society of London confirmed this relation in 1888 reporting that 36 % of the patients with myxedema also had insanity symptoms. Committee report described some degree of mental disturbance, ranging from irritability and agoraphobia to dementia and melancholia in almost all untreated patients with hypothyroidism. On account of the insidious development with minor and often diffuse complaints related to hypothyroidism at its presentation, diagnosis may be considerably delayed. Isolated case reports of hypothyroid patients presenting with psychiatric manifestations continue to appear in the literature [3].

In 1949, Asher described the association between hypothyroidism and insanity in 14 clinical cases, named 'myxedema madness' and warned that a melancholic state, in the presence of hypothyroidism, would be reverted with the

E. Elmaghraby, MRC Psych
Military Medical Academy,
Ehsan Abdelkadoos St. Abasseia, Cairo, Egypt
e-mail: nasirmaghraby@hotmail.com

S.K. Imam, S.I. Ahmad (eds.), *Thyroid Disorders: Basic Science and Clinical Practice*,
DOI 10.1007/978-3-319-25871-3_15

corrective utilization of thyroid hormones (TH). This observation encouraged clinicians to experience the efficacy of these hormones in the treatment of depression [4].

Thyroid hormone is required for the metabolic activity of every cell in the body. When patients experience symptoms related to abnormal functioning of the hypothalamic-pituitary-thyroid axis, psychiatrists often are the first professionals they consult. Diagnosis of thyroid disorders is based on biochemical and clinical data which might not be congruent. Clinical symptoms of hypothyroidism, for example, are notoriously variable. Severe biochemical hypothyroidism may be associated with mild clinical symptoms, whereas mild biochemical hypothyroidism may be associated with severe symptoms [5].

Mental state examination of a hypothyroid patient may reveal a broad spectrum of dysfunction, ranging from mild attention impairment to a significant agitated delirium or psychosis.

Patients with thyrotoxicosis may experience behavioral and personality changes, such as psychosis, agitation, and depression. Less overt manifestations that are more common in less severe thyrotoxicosis include anxiety, restlessness, irritability, emotional labiality and insomnia [6].

Consequently psychiatric manifestations of thyroid dysfunction diverge much (see Table 15.1 below). They could be classified globally into mood, cognitive, psychotic and anxiety disorders. In this chapter, those psychiatric manifestations or disorders will be detailed and clarified. The neurophysiological basis and possible mechanisms for psychiatric symptoms will be discussed. Management and outcome of such disorders will be covered as well.

Table 15.1 Psychiatric disorders related to thyroid dysfunction

Psychiatric disorder	Type
Mood disorders	Major depressive disorder
	Dysthymia
	Atypical depression
Bipolar disorder	Type I and type II
	Cyclothymia
Anxiety disorder	Generalized anxiety disorder
	Social phobia
	Panic disorder
	Phobias
Psychotic disorder	Schizophrenia
	Schizophreniform disorder,
	Schizoaffective disorder,
	Brief psychotic disorder,
	Delusional disorder,
	Chronic hallucinatory psychosis
Cognitive disorder	Attention, concentration, memory, problem solving etc

Basic Concepts and Terminology

Thyroid dysfunctions could be classified globally as hypo or hyper function of thyroid. Both conditions could be associated with a wide range of psychiatric symptoms and clinical presentation. In psychiatry the term mental disorder and mental illness are used as synonyms. Psychiatry deals with disorders rather than diseases of mind. A disorder will be defined generically as something actually wrong with a subject. It might be a condition, an abnormality, a sign or a symptom. On the other hand, disease is a definite pathological process having a characteristic set of signs and symptoms [7].

Psychiatry also deals with spectrum disorder which includes a range of disorders containing core manifestations in their clinical presentation. A spectrum disorder is a mental disorder that includes a range of linked conditions. The different elements of a spectrum either have a similar appearance or are thought to be caused by the same underlying mechanism. The spectrum may represent a range of severity, comprising relatively "severe" mental disorders through to relatively "mild and nonclinical deficits" [8, 9].

Neurophysiology of Psychiatric Disorders

Mood regulation involve the medial prefrontal cortex and closely related areas in the medial and caudolateral orbital cortex, amygdala, hippocampus, and ventromedial parts of the basal ganglia, The medial prefrontal cortex is part of a larger "default system" of cortical areas that include the dorsal prefrontal cortex, mid- and posterior cingulated cortex, anterior temporal cortex, and entorhinal and parahippocampal cortex. Dysfunctions within and between structures in this circuit may induce disturbances in emotional behavior and other cognitive aspects of depressive syndromes in humans [10].

Norepinephrine, serotonin, dopamine and acetylcholine are involved with mood regulation. The limbic cortex is linked with both the neocortex, which subserves higher symbolic functions, the midbrain and lower brain centers, which are involved in autonomic control, hormonal production, and sleep and wakefulness. Nor epinephrine-containing neurons are involved in many of the functions that are profoundly disturbed in melancholia, including mood, arousal, appetite, reward, and drives. Other neurotransmitters that mediate such functions are the catecholamine dopamine, especially important for psychomotor activity, and the indoleamine serotonin, involved in mood and sleep and inhibitory control. Cholinergic neurons, secreting acetylcholine at their dendritic terminals, are generally antagonistic in function to catecholaminergic neurons [11].

Anxiety disorders have been linked to disrupted functional connectivity of the amygdala and it's processing of fear and anxiety. Sensory information enters the amygdala through the nuclei of the basolateral complex (consisting of lateral, basal and accessory basal nuclei) [12].

The three major neurotransmitters associated with anxiety on the bases of animal studies and responses to drug treatment are nor epinephrine, serotonin, and gamma amino butyric acid (GABA). Much of the basic neuroscience information about anxiety comes from animal experiments involving behavioral paradigms and psychoactive agents.

In **Schizophrenia,** studies using neurophysiologic tests and brain imaging such as MRI and PET to examine the functional differences in brain activity have shown that differences seem to most commonly occur in frontal lobes, hippocampus and temporal lobes [13].

As regards cognitive functions, brain areas such as the prefrontal cortex, the hippocampus, the amygdale and the mammillary bodies are thought to be involved in certain kinds of memory and cognition. For example, the hippocampus is believed to be involved in spatial learning and declarative learning. Damage to certain areas in patients and animal models and subsequent memory deficits is a primary source of information. The dorsolateral prefrontal and posterior parietal cortex are two components of the cortical network controlling attention, working memory and executive function [14].

Acetylcholine, norepinephrine, serotonin, GABA, histamine, adenosine, nitric oxide and choleystokinin play role in memory and learning in animals.

Mood Disorders

Mood disorder is a group of diagnoses where a disturbance in the person's mood is hypothesized to be the main underlying feature. They are broadly classified into unipolar and bipolar disorder. In unipolar depression there are episodes of depressive symptoms while in Bipolar disorders there are episodes of depression and others of mania or hypomania [15].

Mood is defined as Pervasive and sustained feeling tone that is experienced internally and that in the extreme, can markedly influence virtually all aspects of a person's behavior and perception of the world. While affect is the subjective and immediate experience of emotion attached to ideas or mental representations of objects. Affect has outward manifestations that can be classified as restricted, blunted, flattened, broad, labile, appropriate or inappropriate.

Patients with thyroid disturbance and psychiatric symptoms most often are diagnosed with mood changes usually related to depressive-spectrum [5]. Depressive affect has been reported as a frequent association with hypothyroidism and a regular feature of early cases of hypothyroidism [16].

Several of the metabolic and behavioral changes seen in hypothyroidism are common to depression, suggesting that changes in the pituitary–thyroid system may play a role in the modulation of mood [17].

Patients with subclinical hypothyroidism have higher prevalence of depression than the general population and it has been proposed that this clinical entity shares with overt hypothyroidism the capability of causing depression, being considered one of the main risk factors in non-elderly women with 56 % prevalence of life time depression in this population as compared to 20 % in the euthyroid population [18].

In another study by Haggert and Prange reported that 15–20 % of depressed patients show subclinical hypothyroidism and also show poor response to antidepressant therapy [19]. In case of refractory depression are these rates are even higher.

Howland, in his review of six studies, found a mean rate of 52 % as compared to 8–17 % in general population and concluded that subclinical hypothyroidism is significantly associated with refractory depression [20].

In a study of twins, autoimmune thyroiditis was related to bipolar disorder and the genetic tendency to develop bipolar disorder. The authors suggest that autoimmune thyroiditis, using the marker of thyroperoxidase antibodies, is a possible endophenotype for bipolar disorder [21].

Another study evaluating outpatients with bipolar disorder found thyroid autoimmunity to be highly prevalent. The presence of thyroperoxidase antibodies appeared to be an independent risk factor for the development of hypothyroidism, particularly in women with bipolar disorder [22].

Thyroid dysfunction is more common in patients with rapid cycling bipolar disorder (i.e., having 4 or more mood swings or episodes in a 12-month period) or mixed states (i.e., an episode that simultaneously presents symptoms of both depression and mania) than in patients with classic mania [23].

Levothyroxine may decrease the severity and frequency of manic and depressive episodes [24].

In addition, triiodothyronine has been effectively used as an augmentation agent in treatment-resistant bipolar depression [25].

While hyperthyroidism is typically associated with mania, there are case reports of mania or hypomania associated with hypothyroidism. These reports typically occurred in young women of reproductive age; however, late-onset mania associated with hypothyroidism in an elderly woman has been reported [26, 27].

Mood Disorders could occur with either hypo or hyper function of thyroid gland. In DSM.5 they are classified as mood disorder due to another medical condition [28].

Several studies have suggested that mild symptoms of hypothyroidism are commoner and scores on measures of depression and anxiety higher in patients with subclinical hypothyroidism than in age-matched controls. These findings, however, are inconsistent with other studies that have found no significant differences . Mild hypothyroidism is also more frequent in rapid cycling bipolar disorder, occurring in up to 25 % of cases. Thyroxin supplementation of established treatment for bipolar disorder has been shown to reduce the number of episodes.

In a large epidemiological study involved 30,175 individuals, no associations were found between antithyroid antibodies and depression or anxiety [29].

Generally hypothyroid patients usually meet several criteria for a major depressive episode—such as concentration difficulties, lassitude, low libido, and sometimes pessimism or sadness. Symptoms improve after sustained thyroid hormone replacement therapy [30]. In one study no statistical association between thyroid dysfunction and the presence of depression or anxiety disorder was found [31].

While another study showed association between estimated free thyroxine level and severity of depression [32].

Antidepressant Effects on Thyroid Function

Associations between lithium, the gold-standard for treatment of bipolar disorder, and thyroid function have been recognized for some time. A review of the literature found that Inhibition of thyroid hormone release is critical for the development of hypothyroidism and goiter; Hypothyroidism may occur in the early years of lithium use, in middle-aged women, and when thyroid autoimmunity is present; The outcome of thyroid dysfunction in patients who have been on lithium for many years is not greatly different from that observed in the general population, and Hyperthyroidism and thyroid cancer are uncommon during treatment with lithium. The authors recommend that thyroid function tests to be performed at baseline prior to lithium initiation and repeated after 1 year. An annual TSH may then be sufficient to detect hypothyroidism. Thyroid function abnormalities are not a contraindication to lithium treatment and lithium should not be discontinued if thyroid abnormalities occur [33].

A recent nested, matched, case–control study of patients with bipolar disorder and incident hypothyroidism found that lithium, carbamazepine and valproate increased the risk for hypothyroidism. Combination of agents (especially lithium and valproate) further heightened risk for hypothyroidism. Based on these results, the authors recommend regular monitoring of thyroid function and monotherapy of mood stabilizers for treatment of bipolar disorders [34].

Psychosis

Psychosis refers to an abnormal condition of the mind, and is a generic psychiatric term for a mental state often described as involving a "loss of contact with reality. The term "psychosis" is very broad and can mean anything from relatively normal aberrant experiences through to the complex and catatonic expressions of schizophrenia and bipolar disorder [35].

Patients with thyroid dysfunction may develop a spectrum of psychotic presentation e.g., schizophrenia, schizoaffective disorder and delusional disorder.

Very occasionally in treatment of hyperthyroidism the initiation of treatment is accompanied by the emergence of psychotic disorder, which interestingly usually takes the form of mania. Josephson and Mackenzie (1980) referred to 18 examples in the literature, 12 being manic illnesses and the others mixed affective or depressive disorders [36].

The symptoms usually began within 4–7 days of starting thyroxin treatment, resolving over 1–2 weeks irrespective of further therapeutic intervention. All recovered completely. Such patients often had a personal or family history of psychiatric disorder and had frequently been depressed or delusional prior to starting treatment [37].

Psychosis is an uncommon association of hyperthyroidism, which may occasionally be the presenting feature and lead directly to psychiatric referral. A study of thyrotoxic psychosis from New Zealand suggested that in contemporary practice approximately 1 % of thyrotoxic patients are first diagnosed with a major psychiatric illness [38].

The diagnostic distinctions between the affective and schizophrenic reactions are often blurred, and an admixture of organic psychiatric features is relatively common.

Cognitive Changes

Cognitive functions is a broad term which encompass a variety of integrated brain functions e.g., attention, concentration, memory, perception, language, information processing, orientation and decision making. Initially in thyroid dysfunctions cognitive changes are non-specific and ill-defined. Cognitive disturbances include the inability to concentrate, poor attention, bradyphrenia, calculation difficulties and difficulty understanding complex questions. Memory is often affected from an early stage, with failure to register events and forgetfulness for day-to-day events. Memory for remote events may also deteriorate in chronic cases. Psychomotor retardation is seen and fatigability ability is conspicuous. Elderly patients may have a less activated presentation with depression and lethargy, so-called apathetic thyrotoxicosis . In one review of elderly patients with hyperthyroidism, dementia and confusion were found in 33 and 18 % of patients respectively [39].

Studies in younger individuals with newly-diagnosed hyperthyroidism have found lower cognitive scores compared with controls [40, 41].

With chronic thyroid dysfunctions, the ability to perform everyday routine tasks is decreased and such tasks take a progressively longer time to be completed. Patients become less concerned about and less responsive to others, and there is marked inability to sustain mental exertion. The patient also becomes less capable of learning and performing new tasks. Speech is reduced and perseverations are frequently seen. Alterations in the accuracy of perception may also develop [5].

Acute organic reactions accompany 'thyroid crises' and show the typical picture of delirium, usually are accompanied by fever. They were formerly one of the commonest forms of major mental illness encountered in the disease, but are now very rare because of modern methods of treatment. They constitute a grave emergency and warrant urgent intervention [3, 42].

In a study included 1,327 adolescents 13–16 years old in the United States, subclinical hypothyroidism, subclinical hyperthyroidism and euthyroid groups were defined. Cognitive performance was assessed using the subscales of the Wide Range Achievement Test-Revised (WRAT-R) and the Wechsler Intelligence Scale for Children-Revised (WISC-R). Results showed that subclinical hypothyroidism was found in 1.7 % and subclinical hyperthyroidism was found in 2.3 % of the adolescents. Cognitive assessment scores on average tended to be lower in adolescents with subclinical hyperthyroidism and higher in those with subclinical hypothyroidism than the score for the euthyroid group. Adolescents with subclinical hypothyroidism had significantly better scores in block design and reading than the euthyroid subjects even after adjustment for a number of variables including sex, age and family income level. It was concluded that subclinical hypothyroidism was associated with better performance in some areas of cognitive functions while subclinical hyperthyroidism could be a potential risk factor [40].

Anxiety Disorders

Anxiety disorders are a category of mental disorders characterized by feelings of anxiety and fear, where anxiety is a worry about future events and fear is a reaction to current events. These feelings may cause physical symptoms, such as a racing heart and shakiness.

Anxiety disorder is characterized by at least 6 months of pervasive and excessive anxiety; recurring worry about common events; and physical symptoms, such as muscle tension, insomnia, and fatigue [43].

Anxiety disorders are common in the setting of medical disease and are associated with several types of psychosomatic presentations [44].

Generalized anxiety has been reported in 80 % of those who have hyperthyroidism. An association with panic disorder and the earlier 'atypical organic brain syndrome' and 'organic anxiety syndrome' has been described as well [45, 46].

Mechanism of Psychiatric Disorders Associated with Thyroid Dysfunction

The question of whether the cerebral hypometabolism seen in hypothyroidism is a consequence of a direct action of thyroid hormones on neurons or is secondary to altered cerebral blood flow remains unanswered and will perhaps await the development of techniques to directly measure CNS thyroid metabolism *in vivo*. Nevertheless, the associated mental symptomatology can be largely ascribed to changes in cerebral metabolism, regardless of cause. Cases of major affective disorder and schizophrenia are likely to be determined by both organic factors, genetic and environmental factors. In the rare examples where organic features are entirely absent from the mental state, the cerebral metabolic defect has probably served merely as a precipitant. However, the situation is not entirely straightforward, since patients with purely depressive symptomatology with no evidence of hypothyroidism have been found to respond to thyroxine, often after other forms of treatment have failed entirely [47].

Psychiatric Management

Management starts by establishing and maintaining a therapeutic alliance with the patient and complete psychiatric assessment should be done. It is important to evaluate the safety of the patient and establish the appropriate setting for treatment.

This is followed by evaluating types and severity of functional impairment with quality of life of the patient. Coordination of the patient's care with other clinicians should be arranged. It is central to define the goals of the treatment and to monitor the patient's psychiatric status. It is also vital to keep an eye on the patient's adherence to the treatment plan and to overcome the obstacles which diminish compliance. Providing education to the patient and, when appropriate, to the family is crucial and mandatory in determining the success of the management plan.

In psychiatry the management plan usually go through three consecutive phases. The acute phase followed by continuation and maintenance phases. Treatment in the acute phase should be aimed at inducing remission of the major depressive episode and achieving a full return to the patient's baseline level of functioning [48].

During the continuation phase of treatment, the patient should be carefully monitored for signs of possible relapse. Systematic assessment of symptoms, side effects, adherence, and functional status is essential and may be facilitated through the use of clinician- and/or patient administered rating scales.

Maintenance therapy should also be considered for patients with additional risk factors for recurrence, such as the presence of residual symptoms, ongoing psychosocial stressors, early age at onset, and family history of mood disorders.

It is important to recognize and address the potential interplay between Psychiatric disorder and thyroid dysfunction. Communication with other clinicians who treat the patient is recommended. The clinical assessment should include identifying any potential interactions between medications used to treat depression and those used to treat thyroid dysfunction. In addition, the psychiatrist should consider the effects of prescribed psychotropic medications on the patient's general medical conditions, as well as the effects of interventions for such disorders on the patient's psychiatric condition.

Drugs used to treat seizures including carbamazepine, oxcarbazepine, phenobarbital, primidone and phenytoin can increase the metabolism of levothyroxine and would require larger doses of the drug. The selective serotonin reuptake inhibitor (SSRI) sertraline widely prescribed for depression, has been associated with a decrease in the effect of levothyroxine. Further studies are needed on this, and on any similar effects of other SSRIs. Levothyroxine increases receptor sensitivity to catecholamines thus accelerating the response to tricyclic antidepressants. St. John's wort(antidepressant) is also an enzyme inducer. One study found that it may increase levothyroxine metabolism. Taking the two drugs should be avoided, since it may cause hypothyroidism [49].

Lithium is used as an integral component in the management of acute mania, unipolar and bipolar depressive disorder. It is also used as long-term prophylaxis of bipolar disorders. Thyroid abnormalities associated with lithium treatment have been widely reported in the medical literature over the last five decades. These include hypothyroidism, hyperthyroidism, unmasking or induction of autoimmune thyroiditis and goiter [50, 51].

Despite adequate therapy with thyroxine and TSH within the desired range, many hypothyroid patients complain of persistent lethargy and other persisting psychological symptoms. A randomized clinical trial has suggested that combined therapy with tri-iodothyronine and thyroxine leads to improved cognitive performance, mood and physiological well-being compared with treatment with thyroxine alone [52].

However, subsequent randomized clinical trials have failed to replicate these findings, leading to suggestions that it is perhaps only patients with complete absence of thyroid function alone who may benefit from combined therapy [53, 54].

Optimum treatment of persistent psychological symptoms and mood disturbance therefore currently remains unclear.

Outcome of Mental Disturbances

The treatment of hypothyroidism is usually highly rewarding, with behavioral disturbances responding well to adequate thyroxin therapy, although supplementation with an antidepressant or neuroleptic is often initially helpful. The great majority of patients with serious psychiatric developments can also be expected to respond, even those with overt dementia, provided too long an interval has not elapsed. The same apply for the treatment of hyperthyroidism where results are generally good, with resolution of emotional disorder as the patient is rendered euthyroid. Sometimes, however, emotional instability persists, and in most cases is probably attributable to premorbid tendencies. It has been observed that the depression and anxiety resolved in the great majority of cases with antithyroid treatment alone. Occasionally, however, additional psychotropic medication may be necessary.

Acute organic and affective psychoses usually also respond rapidly as the Thyrotoxicosis comes under control. Schizophrenic psychoses may run a more variable course, but as with other psychoses in which a precipitating cause is apparent the prognosis will usually be better than for schizophrenia that arises spontaneously. Additional measures in the form of antipsychotic, antidepressant medication or electroconvulsive therapy may be necessary in psychotic disorders, and particularly so when organic features are absent from the mental state [5].

Conclusion

Mental disorders related to thyroid dysfunction are diverse and variable. They include mood, anxiety, psychotic and cognitive disorders. These could arise with both hypo and hyperfunction of thyroid. Mental symptomatology can be largely ascribed to changes in cerebral metabolism, regardless of cause.

The outcome is generally good when thyroid is treated. The addition of psychotropic medication and other psychiatric interventions could be helpful as well.

References

1. Esposito S, Prange Jr AJ, Golden RN. The thyroid axis and mood disorders: overview and future prospects. Psychopharmacol Bull. 1997;33(2):205–17.
2. Pearce JMS. Myxoedema and Sir William Withey Gull (1816–1890). J Neurol Neurosurg Psychiatry. 2006;77(5):639.
3. Harrison NA, Michael D, Kopelman MD. Endocrine diseases and metabolic disorders. In: LISHMAN'S organic psychiatry: a textbook of neuropsychiatry. 4th ed. Wiley-Blackwell p. 628–35.
4. Jackson IMD, Asamoah EO. Thyroid function in clinical depression: insights and uncertainties. Thyroid Today. 1999;22(2):1–11.
5. Thomas DG Jr. Identifying hypothyroidism's psychiatric presentations. Curr Psychiatry. 2006;5:98–117.
6. Stern RA, Robinson B, Thorner AR, et al. A survey study of neuropsychiatric complaints in patients with Graves' disease. J Neuropsychiatry Clin Neurosci. 1996;8:181–5.
7. Kraemer HC. Evaluating medical tests: objective and quantitative guidelines. Newbury Park: SAGE Publications; 1992. p. 151–8.
8. Maser JD, Akiskal HS. "Spectrum concepts in major mental disorders". Psychiatr Clin North Am. 2002;25: xi–xiii.
9. Angst J, Merikangas K. "The depressive spectrum: diagnostic classification and course". J Affect Disord. 1997;45:31–9; 39–40.
10. Wayne C, Joseph L, Maura L. Implications for neurocircuitry models of depression. Brain Struct Funct. 2008;213:93–118.
11. Kandel ER. Disorders of mood: depression, mania and anxiety disorders. J Prin Neural Sci. 2000; 1209–26 chapter 61.
12. Etkin A, Katherine E, Alan F, et al. Disrupted amygdalar subregion functional connectivity and evidence of a compensatory network in generalized anxiety disorder. Arch Gen Psychiatry. 2009;66:1361–72.
13. Green MF. Schizophrenia revealed: from neurons to social interactions. New York: W.W Norton; 2001. p. 207.
14. Fumi K, Xue-Lian Q, Travis M, et al. Differences in intrinsic functional organization between dorsolateral prefrontal and posterior parietal cortex. Cereb Cortex. 2014;24:2334–49.
15. Kennedy SH. Core symptoms of major depressive disorder: relevance for diagnosis and treatment. Dialogues Clin Neurosci. 2008;10:271–7.
16. Whybrow P, Prange TR. Mental changes accompanying thyroid gland dysfunction. Arch Gen Psychiatry. 1969;20:48–63.
17. Braverman LE, Utiger RD. Werner and Ingbar's the thyroid: a fundamental and clinical text. 8th ed. Philadelphia: Lippincott Williams & Wilkins; 2000. p. 837–42.
18. Haggerty JJ, Stern RA, Mason GA, et al. Subclinical hypothyroidism: a modifiable risk factor for depression? Am J Psyciatry. 1993;150:508–10.
19. Haggerty JJ, Prange AJ. Borderline hypothyroidism and depression. Ann Rev Med. 1995;46:37–46.
20. Howland RH. Thyroid dysfunction in refractory depression: implications for pathophysiology and treatment. J Clin Psychiatry. 1993;54:47–54.
21. Vonk R, van der Schot AC, Kahn RS, Nolen WA, Drexhage HA. Is autoimmune thyroiditis part of the genetic vulnerability (or an endophenotype) for bipolar disorder. Biol Psychiatry. 2007;62:135–40.

22. Kupka RW, Nolen WA, Post RM, et al. High rate of autoimmune thyroiditis in bipolar disorder: lack of association with lithium exposure. Biol Psychiatry. 2002;51:305–11.
23. Chang KD, Keck PE, Stanton SP, McElroy SL, Strakowski SM, Geracioti TD. Differences in thyroid function between bipolar manic and mixed states. Biol Psychiatry. 1998;43:730–3.
24. Bauer MS, Whybrow PC. Rapid cycling bipolar affective disorder. Treatment of refractory rapid cycling with high-dose levothyroxine: a preliminary study. Arch Gen Psychiatry. 1990;47:435–40.
25. Moret C. Combination/augmentation strategies for improving the treatment of depression. Neuropsych Dis Treat. 2005;1:301–9.
26. Kelly T, Lieberman DZ. The use of triiodothyronine as an augmentation agent in treatment-resistant bipolar II and bipolar disorder NOS. J Affect Disord. 2009;116:222–6.
27. Tor PC, Lee HY, Fones CL. Late-onset mania with psychosis associated with hypothyroidism in an elderly Chinese lady. Singapore Med J. 2007;48:354–7.
28. American Psychiatric Association. Diagnostic and statistical manual of mental disorders, 4th ed, text revision. Washington, DC: American Psychiatric Association; 2000.
29. Engum A, Bjøro T, Mykletun A, Dahl AA. Thyroid autoimmunity, depression and anxiety; are there any connections? An epidemiological study of a large population. J Psychosom Res. 2005;59:263–8.
30. Hennessey JV, Jackson IM. The interface between thyroid hormones and psychiatry. Endocrinologist. 1996;6:214–23.
31. Engum A, Bjøro T, Mykletun A, Dahl AA. An association between depression, anxiety and thyroid function: a clinical fact or an artefact? Acta Psychiatr Scand. 2002;106:27–34.
32. Kolakowsk T, Swigar ME. Thyroid function in depression and alcohol abuse: a retrospective study. Arch Gen Psychiatry. 1977;34:984–8.
33. Bocchetta A, Loviselli A. Lithium treatment and thyroid abnormalities. Clin Pract Epidemiol Ment Healt. 2006;2:23.
34. Gau CS, Chang CJ, Tsai FJ, Chao PF, Gau SS. Association between mood stabilizers and hypothyroidism in patients with bipolar disorders: a nested, matched case-control study. Bipolar Disord. 2010;12: 253–63.
35. Gelder MG, Mayou R, Geddes J. Psychiatry. New York: Oxford University Press; 2005. p. 12.
36. Josephson AM, Mackenzie TB. Thyroid-induced mania in hypothyroid patients. Br J Psychiatr. 1980; 137:222–8.
37. Benjamin JS, Harold IK, Virginia AS. Kaplan & Sadock's synopsis of psychiatry: behavioral sciences/ clinical psychiatry. 10th ed. Philadelphia: Lippincott Williams & Wilkin; 2007.
38. Brownlie BEW, Rae AM, Walshe JWB, et al. Psychoses associated with thyrotoxicosis: 'thyrotoxic psychosis'. A report of 18 cases, with statistical analysis of incidence. Eur Endocrinol. 2000;142:438–44.
39. Martin FI, Deam DR. Hyperthyroidism in elderly hospitalised patients. Clinical features and treatment outcomes. Med J Aust. 1996;164:200–3.
40. Wu T, Flowers JW, Tudiver F, et al. Subclinical thyroid disorders and cognitive performance among adolescents in the United States. BMC Pediatr. 2006;6:12.
41. Schlote B, Schaaf L, Schmidt R, et al. Mental and physical state in subclinical hyperthyroidism: investigations in a normal working population. Biol Psychiatry. 1992;32:48–56.
42. Román GC, Ghassabian A, Bongers-Schokking JJ, et al. Association of gestational maternal hypothyroxinemia and increased autism risk. Ann Neurol. 2013;74:733–42.
43. Patel G, Fancher TL. Generalized anxiety disorder. Ann Intern Med. 2013;159:ITC6–1.
44. Fava GA, Porcelli P, Rafanelli C, et al. The spectrum of anxiety disorders in the medically ill. J Clin Psychiatry. 2010;71:910–4.
45. Kathol RG, Turner R, Delahunt J. Depression and anxiety associated with hyperthyroidism: response to antithyroid therapy. Psychosomatics. 1986;27:501–5.
46. Jadresic DP. Psychiatric aspects of hyperthyroidism. J Psychosom Res. 1990;34:603–15.
47. Bauer M, Hellweg R, Graf KJ, et al. Treatment of refractory depression with high dose thyroxine. Neuropsychopharmacology. 1998;18:444–55.
48. American Psychiatric Association. Practice guideline for the treatment of patients with bipolar disorder (revision). Am J Psychiatry. 2002;159:1–50.
49. Mitchell L. Evaluation of the association between St. John's wort and elevated thyroid-stimulating hormone. Pharmacotherapy. 2001;21:1574–8.
50. Kibirige D, Luzinda K, Ssekitoleko R. Spectrum of lithium induced thyroid abnormalities: a current perspective. Thyroid Res. 2013;6(1):3.
51. Barbesino G. Drugs affecting thyroid function. Thyroid. 2010;20:763–70.
52. Bunevicius R, Kazanavicius G, Zalinkevicius R, et al. Effects of thyroxine as compared with thyroxine plus triiodothyronine in patients with hypothyroidism. N Engl J Med. 1999;340:424–9.
53. Clyde PW, Harari AE, Getta EJ, et al. Combined levothyroxine plus liothyronine compared with levothyroxine alone in primary hypothyroidism. A randomized controlled trial. JAMA. 2003;290: 2952–8.
54. Cooper DS. Combined T4 and T3 therapy: back to the drawing board. JAMA. 2003;290:3002–4.

Thyroid Dysfunction and Arrhythmias

16

Sonia Marrakchi Meziou, Faouzi Kanoun, Dania Idriss Marrakchi, Ikram Kammoun, and Salem Kachboura

Abstract

Context: Arrhythmia is a major cause of morbidity and mortality in Europe and in the United States. The aim of this review article was to assess the results of the prospective studies that evaluated the risk of arrhythmia in patients with overt and subclinical thyroid disease and discuss the management of this arrhythmia.

Evidence Acquisition: Reports published with the following search terms were searched: thyroid, hypothyroidism, hyperthyroidism, subclinical hyperthyroidism, subclinical hypothyroidism, levothyroxine, triiodothyronine, antithyroid drugs, radioiodine, deiodinases, atrial flutter, supraventricular arrhythmia, ventricular arrhythmia, ventricular tachycardia, ventricular fibrillation, torsade de pointe, amiodarone and atrial fibrillation. The investigation was restricted to reports published in English.

Evidence Synthesis: The outcome of this analysis suggests that patients with untreated overt thyroid dysfunction are at increased risk of arrhythmia.

Conclusions: The timely recognition and effective treatment of thyroid dysfunction in patients with arrhythmia is mandatory because the long-term and prognosis of arrythmias may be improved with the appropriate treatment of thyroid dysfunction.

S. Marrakchi Meziou, MD (✉) • I. Kammoun
S. Kachboura
Cardiology Department, Abderrahman Mami Hospital, Ariana, Tunisia
e-mail: marrakchi.sonia@yahoo.fr

F. Kanoun
Endocrinology Department, La Rabta Hospital, Tunis, Tunisia

D. Idriss Marrakchi
Department of Molecular Biology, University Manar 2 of Tunis, Tunis, Tunisia

Abbreviations

AF	Atrial fibrillation
AIT	Amiodarone-induced thyrotoxicosis
AP	Action potential
EAD	Early afterdepolarization
ECG	Electrocardiogram
FT4	Free thyroxine
*I*K	Delayed rectifier potassium current

S.K. Imam, S.I. Ahmad (eds.), *Thyroid Disorders: Basic Science and Clinical Practice*,
DOI 10.1007/978-3-319-25871-3_16

LQTS	Long QT syndrome
PLB	Phospholamban
PVs	Pulmonary veins
SERCA2	Calcium-activated adenosine triphosphatase
SR	Sarcoplasmic reticulum
SR Ca^{2+}-ATPase	Sarcoplasmic reticulum calcium pumps
T3	Triiodothyronine
TdP	Torsade de pointes
TH	Thyroid hormone
TSH	Thyroid stimuling hormone
UFH	Unfractionated heparin
VF	Ventricular fibrillation
VPB	Ventricular premature beats
VT	Ventricular tachycardia

Introduction

The most common clinical manifestations of thyrotoxic heart disease are heart rate disorders, in particular, sinus tachycardia and atrial fibrillation, which presents in 28 % of patients [1]. Typical arrhythmias found in hyperthyroidism are atrial premature contractions or atrial fibrillation, the latter occurring in 9–22 % of patients [2]. Conversely, ventricular premature contractions are rare in this setting, and if present, their frequency is not decreased after treatment [3]. Malignant ventricular arrhythmias such as ventricular tachycardia or fibrillation, which are potentially fatal, are exceptional [4] and usually occur only in patients with marked heart failure or associated cardiac disease [5]. Surprisingly, there have been few population-based studies examining the long-term influence of thyroid disease and its treatment on morbidity and mortality [6].

Genomic Action of Thyroid Hormone on Heart

Thyroid hormone exerts a broad range of effects on development, growth, and metabolism. The clinical manifestations of thyroid hormone excess and deficiency are dramatic examples of the myriad actions of the hormone. Thyroxine (T_4), the primary secretory product of the thyroid, is relatively inactive and is converted to the active hormone, triiodothyronine (T_3), by the enzyme thyroxine 5′-deiodinase. The actions of thyroid hormone are primarily the result of the interaction of T_3 with nuclear receptors for T_3 that bind to regulatory regions of genes (thyroid hormone-response elements) and modify their expression [7]. These receptors have been cloned, and there has been considerable progress in unraveling the various mechanisms by which thyroid hormone regulates gene expression [8].

The clinical findings in hypothyroidism and hyperthyroidism are the net result of the actions of products of a variety of genes whose expression is directly or indirectly regulated by T_3. There are markers of thyroid hormone action that can be monitored clinically and that provide information about the ability of T_3 to regulate a gene product. Thyroid hormone excess reduces systemic vascular resistance, enhances cardiac contractility, and has a positive chronotropic effect [9]. Thyroid hormone deficiency has the opposite effects: it increases systemic vascular resistance, decreases contractility, and slows the heart rate. These changes in cardiac function are the result of both regulation of cardiac-specific genes by T_3 [10] and changes in hemodynamic function induced by T_3 [11]. The contractile properties of the heart are dependent on the relative amounts of the products of the various myosin genes [8, 12]. Thyroid hormone exerts marked effects on cardiac contractility through changes in the expression of thyroid hormone-responsive genes as well as through alterations in function of important regulatory proteins [1, 2]. It has been demonstrated that a variety of proteins in the cardiac myocyte, including the α- and β-myosin heavy chains, β-adrenergic receptors, sarcoplasmic reticulum (SR) calcium-activated adenosine triphosphatase (SERCA2), and phospholamban (PLB), calcium transporter proteins are regulated by thyroid hormone [12, 13]. The classically described cellular actions of thyroid hormone are mediated by nuclear triiodothyronine (T3) receptors that function to regulate the expression of specific cardiac genes [8, 10] such as plasma membrane sodium potassium ATPase [14] and voltage-activated K1 channel genes including Kv4.2, Kv4.3, and Kv1.5 [15].

In the ventricle, the transcription of the beta myosine heavy chain (β-MHC) antisense (AS) gene appears to be associated with and linked to the transcription of the α-MHC gene; both are induced in the presence of T3. However, in atria this expression appears to be uncoupled. As observed in the ventricles, the expression of the β-MHC AS gene in the atria is inversely correlated, while the expression of the α-MHC gene is not thyroid hormone responsive and highly expressed in all thyroid states. This observation demonstrates for the first time that the previously identified shared promoter region that lies in the intergenic region between the b-MHC and a-MHC genes is differentially regulated in a tissue-specific manner [10]. Exploration of the differences in cofactors and potential epigenetic influences in this shared intergenic promoter region in atria and ventricles may provide additional information regarding the potential mechanism by which T3 influences the MHC genes in the human heart [12].

Non Genomic Action of Thyroid Hormone on Heart

In addition to the well-characterized nuclear effects of thyroid hormone, some cardiac responses to thyroid hormone appear to be mediated through non genomic mechanisms [16], as suggested by relatively rapid onset of action-faster than can be accounted for by changes in gene expression and protein synthesis and failure to be affected by inhibitors of gene transcription. The significance of these diverse actions remains to be established, but may explain the ability of acute T3 to alter cardiovascular hemodynamics. They may alter the functional proprieties of membrane ion channels and pumps, including the sodium channel and inward rectifying potassium current (IK) [17].

Electrophysiology and Mechanism of Action of T3 on the Atria

Thyroid hormones have profound effects on the cardiovascular system. The mechanism of pacemaker activity in adult cardiac tissue is increasingly well documented. Although there is some controversy regarding the relative contributions of various ionic currents, it is becoming clear that a variety of ionic currents are responsible for pacemaker activity in various regions of the heart. Sun et al. [18] demonstrated through electrophysiological recordings that thyroid hormone increases the pacemaker rate of these myocytes by increasing the slope of spontaneous depolarization. Under voltage clamp conditions, Sun et al. focused on several ionic currents that may be involved in pacemaker activity in atrial cells, including *I*Ca, *I*f and *I*Na/Ca. of the ionic currents studied, the electrogenic Na+–Ca2+ exchange current was the only candidate to be changed by T3 and which may have altered the slope of spontaneous depolarization. They suggest that, of the ionic currents studied, T3 might accelerate diastolic depolarization and pacemaker activity (at least in part) by an up-regulation of the Na+–Ca2+ exchanger.

Several ionic currents may contribute to pacemaker activity in this tissue, including *I*f, the delayed rectifier potassium current (*I*K) [19–21], both the L-type (*I*Ca,L) and T-type (*I*Ca,T) calcium currents [20] and a background Na+ current (*I*b) [19]. The electrogenic Na+–Ca2+ exchanger, triggered as a result of SR Ca2+ release, may also contribute to the initial phases of diastolic depolarization in the sinoatrial (SA) node [22]. Thus, the positive chronotropic action of thyroid hormones is potentially caused by modulation of any of these electrogenic ion conductances and/or by alterations in intracellular calcium homeostasis.

Early experimental studies of thyroid hormone effects on transmembrane potentials of sinoatrial node cells and atrial muscle cells showed an increased rate of diastolic depolarization and decreased duration of action potential in thyrotoxic animals, suggesting that conductance of K1 ions may be altered [23, 24].

Electrophysiology and Mechanism of Action of T3 on the Ventricles

Recent evidence has shown that thyroid hormones exert effects on the cardiovascular system that are not mediated by alterations in gene expression. Sakaguchi and co-workers [25] showed that T3 caused a shortening of the action potential duration in guinea pig ventricular myocytes by increasing whole cell inward rectifier potassium current (*I*K1).

In the rat ventricular myocyte, two primary depolarization-activated outward currents are important in regulating action potential duration: the Ca21-independent transient outward K1 current (*I*to) and a slowly inactivating K1 current (*I*K) [26].

Although thyroid hormone has been shown to regulate the expression of numerous cardiac-specific genes, Sun et al. [27] show that T3 shortens the action potential duration (APD) in hypothyroid rats due at least in part to the increase of the delayed rectifier current *I*K. The *I*to appears to be regulated by thyroid hormone at the transcriptional level, whereas the *I*K is regulated by a nongenomic mechanism of action.

Relation Between Thyroid Hormone and Adrenergic System

Many of the cardiovascular manifestations of thyroid hormone excess resemble those produced by sympathoadrenal stimulation. Since plasma catecholamine levels and turnover rates are not increased in hyperthyroidism [28], it has been argued that the effects of thyroid hormone result partly from increased responsiveness to catecholamines. This hypothesis is supported by studies that indicate that β-aderenergic receptor (βAR) number and sensitivity are increased in isolated hearts and cultured cells from experimental animals (most often the rat) treated with thyroid hormone [29, 30]. The influence of thyroid hormone on adrenergic responsiveness is particularly controversial in large animals and humans but Brian et al. [31] suggest that the cardiac mechanical effects of hyperthyroidism cannot be explained by enhanced sensitivity to catecholamines. Despite significant increases in basal heart rate and rates of left ventricular (LV) contraction and relaxation, the response to β-adrenergic agonists was not increased in hyperthyroid baboons. Increased basal indices of LV contraction and relaxation in this model are more clearly related to changes in myosin heavy chain isoform expression and the relative abundance of the sarcoplasmic reticulum (SR) calcium pumps (SR Ca^{2+}-ATPase) and its phosphoprotein inhibitor, phospholamban, although other thyroid hormone–mediated effects, such as those reported for L-type calcium channels and Na^+/K^+-ATPase pumps cannot be excluded.

Thyroid hormone potentiates the effect of adrenergic system on heart. Catecholamine levels are either normal or decreased in thyrotoxicosis. Facilitation of action of catecholamines is by increasing tissue sensitivity by increased transcription of beta adrenergic receptors and structural similarity to catecholamines. Hyperthyroidism is associated with reduced vagal activity and reduced heart rate variability which can persist despite restoration of euthyroidism [32]. Ojamaa et al. [33] indicate that an analysis confined to the changes in 13-adrenergic receptor expression is insufficient to ascertain the role of catecholamines as mediators of thyroid hormone--dependent effects on cardiac autonomic responsiveness. It is important to consider all three components, the β3-adrenergic receptor, G-coupled protein, and catalytic subunit expression, in assessing adrenergic responsiveness of target tissues.

Mechanism Underlying the Effect of Thyroid Hormone (TH) on the Arrhythmogenesis

Thyroid hormone has been shown to have several cardiovascular effects, and hyperthyroidism has been known to be an important factor in the etiology of atria and ventricles arrhythmias [5]. In fact, there are always three main ingredients required for the production of a clinical arrhythmia: (1). the arrhythmogenic substrate; (2). the trigger factor; (3). the modulation factors of which the most common is the autonomic nervous system [34]. The cardiovascular manifestations of thyroid dysfunction is due to three potential mechanisms by which thyroid hormones might exert their cardiovascular actions by direct effects at the cellular level, by interacting with the sympathetic nervous system, through alterations of the peripheral circulation and energy metabolism [5]. Thyroid hormones have been shown to alter cardiac excitability, which may lead to arrhythmias [8].

Effects of Thyroid Hormones Excess on the Atrias

Hyperthyroidism has been known to be an important factor in the etiology of paroxysmal atrial fibrillation (AF) [5]. The pathogenesis of AF in these patients is postulated to result from shortening of the action potential (AP) duration in the atrial myocardium from excess thyroid hormone facilitating formation of multiple reentry circuits [35, 36]. Graves' disease is one of the most common causes of hyperthyroidism. The prevalence of AF in patients with Graves' disease, as in all other forms of hyperthyroidism, increases with age [36]. Shortening of the AP duration also decreases the refractoriness of cardiomyocytes, which may facilitate the maintenance of multiple reentrant circuits in heart. Using voltage clamp methods, several ionic currents have been investigated in cardiomyocytes. Calcium currents and delayed rectified potassium currents of ventricular cardiomyocytes were increased in hyperthyroidism [37]. Moreover, transient outward potassium currents and inward rectified currents have also been demonstrated to be increased in hyperthyroid ventricular cardiomyocytes [36].

Pulmonary veins (PVs) have been demonstrated to be important sources of ectopic beats with the initiation of paroxysmal AF or the foci of ectopic atrial tachycardia and focal AF [38]. Previous studies have demonstrated that PVs have pacemaker cells in several species [39]. Thyroid hormone changes the electrophysiological activity of the Pulmonary vein cardiomyocytes. Increased automaticity and enhanced triggered activity may increase the arrhythmogenic activity of PVs in hyperthyroidism [36]. Chen et al. suggest in their study that the electrophysiological features of paroxysmal AF associated with hyperthyroidism are essentially different from those of lone paroxysmal AF. In patients with paroxysmal AF and hyperthyroidism, a shortening of the refractory period in association with a facilitation of the atrial conduction delay could be expected to increase the propensity for AF, and a pre-existent arrhythmogenic substrate might not be essential to the genesis of AF. These findings suggest that the agents that prolong the atrial effective refractory period are effective against AF in patients with hyperthyroidism [40].

Effects of Thyroid Hormones Excess on the Ventricles

The onset of tachycardia or ventricular fibrillation (VF) has been reported within a thyrotoxic storm [41]. The presentation of these arrhythmias in the initial phase of the disease is much less common, and only a few isolated cases are described in the scientific literature. The majority [42, 43] occur in the context of thyrotoxic periodic paralysis with severe hypokalemia [44]. There has been an occasional patient in whom the ventricular arrhythmia were related to coronary spasm [45].

Nevertheless, the shortening of the Q–T interval and the effect of TH on the autonomic nervous system may affect ventricular arrhythmogenesis [46]. TH interacts with the sympathetic nervous system by altering responsiveness to sympathetic stimulation presumably by modulating adrenergic receptor function and/or density [5]. The density of myocardial adrenergic binding sites has been shown to be enhanced by chronic as well as acute treatment with thyroid hormone in hypothyroidism [47]. Thyroid hormone, in addition, induces a rate-dependent lengthening of the Purkinje fiber action potential while ventricular action potential shortens [48]. Consequently, these differences can enhance dispersion of myocardial repolarization and facilitate re-entrant arrhythmias including ventricular fibrillation (VF) [49]. It should also be noted that hyperthyroidism may affect myocardial electrical stability [50] due to increased excitability linked to triggered activity [51] resulting in ventricular premature beats (VPB) [52] that often initiate malignant arrhythmias [53].

On the other hand, it has been suggested that hypothyroidism might confer a protection against arrhythmias because they are rarely encountered in hypothyroid patients. Only atrioventricular blocks, sinus bradycardia, and rare episodes of "torsade de pointes" have been reported to be associated with clinical hypothyroidism [3]. In an animal model of ventricular fibrillation, hypothyroidism has been shown to increase the fibrillatory threshold of the ventricles [5].

In humans, the prolongation of the QTc interval encountered in hypothyroid patients is similar to that seen in euthyroid patients on class III antiarrhythmic agents [54]. In this regard, it has been suggested that the antiarrhythmic effect of amiodarone parallels its blocking effect on the peripheral thyroid hormone metabolism, suggesting that tissue hypothyroidism may have some antiarrhythmic properties [55]. However, this concept has been challenged by several observations. Tri-iodothyronine T3 administration to euthyroid patients treated with amiodarone for benign atrial or ventricular arrhythmias does not increase the frequency of arrhythmias [52]. In patients with hypothyroidism, thyroid replacement therapy did not increase significantly the frequency of benign atrial or ventricular premature beats [56].

Many patients with overt hypothyroidism have Q–T interval lengthening, which reflects the prolonged ventricular action potential due to electrical remodeling [57]. It renders the heart prone to ventricular arrhythmias, such as potentially lethal polymorphic tachycardia "Torsade de Pointes" [58]. The incidence of arrhythmia precedes the occurrence of early after depolarization (EAD) usually triggered in the setting of hypokalemia. EAD-induced triggered responses are traditionally thought to be involved in the generation of ventricular arrhythmias under long Q–T conditions. Dispersion of ventricular refractoriness resulting from heterogeneous myocardial structural remodeling [59] predisposes to Q–T dispersion and consequently to ventricular arrhythmias particularly in patients with subclinical hypothyroidism that are treated with L-thyroxine [60]. Furthermore, in hypothyroidism an atrioventricular block of different degrees may occur [61]. Nevertheless, the VF incidence is reduced in hypothyroidism [62] depression of TH levels seems to be beneficial in patients with angina and acute myocardial infarction [53, 63].

Finally, thyroid hormones may trigger arrhythmias mostly at the level of the atria, and there is some evidence that tissue hypothyroidism may increase the fibrillation threshold of the ventricles. However, there are no clear data in humans indicating that hypothyroidism confers a protection against ventricular or atrial arrhythmias [5].

Supraventricular Arrhythmia

Atrial Arrhythmia

The atrial arrhythmia includes AF, atrial flutter and atrial tachycardia. Atrial fibrillation is the most frequent atrial arrhythmia. Hyperthyroidism has been associated with atrial tachyarrhythmias [64] and with sustained AF occurring in 20–30 % of patients even after return to the euthyroid state [64]. The risk of atrial fibrillation or flutter in hyperthyroidism was higher in men than in women, and the risk of atrial fibrillation in hyperthyroidism increased by increasing age during the age range of 20–89 years. The presence of ischemic heart disease, congestive heart failure, and heart valve disease was also associated with an increased risk of atrial fibrillation [65].

We could not differentiate atrial fibrillation from atrial flutter because in the literature and a lot of articles didn't differentiate the two arrhythmias. In fact, they had the same ICD-10 code [66]. In other hand, there is a low proportion of patients with pure atrial flutter these represent approximately 5 % of the recorded cases [37–39, 67].

Hyperthyroidism

Thyrotoxicosis is a common disorder with a prevalence of 3 % in females and 0.3 % in males in iodine-replete areas such as the United Kingdom and the United States [68]. It is known to induce many cardiovascular effects such as sinus tachycardia, systolic hypertension, changes in ventricular systolic and diastolic function, and predisposition to dysrhythmias, especially AF [6]. The prevalence of AF in patients with hyperthyroidism ranges between 2 and 20 %, and the risk is approximately sixfold greater than normal population [69].

The first step in the management of atrial fibrillation, despite the cause, is to control the ventricular response. β-blockers are one of the mainstays of treatment of AF in the setting of hyperthyroidism [69]. Selective or non-selective β-blockers can provide rapid symptom relief by reducing the ventricular rate, but these agents are unlikely to convert AF to sinus rhythm as they have little effect on hyperthyroidism, the primary cause of cardiac stimulation and AF. Therefore, restoration of euthyroidism by radioiodine or anti-thyroid drugs is the ultimate treatment of choice for long-term AF management in this setting. Successful treatment of hyperthyroidism with either radioiodine or thioureas is associated with a reversion to sinus rhythm in a majority of patients within 2–3 months [70]. Zhen-Hu Zhou et al. demonstrated in their study that after euthyroidism or hypothyroidism states were achieved, very frequent paroxysmal AF were observed and no recurrence was noted at the end of the follow-up. Persistent AF, however, spontaneously converted to sinus rhythm in only 40 % of the patients, but persistent AF continued in the remaining patients. Further analysis showed that older age (>55 years) and a long duration of hyperthyroidism of more than 5 years, and a long duration of pre-treatment AF are independent predictors for continued AF following the successful treatment of hyperthyroidism [71]. In other hand, Xiao et al. suggested that Blockade of angiotensin II could improve abnormal atrial electrophysiological properties and further reduce AF vulnerability by extenuating ion channel, gap junction and structural remodeling in experimental thyrotoxic rabbits [72].

The management strategies for persistent AF following hyperthyroidism treatment are not entirely clear. The current recommendations are that after the patient has been rendered chemically euthyroid, electrical or pharmacological cardioversion should be attempted [69].

Elective cardioversion for persistent AF is highly effective and sinus rhythm maintenance rates are greater than 50 % over 10 years. The addition of anti-arrhythmic drugs may also help to maintain sinus rhythm in these patients [73]. Bepridil is as beneficial treatment to convert AF for the patients with hyperthyroidism-induced persistent AF as it is for the patients with AF due to other causes [74]. Yo Kunii et al. showed that bepridil converted hyperthyroidism-induced persistent AF to sinus rhythm as much as it does after a long duration of AF due to other causes, and the sinus rhythm maintenance rate was very high. Bepridil is very beneficial medicine for the patient of hyperthyroidism-induced AF, however, it should be used with caution, and frequent or continuous ECG monitoring is necessary, to avoid serious side effects [74].

Subclinical Hyperthyroidism and Atrial Fibrillation

Sub clinical hyperthyroidism is defined as low serum thyrotropin concentration in an asymptomatic patient with normal serum T3 and T4 concentration. It has a prevalence of 0.5–3.9 % in adults [75]. The prevalence of atrial fibrillation in patients with low serum thyrotropin concentration was 13.3 % compared to 2.3 % in persons with normal values. The relative risk of atrial fibrillation in subjects with low serum thyrotropin and normal free T3, T4 values compared to those with normal serum thyrotropin was 5.2 [32]. Osturk et al. [76] showed that left atrial mechanical and electromechanical function in subclinical thyroid disorders was impaired. TSH was an independent determinant of interatrial delay. Prolonged atrial electromechanical coupling time and impaired mechanical atrial functions may be related to the increased incidence of arrhythmias.

Hypothyroidism and Subclinical Hypothyroidism

Hypothyroidism is associated with cardiovascular risk factors, subclinical cardiovascular disease, and overt cardiovascular disease, all of which predispose to AF. Subclinical hypothyroidism was common. In fact, the prevalence was

4–8 % in people older than 60 years of age. Subclinical hypothyroidism has some clinical consequences like an increase in the prevalence of atria fibrillation [77]. However, Klemperer et al. [78] found that perioperative T3 administration in Cardiopulmonary bypass in euthyroid patients decreased the incidence and need for treatment of postoperative atrial fibrillation. This finding still unexplained. Kim et al. [79] did not identify a significant association between hypothyroidism and 10-year risk of incident AF in a community-based study from the Framingham heart study.

Euthyroid Range in Older Adults

Cappola et al. [80] examined the relationship between thyroid function testing within the euthyroid range and outcomes encompassing the cardiovascular system in cohort of community-dwelling individuals aged 65 years and older. They found increased risk of atrial Fibrillation at higher concentrations of FT4 and they suggested that there is no optimal set of thyroid function tests within current reference ranges to reflect the euthyroid ideal in the age group. Cappola et al. [80] proposed that the optimal TSH may need to be higher in older people than the currently defined references ranges.

Should We Anticoagulate and Attempt Cardioversion in Those with AF?

Anticoagulation of patients with hyperthyroidism and AF is controversial [81] as the risk for systemic thromboembolic events in the setting of thyrotoxicosis is not well defined [82], and anticoagulation drugs such as warfarin, are associated with a significant risk of bleeding complications and other side effects [82]. There are beliefs that in patients with hyperthyroidism it is advancing age rather than the presence of AF that is the main risk factor [81] for a thromboembolic event, and in younger patients without organic heart disease, hypertension, or other independent risk factors for embolization, the benefits of anticoagulation may actually be outweighed by the risks [69]. In our knowledge, no interaction between thyroid function and unfractionated heparin (UFH) has been documented, however Badawi [83] reported an interaction between thyroid function and UFH. Nakazawa et al. [84] suggested that spontaneous reversion of atrial fibrillation to sinus rhythm is highly unlikely if the duration of atrial fibrillation before the euthyroid state is achieved exceeds 13 months, or if it is still present after the patient has been in a euthyroid state for 4 months, Cardioversion should be performed at about the 16th week after the euthyroid state is achieved.

Arrhythmia and Amiodarone-Induced Hyperthyroidism

Amiodarone is the most commonly used antiarrhythmic drug worldwide [85]. It is effective in the treatment of both supraventricular and ventricular tachyarrhythmias and has the added advantage of being well tolerated in patients with both normal and impaired left ventricular systolic function [85]. The majority of patients (>70 %) on amiodarone will remain euthyroid. However, treatment may lead to either amiodarone-induced hypothyroidism (AIH) or amiodarone-induced thyrotoxicosis (AIT), with AIH more common in iodine-sufficient populations and AIT in iodine-deficient populations [86].

Amiodarone-induced thyroid dysfunction occurs in 15–20 % of amiodarone-treated patients [87]. Amiodarone-induced hypothyroidism (AIH) does not pose relevant problems, is easily controlled by L-thyroxine replacement, and does not require amiodarone withdrawal. Most frequently, AIH develops in patients with chronic autoimmune thyroiditis. Amiodarone-induced thyrotoxicosis (AIT) is most frequently due to destructive thyroiditis (type 2 AIT) causing release of thyroid hormones from the damaged, but otherwise substantially normal gland. Less frequently AIT is a form of hyperthyroidism (type 1 AIT) caused by the iodine load in a diseased gland (nodular goiter, Graves' disease). A clear-cut differentiation between the two main forms is not always possible, despite recent diagnostic advances. As a matter of fact, mixed or indefinite forms do exist, contributed to by both thyroid damage and increased thyroid hormone synthesis. Treatment of type 1 (and mixed forms) AIT is based on the use of thionamides, a short course of potassium perchlorate and, if treatment is not rapidly effective, oral glucocorticoids. Glucocorticoids are the first-line treatment for type 2 AIT. Amiodarone should be discontinued, if feasible from a cardiac standpoint. Continuation of amiodarone has recently been associated with a delayed restoration of euthyroidism and a higher chance of recurrence after glucocorticoid withdrawal. Whether amiodarone treatment can be safely reinstituted after restoration of euthyroidism is still unknown. In rare cases of AIT resistance to standard treatments, or when a rapid restoration of euthyroidism is advisable, total thyroidectomy represents a valid alternative. Radioiodine treatment is usually not feasible due to the low thyroidal iodine uptake [4]. Dronedarone was approved in 2009 for the treatment of patients with atrial fibrillation. Like amiodarone, dronedarone is a benzofuran derivative with similar electrophysiologic properties. In contrast to amiodarone, however, dronedarone is structurally devoid of iodine and has a notably shorter half-life. Dronedarone proved to be associated with significantly fewer adverse effects than amiodarone, making it a more attractive choice for patients with atrial fibrillation or flutter, who are at risk of developing amiodarone-induced thyroid dysfunction [88].

Other Supraventricular Arrhythmia

Biondi et al. [46] reported the possibility that thyroid hormones may also induce other kinds of supraventricular arrhythmias not frequently described in hyperthyroid patients, such as reentrant atrioventricular (A-V) nodal tachycardia. This report also showed that reentrant A-V nodal tachycardia may be triggered by thyroid hormone in predisposed subjects. The reentrant A-V nodal tachycardia is a relatively common cause of regular, narrow QRS complex tachycardia, and it is more prevalent in women than in men with a ratio of 7:1 respectively [89]. Epidemiologically, it must be emphasized that both thyroid disease and reentrant A-V nodal tachycardia are highly prevalent in females.

In patients with reentrant A-V nodal tachycardia, at least two functionally distinct A-V nodal conduction patterns are demonstrable [90, 91]. One pathway, referred to as the fast pathway, is characterized by rapid conduction velocity and relatively long refractoriness. The second or slow pathway typically shows slow conduction velocity and short refractoriness. During sinus rhythm, the electric impulse is expected to reach the His bundle and the ventricle preferentially over the faster-conducting pathway with the frequent evidence of a short P-R interval. A-V nodal reentry of the common type (slow-fast) is typically initiated by an atrial premature beat that conducts down only through the slow pathway because of functional block of the fast pathway, and reenters back through the fast pathway because of recovery of its excitability. Conceivably, thyroid hormones might increase the occurrence of reentrant A-V nodal tachycardia in predisposed subjects because of the enhancement of atrial excitability, with consequent increase of the number of atrial premature beats and the shortening of the refractory period of the conducting tissues. Thus, reentrant A-V nodal tachycardia might be triggered in patients in whom L-T4 is exogenously administered to lower TSH [46].

Abbasoglu et al. [92] reported a case of Neonatal thyrotoxicosis with concurrent supraventricular tachycardia caused by the transplacental passage of thyroid stimulating immunoglobulins from mothers with Graves' disease. The heart rate was between 260 and 300 beats/min. Matthew et al. [93] described a case of 43 year old woman who presented in supraventricular tachycardia and acute pulmonary edema and died without any evident cause of mortality. At autopsy the significant positive macroscopic findings were confined to the lungs (acute pulmonary edema) and thyroid (diffusely enlarged). Histology revealed features typical of Graves' disease while post mortem thyroid function tests supported a diagnosis of thyrotoxic crisis in the setting of undiagnosed Graves' disease.

Ventricular Arrhythmia

In contrast to high incidence of atrial arrhythmias in the hyperthyroid status, the ventricular arrhythmias are uncommon and found with a frequency similar to that in the normal population [3, 6, 89, 90]. It is likely because VF is exceptional in those with elevated TH without cardiomyopathy [41, 94, 95]. Thus, the occurrence of ventricular arrhythmias in thyrotoxic subjects during and after antithyroid therapy is rare [3, 6]. However, VF may occur in those with associated heart disease or heart failure of various etiology [5, 26].

Hyperthyroidism

Ventricular tachycardia (VT) is one of the major causes of death in patients with structural heart disease. Electrical storm (ES) is defined as hemodynamically significant VT occurring at least three times over a 24-h period and requiring delivery of direct current shocks [96]. Determining the etiology of extrastimulus ES is quite challenging and requires detailed evaluation of the patient. The etiology of ES varies and includes enhanced sympathetic tone, myocardial ischemia, electrolyte imbalance, endocrine disorders (pheochromocytoma, thyrotoxycosis, etc.), genetic abnormalities (Brugada syndrome, long-QT syndrome, arrhythmogenic right ventricular dysplasia, etc.). Tachycardia during ES might be monomorphic or polymorphic. Polymorphic ES without QT prolongation is frequently associated with myocardial ischemia [97].

Subclinical Hyperthyroidism

Subclinical hyperthyroidism exerts many significant effects on the cardiovascular system; it is usually associated with a higher heart rate and a higher risk of supraventricular arrhythmias, and with an increased left ventricular mass, often accompanied by an impaired diastolic function and sometimes by a reduced systolic performance on effort and decreased exercise tolerance. It is well known that these abnormalities usually precede the onset of a more severe cardiovascular disease, thus potentially contributing to the increased cardiovascular morbidity and mortality observed in these patients [98]. To our knowledge, the literature has not reported ventricular arrhythmias caused by subclinical hyperthyroidism.

Hypothyroidism

It is well known that an excess or deficit of thyroid hormones affects the cardiovascular system. A typical ECG in hypothyroidism shows bradycardia, a low voltage of the QRS complexes, elongation of the QT and flattening or inverting of the T waves. However, less well known is the fact that hypothyroidism may be the cause of atrioventricular blocks and of acquired long QT syndrome (LQTS). Only few publications reported life-threatening by possibility of torsade de pointes (TdP) type tachycardia and ventricular fibrillation occurring in patients with prolonged QT syndrome in the course of hypothyroidism [99].

Profound hypothyroidism and decreased expression of tri-iodothyronine in the heart cells may cause a worsening of cardiac contractility, a decreasing heart rate and a slowing down of the conduction of electrical stimuli in the heart muscle. This may be the reason for bradycardia and elongation of the QT interval and, in consequence, life-threatening arrhythmias may occur, for example TdP-type tachycardia. Decreased triiodothyronine expression and electrolyte disorders such as moderate hypokalaemia and hypocalcaemia probably prompted LQTS and shock in this case [99]. It is important to note that amiodarone was not sufficiently effective to prevent recurrent ventricular arrhythmias. Few publications reported that lidocaine or bretylium tosylate may interrupt this kind of paroxysmal tachycardia and endocavitary electrode stimulation [62].

Hypothyroidism may be the cause of life-threatening arrhythmias secondary to acquired long QT syndrome. Ventricular electrostimulation was a life-saving procedure in this case of prolonged QT syndrome. The use of temporary ventricular electrostimulation protected the patient against dangerous ventricular arrhythmias, while balancing the deficiency of thyroid hormones and electrolytes [31].

Subclinical Hypothyroidism

Subclinical hypothyroidism is a common disorder characterized by elevated serum thyroid-stimulating hormone, normal free thyroxine and free triiodothyronine levels. Its prevalence reportedly ranges between 1.3 and 17.5 %, depending on age, gender and the amount of iodine exposure [100]. Bakiner et al. detected prolonged QT intervals and increased QTc among their subclinical hypothyroid cases. The prolongation remained significant for the whole group, as well as within the subgroups. There was a positive correlation between TSH levels and QTc. Return of serum TSH levels from 110 mIU/l to values within the reference range resulted in normalization of QTc. Such an outcome for patients with TSH between 5 and 10 mIU/l remains to be investigated [101]. TSH concentration has a role in ventricular inhomogeneity and, therefore, subclinical hypothyroidism may predispose to ventricular arrhythmias [60].

Conclusion

Thyroid hormones may trigger arrhythmias mostly at the level of the atria. The incidence of cardiac arrhythmias is in relation to the altered thyroid status. It appears that hypothyroidism is mostly associated with reduced probability of cardiac arrhythmias unlike hyperthyroidism that increases a risk notably for atrial and to a lesser extent ventricular arrhythmias that occur particularly in a cardiomyopathic heart. The long-term arrhythmia depends of the precocity of thyroid disease treatment and cardiomyopathic heart.

References

1. Sawin CT, Geller A, Wolf PA, Belanger AJ, Baker E, Bacharach P, et al. Low serum thyrotropin concentrations as a risk factor for atrial fibrillation in older persons. N Engl J Med. 1994;331(19):1249–52.
2. Golf S, Løvstad R, Hansson V. Beta-adrenoceptor density and relative number of beta-adrenoceptor subtypes in biopsies from human right atrial, left ventricular, and right ventricular myocard. Cardiovasc Res. 1985;19(10):636–41.
3. Von Olshausen K, Bischoff S, Kahaly G, Mohr-Kahaly S, Erbel R, Beyer J, et al. Cardiac arrhythmias and heart rate in hyperthyroidism. Am J Cardiol. 1989;63(13):930–3.
4. Roffi M, Cattaneo F, Brandle M. Thyrotoxicosis and the cardiovascular system. Minerva Endocrinol. 2005;30(2):47–58.
5. Polikar R, Burger AG, Scherrer U, Nicod P. The thyroid and the heart. Circulation. 1993;87(5):1435–41.
6. Osman F, Gammage MD, Sheppard MC, Franklyn JA. Clinical review 142: cardiac dysrhythmias and thyroid dysfunction: the hidden menace? J Clin Endocrinol Metab. 2002;87(3):963–7.
7. Glass CK, Holloway JM. Regulation of gene expression by the thyroid hormone receptor. Biochim Biophys Acta. 1990;1032(2–3):157–76.
8. Brent GA. The molecular basis of thyroid hormone action. N Engl J Med. 1994;331(13):847–53.
9. Woeber KA. Thyrotoxicosis and the heart. N Engl J Med. 1992;327(2):94–8.
10. Dillmann WH. Biochemical basis of thyroid hormone action in the heart. Am J Med. 1990;88(6):626–30.
11. Klein I, Ojamaa K, Samarel AM, Welikson R, Hong C. Hemodynamic regulation of myosin heavy chain gene expression. Studies in the transplanted rat heart. J Clin Invest. 1992;89(1):68–73.
12. Danzi S, Klein S, Klein I. Differential regulation of the myosin heavy chain genes alpha and beta in rat atria and ventricles: role of antisense RNA. Thyroid Off J Am Thyroid Assoc. 2008;18(7):761–8.
13. Ojamaa K, Kenessey A, Klein I. Thyroid hormone regulation of phospholamban phosphorylation in the rat heart. Endocrinology. 2000;141(6):2139–44.
14. Liu B, Huang F, Gick G. Regulation of Na, K-ATPase beta 1 mRNA content by thyroid hormone in neonatal rat cardiac myocytes. Cell Mol Biol Res. 1993;39(3):221–9.
15. Ojamaa K, Sabet A, Kenessey A, Shenoy R, Klein I. Regulation of rat cardiac Kv1.5 gene expression by thyroid hormone is rapid and chamber specific. Endocrinology. 1999;140(7):3170–6.
16. Davis PJ, Davis FB, Lin H-Y, Mousa SA, Zhou M, Luidens MK. Translational implications of nongenomic actions of thyroid hormone initiated at its integrin receptor. Am J Physiol Endocrinol Metab. 2009;297(6):E1238–46.

17. Bonow RO, Mann DL, Zipes DP, Libby P. Braunwald's heart disease: a textbook of cardiovascular medicine. Philadelphia: Elsevier Health Sciences; 2011. 11033 p.
18. Sun ZQ, Ojamaa K, Nakamura TY, Artman M, Klein I, Coetzee WA. Thyroid hormone increases pacemaker activity in rat neonatal atrial myocytes. J Mol Cell Cardiol. 2001;33(4):811–24.
19. Hagiwara N, Irisawa H, Kasanuki H, Hosoda S. Background current in sino-atrial node cells of the rabbit heart. J Physiol. 1992;448:53–72.
20. Hagiwara N, Irisawa H, Kameyama M. Contribution of two types of calcium currents to the pacemaker potentials of rabbit sino-atrial node cells. J Physiol. 1988;395:233–53.
21. Kodama I, Boyett MR, Nikmaram MR, Yamamoto M, Honjo H, Niwa R. Regional differences in effects of E-4031 within the sinoatrial node. Am J Physiol. 1999;276(3 Pt 2):H793–802.
22. Hüser J, Blatter LA, Lipsius SL. Intracellular Ca2+ release contributes to automaticity in cat atrial pacemaker cells. J Physiol. 2000;524(Pt 2):415–22.
23. Kiehn J, Karle C, Thomas D, Yao X, Brachmann J, Kübler W. HERG potassium channel activation is shifted by phorbol esters via protein kinase A-dependent pathways. J Biol Chem. 1998;273(39): 25285–91.
24. Johnson PN, Freedberg AS, Marshall JM. Action of thyroid hormone on the transmembrane potentials from sinoatrial node cells and atrial muscle cells in isolated atria of rabbits. Cardiology. 1973;58(5): 273–89.
25. Sakaguchi Y, Cui G, Sen L. Acute effects of thyroid hormone on inward rectifier potassium channel currents in guinea pig ventricular myocytes. Endocrinology. 1996;137(11):4744–51.
26. Apkon M, Nerbonne JM. Characterization of two distinct depolarization-activated K+ currents in isolated adult rat ventricular myocytes. J Gen Physiol. 1991;97(5):973–1011.
27. Sun ZQ, Ojamaa K, Coetzee WA, Artman M, Klein I. Effects of thyroid hormone on action potential and repolarizing currents in rat ventricular myocytes. Am J Physiol Endocrinol Metab. 2000;278(2): E302–7.
28. Levey GS, Klein I. Catecholamine-thyroid hormone interactions and the cardiovascular manifestations of hyperthyroidism. Am J Med. 1990;88(6):642–6.
29. Williams LT, Lefkowitz RJ, Watanabe AM, Hathaway DR, Besch Jr HR. Thyroid hormone regulation of beta-adrenergic receptor number. J Biol Chem. 1977;252(8):2787–9.
30. Morkin E, Flink IL, Goldman S. Biochemical and physiologic effects of thyroid hormone on cardiac performance. Prog Cardiovasc Dis. 1983;25(5): 435–64.
31. Hoit BD, Khoury SF, Shao Y, Gabel M, Liggett SB, Walsh RA. Effects of thyroid hormone on cardiac beta-adrenergic responsiveness in conscious baboons. Circulation. 1997;96(2):592–8.
32. Jayaprasad N, Francis J. Atrial fibrillation and hyperthyroidism. Indian Pacing Electr J. 2005; 5(4):305–11.
33. Ojamaa K, Klein I, Sabet A, Steinberg SF. Changes in adenylyl cyclase isoforms as a mechanism for thyroid hormone modulation of cardiac beta-adrenergic receptor responsiveness. Metabolism. 2000;49(2):275–9.
34. Farre J. Philippe Coumel: a founding father of modern arrhythmology. Europace. 2004;6(5):464–5.
35. Freedberg AS, Papp JG, Williams EM. The effect of altered thyroid state on atrial intracellular potentials. J Physiol. 1970;207(2):357–69.
36. Chen Y-C, Chen S-A, Chen Y-J, Chang M-S, Chan P, Lin C-I. Effects of thyroid hormone on the arrhythmogenic activity of pulmonary vein cardiomyocytes. J Am Coll Cardiol. 2002;39(2):366–72.
37. Rubinstein I, Binah O. Thyroid hormone modulates membrane currents in guinea-pig ventricular myocytes. Naunyn Schmiedebergs Arch Pharmacol. 1989;340(6):705–11.
38. Haïssaguerre M, Jaïs P, Shah DC, Takahashi A, Hocini M, Quiniou G, et al. Spontaneous initiation of atrial fibrillation by ectopic beats originating in the pulmonary veins. N Engl J Med. 1998;339(10): 659–66.
39. Chen YJ, Chen SA, Chen YC, Yeh HI, Chan P, Chang MS, et al. Effects of rapid atrial pacing on the arrhythmogenic activity of single cardiomyocytes from pulmonary veins: implication in initiation of atrial fibrillation. Circulation. 2001;104(23):2849–54.
40. Komiya N, Isomoto S, Nakao K, Hayano M, Yano K. Electrophysiological abnormalities of the atrial muscle in patients with paroxysmal atrial fibrillation associated with hyperthyroidism. Clin Endocrinol (Oxf). 2002;56(1):39–44.
41. Jao YTFN, Chen Y, Lee W-H, Tai F-T. Thyroid storm and ventricular tachycardia. South Med J. 2004;97(6):604–7.
42. Boccalandro C, López-Penabad L, Boccalandro F, Lavis V. Ventricular fibrillation in a young Asian man. Lancet. 2003;361(9367):1432.
43. Fisher J. Thyrotoxic periodic paralysis with ventricular fibrillation. Arch Intern Med. 1982;142(7): 1362–4.
44. Muñoz-Camacho JF, Sagristá-Sauleda J. Malignant ventricular arrhythmias as the initial manifestation of hyperthyroidism. Rev Esp Cardiol Engl Ed. 2007;60(4):449–50.
45. Wei JY, Genecin A, Greene HL, Achuff SC. Coronary spasm with ventricular fibrillation during thyrotoxicosis: response to attaining euthyroid state. Am J Cardiol. 1979;43(2):335–9.
46. Biondi B, Fazio S, Coltorti F, Palmieri EA, Carella C, Lombardi G, et al. Clinical case seminar: reentrant atrioventricular nodal tachycardia induced by levothyroxine. J Clin Endocrinol Metab. 1998;83(8):2643–5.
47. Gross G, Lues I. Thyroid-dependent alterations of myocardial adrenoceptors and adrenoceptor-mediated responses in the rat. Naunyn Schmiedebergs Arch Pharmacol. 1985;329(4):427–39.

48. Jaeger JM, Houser SR, Freeman AR, Spann Jr JF. Effect of thyroid hormone on canine cardiac Purkinje fiber transmembrane potential. Am J Physiol. 1981;240(6):H934–40.
49. Qu Z, Weiss JN. Dynamics and cardiac arrhythmias. J Cardiovasc Electrophysiol. 2006;17(9):1042–9.
50. Meo SD, de Martino RP, Piro MC, De Leo T. Electrophysiological properties of the hyperthyroid rat heart. Arch Int Physiol Biochim Biophys. 1994;102(2):153–9.
51. Buscemi S, Verga S, Cottone S, Andronico G, D'Orio L, Mannino V, et al. Favorable clinical heart and bone effects of anti-thyroid drug therapy in endogenous subclinical hyperthyroidism. J Endocrinol Invest. 2007;30(3):230–5.
52. Polikar R, Goy JJ, Schlapfer J, Lemarchand-Beraud T, Biollaz J, Magnenat P, et al. Effect of oral triiodothyronine during amiodarone treatment for ventricular premature complexes. Am J Cardiol. 1986; 58(10):987–91.
53. Tribulova N, Knezl V, Shainberg A, Seki S, Soukup T. Thyroid hormones and cardiac arrhythmias. Vascul Pharmacol. 2010;52(3–4):102–12.
54. Surawicz B, Mangiardi ML. Electrocardiogram in endocrine and metabolic disorders. Cardiovasc Clin. 1977;8(3):243–66.
55. Nademanee K, Singh BN, Hendrickson JA, Reed AW, Melmed S, Hershman J. Pharmacokinetic significance of serum reverse T3 levels during amiodarone treatment: a potential method for monitoring chronic drug therapy. Circulation. 1982;66(1): 202–11.
56. Polikar R, Feld GK, Dittrich HC, Smith J, Nicod P. Effect of thyroid replacement therapy on the frequency of benign atrial and ventricular arrhythmias. J Am Coll Cardiol. 1989;14(4):999–1002.
57. Di Meo S, Venditti P, De Leo T. Effect of iodothyronines on electrophysiological properties of rat papillary muscle fibres. Horm Metab Res. 1997;29(5): 225–30.
58. Schenck JB, Rizvi AA, Lin T. Severe primary hypothyroidism manifesting with torsades de pointes. Am J Med Sci. 2006;331(3):154–6.
59. Fredlund BO, Olsson SB. Long QT interval and ventricular tachycardia of « torsade de pointe » type in hypothyroidism. Acta Med Scand. 1983;213(3):231–5.
60. Unal O, Erturk E, Ozkan H, Kiyici S, Guclu M, Ersoy C, et al. Effect of levothyroxine treatment on QT dispersion in patients with subclinical hypothyroidism. Endocr Pract Off J Am Coll Endocrinol Am Assoc Clin Endocrinol. 2007;13(7):711–5.
61. LEE JK, LEWIS JA. Myxoedema with complete A-V block and Adams-Stokes disease abolished with thyroid medication. Br Heart J. 1962;24: 253–6.
62. Chess-Williams R, Coker SJ. Ventricular fibrillation is reduced in hypothyroid rats with enhanced myocardial alpha-adrenoceptor responsiveness. Br J Pharmacol. 1989;98(1):95–100.
63. Friberg L, Werner S, Eggertsen G, Ahnve S. Rapid down-regulation of thyroid hormones in acute myocardial infarction: is it cardioprotective in patients with angina? Arch Intern Med. 2002;162(12):1388–94.
64. Epstein FH, Klein I, Ojamaa K. Thyroid hormone and the cardiovascular system. N Engl J Med. 2001;344(7):501–9.
65. Frost L, Vestergaard P, Mosekilde L. Hyperthyroidism and risk of atrial fibrillation or flutter: a population-based study. Arch Intern Med. 2004;164(15): 1675–8.
66. Frost L, Vestergaard P. Alcohol and risk of atrial fibrillation or flutter: a cohort study. Arch Intern Med. 2004;164(18):1993–8.
67. Frost L, Vestergaard P, Mosekilde L, Mortensen LS. Trends in incidence and mortality in the hospital diagnosis of atrial fibrillation or flutter in Denmark, 1980–1999. Int J Cardiol. 2005;103(1):78–84.
68. Tunbridge WM, Evered DC, Hall R, Appleton D, Brewis M, Clark F, et al. The spectrum of thyroid disease in a community: the Whickham survey. Clin Endocrinol (Oxf). 1977;7(6):481–93.
69. Klein I, Danzi S. Thyroid disease and the heart. Circulation. 2007;116(15):1725–35.
70. Nakazawa H, Lythall DA, Noh J, Ishikawa N, Sugino K, Ito K, et al. Is there a place for the late cardioversion of atrial fibrillation? A long-term follow-up study of patients with post-thyrotoxic atrial fibrillation. Eur Heart J. 2000;21(4):327–33.
71. Zhou Z-H, Ma L-L, Wang L-X. Risk factors for persistent atrial fibrillation following successful hyperthyroidism treatment with radioiodine therapy. Intern Med Tokyo Jpn. 2011;50(24):2947–51.
72. Xiao P, Gao C, Fan J, Du H, Long Y, Yin Y. Blockade of angiotensin II improves hyperthyroid induced abnormal atrial electrophysiological properties. Regul Pept. 2011;169(1–3):31–8.
73. Shimizu T, Koide S, Noh JY, Sugino K, Ito K, Nakazawa H. Hyperthyroidism and the management of atrial fibrillation. Thyroid Off J Am Thyroid Assoc. 2002;12(6):489–93.
74. Kunii Y, Uruno T, Matsumoto M, Mukasa K, Noh J, Ito K, et al. Pharmacological conversion of atrial fibrillation in the patients of Graves' disease. Tokai J Exp Clin Med. 2012;37(4):107–12.
75. Bagchi N, Brown TR, Parish RF. Thyroid dysfunction in adults over age 55 years. A study in an urban US community. Arch Intern Med. 1990;150(4): 785–7.
76. Ozturk S, Dikbas O, Baltacı D, Ozyasar M, Erdem A, Ayhan SS, et al. Evaulation of atrial conduction abnormalities and left atrial mechanical functions in patients with subclinical thyroid disorders. Endokrynol Pol. 2012;63(4):286–93.
77. Sawin CT. Subclinical hypothyroidism in older persons. Clin Geriatr Med. 1995;11(2):231–8.
78. Klemperer JD, Klein IL, Ojamaa K, Helm RE, Gomez M, Isom OW, et al. Triiodothyronine therapy lowers the incidence of atrial fibrillation after cardiac operations. Ann Thorac Surg. 1996;61(5):1323–7.

79. Kim E-J, Lyass A, Wang N, Massaro JM, Fox CS, Benjamin EJ, et al. Relation of hypothyroidism and incident atrial fibrillation (from the Framingham Heart Study). Am Heart J. 2014;167(1):123–6.
80. Cappola AR, Arnold AM, Wulczyn K, Carlson M, Robbins J, Psaty BM. Thyroid function in the euthyroid range and adverse outcomes in older adults. J Clin Endocrinol Metab. 2015;100(3):1088–96.
81. Petersen P, Hansen JM. Stroke in thyrotoxicosis with atrial fibrillation. Stroke J Cereb Circ. 1988; 19(1):15–8.
82. Fuster V, Rydén LE, Cannom DS, Crijns HJ, Curtis AB, Ellenbogen KA, et al. 2011 ACCF/AHA/HRS focused updates incorporated into the ACC/AHA/ESC 2006 guidelines for the management of patients with atrial fibrillation: a report of the American College of Cardiology Foundation/American Heart Association Task Force on Practice Guidelines developed in partnership with the European Society of Cardiology and in collaboration with the European Heart Rhythm Association and the Heart Rhythm Society. J Am Coll Cardiol. 2011;57(11):e101–98.
83. Badawi O. Possible effect of thyroid function on anticoagulant response to unfractionated heparin. Pharmacotherapy. 2006;26(2):285–8.
84. Nakazawa HK, Sakurai K, Hamada N, Momotani N, Ito K. Management of atrial fibrillation in the post-thyrotoxic state. Am J Med. 1982;72(6):903–6.
85. Singh BN. Amiodarone as paradigm for developing new drugs for atrial fibrillation. J Cardiovasc Pharmacol. 2008;52(4):300–5.
86. Narayana SK, Woods DR, Boos CJ. Management of amiodarone-related thyroid problems. Ther Adv Endocrinol Metab. 2011;2(3):115–26.
87. Bogazzi F, Tomisti L, Bartalena L, Aghini-Lombardi F, Martino E. Amiodarone and the thyroid: a 2012 update. J Endocrinol Invest. 2012;35(3):340–8.
88. Cohen-Lehman J, Dahl P, Danzi S, Klein I. Effects of amiodarone therapy on thyroid function. Nat Rev Endocrinol. 2010;6(1):34–41.
89. Ganz LI, Friedman PL. Supraventricular tachycardia. N Engl J Med. 1995;332(3):162–73.
90. Denes P, Wu D, Dhingra RC, Chuquimia R, Rosen KM. Demonstration of dual A-V nodal pathways in patients with paroxysmal supraventricular tachycardia. Circulation. 1973;48(3):549–55.
91. Rosen KM, Mehta A, Miller RA. Demonstration of dual atrioventricular nodal pathways in man. Am J Cardiol. 1974;33(2):291–4.
92. Abbasoğlu A, Ecevit A, Tuğcu AU, Erdoğan L, Kınık ST, Tarcan A. Neonatal thyrotoxicosis with severe supraventricular tachycardia: case report and review of the literature. J Pediatr Endocrinol Metab. 2015;28(3–4):463–6.
93. Lynch MJ, Woodford NWF. Sudden unexpected death in the setting of undiagnosed Graves' disease. Forensic Sci Med Pathol. 2014;10(3):452–6.
94. Colzani RM, Emdin M, Conforti F, Passino C, Scarlattini M, Iervasi G. Hyperthyroidism is associated with lengthening of ventricular repolarization. Clin Endocrinol (Oxf). 2001;55(1):27–32.
95. Davison ET, Davison MJ. Triiodothyronine (T3) toxicosis with hypokalemic periodic paralysis and ventricular tachycardia. J Electrocardiol. 1995;28(2): 161–4.
96. Dorian P, Cass D. An overview of the management of electrical storm. Can J Cardiol. 1997;13 (Suppl A):13A–7.
97. Erdogan HI, Gul EE, Gok H, Nikus KC. Therapy-resistant ventricular tachycardia caused by amiodarone-induced thyrotoxicosis: a case report of electrical storm. Am J Emerg Med. 2012;30(9):2092.e5–e7.
98. Biondi B, Palmieri EA, Klain M, Schlumberger M, Filetti S, Lombardi G. Subclinical hyperthyroidism: clinical features and treatment options. Eur J Endocrinol. 2005;152(1):1–9.
99. Chojnowski K, Bielec A, Czarkowski M, Dmowska-Chalaba J, Kochanowski J, Wasowska A. Repeated ventricular. Cardiol J. 2007;14(2):198–201.
100. Samuels MH. Subclinical thyroid disease in the elderly. Thyroid Off J Am Thyroid Assoc. 1998; 8(9):803–13.
101. Bakiner O, Ertorer ME, Haydardedeoglu FE, Bozkirli E, Tutuncu NB, Demirag NG. Subclinical hypothyroidism is characterized by increased QT interval dispersion among women. Med Princ Pract. 2008;17(5):390–4.

Part III

Pregnancy and Thyroid Dysfunction

Pregnancy and Hypothyroidism 17

Aqiba Sarfaraz

Abstract

Pregnancy is a state that causes massive physiological stress on both the mother and the fetus. When pregnancy is associated with endocrine disorders such as hypothyroidism, the risk for maternal and fetal adverse outcomes can be enormous. While a lot of attention has been focused on the adverse fetal outcomes consequent to hypothyroidism, it is being gradually directed towards the adverse maternal outcomes. Timely diagnosis and treatment of thyroid disorders in pregnancy is very important. Subclinical hypothyroidism also needs to be detected and treated to prevent adverse outcomes. Symptoms of SCH may vary from being asymptomatic to having mild nonspecific symptoms. This condition occurs in 3–8 % of the general population. It is more common in women than men, and its prevalence increases with age. In patients with SCH, 80 % have a serum TSH of less than 10 mIU/L. The most important implication of SCH is high likelihood of progression to clinical hypothyroidism during pregnancy and these patients needs thyroxine replacement during pregnancy to reduce adverse fetal outcomes. The risk of progression to overt hypothyroidism is related to a number of factors including initial serum TSH concentration, presence of auto antibodies (anti TPO), family history and presence of goiter. Women who already on thyroxine prior to pregnancy usually need to increase their daily dosage, on an average, by 30–50 % above preconception dosage.

Introduction

Thyroid disease is second only to diabetes mellitus as the most common endocrinopathy that occurs in women during their reproductive years. Symptoms of thyroid disease often mimic common symptoms of pregnancy, making it challenging to identify. Poorly controlled thyroid disease is associated

A. Sarfaraz
Department of Diabetes and Endocrinology, Liaquat National Hospital and Medical College, Karachi, Pakistan
e-mail: draqiba@hotmail.com

S.K. Imam, S.I. Ahmad (eds.), *Thyroid Disorders: Basic Science and Clinical Practice*, DOI 10.1007/978-3-319-25871-3_17

with adverse outcomes during pregnancy, and treatment is an essential part of prenatal care to ensure maternal and fetal well-being.

While a lot of attention has been focused on the adverse fetal outcomes consequent to hypothyroidism, it is being gradually directed towards the adverse maternal outcomes. Subclinical hypothyroidism also needs to be detected and treated to prevent adverse outcomes [1].

Since the treatment of hypothyroidism is easy, timely detection and treatment of the disorder could reduce the burden of adverse fetal and maternal outcomes. Thyroid disease in pregnancy can affect the health of the mother as well as the child before and after delivery. The harmful effects of thyroid dysfunction can also extend beyond pregnancy and delivery to affect neuro-intellectual development in the early life of the child [2].

Thyroid gland influences almost all of the metabolic processes in our body. Thyroid disorders can range from a small and harmless goiter (enlarged gland) that needs no treatment to life-threatening cancer. The most common thyroid problems involve abnormal production of thyroid hormones. Excessive amount of thyroid hormone results in a condition known as hyperthyroidism. Insufficient hormone production leads to hypothyroidism. Although the effects can be unpleasant or uncomfortable, most thyroid problems can be managed well if properly diagnosed and treated. This review will mainly focus on hypothyroidism during pregnancy.

Physiologic Changes in Thyroid Function During Pregnancy

Pregnancy has a profound impact on the thyroid gland and thyroid function. The gland increases 10 % in size during pregnancy in iodine-replete countries and by 20–40 % in areas of iodine deficiency. Production of thyroxine (T_4) and triiodothyronine (T_3) increases by 50 %, along with a 50 % increase in the daily iodine requirement. These physiological changes may result in hypothyroidism in the later stages of pregnancy in iodine-deficient women who were euthyroid in the first trimester. The range of thyrotropin (TSH), under the impact of placental human chorionic gonadotropin (hCG), is decreased throughout pregnancy with the lower normal TSH level in the first trimester being defined as an upper limit of 2.5 mIU/L [3] See Table 17.1.

The most notable change is the increase in thyroxine-binding globulin (TBG). This begins early in the first trimester, plateaus during mid gestation, and persists until shortly after delivery. This is due to stimulation of TBG synthesis by elevated maternal estrogen levels, and more importantly, due to a reduced hepatic clearance of TBG because of estrogen-induced sialylation [4]. This increased TBG concentration leads to an expansion of the extra-thyroidal pool and results in elevated total T3 and T4 levels. T4 metabolism is enhanced in the second and third trimesters, due to a rise in placental type II and type III deiodinases, which convert T4 to T3 and T4 to reverse T3. Plasma iodide levels decrease due to both increased thyroxine metabolism and increased renal iodide clearance [5]. All these changes lead to an increase in the size of the thyroid gland in 15 % of pregnant women, which returns to normal in the post-partum period. Serum hCG has intrinsic thyrotropic activity, which increases after fertilization and peaks at 10–12 weeks. Hence, in the first trimester, free T3 and T4 levels increase slightly and TSH levels decrease in the first trimester with a readjustment in the second and third trimesters, when hCG levels decrease. As a consequence, cut-offs to determine hypothyroidism in pregnancy are different in the first trimester and the rest of the pregnancy. See table [3, 6].

Table 17.1 Trimester-specific reference ranges of thyroid function tests

Test	First trimester	Second trimester	Third trimester
Thyroid stimulating hormone (TSH) miu/l	0.1–2.5	0.2–3.0	0.3–3.0
Total thyroxine (T4) μg/dl	6.5–10.1	7.5–10.3	6.3–9.7
Free thyroxine (FT4) ng/dl	0.8–1.2	0.6–1.0	0.5–0.8
Total triiodothyronine (T3) ng/dl	97–149	117–169	123–162
Free triiodothyronine (FT3) pg/ml	4.1–4.4	4.0–4.2	Not available

Thyroid Function and the Fetus

The fetal thyroid begins concentrating iodine at 10–12 weeks of gestation and is controlled by pituitary TSH by approximately 20 weeks of gestation. Fetal serum levels of TSH, TBG, FT_4, and free triiodothyronine (FT_3) increase throughout gestation, reaching mean adult levels at approximately 36 weeks of gestation [7]. Thyroid stimulating hormone does not cross the placenta, and only small amounts of thyroxine (T_4) and triiodothyronine (T_3) cross the placenta. In neonates with congenital hypothyroidism, enough maternal thyroid hormone crosses the placenta to prevent the overt stigmata of hypothyroidism at birth and maintain cord blood thyroid hormone levels at 25–50 % of normal [8]. However, thyrotropin releasing hormone (TRH), iodine, and TSH receptor immunoglobulins do cross the placenta, as do the thioamides propylthiouracil (PTU) and methimazole.

Subclinical Hypothyroidism During Pregnancy

Subclinical hypothyroidism (SCH) is biochemically diagnosed when there is a persistently high TSH level, while circulating free thyroid hormone levels are within range [9, 10]. Other terms for this condition are mild hypothyroidism, early thyroid failure, preclinical hypothyroidism, and decreased thyroid reserve [11]. Thyroid diseases are one of the most common endocrine disorders and most prevalent in iodine deficient areas. During the first trimester, approximately one in ten pregnant women develop antibodies to TPO or to thyroglobulin, and hypothyroidism develops in roughly 16 % of these women. The prevalence of hypothyroidism in pregnancy is around 2.5 % according to the Western literature [12].

There are a few reports of prevalence of subclinical hypothyroidism during pregnancy from India with prevalence rates ranging from 4.8–11 % [13, 14].

Data on the prevalence of thyroid dysfunction during pregnancy is lacking in Asian-Indian population. There is insufficient evidence to recommend the use of one intervention for clinical or SCH pre pregnancy or during pregnancy over another, for improving maternal, fetal, neonatal and childhood outcomes. Thyroid hormone disturbances have known to have adverse effect in pregnancy outcomes. That is why thyroid function assessment is relevant in reproductive dysfunction [15]. One review of literature revealed that SCH increased the rate of miscarriage/fetal death and later it adversely affects the cognitive development of offspring [16–18].

Though universal screening for thyroid hormone abnormalities in pregnancy is not routinely recommended at present, but thyroid function must be assessed in those having reproductive dysfunction and must be treated appropriately. Although it is evident from current literature that pregnancy outcomes are worse in women with overt hypothyroidism versus SCH. Studies done in individuals with SCH showed an increased risk of preterm birth, miscarriage, severe preeclampsia and impaired cognitive development in children [19].

Thyroid Autoimmunity and Subclinical Hypothyroidism

It has been observed that the autoimmune thyroid disease without overt hypothyroidism is associated with a higher miscarriage rate. One study done by Negro et al showed that euthyroid Caucasian women with positive anti – thyroid peroxidase (anti-TPO) antibodies who were treated with LT4 during the first trimester had lower miscarriage rates than those who were not treated. These women also had lower rates of premature delivery, comparable to rates in women without thyroid antibodies [20].

In a meta-analysis of 3 studies involving 220 women with subclinical hypothyroidism or thyroid autoimmunity who were undergoing assisted reproduction technologies, Velkeniers et al concluded that treatment with LT4 should be recommended to improve pregnancy outcomes [21]. In this meta-analysis, LT4 treatment resulted in a significantly higher delivery rate and a significantly lower miscarriage rate. Such findings, if confirmed by sufficient data, would provide an indication for treating Euthyroid pregnant women who have thyroid antibodies.

Hypothyroidism in Pregnancy

The prevalence of hypothyroidism during pregnancy is estimated to be 0.3–0.5 % for overt hypothyroidism and 2–3 % for subclinical hypothyroidism. Autoimmune thyroiditis is the commonest cause of hypothyroidism during pregnancy [22]. Other causes include radioiodine ablation of thyroid while treating hyperthyroidism or thyroid cancer, surgery of the thyroid tumors and rarely, central hypothyroidism. On the other hand, globally, iodine deficiency still remains one of the leading causes of hypothyroidism, both overt and subclinical [1].

Feto-maternal Risk

Women with hypothyroidism have decreased fertility; even if they conceive, risk of abortion is increased, and risk of gestational hypertension, anemia, abruptio placenta and postpartum hemorrhage is increased [23].

The risk of these complications is greater in women with overt than subclinical hypothyroidism. Untreated maternal hypothyroidism can lead to preterm birth, low birth weight, and respiratory distress in the neonate. Enough evidence has accumulated over the years about the role of thyroxine in normal development of the fetal brain [1]. Various studied proved that children born to mothers with hypothyroidism had a significantly increased risk of impairment in intelligence quotient (IQ) scores, neuropsychological developmental indices and learning abilities. Children born to untreated hypothyroid women had an IQ score that was seven points below the mean IQ of children born to healthy women and women given thyroxine supplements. This risk applies to children born not only of untreated women, but also women with suboptimal supplementation [24].

Adverse outcome of hypothyroidism in pregnancy can be summarized as follows;

- Increased risk of spontaneous abortion
- Preeclampsia
- Low birth weight
- Impaired cognitive development in the fetus
- Fetal mortality
- Postpartum hemorrhage
- Anemia

Screening

Despite the possibility of poor fetal outcomes, routine screening for thyroid dysfunction is not performed in the United States and remains a controversial topic [25–27].The Endocrine Society recommends screening only pregnant women at high risk of thyroid disease using serum TSH measurement [2, 3].

Hypothyroidism commonly manifests as a slowing in physical and mental activity but may be asymptomatic. Symptoms and signs of this disease are often subtle and neither sensitive nor specific. Classic signs and symptoms such as cold intolerance, puffiness, decreased sweating, and coarse skin may not be present as commonly as was once believed. See chap. 17 for clinical manifestation of hypothyroidism.

Diagnosis

Thyroid function tests are the mainstay. Serum TSH elevation indicates primary hypothyroidism. Free thyroxine (FT4) and free triiodothyronine (FT3) levels are estimated, as total hormone levels are elevated due to changes in TBG levels.

Indications for Thyroid Testing in Pregnancy [28]

History of thyroid dysfunction
Family history of autoimmune thyroid disease
High-dose neck radiation
Postpartum thyroid dysfunction
Previous delivery of infant with thyroid disease
Type 1 diabetes mellitus

Treatment

Thyroxine Replacement

Administration of levothyroxine is the treatment of choice for maternal hypothyroidism. Pregnant women need larger doses due to the rapid rise in TBG levels resulting from the physiological rise in estrogen, the increased placental transport and metabolism of maternal T4 and the increased distribution volume of thyroid hormones. During pregnancy, the full replacement thyroxine dose is around 2–2.4 μg/kg/day. In severe hypothyroidism, for the first few days, a thyroxine dose twice the estimated final replacement daily dose may be given, to rapidly normalize the extra thyroidal thyroxine pool before reducing to the final replacement dose. Women who already on thyroxine prior to pregnancy usually need to increase their daily dosage, on an average, by 30–50 % above preconception dosage. Dose of thyroxine also depends on the etiology of hypothyroidism with disorders with very little residual tissue, like radioiodine ablation and extensive thyroid surgery requiring a greater increment in thyroxine dosage than women with Hashimoto's thyroiditis, who usually have some residual thyroid tissue.

LT4 should not be taken with vitamin preparations containing iron and calcium. After delivery, the LT4 dose can be reduced to the prepregnancy level, and TSH should be checked in 6 weeks.

In a study of 77 pregnant women with newly diagnosed subclinical (64 women) or overt (13 women) hypothyroidism, Abalovich et al determined the specific levothyroxine (LT4) dosages required to return these patients to a euthyroid state. The investigators found that the most successful dosages, mentioned below, varied according to baseline levels of thyroid stimulating hormone [29, 30]:

Subclinical hypothyroidism (TSH 4.2 mIU/L or less): 1.2 μg/kg/day
Subclinical hypothyroidism (TSH >4.2–10 mIU/L): 1.42 μg/kg/day
Overt hypothyroidism: 2.33 μg/kg/day

These dosages proved appropriate in 89 % and 77 % of patients with subclinical or overt hypothyroidism, respectively, and were recommended by the study's authors for pregnant patients with hypothyroidism that has been newly diagnosed during pregnancy.

Iodine Replacement

In addition, iodine demands are higher with pregnancy and lactation. Iodine needs rise from approximately 150 μg/day in the nonpregnant woman to 240–290 μg/day with pregnancy and lactation. Guidelines from the American Thyroid Association recommend that all pregnant and lactating women ingest a minimum of 250 mg iodine daily—optimally, in the form of potassium iodide, to ensure consistent delivery [3]. Recently researchers analyzed clinical data to determine the cost of iodine supplementation for pregnant women; they then compared the costs to the money saved from both a health and societal perspective after the heightened IQ that can accompany supplementation. They found that iodine supplementation could result in a net gain of 1.22 IQ points, saving about $308 per pregnant woman in health costs and $6,925 in societal costs [31, 32].

Monitoring Thyroid Status During Pregnancy

For pregnant women with previously diagnosed hypothyroidism, serum TSH levels should be measured every 3–4 weeks during the first half of pregnancy and every 6–10 weeks thereafter. The dose of thyroxine should be adjusted so as to keep the serum TSH below 2.5 mIU/L. TSH and free T4 levels should be measured 3–4 weeks after every dosage adjustment [12].

Serum free T4 and TSH levels should be measured 1 month after the initiation of treatment. The thyroxine dose should be titrated to reach a serum TSH value less than 2.5 mIU/l, while maintaining free T4 levels in the high normal range. Women should be followed up every

4–6 weeks with free T4 and TSH value, till delivery, to facilitate periodic adjustment of LT4 supplementation. If hypothyroidism has not been diagnosed until the end of the first trimester, offspring may display impairment in final intellectual and cognitive abilities, thus underscoring the importance of early diagnosis and treatment.

Prognosis

- Prognosis for mother and fetus is excellent with appropriate treatment.
- However, there is a small increase in stillbirth rate and fetal assessment in the third trimester is necessary.
- Recent research has suggested an increased risk of neurocognitive difficulties in children of women with hypothyroidism, even with a euthyroid fetus, as maternal thyroid hormone is needed for neuronal development until 12–13 weeks.

Preconception Counseling

Women with hypothyroidism should be counseled about the importance of achieving euthyroidism before conception because of the risk of decreased fertility and miscarriage. They must also understand the importance of immediate monitoring at the onset of pregnancy, because by the first prenatal visit, many of these patients will already have an elevated TSH level consistent with uncontrolled hypothyroidism. Euthyroid women who are taking a stable dosage of levothyroxine should be counseled to notify their physician and independently increase their medication by two additional doses per week after a missed menstrual cycle or positive home pregnancy test. In a study of 48 women treated for hypothyroidism with a normal prepregnancy serum TSH level, increasing levothyroxine by two doses per week prevented maternal TSH elevation above 2.5 mIU/L and above 5 mIU/L in 85–100 % of patients, respectively, with only two patients requiring a subsequent dose reduction [33].

Summary of Recommendations

1. Evidence is insufficient to recommend for or against routine screening for antithyroid antibodies among women with miscarriage, or universal TSH screening in the first trimester. However, screening for FT_4 level is not recommended.
2. In the first trimester, normal range for TSH level is 0.1–2.5 mIU/L; this level increases to 0.2–3.0 mIU/L in the second trimester and 0.3–3.0 mIU/L in the third trimester.
3. Oral levothyroxine is indicated for women with overt hypothyroidism, which is associated with greater risks for fetal loss and premature birth, and for those with subclinical hypothyroidism who test positive for TPO antibodies.
4. Women who are already receiving thyroid replacement therapy should increase their dose by 25–30 % when they become pregnant.
5. Women with subclinical hypothyroidism in pregnancy who are not initially treated should be monitored for progression to overt hypothyroidism. Serum thyroid-stimulating hormone (TSH) and free thyroxine (FT_4) levels should be measured approximately every 4 weeks until 16–20 weeks' gestation and at least once between 26 and 32 weeks' gestation.
6. During pregnancy and lactation, the minimal suggested daily recommended allowance for iodine is 250 μg. The risk for fetal hypothyroidism may increase when total daily iodine intake from diet and/or supplements is or exceeds 500 μg.
7. Pregnant women should not undergo radioactive iodine thyroid scanning, but fine-needle aspiration of thyroid nodules may be performed if indicated.

Conclusion

Thyroid disease is one of the most common endocrine disorders affecting women of reproductive age, and when untreated during pregnancy is associated with an increased risk of miscarriage, placental abruption, hypertensive disorders, and growth restriction. Women with autoimmune thyroid dysfunction who are euthyroid in early pregnancy also carry a significant risk of developing hypothyroidism progressively during gestation, despite a marked reduction in antibody titers. Hypothyroidism results from the reduced ability of the gland to adjust to the changes in thyroid physiology associated with pregnancy. At the individual level, progression to subclinical hypothyroidism was broadly predictable on the basis of serum TSH levels and TPO-Ab titers in the first trimester. Hence, these parameters provide useful markers to identify women who carry a higher risk, allowing for a close monitoring of thyroid function during pregnancy and the administration of L-T4 in specific cases. Current guidelines recommend targeted screening of women at high risk, including those with a history of thyroid disease, type 1 diabetes mellitus, or other autoimmune disease. In women with hypothyroidism, levothyroxine is titrated to achieve a goal serum thyroid-stimulating hormone level less than 2.5 mIU/L. The corner stone treatment for hyporthyroidism is the thyroxine replacement, with a goal of maintaining a trimester specific serum TSH level. Appropriate management results in improved outcomes, demonstrating the importance of proper diagnosis and treatment.

References

1. Sahay RK, Nagesh VS. Hypothyroidism in pregnancy. Indian J Endocrinol Metab. 2012;16(3):364–70.
2. Okosieme OE, Marx H, Lazarus JH. Medical management of thyroid dysfunction in pregnancy and the postpartum. Expert Opin Pharmacother. 2008;9(13):2281–93.
3. Stagnaro-Green A, Abalovich M, Alexander E, et al. American Thyroid Association Taskforce on Thyroid Disease During Pregnancy and Postpartum. Guidelines of the American Thyroid Association for the diagnosis and management of thyroid disease during pregnancy and postpartum. Thyroid. 2011;21(10):1081–125.
4. Ain KB, Mori Y, Refetoff S. Reduced clearance rate of thyroxine-binding globulin (TGB) with increased sialylation: a mechanism for estrogen-induced elevation of serum TBG concentration. J Clin Endocrinol Metab. 1987;65:689–702.
5. Soldin OP, Tractenberg RE, Hollowell JG, et al. Trimester-specific changes in maternal thyroid hormone, thyrotropin, and thyroglobulin concentrations during gestation: trends and associations across trimesters in iodine sufficiency. Thyroid. 2004;14:1084–90.
6. Abbassi-Ghanavati M, Greer LG, Cunningham FG. Pregnancy and laboratory studies: a reference table for clinicians. Obstet Gynecol. 2010;15(2 pt 1):387; Obstet Gynecol. 2009;114(6):1326–31.
7. Thorpe-Beeston JG, Nicolaides KH, Felton CV, et al. Maturation of the secretion of thyroid hormone and thyroid-stimulating hormone in the fetus. N Engl J Med. 1991;324:532–6.
8. Utiger RD. Maternal hypothyroidism and fetal development [letter]. N Engl J Med. 1999;341:601–2.
9. Biondi B, Cooper DS. The clinical significance of subclinical thyroid dysfunction. Endocr Rev. 2008; 29:76–131.
10. Cooper DS, Biondi B. Subclinical thyroid disease. Lancet. 2012;379:1142–54.
11. Cooper DS. Subclinical hypothyroidism. N Engl J Med. 2001;345:260–5.
12. LeBeau SO, Mandel SJ. Thyroid disorders during pregnancy. Endocrinol Metab Clin North Am. 2006;35:117–36.
13. Nambiar V, Jagtap VS, Sarathi V, et al. Prevalence and impact of thyroid disorders on maternal outcome in Asian-Indian pregnant women. J Thyroid Res. 2011;2011:429097.
14. Sahu MT, Das V, Mittal S, Agarwal A, Sahu M. Overt and subclinical thyroid dysfunction among Indian pregnant women and its effect on maternal and fetal outcome. Arch Gynecol Obstet. 2010;281:215–20.
15. Sarkar D. Recurrent pregnancy loss in patients with thyroid dysfunction. Indian J Endocrinol Metab. 2012;16 Suppl 2:S350–1.
16. Haddow JE, Palomaki GE, Allan WC, et al. Maternal thyroid deficiency during pregnancy and subsequent neuropsychological development of the child. N Engl J Med. 1999;341(8):549–55.
17. Casey BM, Dashe JS, Wells CE, et al. Subclinical hypothyroidism and pregnancy outcomes. Obstet Gynecol. 2005;105:239–45.
18. Glinoer D, Soto MF, Bourdoux P, et al. Pregnancy in patients with mild thyroid abnormalities: maternal and neonatal repercussions. J Clin Endocrinol Metab. 1991;73:421–7.
19. Li Y, Shan Z, Teng W, Yu X, Li Y, Fan C, et al. Abnormalities of maternal thyroid function during pregnancy affect neuropsychological development of

their children at 25–30 months. Clin Endocrinol (Oxf). 2010;72:825–9.
20. Negro R, Formoso G, Mangieri T, et al. Levothyroxine treatment in euthyroid pregnant women with autoimmune thyroid disease: effects on obstetrical complications. J Clin Endocrinol Metab. 2006;91(7):2587–91.
21. Velkeniers B, Van Meerhaeghe A, Poppe K, et al. Levothyroxine treatment and pregnancy outcome in women with subclinical hypothyroidism undergoing assisted reproduction technologies: systematic review and meta-analysis of RCTs. Hum Reprod Update. 2013;19(3):251–8.
22. Klein RZ, Haddow JE, Faix JD, Brown RS, Hermos RJ, Pulkkinen A, et al. Prevalence of thyroid deficiency in pregnant women. Clin Endocrinol (Oxf). 1991;35:41–6.
23. Abalovich M, Gutierrez S, Alcaraz G, Maccallini G, Garcia A, Levalle O. Overt and subclinical hypothyroidism complicating pregnancy. Thyroid. 2002;12:63–6.
24. Rovet JF. Neurodevelopmental consequences of maternal hypothyroidism during pregnancy (abstract 88;annual meeting of the American Thyroid Association). Thyroid. 2004;14:710.
25. Blat AJ, Nakamoto JM, Kaufman HW. National status of testing for hypothyroidism during pregnancy and postpartum. J Clin Endocrinol Metab. 2012;97(3):777–84.
26. Allan WC, Haddow JE, Palomaki GE, et al. Maternal thyroid deficiency and pregnancy complications: implications for population screening. J Med Screen. 2000;7:127–30.
27. Vaidya B, Anthony S, Bilous M, et al. Detection of thyroid dysfunction in early pregnancy: universal screening or targeted high-risk case finding? J Clin Endocrinol Metab. 2007;92:203–7.
28. De Groot L, Abalovich M, Alexander EK, et al. Management of thyroid dysfunction during pregnancy and postpartum: an endocrine society clinical practice guideline. J Clin Endocrinol Metab. 2012;97(8):2543–65.
29. Beverly MS, Bridget AK, Anita VH, et al. Five-Year follow-up for women with subclinical hypothyroidism in pregnancy. J Clin Endocrinol Metab 2013;98:E1941–E1945.
30. Abalovich M, Vazquez A, Alcaraz G, et al. Adequate levothyroxine doses for the treatment of hypothyroidism newly discovered during pregnancy. Thyroid. 2013;23(11):1479–83.
31. Monahan M, et al. Costs and benefits of iodine supplementation for pregnant women in a mildly to moderately iodine-deficient population: a modelling analysis. Lancet Diabetes Endocrinol. 2015;3:715–22. doi:10.1016/S2213-8587(15)00212-0.
32. Pearce E. Iodine deficiency in pregnant women in the UK: the costs of inaction. Lancet Diabetes Endocrinol. 2015;3:671–2. doi:10.1016/S2213-8587(15)00228-4.
33. Yassa L, Marqusee E, Fawcett R, Alexander EK. Thyroid hormone early adjustment in pregnancy (the THERAPY) trial. J Clin Endocrinol Metab. 2010;95(7):3234–41.

Pregnancy and Hyperthyroidism

18

Aisha Sheikh

Abstract

Hyperthyroidism during pregnancy is coupled with diagnostic and treatment dilemmas since there are several causes of hyperthyroidism during pregnancy including Gestational Transient Thyrotoxicosis (GTT) which is a self- limiting condition. The symptoms of pregnancy mimic that of hyperthyroidism, thus cannot be entirely relied upon. The lack of consensus on the lower limit of Thyroid Stimulating Hormone (TSH) during pregnancy and lack of universal availability of trimester-specific reference ranges for thyroid function tests in most of laboratories; add more to diagnostic confusion. Any unnecessary treatment with anti-thyroid drugs can lead to adverse effects on the fetus, same is true for uncontrolled hyperthyroidism. All this calls for vigilance in diagnosing and managing pregnancy complicated by hyperthyroidism.

Introduction

The prevalence of Hyperthyroidism in pregnancy ranges from 0.1 to 0.4 % [1, 2]. Untreated hyperthyroidism during pregnancy can compromise fetal growth [2, 3]. There are several causes of Hyperthyroidism during pregnancy and it is important to know the etiology in a particular patient since management differs accordingly [1, 2, 4–6] (Table 18.1).

A. Sheikh, MBBS, FCPS
Section of Endocrinology, Department of Medicine,
The Aga Khan University Hospital,
Stadium Road, Karachi 74800, Pakistan
e-mail: aisha.sheikh@aku.edu

Clinical Features of Hyperthyroidism During Pregnancy

Physiologic changes of pregnancy owing to decreased peripheral vascular resistance, vasodilation and tachycardia, may suggest thyrotoxicosis [1, 4, 7]. Due to the increased basal metabolic rate during pregnancy particularly in the second and third trimester, heat intolerance, tachycardia and increased perspiration are common and not suggestive of hyperthyroid state [2]. However; anxiety, tremors, weight loss despite increased appetite may suggest hyperthyroidism. A goiter with bruit and ophthalmopathy suggest Graves' disease [8].

S.K. Imam, S.I. Ahmad (eds.), *Thyroid Disorders: Basic Science and Clinical Practice*,
DOI 10.1007/978-3-319-25871-3_18

Table 18.1 Causes of hyperthyroidism in pregnancy [1, 4, 6]

Causes	Prevalence
Graves' Disease (TSH-receptor autoantibodies)	0.1–1 % of pregnancies Clinical – 0.4 % Subclinical – 0.6 %
hCG-induced thyrotoxicosis Gestational Transient thyrotoxicosis Hyperemesis gravidarum Multiple gestation Hydatidiform mole or Choriocarcinoma	1–3 %
Autonomous thyroid hormone secretion: Toxic nodule Toxic multinodular goiter Genomic activating TSH-receptor mutation [9]	Rare
Destruction of follicles with release of thyroid hormone Subacute painful thyroiditis (Granulomatous, de Quervain's, viral infection) Silent painless thyroiditis (autoimmunity) Acute thyroiditis (bacterial infection)	
Extrathyroidal sources of thyroid hormone Overtreatment with thyroid hormone Factitious intake of thyroid hormone Functional thyroid cancer metastases Struma ovarii'	

Table 18.2 Complications of hyperthyroidism in pregnancy [1, 2, 4, 6]

Fetal/neonatal:
Spontaneous miscarriage
Fetal growth restriction and Low birth weight – tenfolds higher frequency with poorly controlled hyperthyroidism [10]
Fetal thyroid hyperfunction or hypofunction caused by TRAbs
Fetal goiter from excessive anti-thyroid drug treatment
Neonatal thyrotoxicosis
Premature labor
Increase perinatal mortality – fetal death or still birth occurred in 5.6 % of pregnant women with hyperthyroidism with or without treatment [11]
Maternal:
Preeclampsia
Heart failure – 13 cases of heart failure in 150 pregnant women with hyperthyroidism is reported [12]
Thyroid storm – rare but when it does occur it is due to the combined effects of hyperthyroidism and pregnancy
Maternal mortality

TRAbs thyrotropin receptor antibodies

Impact of Hyperthyroidism During Pregnancy

Poorly controlled hyperthyroidism complicating pregnancy can lead to multitude of maternal and fetal effects (Table 18.2).

Diagnosis of Hyperthyroidism During Pregnancy

Maternal hyperthyroidism is defined as low or suppressed TSH level in the presence of high Free Thyroxine level (FT4) based on trimester-specific

Table 18.3 Characteristics of GTT and Graves' disease in pregnancy

Gestational transient thyrotoxicosis (GTT)	Graves' hyperthyroidism
No specific relation to family history of Graves' or other autoimmune disorders	Family history of Graves' disease might be present,
Diagnosed in first trimester	Diagnosed at any time during pregnancy, but more often in early pregnancy
No symptoms or signs before pregnancy	Symptoms and signs might have been present already before pregnancy
More common with hyperemesis	No specific relation to hyperemesis
More common with multiple gestation	No specific relation to multiple gestation
Not associated with other manifestations of Graves' disease	Other manifestations might be present (orbitopathy, diffuse goiter)
Often mild or absent clinical signs of hyperthyroidism	Any degree of clinical hyperthyroidism can be present
Not associated with TSH-receptor antibodies and TPO antibodies	Measurable TRAbs and TPO antibodies in most patients
Course of disease usually self-limiting	Course of disease unpredictable

Adapted from Cooper and Laurberg [6]. Reprinted from the Lancet, with permission from Elsevier

and method-specific reference ranges [2, 4]. The lower limit of TSH during pregnancy is still ill-defined with studies reporting lower normal TSH at 0.03 or 0.08 mIU/L [13, 14]. The American Thyroid Association (ATA) suggests that a TSH that is within detection is unlikely to be clinically significant as subclinical hyperthyroidism is not associated with adverse pregnancy outcomes [4, 15]. The total T4 and total Triiodothyronine (T3) levels during pregnancy are 1.5 folds higher than in non-pregnant women due to thyroxine binding globulin (TBG) excess [1, 3, 4]. In clinical practice if the trimester specific reference ranges are not available then besides the TSH and FT4 levels one has to rely on total T3 and total T4 levels as well to confirm or refute the diagnosis of hyperthyroidism in pregnancy [6]. Alternatively, thyroid-binding globulin or another measure of T4-binding (e.g. T3 resin uptake test) can be done and used to adjust the total T3 and T4 values obtained to correspond to the non-pregnant range [16].

Establishing the Cause of Hyperthyroidism During Pregnancy

The main differential is either the Graves' disease or GTT as other causes of hyperthyroidism are rare in pregnancy. If is important to differentiate between the two conditions as the management, outcomes and clinical course of both differ.

The thyroidal T3 production is high in Graves' and serum T3 or free T3 concentrations are typically more raised than serum T4 or free T4 concentrations [17]. However, GTT is unique in many ways i.e. absence of prepregnancy thyrotoxic symptoms, lack of thyrotorpin receptor antibodies (TRAbs), absence of a goiter with bruit, and absence of Graves' Ophthalmopathy (Table 18.3).

Radionuclide imaging is contraindicated in pregnancy [4]. Thyroid ultrasound with Doppler flow may help to distinguish Graves' disease from painless or postpartum thyroiditis [19] However, the utility of thyroid ultrasound with Doppler in diagnosing hCG-mediated hyperthyroidism is unknown.

Women who have a history of Graves' disease in past whether they are in remission [following antithyroid drug (ATD) use] or had received a definitive treatment [Radioactive iodine (RAI) treatment or thyroidectomy] and now are on L-thyroxine replacement should undergo thyroid function testing either at preconception period or in early antenatal period [6, 7].

Gestational Transient Thyrotoxicosis

Gestational Transient Thyrotoxicosis or GTT can be caused by excessive stimulation of thyroid gland induced by elevated human chorionic gonadotropin (hCG). hCG is a glycoprotein that shares a common alpha subunit with TSH and thus acts as a TSH agonist. In GTT the hCG concentrations are generally higher than 200,000 IU/L [2, 4].

Risk factors for GTT include hyperemesis gravidarum, multiple gestations, hydatiform mole, and choriocarcinoma [20, 21]. Biochemical results show a suppressed TSH with an elevated FT4/ Total T4 levels similar to Graves' Disease.

GTT presents in the 1st trimester at a time when peak levels of hCG are evident and characteristically resolves spontaneously by mid-trimester as hCG levels decline. Usually GTT is seen in women with Hyperemesis Gravidarum (vomiting, dehydration, weight low of >5 % body weight, ketonuria and hospitalization and intravenous hydration) but can be seen in women with morning sickness. A state of thyrotoxicosis is seen in about 50 % of patients with hyperemesis gravidarum [22–25].

As GTT resolves spontaneously, there is no need to treat these women with Antithyroid drugs (ATDs) [4–6]. ATDs can potentially induce maternal hypothyroidism which can have deleterious effects on fetal development and viability. It is therefore crucial to differentiate GTT from Graves' disease as only Graves's disease will need ATDs. If a woman is very symptomatic then small doses of beta-blockers can be given for a short while [4, 6]. Supportive management for hyperemesis gravidarum is the mainstay of therapy and hospitalization may be required in severe cases [26].

A woman with GTT needs to be followed up with Thyroid Function tests done at an interval of 3–4 weeks and by mid-gestation these show a trend towards euthyroidism along with symptomatic improvement i.e. hyperemesis subsides and the woman starts to regain her weight. FT4 concentrations tend to show a progressive decline while the TSH may remain partially or totally suppressed for several weeks [25].

Graves' Disease

Graves' disease is the most common cause of hyperthyroidism in women of childbearing age. The incidence is roughly 55–80 cases per 100,000 per year in women older than 30 years. While the risk is much lower in women younger than 20 years; an incidence of 35–50 cases per 100,000 per year is reported in women aged 20–29 years [27, 28]. Thus, the risk of a woman getting pregnant with Graves' hyperthyroidism is 1.3 % at age 40 years and 0.5 % at age 30 years [6].

Pre-pregnancy Counseling

All women with Hyperthyroidism should avoid conception till their hyperthyroidism is well under control as uncontrolled thyrotoxicosis can lead to wide array of maternal and fetal complications [4, 29] (Table 18.4). Well before conception, the woman is offered a definitive treatment of her thyrotoxicosis either with surgery or radioactive iodine (RAI) ablation and alternatively she may wish to continue with ATDs. The pros and cons of each of these management options should be thoroughly discussed with the woman that will help her in making the decision [4, 6].

Radioactive Iodine Ablation or Surgery

A woman who opts for RAI ablation needs to understand that:

- Before getting the RAI, a proof of negative pregnancy test should be available at least within 48 h before the RAI treatment.
- After RAI, she needs to avoid conception for at least 6 months and let the L-thyroxine replacement be sufficient enough to bring the TSH within a normal range required for conception i.e. ≤2.5 mIU/L (range 0.3–2.5 mIU/L) [4].

If the woman has high titres of TRAbs, the titres are likely to rise after RAI treatment for 1 year and remain elevated for several years before finally disappearing [30]. In a 5 year prospective randomized study, medical therapy with ATDs and surgery was followed by a gradual decline in TRAb in serum, with the disappearance of TRAb in 70–80 % of the patients after 18 months. On the other hand, RAI led to a 1-year long worsening of autoimmunity against

Table 18.4 Effects of poorly treated hyperthyroidism in pregnancy

Clinical	Mother	Pregnancy	Fetus	Neonate
Untreated/ inadequate	Congestive cardiac failure Pre-eclampsia/toxemia Thyroid storm	Miscarriage Abruptio Post-partum thyroid disease	Hyperthyroidism Goiter Death	Primary hyperthyroidism Secondary hyperthyroidism
Antithyroid drugs			Hypothyroidism Goiter	Transient hyperthyroidism
Surgery + L-thyroxine	Hypothyroidism		Hyperthyroidism (TRAb)	Hyperthyroidism (TRAb)
RAI+ L-thyroxine	Hypothyroidism		Hyperthyroidism (TRAb)	Hyperthyroidism (TRAb)
Previous ATDs	Relapse post-partum			

Adapted from Laurberg et al. [18]

the TSH receptor, and the number of patients entering remission of TSH-receptor autoimmunity with the disappearance of TRAb from serum during the following years was considerably lower than with the other types of therapy [31]. So if the woman has high levels of TRAb and she is planning pregnancy in near future; surgery could be a better option as this will reduce the TRAbs earlier than RAI.

Antithyroid Drugs [4, 6, 29]

If the woman chooses to opt for ATDs then she should be counseled about:

- The ideal time to conceive is when hyperthyroidism is well controlled preferably with small doses of ATDs.
- The risks (maternal and fetal) associated with both ATDs should be discussed.
- She will be switched to Propylthiouracil during the 1st trimester of pregnancy to reduce the risk to fetus. However, she will be switched back to Carbimazole/methimazole after 1st trimester of pregnancy to avoid PTU associated hepatotoxicity in mother.

Incidence of Hyperthyroidism During Pregnancy

Maternal hyperthyroidism is reported to occur at a frequency of around 0.2 %. The incidence of hyperthyroidism fluctuates widely in and around pregnancy. The overall incident ratio of maternal hyperthyroidism from Danish nationwide registers is reported as 65/100,000/year. This incident ratio was high in first 3 months of pregnancy [incidence rate ratio (IRR) vs the remaining study period: 1.50 (95 % CI 1.09–2.06]), very low in last 3 months of pregnancy [0.26 (0.15–0.44)] and reached the highest level 7–9 months post-partum [3.80 (2.88–5.0)]. Such particular pattern was not observed for other diseases of autoimmune origin [32].

Poorly controlled thyrotoxicosis is associated with miscarriages, pregnancy induced hypertension, intrauterine growth restriction, prematurity, low birth weight, still birth, maternal congestive heart failure and thyroid storm (Tables 18.2 and 18.4).

Treating Graves' Disease in Pregnancy

During pregnancy ATDs are the ideal treatment for Graves' Disease. ATDs reduce thyroid hormone synthesis by virtue of reducing iodine organification and coupling of mono- and diiodotyrosine. In non-pregnant individuals the most frequently encountered side effects are allergic reactions occurring in 3–5 % of patients [8]. The rare side effects are agranulocytosis and PTU associated hepatotoxicity [8].

During pregnancy there is a risk of teratogenic effects with the use of ATDs especially

Carbimazole/methimazole (CMZ/MMI) [33]. CMZ/MMI exposure at the time of embryogenesis can lead to congenital malformations. Generally it is associated with aplasia cutis or a rare "MMI embryopathy" consisting of esophageal or choanal atresia, dysmorphic facies and omphalomesenteric anomalies [34–36]. Such complications however are not reported with the use of PTU yet there is possible association of birth defect in the face and neck region (periauricular and branchial sinus/fistula/cyst) and in the urinary system (single cyst of kidney and hydronephrosis). In a study from Denmark; the adjusted Hazard Ratio of having a birth defect in the face and neck region was 4.92 (95 % CI 2.04–11.86) and in the urinary system 2.73 (1.22–6.07) [37]. These defects tend to be less severe than the defects observed after CMZ/MMI exposure [38]. Infants of mothers with diagnosed thyrotoxicosis or ATD use during pregnancy; were more likely to be preterm and admitted to the neonatal intensive care unit [39]. The frequency of PTU associated hepatotoxicity was 1.8 per 1000 delivered pregnancies [39]. Due to PTU-associated hepatotoxicity, the FDA advisory committee has recommended limiting its use to 1st trimester of pregnancy, in those who are allergic to MMI/CMZ and in the management of thyroid storm [4, 5, 8, 40]. Similarly if PTU is not available or the patient is intolerant of PTU, it is acceptable to proceed with MMI/CMZ in the lowest possible effective dose [6].

It is important to bear in mind that the risk of complications in an untreated or undertreated hyperthyroid patient far outweighs the small and potential risk associated with maternal ATD use [10]. Thus, it is important to treat Graves' disease in pregnancy [7].

It is prudent to get a baseline Complete Blood Count and Liver function tests before starting ATDs [8]. Patients need to be advised that in the event of fever, pharyngitis or oral ulcers they should get their White Cell Count and report to their doctor [8]. If there is any evidence of agranulocytosis, then the ATD has to be stopped immediately and should not be replaced by the other ATD since these drugs exhibit cross reactivity [8, 41]. Similarly if the patient develops nausea, vomiting, jaundice, upper abdominal pain then liver function tests should be done [8].

The initial doses of ATDs depend upon the severity of hyperthyroidism but usually these are started at a lower dose as compared to a non-pregnant individual [4–6]. CMZ is the precursor of MMI and is converted to MMI rapidly in serum. (10 mg of CMZ is metabolized to approximately 6 mg of MMI). Generally the initial doses could vary from MMI 5–15 mg/day; CMZ 10–15 mg/day; or PTU 50–300 mg/day. MMI or NMZ can be given in once daily dose while PTU should be given in divided doses [4–6, 8].

If the woman is overtly symptomatic then Beta adrenergic blocking agents like propranolol 10–40 mg every 6–8 hourly can be given to control symptoms. Depending upon the clinical condition, the drug should then be tapered off over next 2–6 weeks [4–6]. Beta blockers can lead to fetal intrauterine growth restriction, fetal bradycardia and neonatal hypoglycemia thus long-term use during pregnancy should be avoided [4–6].

Use of Block-replace regimen is contraindicated in pregnancy as it can lead to fetal hypothyroidism. The only exception is for treatment of fetal hyperthyroidism [4].

Monitoring a Pregnant Woman on ATDs (Table 18.5)

ATDs cross the placenta and can lead to fetal hypothyroidism thus the aim of treating hyperthyroidism during pregnancy is to keep the lowest possible doses of ATDs to keep the FT4 values at, or just above the trimester specific reference range [4, 42]. Avoiding over treatment can reduce the occurrence of fetal hypothyroidism and fetal goiter [4–6]. If the trimester and method-specific reference ranges are not available for different populations, thus in such situations the ATA suggests to rely on the non-pregnant FT4 reference range for ATD dose adjustment [4].

The rationale for keeping the FT4 around the upper limit of normal is twofolds [4–6]:

1. The available evidence suggests that subclinical hyperthyroidism is not associated with adverse maternal or fetal effects.
2. Keeping the lowest possible maternal ATD dose reduces the trans-placental passage of the ATD and thus reduces the risk of fetal/neonatal hypothyroidism [33, 42].

Table 18.5 Graves' hyperthyroidism in pregnancy and the balance between maternal and fetal thyroid function

1. TSH-receptor stimulating antibodies (TRAbs) produced in the mother and inducing maternal hyperthyroidism pass the placenta, and they stimulate the fetal thyroid
2. If the mother has an intact thyroid, her thyroid function mirrors the thyroid function of the fetus
3. Antithyroid drugs (methimazole/carbimazole or propylthiouracil) pass the placenta and induce a block of both the maternal and the fetal thyroid hormone production
4. At a given dose of propylthiouracil or methimazole/carbimazole the block of fetal thyroid is more effective than of the maternal thyroid
5. During antithyroid drug therapy the thyroid function of the mother should be kept around or slightly above the upper normal to avoid fetal hypothyroidism in the last part of pregnancy
6. Thyroid hormones only pass the placenta barrier to a very limited degree
7. A combination of antithyroid drug and L-thyroxine given to the mother to keep her euthyroid (block + replace therapy) may mask fetal hypothyroidism induced by the antithyroid drugs
8. The combination of block (of fetal thyroid) + replacement (of the hypothyroid mother) is only appropriate in a hypothyroid mother (after previous surgery or radioiodine therapy for Graves' hyperthyroidism) with a hyperthyroid fetus from persistent maternal production of TSH-receptor stimulating antibodies

Adapted from Laurberg et al. [18]

FT4 and TSH should be measured every 2–4 weeks at initiation of therapy. Generally it takes 2–6 weeks for thyroid function tests to improve and at that time the dose can be cut by 50 % in many patients [4, 6]. Thereafter, FT4 levels should be checked at 2–4 weekly intervals and ATD dose should be adjusted accordingly [6]. TSH may remain suppressed longer and thus FT4 remains the best test to help with ATD dose adjustment during pregnancy [4, 6]. Normalizing the TSH is not the goal of treatment as it will lead to fetal goiter and fetal hypothyroidism [4]. Serum total T3 monitoring is not recommended as normalization of T3 can lead to elevated serum TSH in the neonate at birth [4]. The only exception is T3-toxicosis in the setting of a nodular goiter. However, the optimum maternal T3 concentration that controls maternal hyperthyroidism with minimal fetal thyroidal exposure is unknown [6].

Natural Course of Graves' Disease During Pregnancy

Graves' disease tends to exacerbate during the first trimester of pregnancy in some women. This deterioration in clinical features of Graves' disease in first trimester may occur due to stimulation of thyroid both by hCG and TRAb [43]. A high TBG state may also contribute to deterioration. Later on, there is a trend towards gradual improvement in the second and third trimester of pregnancy due to falling titres of TRAb and possible presence of thyroid receptor blocking antibodies [44, 45]. This calls for ATD dose reduction accordingly; some 20–30 % of women can go off their ATDs in third trimester [42]. However, women with very high TRAbs should be continued on their ATDs [6]. After delivery, generally an exacerbation of Graves' Disease is seen, thus it is prudent to closely follow the woman with FT4 levels in the postpartum period and make ATD dose adjustments accordingly.

Thyroidectomy for Graves' Disease During Pregnancy

Thyroidectomy is rarely indicated during pregnancy but following are the indications for thyroidectomy [4–6]:

- If the woman is having allergies or intolerance to both ATDs.
- If both ATDs are contraindicated.
- If the woman requires persistently high doses of ATDs and still remain poorly controlled threatening her health.
- If the woman is having compliance issue with intake of ATD.

The relatively safe time for thyroidectomy is the second trimester of pregnancy. The decision should be made in close consultation of the surgeon and obstetrician. The woman should be properly counseled about the need of thyroidectomy is her clinical situation [6]. Beta blockers and short course of potassium iodide solution (50–100 mg/day) is recommended in preparation for surgery [4]. Maternal TRAbs levels should be tested at the time of surgery which will help in risk assessment of fetal hyperthyroidism [6]. TRAb disappears slowly after surgical thyroidectomy, with only about half of the patients being TRAb negative after a year [31]. Thus, a woman may have undergone thyroidectomy and is off ATDs and now receiving L-thyroxine but due to her high TRAb, the fetus may be hyperthyroid [18]. All this calls for a systematic and careful follow-up evaluation of the fetal thyroid state.

Radioactive iodine treatment is contraindicated in pregnancy because it destroys the fetal thyroid gland, resulting in permanent hypothyroidism in the newborn [2, 4].

Metarnal TRAb and Its Impact on the Fetus

TRAb are present in over 95 % of patients with active Graves' Disease and even following RAI ablation; TRAb remains elevated for many months [31]. High titres of TRAb can lead to fetal or neonatal hyperthyroidism [46–48]. TRAb determination is advisable in following condition [4–6]:

- Maternal active hyperthyroidism
- Past history of treatment with RAI or thyroidectomy for Graves' disease
- Past history of delivering an infant with hyperthyroidism
- Thyroidectomy during pregnancy for treatment of Graves' Disease

Fetal and Neonatal Hyperthyroidism

The prevalence of fetal or neonatal hyperthyroidism is 1–5 % in women with active or past history of Graves' disease but if remains unrecognized or untreated then it is associated with increased fetal and neonatal morbidity and mortality [47]. In a study from Japan; in women who had received RAI in the past for severe and intractable Graves' disease; an incidence of neonatal hyperthyroidism as high as 11.3 % is reported [48]. Mothers who have had received RAI in the past for severe and intractable Graves' disease are more likely to exhibit higher TRAb titres in pregnancy and subsequent risk of neonatal hyperthyroidism. Still others have reported a 30 % occurrence of neonatal hyperthyroidism in TRAb positive women [48, 49].

TRAb titres decrease with the progression of pregnancy. It is recommended to test for serum TRAb at 24–28 weeks of gestation and if the levels are elevated three times the upper limit of normal then close fetal monitoring by fetal medicine physicians should be done [4, 6].

Fetal Monitoring in a Woman with Graves's Disease

In most cases, the diagnosis of fetal hyperthyroidism should be made on clinical grounds based on maternal history, serum TRAb levels, and fetal ultrasonography.

Fetal surveillance with serial ultrasound examinations may be performed for the assessment of gestational age, fetal viability, amniotic fluid volume, fetal anatomy, and detection of malformations. Fetal well-being may be compromised in the presence of elevated TRAb, uncontrolled hyperthyroidism, and pre-eclampsia [4–6].

Signs of potential fetal hyperthyroidism that may be detected by ultrasonography include fetal tachycardia (>160 beats/min, persistent for over 10 min), intrauterine growth restriction, presence of fetal goiter (the earliest sonographic sign of fetal thyroid dysfunction), accelerated bone maturation, signs of congestive heart failure, and fetal hydrops [6, 47]. A team approach is recommended for the management of these patients. The team should include an experienced obstetrician or maternal–fetal medicine specialist, neonatologist, and anesthesiologist.

In extremely rare circumstances; cordocentesis or umbilical cord sampling can be performed to detect whether the fetus is hypothyroid or hyperthyroid [4, 6]. The indications are for a woman who is having high TRAb and is being treated with ATDs and fetal goiter is visualized on ultrasonography but the thyroid status of the fetus is undetermined [4, 6]. Cordocentesis carries significant fetal morbidity and mortality so should be offered and performed only in appropriate setting.

None of the infants born to TRAb negative mothers develop neonatal hyperthyroidism. At birth, taking a cord blood sample for TRAb estimation in the neonate helps in risk prediction for development of neonatal hyperthyroidism [50, 51]. FT4 measurement at birth should be repeated between days 3 and 5 (and by day 7 at the latest); rapid FT4 elevation during the first postnatal week is predictive of hyperthyroidism and warrants ATD therapy [52].

ATDs Use in Lactation

Both ATDs are secreted in human milk. In general, there is no evidence to advice mothers against breast-feeding when taking antithyroid drugs [53]. Moderate dose of ATDs are safe in lactating mothers. MMI/CMZ stay as first line agents with doses up to 20–30 mg/day; while PTU as second line with doses up to 300 mg/day during lactation [54]. Mothers should be advised to take their ATD in divided doses and immediately following each feed. The American Academy of Pediatrics has approved both PTU and CMZ/MMI for use by lactating mothers; doses of less than 20 mg of MMI are safe [55].

Graves' Disease in Post-partum Period

During the post-partum period, woman with Graves' disease needs careful monitoring as there is increased incidence of relapse of Graves' hyperthyroidism in women who have had a pregnancy after previous ATD withdrawal compared to those women who did not become pregnant following their ATD withdrawal [56, 57]. The relapse of Graves' hyperthyroidism occurs between 4 and 8 months post-partum and relapse is expected in 84 % of women after a pregnancy [58].

Conclusion

Uncontrolled hyperthyroidism in pregnancy is associated with adverse maternal and fetal outcomes. Wherever available; trimester-specific and method-specific reference ranges for thyroid function tests should be used. It is important to differentiate between the two common causes of hyperthyroidism in pregnancy i.e. GTT and Graves' disease as the former condition is largely self-limiting and requires only supportive care. ATDs stay as the first line treatment for Graves' disease during pregnancy, PTU in the first trimester and CMZ/MMI for rest of gestation. It is important to keep the lowest possible doses of ATDs to keep the FT4 at or just above the reference range. TSH may remain suppressed throughout pregnancy thus ATD dose adjustment should be done mainly on the basis of 2–4 weekly FT4 levels. Maternal TRAbs estimation in the third trimester helps in assessing the risk of fetal and neonatal hyperthyroidism. There is a risk of Graves' disease relapse in the post-partum period.

References

1. Melmed S, Polonsky KS, Larsen PR, et al. Melmed: Williams textbook of endocrinology. 12th ed. Philadelphia: Elsevier Saunders; 2011.
2. Marx H, Amin P, Lazarus JH. Hyperthyroidism and pregnancy. BMJ. 2008;336:663–7.
3. Lazarus JH. Thyroid function in pregnancy. Br Med Bull. 2011;97:137–48.
4. Stagnaro-Green A, Abalovich M, Alexander E, et al. Guidelines of the American Thyroid Association for the diagnosis and management of thyroid disease during pregnancy and postpartum. Thyroid. 2011;21:1081–125.
5. De Groot L, Abalovich M, Alexander EK, et al. Management of thyroid dysfunction during pregnancy and postpartum: an Endocrine Society clinical practice guideline. J Clin Endocrinol Metab. 2012;97:2543–65.
6. Cooper DS, Laurberg P. Hyperthyroidism in pregnancy. Lancet Diabetes Endocrinol. 2013;1:238–49.
7. Negro R, Stagnaro-Green A. Clinical aspects of hyperthyroidism, hypothyroidism, and thyroid screening in pregnancy. Endocr Pract. 2014;20(6):597–607.

8. Bahn RS, Burch HB, Cooper DS, et al. Hyperthyroidism and other causes of thyrotoxicosis: management guidelines of the American Thyroid Association and American Association of Clinical Endocrinologists. Endocr Pract. 2011;17(3):e1–65.
9. Rodien P, Brémont C, Sanson ML, et al. Familial gestational hyperthyroidism caused by a mutant thyrotropin receptor hypersensitive to human chorionic gonadotropin. N Engl J Med. 1998;339:1823–6.
10. Millar LK, Wing DA, Leung AS, et al. Low birth weight and preeclampsia in pregnancies complicated by hyperthyroidism. Obstet Gynecol. 1994;84:946–9.
11. Hamburger JI. Diagnosis and management of Graves' disease in pregnancy. Thyroid. 1992;2(3):219–24.
12. Sheffield JS, Cunningham FG. Thyrotoxicosis and heart failure that complicate pregnancy. Am J Obstet Gynecol. 2004;190:211–7.
13. Dashe JS, Casey BM, Wells CE, et al. Thyroid-stimulating hormone in singleton and twin pregnancy: importance of gestational age-specific reference ranges. Obstet Gynecol. 2005;106(4):753–7.
14. Stricker R, Echenard M, Eberhart R, et al. Evaluation of maternal thyroid function during pregnancy: the importance of using gestational age-specific reference intervals. Eur J Endocrinol. 2007;157(4):509–14.
15. Casey BM, Dashe JS, Wells CE, et al. Subclinical hyperthyroidism and pregnancy outcomes. Obstet Gynecol. 2006;107:337–41.
16. Lee RH, Spencer CA, Mestman JH, et al. Free T4 immunoassays are flawed during pregnancy. Am J Obstet Gynecol. 2009;200(3):e1–6.
17. Laurberg P, Vestergaard H, Nielsen S, et al. Sources of circulating 3,5,3′-triiodothyronine in hyperthyroidism estimated after blocking of type 1 and type 2 iodothyronine deiodinases. J Clin Endocrinol Metab. 2007;92(6):2149–56.
18. Laurberg P, Bournaud C, Karmisholt J, et al. Management of Graves' hyperthyroidism in pregnancy: focus on both maternal and foetal thyroid function, and caution against surgical thyroidectomy in pregnancy. Eur J Endocrinol. 2009;160(1):1–8.
19. Ota H, Amino N, Morita S, et al. Quantitative measurement of thyroid blood flow for differentiation of painless thyroiditis from Graves' disease. Clin Endocrinol (Oxf). 2007;67(1):41–5.
20. Hershman JM. Human chorionic gonadotropin and the thyroid: hyperemesis gravidarum and trophoblastic tumors. Thyroid. 1999;9(7):653–7.
21. Lockwood CM, Grenache DG, Gronowski AM. Serum human chorionic gonadotropin concentrations greater than 400,000 IU/L are invariably associated with suppressed serum thyrotropin concentrations. Thyroid. 2009;19(8):863–8.
22. Montoro M, Spencer C, Jacobson S, et al. Evidence for a physiological role of hCG as a thyroid stimulator: genesis of hyperthyroidism in hyperemesis gravidarum. Clin Res. 1984;32:20A.
23. Rodien P, Jordan N, Lefevre A, et al. Abnormal stimulation of the thyrotrophin receptor during gestation. Hum Reprod Update. 2004;10:95–105.
24. Kimura M, Amino N, Tamaki H, et al. Gestational thyrotoxicosis and hyperemesis gravidarum: possible role of hCG with higher stimulating activity. Clin Endocrinol. 1993;38:345–50.
25. Goodwin TM, Montoro M, Mestman JH, et al. The role of chorionic gonadotropin in transient hyperthyroidism of hyperemesis gravidarum. J Clin Endocrinol Metab. 1992;75:1333–7.
26. Yazbeck CF, Sullivan SD. Thyroid disorders during pregnancy. Med Clin North Am. 2012;96(2): 235–56.
27. Carlé A, Pedersen IB, Knudsen N, et al. Epidemiology of subtypes of hyperthyroidism in Denmark: a population-based study. Eur J Endocrinol. 2011; 164:801–9.
28. Abraham-Nordling M, Byström K, Törring O, et al. Incidence of hyperthyroidism in Sweden. Eur J Endocrinol. 2011;165:899–905.
29. Lazarus JH. Pre-conception counselling in Graves' disease. Eur Thyroid J. 2012(1);1:24–9.
30. Bech K, Nistrup Madsen S. Influence of treatment with radioactive iodine and propylthiouracil on thyroid stimulating immunoglobulins in Graves' disease. Clin Endocrinol (Oxf). 1980;13:417–24.
31. Laurberg P, Wallin G, Tallstedt L, et al. TSH-receptor autoimmunity in Graves' disease after therapy with antithyroid drugs, surgery, or radioiodine: a 5-year prospective randomized study. Eur J Endocrinol. 2008;158(1):69–75.
32. Anderson SL, Olsen J, Carle A, et al. Hyperthyroidism incidence fluctuates widely in and around pregnancy and is at variance with some other autoimmune diseases: a Danish population-based study. J Clin Endocrinol Metab. 2015;100(3):1164–71.
33. Wing DA, Millar LK, Koonings PP, et al. A comparison of propylthiouracil versus methimazole in the treatment of hyperthyroidism in pregnancy. Am J Obstet Gynecol. 1994;170:90–5.
34. Milham SJ, Elledge W. Maternal methimazole and congenital defects in children. Teratology. 1972; 5: 125–6. In: Anderson SL, Laurberg P. Antithyroid drugs and congenital heart defects: ventricular septal defect is part of the methimazole/carbimazole embryopathy. Eur J Endocrinol. 2014;171(5):C1–C3.
35. Foulds N, Walpole I, Elmslie F, et al. Carbimazole embryopathy: an emerging phenotype. Am J Med Genet A. 2005;132A(2):130–5.
36. Douchement D, Rakza T, Holder M, et al. Choanal atresia associated with tracheoesophageal fistula: the spectrum of carbimazole embryopathy. Pediatrics. 2011;128(3):e703–6.
37. Andersen SL, Olsen J, Wu CS, et al. Birth defects after early pregnancy use of antithyroid drugs: a Danish nationwide study. J Clin Endocrinol Metab. 2013;98:4373–81.
38. Andersen SL, Olsen J, Wu CS, et al. Severity of birth defects after propylthiouracil exposure in early pregnancy. Thyroid. 2014;24(10):1533–40.
39. Lo JC, Rivkees SA, Chandra M, et al. Gestational thyrotoxicosis, antithyroid drug use and neonatal

outcomes within an integrated healthcare delivery system. Thyroid. 2015;25(6):698–705.
40. Cooper DS, Rivkees SA. Putting propylthiouracil in perspective. J Clin Endocrinol Metab. 2009;94:1881–2.
41. Ahmed K, Rao S, Simha V. ANCA-positive vasculitis in a patient with Graves' disease: cross-reaction between Propylthiouracil and Methimazole. Endocr Pract. 2010;9:1–11.
42. Momotani N, Noh J, Oyanagi H, et al. Antithyroid drug therapy for Graves' disease during pregnancy. Optimal regimen for fetal thyroid status. N Engl J Med. 1986;315(1):24–8.
43. Tamaki H, Itoh E, Kaneda T, Asahi K, Mitsuda N, Tanizawa O, Amino N. Crucial role of serum human chorionic gonadotropin for the aggravation of thyrotoxicosis in early pregnancy in Graves' disease. Thyroid. 1993;3:189–93.
44. Kung AW, Jones BM. A change from stimulatory to blocking antibody activity in Graves' disease during pregnancy. J Clin Endocrinol Metab. 1998;83:514–8.
45. Amino N, Izumi Y, Hidaka Y, et al. No increase of blocking type anti-thyrotropin receptor antibodies during pregnancy in patients with Graves' disease. J Clin Endocrinol Metab. 2003;88:5871–4.
46. Kamijko K. TSH-receptor antibodies determined by the first, second, and third generation assays and thyroid-stimulating antibody in pregnant patient with Graves' disease. Endocr J. 2007;54(4):619–24.
47. McKenzie JM, Zakarija M. Fetal and neonatal hyperthyroidism and hypothyroidism due to maternal TSH receptor antibodies. Thyroid. 1992;2(2):155–9.
48. Hamada N, Momotani N, Ishikawa N, et al. Persistent high TRAb values during pregnancy predict increased risk of neonatal hyperthyroidism following radioiodine therapy for refractory hyperthyroidism. Endocr J. 2011;58(1):55–8.
49. Krassas GE, Poppe K, Glinoer D. Thyroid function and human reproductive health. Endocr Rev. 2010;31:702–55.
50. Lafranchi SH, Hanna CE. Graves' disease in the neonatal period and childhood. In: Braverman LE, Utiger RD, editors. The thyroid. 9th ed. Philadelphia: Lippincott Williams & Wilkins; 2005. p. 1049–59.
51. Momotani N, Noh JY, Ishikawa N. Effects of propylthiouracil and methimazole on fetal thyroid status in mothers with Graves' hyperthyroidism. J Clin Endocrinol Metab. 1997;82:3633–6.
52. Besancon A, Beltrand J, Le Gac I, et al. Management of neonates born to women with Graves' disease: a cohort study. Eur J Endocrinol. 2014;170:855–62.
53. Karras S, Tzotzas T, Kaltsas T, et al. Pharmacological treatment of hyperthyroidism during lactation: review of the literature and novel data. Pediatr Endocrinol Rev. 2010;8:25–33.
54. Karras S, Krassas GE. Breast feeding and antithyroid drugs: a view from within. Eur Thyroid J. 2012;1:30–3.
55. American Academy of Pediatrics Committee on Drugs. Transfer of drugs and other chemicals into human milk. Pediatrics. 2001;108:776–89.
56. Muller AF, Drexhage HA, Berghout A. Postpartum thyroiditis and autoimmune thyroiditis in women of childbearing age: recent insights and consequences for antenatal and postnatal care. Endocr Rev. 2001;22:605–63.
57. Amino N, Kubota S. Thyroid disease after pregnancy: postpartum thyroiditis. In: Wass JA, Stewart PM, editors. Oxford textbook of endocrinology and diabetes. 2nd ed. Oxford: Oxford University Press; 2011. p. 552–7.
58. Rotondi M, Cappelli C, Pirali B, et al. The effect of pregnancy on subsequent relapse from Graves' disease after a successful course of antithyroid drug therapy. J Clin Endocrinol Metab. 2008;93:3985–8.

Index

S.K. Imam, S.I. Ahmad (eds.), *Thyroid Disorders: Basic Science and Clinical Practice*,
DOI 10.1007/978-3-319-25871-3

Q

R

S

MIX
Papier aus verantwortungsvollen Quellen
Paper from responsible sources
FSC® C105338

If you have any concerns about our products,
you can contact us on
ProductSafety@springernature.com

In case Publisher is established outside the EU,
the EU authorized representative is:
Springer Nature Customer Service Center GmbH
Europaplatz 3, 69115 Heidelberg, Germany

Printed by Libri Plureos GmbH
in Hamburg, Germany